# ADVANCES IN CARDIOVASCULAR RESEARCH, VOLUME 1

# ADVANCES IN CARDIOVASCULAR RESEARCH

Additional books in this series can be found on Nova's website at:

https://www.novapublishers.com/catalog/product_info.php?cPath=23_29&products_id=10197

ADVANCES IN CARDIOVASCULAR RESEARCH

# ADVANCES IN CARDIOVASCULAR RESEARCH, VOLUME 1

LUKAS SCHMITT
AND
TIMM KÖNIG
EDITORS

Nova Biomedical Books
*New York*

For permission to use material from this book please contact us:
Telephone 631-231-7269; Fax 631-231-8175
Web Site: http://www.novapublishers.com



**Library of Congress Cataloging-in-Publication Data**

Advances in cardiovascular research / editors, Lukas Schmitt and Timm König.
p. ; cm.
Includes bibliographical references and index.
ISBN 978-1-60741-720-0 (v. 1 : hardcover : alk. paper)
1. Cardiovascular system--Diseases. I. Schmitt, Lukas. II. König, Timm.
[DNLM: 1. Cardiovascular Diseases--therapy. WG 120 A244 2009]
RC667.A35 2009
362.196'10072--dc22
2009045943

*Published by Nova Science Publishers, Inc. † New York*

# Contents

# Preface

This book presents original research results on the leading edge of cardiovascular research. Each article has been carefully selected in an attempt to present substantial research results across a broad spectrum.

Chapter I - The mitral valve is a complex, specialised connective tissue structure which acts to maintain the forward flow of blood through the left side of the heart. The mitral valve consists of two leaflets, with numerous supporting chordae tendineae. The mitral valve leaflets have a layered structure, with the structural constituents of each layer determined by its functional role. Evidence suggests that the valvular interstitial cells (VICs) which are present within the connective tissue layers of the mitral valve play an active role in mitral valve dynamics, a theory enhanced by the observation of neural structures within the valve tissue. Disease of the heart valves, such as myxomatous mitral valve disease, has been associated with changes in the phenotype of valvular cells and composition of the valvular extracellular matrix (ECM), and continues to have a devastating impact worldwide. Despite valve repair being the preferred initial treatment method to address severe mitral valve disease, valve repair is not feasible in a large number of patients with end-stage valve disease, and replacement of the mitral valve with a biological or mechanical prosthesis is necessary. A number of limitations are associated with conventional prosthetic mitral valves, however, including thromboembolism, life-threatening haemorrhagic complications, limited durability, rejection and transmission of infection. To overcome these limitations, the focus of prosthetic valve research has shifted to the development of living valves with growth and remodelling capabilities through tissue engineering, with many animal studies demonstrating the feasibility of this approach. The present chapter provides a comprehensive review on the development and structure of the mitral valve, particularly relating to its connective tissue and cellular components, while morphological and histological changes in this structure associated with mitral valve disease are also discussed. Potential future treatment modalities for pathological mitral valve disease using tissue-engineered structures are also discussed.

Chapter II - The annual incidence of sudden cardiac deaths in the United States is about 300,000 cases. Ventricular fibrillation (VF) remains an important cause of sudden death both in hospitals and in the community contributing to about half of these cases, although in monitored setting with rapid response times, VF is the presenting rhythm in almost three quarters of these patients. Despite an overall declining trend in the incidence of VF, the management of the arrhythmia remains challenging due to the fact that the event is usually unexpected and almost certainly lethal in the absence of resuscitation within the first few minutes. There has been a dramatic improvement in survival from VF due to the introduction of defibrillation as a part of resuscitation but in a significant proportion of patients, the process of resuscitation proves futile due to lack of return of spontaneous circulation or significant neurological disability caused by cerebral anoxia.

This review article traces the historical evolution in the management of VF from the era when the term cardiopulmonary resuscitation or CPR was coined less than 50 years ago to represent the series of concerted steps to provide life support and thereby minimize tissue hypoxia by maintaining airway, breathing and circulatory systems through airway patency maneuvers and adjuncts, artificial breathing and delivery of oxygen, chest compressions and defibrillation, to the modern era of “cardio-cerebral resuscitation”. There have been significant changes both in the sequence and methodology of these steps and the persons delivering resuscitation. For instance, there were a series of studies in the 1970s demonstrating the importance of early initiation of resuscitation and therefore the concept of “first responder” or “bystander” CPR leading to improved survival and neurological recovery.

There has been a paucity of high level evidence for many of the resuscitation therapies due to the restrictions on human research created by consent legislation and therefore most of the traditional recommendations such as epinephrine, atropine and strength or type of current delivered by defibrillators, are based on animal research or observational studies. Despite this, there have been many radical developments such as the introduction of automated external defibrillators(AEDs), biphasic defibrillation and re-emphasis on chest compressions preceding defibrillation especially in out of hospital arrests, leading to frequent changes in resuscitation guidelines. The importance of the neurological outcome has also led to the 21$^{st}$ century term cardio-cerebral resuscitation. By charting the evolution of the treatment of VF, this review article can help to discern the progress made and also to foment further novel ideas in this field.

Chapter III - Since the first use of basic life support (BLS) and defibrillation in the pre-hospital setting in Belfast in 1966, few would argue that there have been major improvements in the rate of survival for out-of-hospital cardiac arrests. Indeed, until the widespread introduction of BLS and defibrillators to emergency medical service (EMS) vehicles, an out-of-hospital cardiac arrest would mean certain death.

The initial rhythm of a patient in cardiac arrest is predictive of their chances of survival. In this regard, the rhythms with the highest rate of survival to hospital discharge are ventricular fibrillation (VF) and ventricular tachycardia (VT). In the past century the authors have learnt much about VF and VT, with this knowledge forming the bedrock of present day resuscitation guidelines. In the last decade there has been a truly international effort, headed by the International Liaison Committee on Resuscitation (ILCOR), aimed at reducing the mortality from cardiac arrest. This effort has resulted in the publication of the 2005 guidelines for resuscitation. While there is still much to learn, the 2005 guidelines appear to have reduced mortality from VF/VT arrests more than any before.

The concept of providing cardiopulmonary resuscitation (CPR), defibrillation, and advanced cardiac life support, in a timely fashion to reduce mortality from cardiac arrests evolved in the late 1980’s. It was formalised in 1991 by Cummings as the *“Chain of Survival”*. It is the role of EMS, with regards to cardiac arrest, to provide the final critical links in the chain of survival. Aside from this vital function, EMS have been invaluable in enabling an assessment of the impact of the many changes to resuscitation protocols over the years on the mortality rate from cardiac arrest by facilitating research in the pre-hospital domain.

As VF is a more common presenting rhythm in out-of-hospital cardiac arrest and much of their knowledge of VF is relevant to VT, this chapter will focus primarily on VF cardiac arrest. It will begin by examining the birth of modern CPR and the mechanism and epidemiology of cardiac arrest and sudden cardiac death. It will then touch on the evolution of EMS, equipping them to deal with out-of-hospital cardiac arrests like never before and to make a significant contribution to research in this area. This chapter will also examine some of the issues surrounding the research that has lead to our current guidelines for VF cardiac arrests and how these guidelines have been shaped by a concerted international effort headed by ILCOR.

Chapter IV - Cardiac arrest affects more than 250,000 people per year in the USA. Ventricular Fibrillation (VF) is the rhythm observed in up to 40% of the cases, when help arrives. Current guidelines recommend initiation of immediate bystander cardiopulmonary resuscitation (CPR), electrical defibrillation and epinephrine (adrenaline) administration.

Since the restoration of threshold levels of coronary perfusion pressure (CPP) has been found to be the only independent determinant of return of spontaneous circulation (ROSC), the use of a vasopressor agent has been considered indispensable for successful CPR. Epinephrine holds a predominant role as the drug of choice for more than 100 years. However, recent studies have shown that eventhough the use of epinephrine increases the possibility of ROSC, it does not result in higher hospital discharge rates when compared to placebo in VF cardiac arrest setting.

Epinephrine is an endogenous catecholamine which possesses both alpha and beta adrenergic actions. Its beneficial effects are assumed to be primarily due to its $\alpha_2$ action leading to peripheral arteriolar vasoconstriction, increasing thus the aortic pressure and consequently myocardial and cerebral perfusion.

On the other hand, epinephrine's $\alpha_1$, $\beta_1$ and $\beta_2$ actions have serious arrhythmogenic effects originated from the resulting increase of oxygen demands in an already fasting myocardium, the increase of myocardial lactate levels and the decrease of myocardial ATP reserves, increasing thus the severity of post-resuscitation myocardial dysfunction. Furthermore, epinephrine is very sensitive to the effects of acidosis, which is the case in VF setting. Lastly, in cardiac arrest victims, endogenous catecholamine levels have been found to be in extremely elevated concentrations. Therefore, it is possible that almost all the catecholamine receptors have been already been stimulated and an epinephrine administration will not have the expected impact.

The aforementioned data have oriented CPR research to the quest for alternative pharmacologic agents which will either replace epinephrine or attenuate its undesired effects.

Chapter V - Cardiac arrest still remains a daunting medical emergency in Western societies and is the cause of approximately 250,000-600,000 deaths annually in the United States, with ventricular fibrillation being the initial rhythm in 20-38% of cases. Defibrillation is the only treatment available to terminate this life-threatening arrhythmia. This chapter deals initially with the mechanisms of defibrillation, the waveforms and the recommended energy levels of defibrillation. Furthermore, factors influencing transthoracic impedance, which is a major determinant of successful defibrillation, are analysed. Finally, this chapter discusses the use of automated external defibrillators and the early access to defibrillation by lay personnel in out-of-hospital cardiac arrest

Chapter VI - Acute kidney injury (AKI) is common after cardiac surgery with cardiopulmonary bypass (CPB). Previous studies have reported an incidence from 3 to 30% according to the authors and the different criteria considered [1-4]. The percentage of patients with AKI requiring dialysis may vary from 0.5 to 3% according to certain studies [5-12]. Post-operative AKI after cardiac surgery with CPB correlates with an increased length of stay in the intensive care unit (ICU) [5]. It is also associated with a high mortality rate (up to 60%) when dialysis is required [3,5,13]. Risk factors like female gender, diabetes, chronic obstructive pulmonary disease, congestive heart failure, length of surgery and age have been identified [14], and one of the most important factors seems to be chronic renal failure before surgery, even if this last association although requiring further research, has been universally accepted [15].

Recently, studies have demonstrated the association of genetic polymorphisms with a risk of renal injury. The genetic variants identified are associated with increases in renal inflammatory response through exagerated synthesis in the IL6 protein [16]. There is also genetic predisposition.

AKI in CPB is the consequence of a mixture of several physiopathological phenomena, among which the authors find systemic inflammatory response syndrome (SIRS).

Cardiac bypass surgery activates the inflammatory cascade and leads to systemic inflammatory response syndrome through the phenomenon of ischemia-reperfusion. Indeed, initially, the authors can observe an imbalance between pro- and anti-inflammatory factors as well as between factors of vasoconstriction. Secondly, neutrophils, vascular endothelium and platelets are activated. These events lead to capillary microthrombosis and the elaboration of inflammatory mediators such as IL-6, IL-8 and TNF $\alpha$. These cytokines are both synthetised systemically and locally in the kidney. They are responsible for tubular necrosis, apoptosis, and glomerular injury. Serum creatinine and perioperative urinary output which are routinely used to evaluate the underlying renal status of the patient are not sensitive and specific enough in the detection of the early phases of this condition. New biomarkers, including neutrophil gelatinase, associated lipocalin, interleukin 18 and kidney injury molecule 1 seem promising.

Thus, the authors can hope that a better knowledge of all of the mechanisms leading to acute renal dysfunction after coronary artery bypass and the use of new renal injury biomarkers may reduce the negative consequences of AKI.

Chapter VII - Chronic rheumatic heart disease (CRHD), the most severe sequelae of rheumatic fever (RF), continues to be the most important cause of acquired valvulopathy among children and young adults worldwide, being responsible for approximately 233000 deaths annually. RF is autoimmune sequelae of a group A streptococcal (*Streptococcus pyogenes*) oropharyngeal infection which develops several weeks after sore throat has gone away. Carditis occurs in approximately 50–60% of acute RF cases, and CRHD develops in 30-50% of these patients. Cross-reactive antibodies and autoreactive T-lymphocytes lead to inflammation, cellular infiltration and valvular scarring. All heart valves may be damaged, but the mitral valve is most frequently affected, followed by the aortic valve. The fact that approximately 0.3-3% of the streptococcal oropharyngeal infections cause RF, provides evidence of genetic predisposition to disease development. A number of studies have linked HLA genes to the susceptibility of both RF and CRHD, especially those related to HLA-DR and –DQ loci, but non-HLA genes seem also to be involved in the disease. Molecular mimicry between *S. pyogenes* and human proteins has been proposed as the main factor leading to autoimmunity in RF/CRHD and studies demonstrate that CD4+ T lymphocytes play an important role in the development and maintenance of valve lesions. The cytokines profile observed in rheumatic heart valve specimens suggests a Th1 driven response and an imbalance between proinflammatory (IL-1, IL-6, TNF-alpha) and antiinflammatory (IL-4, IL-10) cytokines in these lesions may also contribute to the development of chronic valvulopathy. In addition, a growing body of evidence supports the hypothesis of ongoing inflammation in CRHD. Elevated serum levels of adhesion molecules, high-sensitive C-reactive protein, advanced oxidation protein products (AOPP) and complement components including mannan-binding lectin (MBL) have been observed in RF/CRHD patients. The deposition of complement in heart tissue of RF/CRHD patients has also been reported. Currently, there is no therapy that shows any benefit in reducing the risk of developing heart lesions in patients with acute RF. Although monoclonal antibodies that block IL-1, IL-6, TNF-alpha and B-lymphocytes are already available and successfully used in the treatment of different autoimmune and inflammatory disorders, there is no report recomending the use of those immunomodulators in RF/CRHD. Here the authors present a review of the current understanding of the underlying mechanisms involved in the pathogenesis of RF and CRHD. The authors also discuss the possibility of immunobiological treatments, based on data available on other autoimmune diseases, such as rheumatoid arthritis, ankylosing spondylitis and systemic lupus erythematosus.

Chapter VIII - The aortic valve leaflet has long been observed to be a composite tri-layered structure. However, in characterizing native tissue function, the leaflet tissue has frequently been assumed to be simply a single membrane with uniform transmural stress. Considering that extracellular matrix components, mechanical loading, and cellularity differ across leaflet layers, more consideration of the layered microstructure is warranted. Such knowledge would lay the foundation for more accurate mathematical models of tissue mechanics, vascularity, and diffusion, as well as for the design and analyses of successful therapies to treat heart valve pathology. This review will summarize the current knowledge regarding the primary extracellular matrix constituents and individual mechanics of each layer, as well as their synergistic roles in whole leaflet function. The aortic valve leaflet consists of the fibrosa, spongiosa, and ventricularis layers, and is surrounded by an endothelial layer. The collagen structure of the fibrosa dominates its mechanical behavior, giving the leaflet tensile strength, but also extensibility and flexibility. The ventricularis serves to open and close the valve through the extensibility and elastic recoil of its elastin network. Situated between the outer layers, the viscous nature of the spongiosa is believed to allow shearing between layers, resist compression, and confer flexibility. An endothelial cell layer surrounds the leaflet, and while it contributes little to aortic valve mechanics directly, endothelial cell function is regulated by shear stress and can influence valvular interstitial cell function. Possible directions of future research on this topic include clarifying the functional role of the spongiosa. Particular importance must be placed on characterizing the interconnecting fibers spanning the spongiosa that connect the fibrosa and ventricularis. Layer-specific matrix organization, interstitial cell phenotype, and proteoglycan and glycosaminoglycan content must also be further investigated.

Chapter IX - Functional morphology of LV myocardium and RA appendage in 48 patients with ICMP was studied based on intraoperative biopsies analysis. In the early postoperative period (1 year) all the patients were divided into 2 groups. Group one was comprised of the patients with positive dynamics of EDI and LV EF, group two – with negative ones. Retrospective analysis of echocardiographical values did not let to reveal predictors of postoperative remodeling of heart in both patients groups. On the contrary, drawing clinical-morphological parallels of negative dynamics in the early postoperative period showed that the presence of diffuse lymphocytic- macrophage inflammatory infiltration of myocardial stroma in combination with pronounced fibrosis, low values of trophic index (TI) (<0,015) and specific volume (SV) of atrial natriuretic peptide granules in atrial cardiomyocytes as well as high values of pericappilar diffusion zone (PDZ) (>1000 mcm) and Kernogan index (KI) (>1,6) of LV myocardium are morphological predictors of postoperative heart remodeling.

Chapter X - Unlike organic mitral regurgitation, so-called “functional” or “secondary” mitral regurgitation (MR) is related to progressive left ventricular dilatation, remodeling, dyssinchrony or distortion involving the mitral apparatus. Thus, there is no primary valve disease and leaflets are basically normal. More in general, valvular function is impaired because of underlying chronic or acute left ventricular dysfunction. As a consequence, functional MR is typically encountered in two clinical scenarios: acute left ventricular failure and chronic cardiomyopathy.

Although the possible causes vary widely, the present chapter will focus on the two most common and best studied etiologies of functional MR: chronic ischemic heart disease with left ventricular dysfunction and non-ischemic, idiopathic dilated cardiomyopathy.

Chapter XI - Pregnancy-Induced Hypertension (PIH) is one of the most common causes of maternal and neonatal mortality. It is a multifactorial disease with genetic and environmental factors involved in its etiology. The authors have carried out molecular epidemiologic research on Japanese subjects in order to identify genetic variants associated with PIH, and to analyze confounding genetic and environmental factors involved in the pathophysiology of PIH. Self-administered questionnaires were returned by the subjects between 1 and 6 months after delivery. The candidate genetic variants were identified by means of a PCR-RFLP method. T235 of *AGT*, C1166 of *AT1* and Asp298 of *NOS3* were respectively associated with PIH, although no significant associations were found between PIH and the common genetic variants of *ACE, FV, MTHFR, B3AR, TNF-A, PAI-1, GSTP1, mEH,* or *LPL*. However, in subgroup analyses, a significant association of the TT genotype of *AGT* was maintained only in women possessing the 4G/4G genotype of *PAI-1*, while that of the GA or AA genotype of *NOS3* was maintained only in women possessing the 5G/5G or 4G/5G genotype, suggesting that there must be at least two kinds of possible pathogenetic pathways for the manifestation of severe PIH.

Furthermore, in analyses using genetic, environmental and lifestyle factors, 9 factors were significantly associated with PIH on univariate analysis, and 5 factors, i.e. "prepregnancy BMI > or = 24 kg/m2", "family history of hypertension", "TT genotype of AGT", "mentally stressful condition during pregnancy," and "salty dishes preferred during pregnancy" were found to be independent and potent risk factors for PIH on multivariate analysis. Dividing the subjects into 2 subgroups according to whether they possessed "TT genotype of AGT" or not, the authors identified acquired risk factors before and during pregnancy for PIH in each of the groups. A multivariate analysis identified "mentally stressful condition" as a potent significant risk factor during pregnancy in the former subgroup. However, there were no significant risk factors concerning "mental stress" in the latter subgroup. Through further exploration of the risk factors associated with PIH, useful insights should emerge for development of new and effective preventive measures for a range of multifactorial diseases.

Chapter XII - The authors have summarized the care management of pregnant women with complete atrioventricular block (CAVB) by reviewing the data from previous literature and their experience including 29 births. The management of patients already implanted with a permanent pacemaker does not involve any risks. Some of the patients without permanent pacemaker may develop syncope due to heart failure during pregnancy. Pre-pregnancy prophylactic placement of a permanent pacemaker is not indicated in all asymptomatic patients; however, for symptomatic patients in the first and second trimesters, permanent pacemaker implantation is the therapy of choice. For symptomatic women with CAVB who present at or near term, temporary pacing at the earliest possible time prior to labor induction should be recommended. Most pregnant women with CAVB who do not require a permanent pacemaker before delivery can be managed safely during labor even without temporary pacing. Elective epidural analgesia and forceps delivery are also important components of the care of patients without permanent pacemaker for maintaining stable maternal hemodynamics.

Chapter XIII - More and more are the evidence that identify hypertensive disorders in pregnancy as an important factor of cardiovascular risk. Compared to women who have had a prior physiological pregnancy the authors can see that those who had pregnancy complicated by hypertensive disorders show an increased predisposition for cardiovascular diseases in the following years, with a higher risk of myocardial infarction and cerebral ictus. The close correlation between hypertensive dysfunction in pregnancy-particularly preeclampsia-and cardiovascular diseases can be in part explained since they have factors of risk in common, such as obesity, diabetes and dyslipidemia, which cause as a whole the so-called "metabolic syndrome".

In addition, the altered endothelial function, *primum movens* of the micro and macro vascular damage, is either present in the metabolic syndrome or in the hypertension in pregnancy. So there are numerous analogies between the two pathologic conditions, and the clinical epidemiological data, almost univocal, shows that hypertension in pregnancy must be considered by the gynaecologist as a factor of risk for women's health, not only during gestation but also to the years to come.

Chapter XIV - In monitoring complex arrhythmias, optical mapping is used to study the signals obtained from the cardiac tissue surface. Most studies have assumed that the fluorescent signal is emitted from the surface layer of cells. However, recent experiments have proved that the optical signal is the averaged response of the transmembrane potential over depth rather than only the surface. It is important to understand how to interpret the measured transmembrane potential resulting from electric stimulation in terms of the fluorescent signal emitted from the tissue. The objective of this chapter is to compare the results of the optical signal from the surface and averaged over depth.

The authors use a computer simulation of the bidomain model of the cardiac tissue and the Beeler-Reuter model of the ion channel kinetics to investigate the difference between the surface and the averaged transmembrane potentials. The bidomain model, which consists of intracellular and extracellular domains, approximates the cardiac tissue as a continuum and is a set of two coupled partial differential equations, solved using numerical methods. The Beeler-Reuter model uses Hodgkin-Huxley-like equations to represent four ionic currents in the cardiac membrane.

The authors use an electrode situated in a bath just above the cardiac tissue to stimulate the tissue, producing an activation wave front and inducing intramural reentry. The authors analyze potentials at the surface and below, and their results indicate that depth-weighted optical signals may provide important information about cardiac activation dynamics, such as the type of reentry, the direction of the propagation, and the spatial distribution of depolarization or repolarization. Their results show that averaging over depth has a significant impact on the interpretation of optical signals and that many of the poorly-understood features of optical mapping signals--such as double-hump action potentials, slow rates of rise and smaller than predicted polarization during the stimulus--can be explained by merely averaging over depth to obtain the optical signal.

Chapter XV - The advancements of cardiac surgery over the last decades led to larger numbers of patients with operated congenital heart diseases surviving into adulthood. The traditional treatment of congenital heart defects in adults has been surgical correction. Percutaneous interventional treatments for such conditions have rapidly advanced in last two decades. The availability of transcatheter devices has revolutionized the management of patients with congenital heart and vascular disease. The adult congenital heart disease patient, at baseline or in need of intervention, presents unique challenges to caregivers.The authors discuss the current applications of interventional treatment in adults with congenital heart defects and conclude that it is safe and feasible, that the indications for this approach to treatment are increasing, that it can be undertaken in patients of any age including high-risk patients.

Chapter XVI - Aortic stenosis is the most frequently occurring valvular heart disease and cardiovascular disease after systemic arterial hypertension and coronary artery disease. Contrary to old assumptions, the coexistence of aortic stenosis and systemic arterial hypertension is highly significant (32 to 50%). In this case, the overloaded left ventricle has to support, at the same time, the increase in pressure due to systemic arterial hypertension as well as the increase in transvalvular pressure gradient due to the aortic stenosis. Knowing which overload is the most significant, valvular or arterial, is a difficult problem. However, this information is essential to determine which medical treatment is more beneficial to the patient: valve replacement or reduction of arterial pressure. Indeed, replacing the native valve while the most significant load supported by the left ventricle is systemic arterial hypertension will not necessarily improve patient's condition. In the same way, reducing arterial pressure in severe aortic stenosis can compromise coronary circulation (mainly if the hypertension results from a significant decrease in arterial compliance). This chapter deals with the interaction between aortic stenosis and systemic arterial hypertension and their combined effect on the left ventricle. More specifically, the impact of systemic arterial hypertension on the assessment of aortic stenosis severity, in terms of transvalvular pressure gradients and effective orifice areas, will be addressed. Then, new parameters such as "valvulo-arterial impedance" and "hypertensive equivalent effective orifice area", introduced to determine the overall load supported by the left ventricle, will be explained and discussed. Furthermore, recommendations on how markers of aortic stenosis severity in hypertensive patients should be interpreted will be issued.

Aortic stenosis (AS) is considered the most common cardiac disease in developed countries after coronary artery disease and systemic arterial hypertension (Braunwald et al. (2001)). It is usually a degenerative disease that produces an obstruction to flow passing from the left ventricle (LV) to the ascending aorta. Its prevalence in industrialized countries ranges between 2 to 7% (Stewart et al. (1997); Lindroos et al. (1993)) and it is responsible for around 100,000 valve replacements and 20,000 deaths per year in North America (Pibarot et al. (2007)). However, only few patients develop an isolated AS. This shows that AS is a component of a more global group of pathologies affecting not only the valve itself but also the proximal arteries. Among all of the pathologies associated with AS, systemic arterial hypertension has a very high prevalence. Systemic arterial hypertension is defined as an abnormal increase in blood pressure (systolic pressure > 140 mmHg and/or diastolic pressure > 90 mmHg). It may result from an increase in systemic arterial resistance (systolo-diastolic hypertension), a decrease in systemic arterial compliance (systolic hypertension), or both.

Table 1 shows the classification of aortic stenosis and hypertension severities as evaluated using systolic pressure, diastolic pressures and effective orifice area, respectively.

Chapter XVII - Median sternotomy with central cannulation is the standard approach to the aortic valve for repair or replacement. Over the last decade, surgical exposure options other than a full sternotomy such as a “J” or “T” partial-sternotomy, or a right "mini” anterior thoracotomy and peripheral cannulation methods have captured the interest of cardiac surgeons in search of a “less invasive, minimal access” approach. Less invasive surgical approaches have reduced peri-operative mortality, ventilatory support time, intensive care unit and hospital stays and total hospital costs. Over the last five years, catheter-based technologies have emerged as viable options for aortic valve replacement in patients previously considered to be too high risk for conventional or minimally invasive aortic valve (MIAV) surgery. Implantation of catheter-mounted prostheses may be performed via the antegrade (femoral vein), retrograde (femoral artery) or transapical (left ventricular apex) route. Each delivery route has potential advantages and disadvantages as well as technical, vascular and mechanical limitations. As technology improves, current and future devices and delivery systems being evaluated should overcome these limitations and provide catheter-based prostheses as a viable therapeutic option for aortic valve replacement.

Chapter XVIII - In this case report authors analyse their own experience in the treatment of aortoenteric fistulas (AEF), consequently to the last technical improvements. They have favoured amongst others, arterial allografts, axillo-femoral bypasses and endografts. For the purpose of this report, their surgical activities between January 1994 and December 2008 have been analysed and obtained datas have proved that allografts are an efficacious technical option for the treatment of AEFs. Extra-anatomical bypasses are an alternative whether a lack of prosthetic material is encountered; endografts, in spite of their wide diffusion in literature, remain a limited and definite indication in few cases or one way to solve a severe haemorrhage, carrying the patients to better conditions to be operated on consequentially.

It is also underlined how the complexity of clinical manifestations of AEFs needs a wide selection of treatments and technical choices available to operators.

Chapter XIX - It is well known that sympathetic nervous system innervation is important in the genesis of ventricular fibrillation. Loss of protective vagal reflex measured using heart rate variability or baroreflex sensitivity is also associated with sudden cardiac death because of reflecting sympathetic hyperinnervation. However, recent studies propose the close relationship between cardiac sympathetic denervation and occurrence of ventricular tachyarrhythmias. Sympathetic hyperinnervation caused by heart diseases or arrhythmogenesis itself results in cardiac sympathetic rejuvenation (hyperplasia, reduced norepinephrine uptake, reduced norepinephrine synthesis, and fetal gene expression) into the heart. Thus, rejuvenated and hyperinnervated neurons progress to cardiac sympathetic nervous system denervation. Recently, these co-existences have been suggested to be a trigger of ventricular tachyarrhythmia. Beta-adrenergic blockade has been shown not only to decrease sudden cardiac death but also to improve cardiac sympathetic nervous system denervation in patients with myocardial ischemia or heart failure. Iodine-123 metaiodobenzylguanidine ($^{123}$I-MIBG) represents an analog of norepinephrine, and $^{123}$I-MIBG scintigraphy can assess the magnitude of catecholamine re-uptake into heart, and impairment of cardiac sympathetic nervous system. Recent investigators and the authors have evaluated using cardiac uptakes of $^{123}$I-MIBG whether cardiac sympathetic nervous system denervation is associated with the occurrence of ventricular tachyarrhythmia and sudden cardiac death. $^{123}$I-MIBG scintigraphy was performed in patients with ventricular tachyarrhythmias, and these patients were followed up. These studies found that the cardiac sympathetic nervous system denervation is predictive of sudden cardiac death in both patients with structural heart disease and idiopathic ventricular tachyarrhythmia. These results may explain that cardiac sympathetic nervous system denervation is one of the triggers of life-threatening ventricular tachyarrhythmias.

Chapter XX – The impact of the fetal environment on the frequency of cardiovascular disorders in adults was first noted in a report by Dr. David Barker. In this seminal report, it was shown that individuals, who were small at birth, had substantially increased risk of death from cardiovascular disease and stroke. This concept has since been coined the 'Barker Hypothesis' and numerous studies and texts have described the phenomenon of fetal imprinting of adult cardiovascular disease. Similar findings have been published by many other investigators, and the main focus of this field of research to date has been on the impact of poor fetal nutrition leading to long term impact on cardiovascular system structure and/or function. Low birth weight has been associated with increased rates of coronary heart disease and the related disorders of stroke, hypertension and type 2 diabetes. Although caloric (and especially protein) restriction leads to reduced fetal growth and development, an additional major cause for delivery of low birth weight infants, particularly preterm infants, is maternal infection and inflammation.[5, 6] Although the mechanisms involved are not well defined, the significance of this problem will expand, as the incidence of preterm birth and the survival of low birth weight babies continues to increase throughout the world.

Chapter XXI – The authors performed a retrospective study on the occurrence of haemostatic disorders in 1381 patients with various malignant tumours between 1996 and 2004. The mean age of the 872 male and 509 female patients was 57.8 (37 to 79) years. In the majority or their patients the authors diagnosed a malignancy of primary pulmonary localisation (1140 patients) including 790 patients with non-small cell lung cancer (NSCLC), mostly adenocarcinoma and squamous cell carcinoma (70 %). In the other cases large cell carcinoma, bronchioloalveolar or mixed type malignant tumour was diagnosed. 68 of the 790 patients with NSCLC were in an operable stage, 346 patients belonged to Stages IIIA and IIIB, while 274 have proven to be of clinical Stage IV.

Of the 350 patients with SCLC, 185 and 165 were of extended or limited clinical stage, respectively. The other patients with tumours of non-bronchopulmonary localisation (n = 241) had advanced, metastasising mammary, colorectal, renal or vesical carcinoma.

Chapter XXII – Purpose: To determine if there is an association between the presence of abdominal aortic aneurysm and the prevalence of ocular pseudoexfoliation syndrome (PEX).

Methods: The authors studied 120 eyes of 60 patients, distributed into two groups according to whether they had been diagnosed with abdominal aortic aneurysm in the past

5 years (n=30) or not (n=30). A complete ophthalmologic examination was performed, classifying patients in whom pseudoexfoliation was found into 3 levels according to its severity, and serum concentrations of folic acid, vitamin B12 and homocysteine were determined.

Results: The prevalence of pseudoexfoliation syndrome in patients with abdominal aortic aneurysm was 3.3% versus 13.3% in the control group. A higher prevalence of ischemic heart disease (50%) was found in the group of patients with pseudoexfoliation than in the rest of the study subjects (7.5%) ($p=0.09$). Mean homocysteine levels in patients without pseudoexfoliation were lower (13.3 µmol/l) than in the group of patients with pseudoexfoliation (31.98 µmol/l) ($p=0.001$).

Conclusions: This study raises the need to screen for hyperhomocysteinemia in patients in whom pseudoexfoliation is detected, because high homocysteine levels could be related to the higher incidence of ischemic heart disease in this patient group. In these cases, treatment with vitamin B group supplements could prevent the development of cardiovascular disease.

In: Advances in Cardiovascular Research, Volume 1
Editors: L. Schmitt, T. Konig, pp. 1-45
ISBN: 978-1-60741-720-0


*Chapter I*

# The Mitral Valve: Development, Structure, Pathology & Tissue Engineering

***Alexander Black[a,*], Brendan M. Corcoran[b], Ruth Heying[c], Stefan Jockenhoevel[d] and Thomas C. Flanagan[e]***

[a]Department of Anatomy, National University of Ireland Galway, Ireland.
[b]Department of Veterinary Clinical Studies, University of Edinburgh, Scotland.
[c]Department of Paediatric Cardiology, UZ Leuven, Belgium.
[d]Department of Applied Medical Engineering, Helmholtz Institute for Biomedical Engineering, Aachen University, Germany.
[e]School of Medicine & Medical Science, Health Sciences Centre, University College Dublin, Ireland.

## Abstract

The mitral valve is a complex, specialised connective tissue structure which acts to maintain the forward flow of blood through the left side of the heart. The mitral valve consists of two leaflets, with numerous supporting chordae tendineae. The mitral valve leaflets have a layered structure, with the structural constituents of each layer determined by its functional role. Evidence suggests that the valvular interstitial cells (VICs) which are present within the connective tissue layers of the mitral valve play an active role in mitral valve dynamics, a theory enhanced by the observation of neural structures within the valve tissue. Disease of the heart valves, such as myxomatous mitral valve disease, has been associated with changes in the phenotype of valvular cells and composition of the valvular extracellular matrix (ECM), and continues to have a devastating impact worldwide. Despite valve repair being the preferred initial treatment method to address severe mitral valve disease, valve repair is not feasible in a large number of patients with end-stage valve disease, and replacement of the mitral valve with a biological or

* Corresponding author: Department of Anatomy, National University of Ireland Galway (NUIG), Newcastle Road, Galway, Ireland, Tel. +353 91 492234, Fax +353 91 494520, E-mail: alexander.black@nuigalway.ie

mechanical prosthesis is necessary. A number of limitations are associated with conventional prosthetic mitral valves, however, including thromboembolism, life-threatening haemorrhagic complications, limited durability, rejection and transmission of infection. To overcome these limitations, the focus of prosthetic valve research has shifted to the development of living valves with growth and remodelling capabilities through tissue engineering, with many animal studies demonstrating the feasibility of this approach. The present chapter provides a comprehensive review on the development and structure of the mitral valve, particularly relating to its connective tissue and cellular components, while morphological and histological changes in this structure associated with mitral valve disease are also discussed. Potential future treatment modalities for pathological mitral valve disease using tissue-engineered structures are also discussed.

# I. Development of the Mitral Valve Apparatus

The process of the development of the mitral valve seems central to proper understanding of the aetiology of valve anomalies and their potential treatment. The mitral valve is a complex arrangement of an annulus and leaflets which are supported by a subvalvular apparatus consisting of papillary muscles and tendinous cords (Figure 1) [Wenink and Gittenberger-de-Groot, 1986; Kanani et al., 2005]. Over time, different aspects of mitral valve development have been investigated and although recent studies bring us closer to the nature of valve formation, it has yet to be fully elucidated [Wenink, 1992; Oosthoek et al., 1998a; Moorman et al., 2003; Kanani et al., 2005].

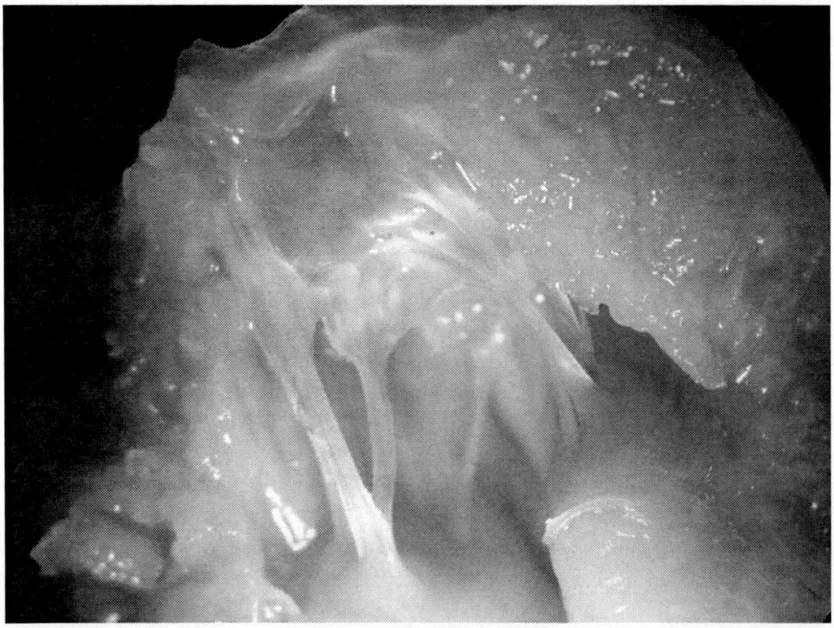

Figure 1. The rat mitral valve *in situ.* The translucence of the leaflets and chordae tendineae of the valve give a false impression of weakness. The relative thinness of the structures comprising the valve is readily apparent.

The mitral valve appears as an intersegmental structure and therefore a brief description of the formation of embryonic cardiac segments is called for.

Mesodermal tissue gives rise to formation of the primary heart tube in week 3 of development. After bending to the right, the primary heart tube consists of an atrial and ventricular loop with the latter developing an inlet and outlet segment [Webb et al., 1998; Moorman et al., 2003]. The atrial and ventricular component of the heart loop is separated by the area of the future atrioventricular (AV) canal. An inner curvature forms in this heart loop prior to the formation of the primary fold. This then fuses in part with the AV groove, a vital structure for the later separation of the future AV and arterial orifices [Wenink et al., 1986].

At this stage, conversion into the four definitive heart chambers is initiated simultaneously [Lamers and Moorman, 2002; Moorman et al., 2003]. At the end of week 4 of development, superior and inferior endocardial cushions are seen forming out of the ventricular wall – these will form the future AV junction [Wenink and Gittenberger-de-Groot, 1986; Kanani et al., 2005]. The superior and inferior endocardial cushions grow towards each other and begin to fuse at 5 weeks of development, dividing the AV canal into a right and left component [Oosthoek et al., 1998a; Lamers and Moorman, 2002; Kanani et al., 2005]. The parts of the fused cushions which remain at the left side of the heart will form the aortic leaflet of the mitral valve. The right sided parts of the fused cushions will form the larger parts of the developing membranous septum.

The larger circumference of the AV canal is supported by the inlet component of the ventricular loop from which the apical part of the developing left ventricle has ballooned [Kim et al., 2001]. The apical part of the developing right ventricle balloons from the outlet part of the ventricular heart tube [Lamers and Moorman, 2002; Moorman et al., 2003].

Ventricular septation begins when the primordium of the muscular ventricular septum appears in week 5 and starts to grow from the heart base towards the AV junction. It leaves a communication between the presumptive right and left ventricle - the interventricular foramen [Webb et al., 2003].

During week 5 of development, endocardial cells situated in the AV junction and ventricles show an epithelial-mesenchymal transformation. In-growths in the ECM are caused by inductive signals originating in the myocardium of the AV junction; this is important for the development of both the AV-valves and membranous part of the interventricular septum. Several factors such as bone morphogenic protein (BMP)-2 and -4, transforming growth factor-ß (TGF-β) -1 and -2 and activin-like kinase-2 play a role [Ng et al., 2004; Somi et al., 2004].

Atrial separation in the area of the AV junction becomes evident when the primary septum grows downwards from the atrial roof and its leading edge, a mesenchymal cap, finally fuses the superior AV endocardial cushion and the mesenchymal tissue of the vestibular spine [Anderson et al., 2003a].

Fusion of the endocardial cushions and septation of the heart are central to the development of the mitral valve apparatus. However, mitral valve formation can only continue after the developing aorta is committed to the left ventricle [Kanani et al., 2005].

Thus, in week 5 of development, the arterial trunks are formed by septation of the solitary outflow tract of the primary heart tube. Two opposing endocardial ridges, also termed outflow cushions, fuse to divide the outlet area into the pulmonary and aortic outflow tract [Anderson et al., 2003b; Kanani et al., 2005]. At the same time, the outflow cushions fuse with the crest of the muscular septum which leads to the aforementioned incorporation of the aorta into the outlet part of the left ventricle, after inferior reorientation of the left AV junction. Closure of the interventricular foramen is now achieved. The aortic root is positioned between the ventricular septum and the fused left ventricular components of the AV cushions. Only later does a definitive fibrous continuity between the aortic leaflet of the mitral valve and the non-coronary and left coronary leaflet of the aortic valve become established.

By week 7 of development, the aortic leaflet of the mitral valve is formed from the left ventricular components of the fused superior and inferior cushion and therefore establishes the first leaflet. A lateral cushion has also been formed and increases in size to occupy two thirds of the circumference of the mitral orifice. This lateral cushion remodels to form longer structures which give origin to the mural leaflet of the developed valve.

Recent investigations reveal that endocardial cushion tissue contributes to the AV junction, the valve leaflets and chordae [De la Cruz et al., 1983; Lamers et al., 1995; Oosthoek et al., 1998a, 1998b]. The endocardial cushions can be distinguished as two different layers by immunohistological staining which remains present in all developmental stages [Oosthoek et al., 1998a]. The so called atrial layer is cell rich and positive for laminin whilst the ventricular layer shows positive type III collagen staining in the extracellular space with a reduction in number of cells present [Oosthoek et al., 1998a]. Fibronectin is predominantly found in the ventricular layer after week 7 of development [Oosthoek et al., 1998a].

Morphologic development continues with the appearance of the papillary muscles. The wall of the left ventricle is built from an outer layer of compact myocardium and an inner trabecular layer [Oosthoek et al., 1998b; Moorman et al., 2003]. By week 5 of development, a prominent muscular ridge composed of thick trabeculae with intertrabecular spaces is visable within the inner layer by electron microscopical examination [Oosthoek et al., 1998b]. This ridge is connected to the ventricular wall and runs from the posterior AV junction around the apex to the anterior AV junction. The anterior edge touches the superior AV cushion and the posterior edge is covered by the inferior cushion - the cushion tissue which gives origin to the aortic leaflet of the mitral valve [Wenink et al., 1986; Oosthoek et al., 1998b].

From week 7, delamination of the ventricular myocardium starts underneath the endocardial cushions of the parietal wall with gaps becoming visible within the myocardium [Oosthoek et al., 1998a, 1998b; Kanani et al., 2005]. Many trabeculae which connect the delaminated myocardium and the left ventricular wall in week 8 condense and further separate from the left ventricular wall in order to form the primordium of the papillary muscles up to week 10.

This implicates that there is no connection between the anterior and posterior part of the ridge and the ventricular wall at this stage of development leading to the characteristic morphology of a solid, freely movable posteromedial and anterolateral papillary muscle [Oosthoek et al., 1998b; Lamers and Moorman, 2002; Kanani et al., 2005]. The papillary muscles are only connected to the ventricular wall at their bases.

Myocardial connections between the delaminated myocardium and the parietal part of the left ventricular wall in the AV region dissolve in week 10 to form ridges of fibrous tissue at the ventricular side of the leaflets which continue in the direction of the chords and papillary muscles. Thus, the lateral cushion tissue of the developing mural leaflet is only attached to the atrial and ventricular myocardium as well as to the tips of the papillary muscles [Oosthoek et al., 1998a, 1998b].

Small gaps develop within the cushion tissue of both developing valve leaflets at the site of attachment to the developing papillary muscles. Following this, the leaflets gradually delaminate from ventricular myocardium and the delaminating myocardial layer below the cushion tissue becomes thinner and fragmented – a characterising stage in formation and liberation of the leaflets [Oosthoek et al., 1998b]. At this stage, the leaflets remain connected to the developing papillary muscles [Oosthoek et al., 1998b; Kanani et al., 2005].

Histologically, an increase in cell density in the ventricular layer of the cushion tissue is seen as well as orientation of cells from the valve annulus towards the developing papillary muscles.

From week 10, interchordal spaces become visible within the ventricular layer of the cushion tissue at the tip of the developing papillary muscles [Oosthoek et al., 1998a, 1998b]. The myocardium separates from the valves and distinct chordae are recognised as thin structures in continuity with the papillary muscles. In this way, the ventricular layer of the cushion tissue remodels into chords, which have been shown in recent studies to derive from cushion tissue only [Oosthoek et al., 1998b].

The development of two valve leaflets and chords attached to the two papillary muscles is now achieved and is clearly visible from week 14. Even with leaflets being only a few millimetres in size, the entire mitral valve apparatus has developed all of its morphologic characteristics [Wenink and Gittenberger-de-Groot, 1986; Oosthoek et al., 1998b; Kanani et al., 2005]. A detailed knowledge of mitral valve formation gives insight to specific mechanisms and timing of maldevelopment which occurs in different mitral valve pathologies [Wenink et al., 1986; Oosthoek et al., 1998b; Kanani et al., 2005].

## II. Histological Anatomy of the Mitral Valve

The histological structure of the valve has received remarkably little attention in its own right. Although some publications appeared in the 1940s and 1960s these are in the German language [e.g. Puff, 1965]. The seminal English language work in the area is therefore that of Gross and Kugel [1931] who studied the human valves. As this is the first publication to offer a histological nomenclature for cardiac valves, subsequent authors tend to refer to this work as a basis for mitral histology.

The mitral leaflets are described as trilaminar structures consisting of a dense connective tissue core of variable consistency covered on both the atrial and ventricular aspects with a layer of endothelium. Later authors prefer to use the term endocardium [Icardo and Colvee, 1995], while others use the two terms interchangeably [Millington-Sanders et al., 1998].

The valve leaflets are regarded as being those structures which commence after the termination of atrial myocardium, a point of some confusion in the past with reference to muscular and vasculature components of the valve – neither of which are deemed present in the normal state [Gross and Kugel, 1931].

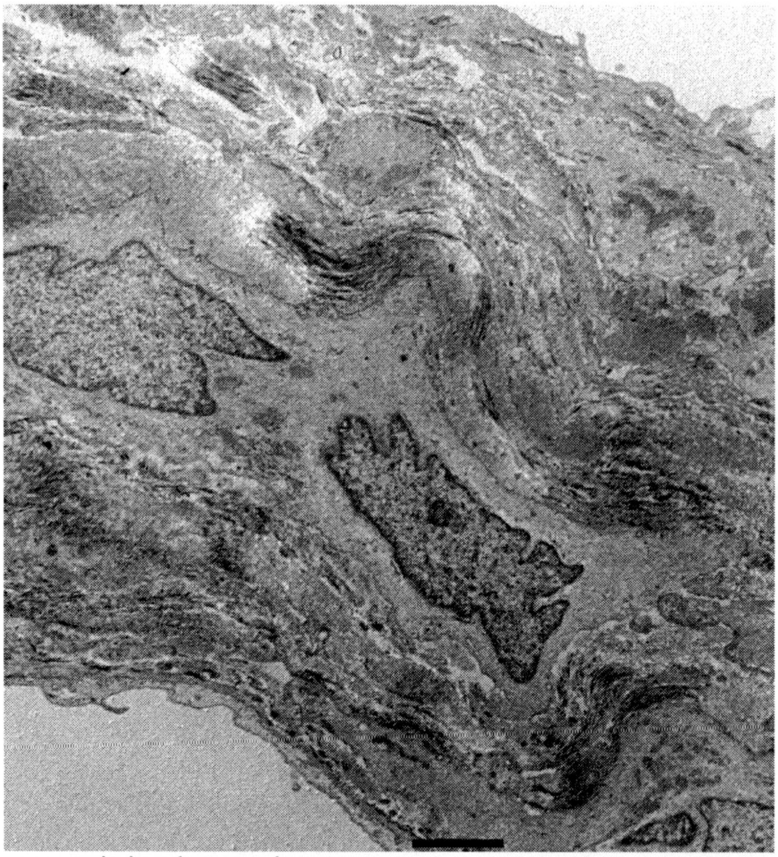

Rat mitral valve; transmission electron microscopy.
Lead citrate and uranyl acetate staining.
Scale bar = 2 μm.

Figure 2. Tranmission electron microscopy of a cross section through a rat mitral leaflet demonstrates the atrial and ventricular endocardial endothelial layers enveloping a connective tissue-rich fibrosa and spongiosa. Obvious in this image are two large valvar interstitial cells. Note the undulating collagen bundles and the surface microappendages of the endothelial cells.

The typical leaflet is essentially an envelope of endocardial endothelium containing connective tissue, connective tissue cells and neural components which hangs off a terminal portion of the annulus fibrosis. This inverted pyramidal area of dense connective tissue has been termed the 'valve ring' [Gross and Kugel, 1931]. The description of the typical leaflet can be made from the atrial through to the ventricular surface in cross-section (Figure 2).

The atrial surface (atrialis) presents a monolayer of flattened endocardium with sparse cytoplasm and moderately dense nuclei. This overlies a mix of loose collagen and elastin fibers, the elastin being thicker on the atrial aspect (Figure 3). A layer of cells regarded as smooth muscle at the time was reportedly situated close to the subendocardium; this may be up to 1/5 of the entire cross sectional (atrial to ventricular) thickness of the anterior leaflet [Gross and Kugel, 1931]. The elastic component is seen in the first two-thirds of the leaflet, being denser at the base and tapering distally. The corresponding ventricular surface (ventricularis) is similar to the atrialis but lies on a more delicate elastic lattice.

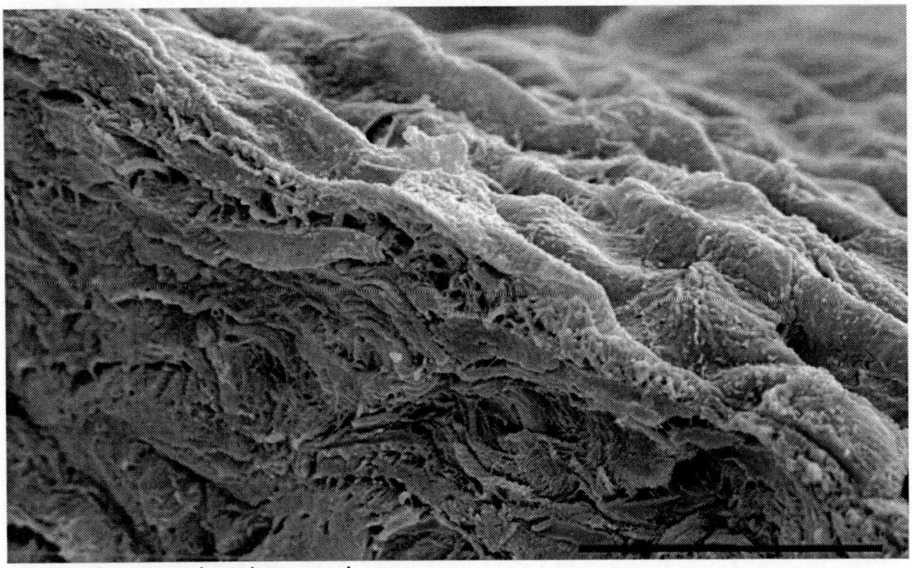

Equine mitral valve; scanning electron microscopy.
Scale bar = 20 µm.

Figure 3. Mitral valve architecture is similar in all mammals. This cross-section through an equine mitral leaflet clearly shows the surface endocardial endothelium overlying a layered arrangement of connective tissues, with elastin scattered throughout the collagen.

The second layer of the valve is termed the zona spongiosa, and consists of a subendothelial layer composed of collagen and elastin interspersed with fibroblast/smooth muscle-like cells which have been variously described as smooth muscle [Gross and Kugel, 1931] and fibroblasts [Cooper et al., 1966]. The spongiosa is less dense in the posterior leaflet, and areas of chordal insertion on both leaflets have abundant collagen with a delicate infiltrate of thin elastic fibrils [Gross and Kugel, 1931].

The final layer is termed the zona fibrosa, and occupies the central zone of the valve, as seen in section. A dense and broad layer, it consists of a tightly organised web of collagen fibres which thins as it approaches the free edge of the leaflet. It may be considered as the collagenous skeleton of the valve. The chordae tendineae are regarded by some as a continuation of the collagenous portion of the fibrosa thus linking the valve 'proper' to the papillary muscles [Gross and Kugel, 1931].

# III. Surface Topographical and Ultrastructural Anatomy of the Mitral Valve

It seems ironic that although there are very few papers dealing with the normal histological structure of the valve, there are many which consider valvar structure with electron microscopy. The term ultrastructure here refers to observations made using transmission electron microscopy (TEM) while the term surface topography refers to those made using scanning electron microscopy (SEM).

The surface topography of the valve will be dealt with first, followed by the internal structure of its constituent cells.

## III.I. Surface Topography of the Mitral Valve

The mitral valve, as outlined above, has a surface covering of endocardial endothelium (EE) and thus this is the cell type observed on the surface of the normal and abnormal valve (Figure 4). Several studies have been carried out using SEM to view the surface of the valve and related endocardial endothelial layers, yet there is little agreement. This seems likely to be due to the range of preparative techniques used and also in part may be due to the range of species studied which includes human [Riddle et al., 1989; Stein et al., 1989; Harasaki et al., 1978; Lim and Boughner, 1977], Japanese and Crab-eating monkey [Harasaki et al., 1975], rat [Andries, 1994], mouse [Icardo et al., 1993], guinea pig [Hill and Folan-Curran, 1993], rabbit [Sarphie, 1982; Iemoto and Kondo, 1982], ferret [Koprla and Nemeseri, 1984], dog [Peine and Low, 1975; Sarphie, 1980; Deck, 1986; Corcoran et al., 2004], cat [Song, 1977] and domestic chicken [Morse et al., 1984].

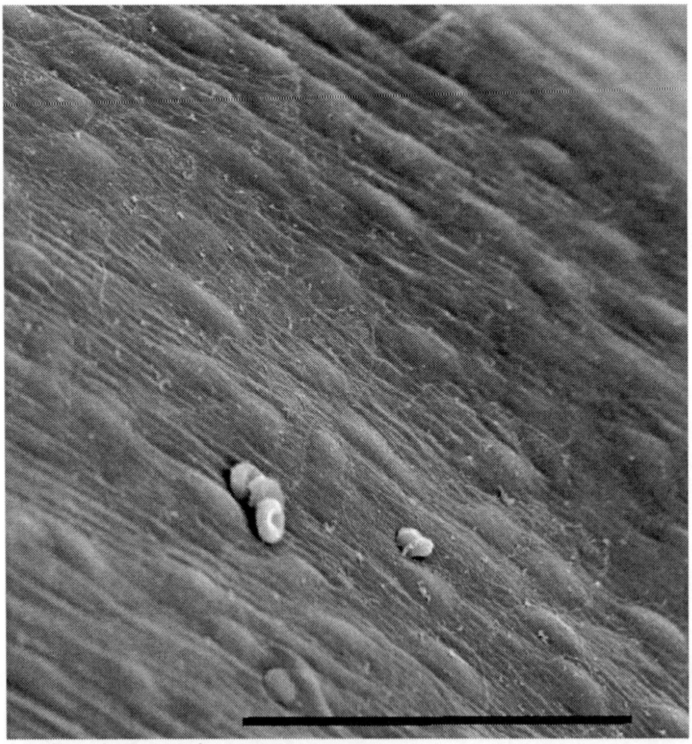

Rat mitral valve; scanning electron microscopy.
Scale bar = 50 μm.

Figure 4. Using scanning electron microscopy, the surface of the mitral valve shows a continuous layer of endocardial endothelium, each cell overlapping its neighbours and producing defined marginal folds. Surface microappendages are also visible, of varying size and morphology. The erythrocytes give an impression of the scale.

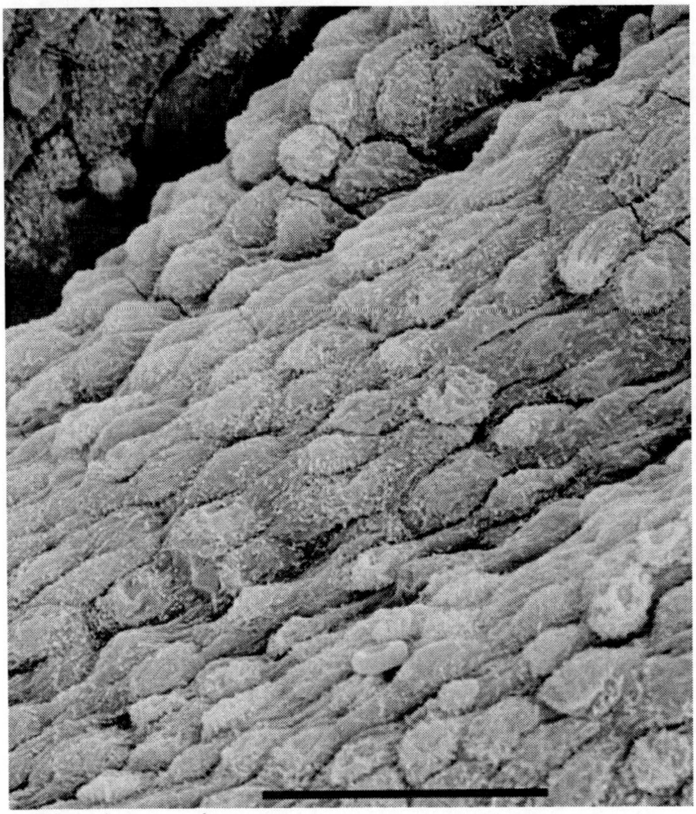

Rat mitral valve; scanning electron microscopy.
Scale bar = 30 μm.

Figure 5. Endocardial endothelial cells align themselves to the underlying collagen of the valve. This produces an ordered appearance on the valvar surface. This specimen demonstrates dense populations of microappendages on the endocardial surface.

The literature agrees on several points regarding EE: it forms a continuous and uninterrupted layer of cells over the entire valve surface (Figure 4). These cells are characterised in all species by a basic polygonal or polyhedral appearance with a raised centre which corresponds to the location of the nucleus. Also present are a variable number of surface projections of very variable morphology (Figure 5).

In the canine, the EE has been described as having a similar morphology over the entire cardiac orifice. Nuclear bulges are regarded as being denser on the valve surface than anywhere else with the remarkably consistent pattern only changing where local conditions dictate. It is reported that there is no change in EE topography during the cardiac cycle with the exception of so-called "systolic furrows" being present between cells during systole and disappearing during diastole; the cardiac cycle was mimicked in one experiment by the addition of $CaCl_2$ and KCl respectively [Peine and Low, 1975]. The same authors observed cell margins which on the AV valves are ribboned along the periphery of each EE cell. The dense population of microappendages seen which included ruffles, blebs and microvilli were assumed to be processing artifact, although as all subsequent groups report these, this seems unlikely. Sarphie [1980] published similar observations on the canine mitral valve and further states that EE of the atrial surface possess more prominent bulges and a denser population of microappendages than the corresponding cells on the ventricular (which are smaller, and thus may be more densely packed). The appearance of microappendages is suggested as being a morphological indicator of synthetic activity. This is supported by Hill and Folan-Curran [1993] in their guinea pig study where an irregular sheet of undulating EE is observed. Margins of cells are outlined by interlacing polyhedral lines around a central nuclear bulge. Cells are similar in size on both sides of the valve with the distal edge of valve possessing more microappendages than either the base or middle region.

The feline valve is said to be also covered with a continuous EE similar to that already outlined. However, some surface pits are seen which have been suggested as being the site of former microappendages [Song, 1977].

The rabbit mitral valve on SEM reveals the general mammalian EE pattern, as does the rat [Andries, 1994] and ferret, although the EE in the latter is reported to be particularly folded [Koprla and Nemeseri, 1984]. That of the rabbit is reported to have ridges of endothelial cells extending from the annulus towards chordal insertion sites, with no major differences between atrial and ventricular surface [Iemoto and Kondo, 1982]. This last point is disputed by Sarphie [1982] who states that the cells of the atrial surface cover a larger surface area and all cells are distinctly oriented, with the transverse axis lying perpendicular to blood flow and the longitudinal axis parallel.

Primate mitral valve, as evidenced by the monkeys Macaca fuscata and M. irus along with humans once again conform to the general plan. Harasaki et al. [1975] using monkeys report mitral EE to be relatively small cells with dimensions of 17x17 μm and of similar shape to all other EE. They also are of the opinion that the marginal folds present are not created by cells overlying one another but by a '...palisade of numerous microvilli'. Cells are covered with microappendages, but mainly situated on the nuclear bulge and were either blunt ended or knob-like. Near the annulus, cells are more squamous in appearance with sparse microvilli. Normal human valves are reported similarly with the exception of possessing a crater-like depression along the marginal fold [Harasaki et al., 1978]. Chordae are also covered with EE which are squamous and even folded in regions [Lim and Boughner, 1977].

The most recent report of SEM observations of mitral EE is on the canine valve. EE cells present prominent nuclear bulges and are arranged in distinct rows. These are most pronounced at the distal zone close to free edge of the valve. EE cells are oriented perpendicular to the free edge if they are located near the edge, but elsewhere remain oriented parallel to it; these observations are in line with previous reports of the EE covering the canine aortic valve [Deck, 1986]: only in one area does cellular orientation veer from this general pattern, on the central portion of the ventricular surface of the aortic valve termed the Nodule of Arantius – a localised thickening of subendocardial collagen [Williams et al., 1995]. Here, the valve receives the initial surge of blood at the initiation of systole and cells are arranged in a swirling pattern [Deck, 1986], taken to be a response to local haemodynamic forces thus supporting the previous suggestion of Peine and Low [1975]. Cells in the middle of valve are more squamous and posses more prominent marginal folds; the perinuclear region contains the densest population of microappendages. Interestingly, cells with less prominent bulges had less microappendages, which may add further support to the theory of microappendages being linked to overall cell activity. The pattern of EE on chordae was similar, with smaller chordae looking similar to the valvar midzone. Large chordae (first order) had all EE helically arranged from the valve edge spiraling towards the appropriate papillary muscle (Figure 6) [Corcoran et al., 2004].

## III.II. Ultrastructure of the Mitral Valve

The TEM appearance of the valve is complex compared with its surface, primarily due to the different cell populations encountered and their inter-relationships. There are four primary elements of the valve: the endocardial endothelium, the fibroblastic-like cell population, the connective tissue structure of the valve and the neuronal elements of the valve. These will be considered in turn.

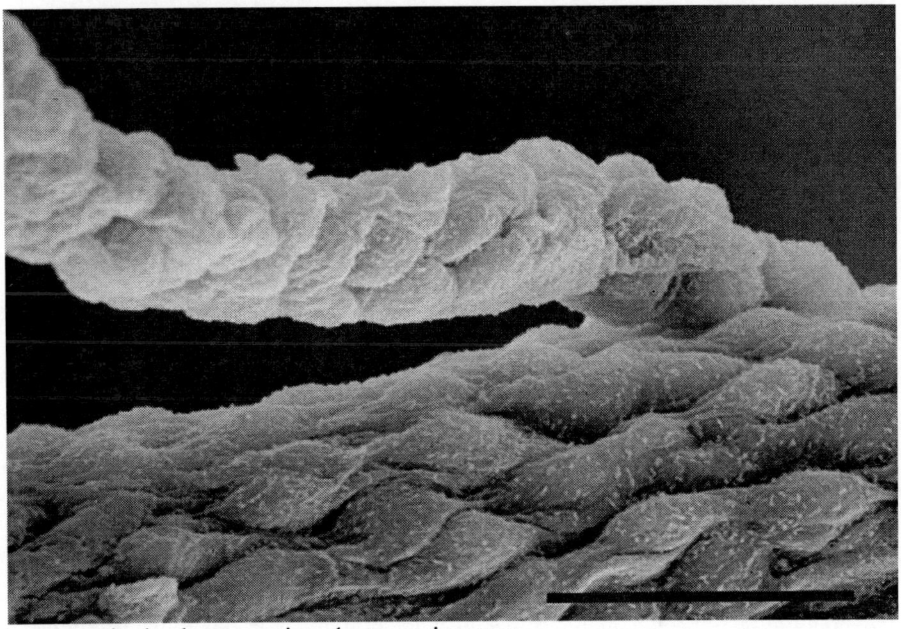

Neonatal canine mitral valve; scanning electron microscopy.
Scale bar = 25 μm.

Figure 6. A small order chorda tendinea inserts into the free edge of a mitral valve leaflet. The endocardial endothelial cells all possess a dense covering of microappendages. Note the near-helical orientation of the chordal endothelium as it mirrors the pattern of the underlying collagen core.

### *III.II.I. Endocardial endothelium (EE)*

The ultrastructural appearance of the EE in several species has been reported. These include chicken [Mitomo et al., 1969], Guinea-pig [Hibbs and Ellison, 1973], monkey [Harasaki et al., 1975; Tsumori and Domoto, 1994], dog [Sarphie and Allen, 1978; Sarphie, 1980], rabbit [Lupu and Simionescu, 1985], cat and rat (Figure 7) [Andries and Brutsaert, 1991; Andries, 1994].

The EE of the chicken mitral valve is of variable size and shape. Cells are squamous as a rule, with average height at the nucleus of 2-4 μm and a total length of approximately 20-40 μm; cells are not fenestrated. The centrally placed nuclei have either an oval or irregular profile, while the cell membrane is also irregular presenting both short and long microappendages on the luminal surface; long projections are more often seen on the ventricular surface.

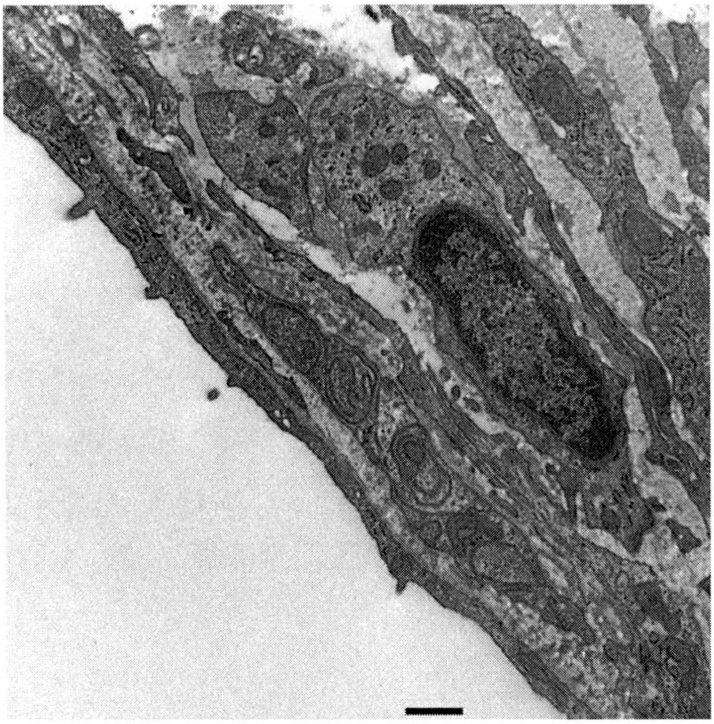

Rat mitral valve; transmission electron microscopy.
Lead citrate and uranyl acetate staining.
Scale bar = 500nm.

Figure 7. The attenuated cytoplasmic processes of an endocardial endothelial cell can be seen at the lower left of the image. Subendothelially, a small caliber unmyelinated nerve is present, in the immediate vicinity of both the endothelial cell and a collection of valvar interstitial cell processes from several different cells which are positioned in a layered fashion throughout the leaflet. All the subendothelial cells are embedded in a connective tissue matrix. It is thought that the interplay between these cell populations is the driving factor in maintenance and function of the valve.

Intercellular junctions may be either simple or complex: simple junctions take the form of cellular overlapping in a linear fashion, whilst others seem to be of an interlocking nature. Some cells have tight junctions or desmosomes. The cytoplasm is pale and organelles are exclusively perinuclear. Small numbers of mitochondria are seen ranging from round to oval. Some lipid droplets are also present. Abundant smooth endoplasmic reticulum (sER) and Golgi apparatus are contained with each endocardial endothelial cell (EEC) along with lysosomes and, rarely, large vacuoles. The cells are somewhat filamentous, with the filaments running parallel to the luminal surface. All aspects of the cell surface contain numbers of pinocytotic vesicles, while the EEC sits on a complete basement membrane which is reported to be better defined on the atrial surface. In the area of coaptation, foot-like cytoplasmic processes are present along the abluminal surface particularly on the ventricular surface side; some of these are regarded as projecting into the basement membrane [Mitomo et al., 1969].

The guinea-pig mitral valve EEC is a layer of thick cells with an irregular luminal surface. These cells are filamentous and tightly packed. The basal lamina underlying cells of the free margin on both sides of leaflet is thickened [Hibbs and Ellison, 1973].

The EEC of the monkey contains numerous pinocytotic vesicles with the free surface presenting microappendages which fold back on themselves. These rejoin the cell surface thus forming a ring-like structure which has been suggested as an entrapment device for elements of the circulating blood, particularly plasma [Harasaki et al., 1975].

In one report, small nerve terminals in monkey mitral valve were seen to terminate in the region of 200 nm away from the EEC. A subendothelial layer of fibroblastic cells was also observed, oriented parallel to the endocardial layer [Tsumori and Domoto, 1994].

One of the most striking aspects of canine mitral valve EEC seems to be their pleiomorphism. Cells of the ventricular surface are larger than the atrial, and they also possess a simple type of junction whereas atrial cells are joined in an irregular and more complex manner [Sarphie and Allen, 1978].

In a follow-on study, canine valves were fixed in different glutaraldehyde solutions which contained a variety of chemicals to ascertain whether there were differences in glycocalyx conformation between the atrial or ventricular surfaces. Solutions contained either Ruthenium Red, Alcian Blue or Cetylpyridium chloride. The latter two solutions also contained Lanthanum nitrate. All the dyes used possess an affinity for glycocalyx constituents. The results obtained indicate that the EE of the ventricular side showed greater affinity for all dyes used, indicating a thicker glycocalyx on this, the outflow, side. This is suggested as being a local reaction to haemodynamic forces [Sarphie, 1980].

The intercellular junctions of rabbit mitral EE were investigated using TEM, Freeze-fracture EM (FF) and the fluorescent tracer 6-carboxyfluorescein; the tracer diffusion between neighbouring cells was viewed using fluorescence microscopy. FF studies revealed large areas of cell membrane along both the luminal and abluminal surfaces. Particles of between 10.46-5.9 μm were observed randomly distributed along all surfaces, although were more common on the luminal aspect. Vesicular stomata were seen as craters with elevated rims on the abluminal surface while those on the luminal surface were papillary in nature: these stomata ranged in size from 25-50 nm in diameter. Some coated pits were also seen, though infrequently. Parajunctional zones, however, were generally free of vesicles. TEM investigation of intercellular junctions revealed most to be occluding junctions, with some possessing an inter-cellular space of approximately 6-8 nm in width. On FF these were seen to possess 1-4 interdigitating ridges with corresponding grooves on the neighbouring cell. Some gap junctions were also observed, and they suggest that these are responsible for cell-cell electrical coupling. Intercellular transport of the fluorescent tracer was seen to occur within 45 s of micro-injection, and was distributed to 3-5 neighbouring cells. These data strongly suggest therefore, that the endocardial layer acts as a functionally integrated unit, rather than as a passive barrier [Lupu and Simionescu, 1985].

Rat endocardium was studied and was determined to be a sheet of polygonal squamous cells, each of which was thickest in the nuclear region and projected into the lumen. Cytoplasm was most abundant in the perinuclear region also, becoming greatly attenuated distal to this area. The majority of cell membrane contains micro-pinocytotic vesicles.

Serial sections reveal the nuclear profile as "saucer-shaped" though it is irregular. The population of organelles is poorly developed with sparse small oval mitochondria containing few cristae. Poorly developed Golgi apparatus and endoplasmic reticulum (ER) are also present as are free ribosomes, although these are low in number. Lysosomes were infrequently encountered.

Intercellular junctions are, in common with other species, complex and variable in morphology. They are reported as being either S, V or wedge-shaped, but may also take the form of simple overlaps. Whilst complex interdigitations were a frequent finding, desmosomes were not encountered.

The complete basement membrane of all EEC showed a frequent infiltration of fine collagen fibrils; in these areas the basement membrane is greatly thickened (increased from a range of 50-70 μm to several hundred). No difference between EEC from any part of the heart or valves was seen [Melax and Leeson, 1967].

In another study, EE was seen to be ‘thick’ in the region of the nucleus and attenuated thereafter [Andries and Brutsaert, 1991]. Cytoplasm contained a variable number of Weibel-Palade bodies dispersed throughout. Multivesicular bodies also found in the periphery – all other organelles similar to that already stated. Threadlike extensions from fibroblast-like subendothelial cells were frequently noted as piercing the EE basal lamina to make close contact with the EE membrane (as narrow as 12 nm) – no gap junctions between them, although electron dense focal adhesions sometimes seen. These intercellular contacts were more common in the cat than in the rat in which species they were exceedingly rare – no other inter-species difference was noted [Andries and Brutsaert, 1991].

Andries [1994] examined many aspects of cat and rat EE. The glycocalyx of EE from both cat and rat was stained by tannic acid which outlined apical pits and others deeper (abluminal) in the cell. No complete transcellular channels were observed. A vast heterogeneity of staining was observed, with some cells staining in the perinuclear region only, whilst others did not exhibit a significant staining in the same area.

Complex intercellular junctions were observed, with marginal folds being created by overlap of two or more cells in the cat EE. Tannic acid infiltrate into these intercellular clefts was seen to terminate at the level of focal adhesions, although a small percentage (4 out of 170 cells examined in detail) of cells did not show such focal contacts. Tight junctions were observed between EE of rat heart. Gap junctions were observed in rat EE as part of intercellular cleft junctional complexes consisting of both gap and tight junctions [Andries, 1994].

Subendothelial cell-cell contacts were not observed in rat EE, but previous observations [Andries and Brutsaert, 1991] on feline EE were supported; although no gap junctions were seen as part of these contacts, it is argued that this does not preclude the existence of intercellular communication due to the presence of cytoplasmic vesicles in both cell types [Andries, 1994].

The presence of microfilament bundles (MFB) was determined via confocal microscopy in rat EE particularly in valves, and is suggested that these filaments (which stain positively for F-actin) may act as stress fibres in response to shear stress which results from haemodynamic flow. It is further postulated that these fibers help EE of the valve to retain cell shape during the constant shape changes experienced during the normally high rate cardiac cycle of the rat [Andries, 1994].

The clotting factor, von Willebrand factor (vWf) is sometimes stored intracellularly in a particular ultrastructural organelle, the Weibel-Palade body. In rat EE, the existence of Weibel-Palade bodies remains uncertain; it is suggested that they are present, although presenting a different structure to the classic rod-shaped tubule-containing granules of up to 0.1 μm in diameter and 3 μm in length [Weibel and Palade, 1964]. The fact that they are presented as specific structures yet bear little morphological relationship to those structures leaves this question entirely open. The presence of vWf in rat EECs is not in doubt however, with specific staining for this factor seen particularly in valve EE in the perinuclear area [Andries, 1994].

Well developed Golgi apparatus were seen in most EE, with up to six stacks of cisternae, although neither the *cis* nor *trans* face could be discerned. ER was also seen, and was preferentially located near the Golgi. Both sER and rough-endoplasmic reticulae (rER) were seen, both being filled with dense material, the composition of which remains unknown.

### *III.II.II. Valvar interstitial cells (VIC)*

The presence of subendothelial cells in the mitral valve has been noted since the early descriptions of Gross and Kugel [1931]. They have been variously described as smooth muscle cells, fibroblasts or a mixture of the two. This section will deal with the ultrastructural characteristics of this cell population.

Cells in the fibrosa of the mitral valve of the chicken are described as spindle-shaped fibroblasts poorly, or not fully differentiated mesenchymal round cells which are arranged parallel to the endothelium. The number of these cells increases in the middle of the valve as seen in atrial-ventricular cross-section. These fibrillar cells have abundant free ribsomes and rER and demonstrate collagenesis [Mitomo et al., 1969].

Typical fibroblasts were seen in the upper (subendothelial) regions of the guinea-pig valve, although in the mid-region and nearing the free edge atypical cells were observed which did not resemble fibroblasts. These cells had a varied morphology but had common features: they possessed abundant Golgi apparatus with a moderate amount of rER. Microtubules and other cytoplasmic filaments were seen in the majority of these cells and the cell membrane exhibited pinocytotic vesicles, which were seen to form a continuous sub-membranous layer. 'Solitary flagella' emanating from the centrioles or basal bodies are also reported for some of this cell population. Lacunae and lysosomes were a frequent finding [Hibbs and Ellison, 1973].

The first reference to this cell population as Interstitial cells seems to be Filip et al. [1986] who studied these cells from human, mouse, rat, Syrian hamster, chinchilla and rabbit valves. The cells are reported as having a similar morphology in all species studied. They are elongated cells with abundant slender cytoplasmic projections which extend throughout the valvar stroma. They connect with each other through these projections and form a three-dimensional interconnected network throughout the valve. They possess characteristics of both fibroblasts and smooth muscle cells (SMCs) as they have an incomplete basement membrane, have attenuated extensions and are make close contact with the ECM of the valve. The cytoplasm has well developed rER cisternae and Golgi apparatus along with a rich population of cytoplasmic filaments (microfilaments and intermediate filaments) (Figure 8). Their similarities to SMCs lie in the fact that they are coupled by gap junctions, contain actin filaments and dense bodies, c-GMP protein kinase, seem to have closely apposed motor nerve terminals and can be induced to contract *in vitro* [Filip et al., 1986].

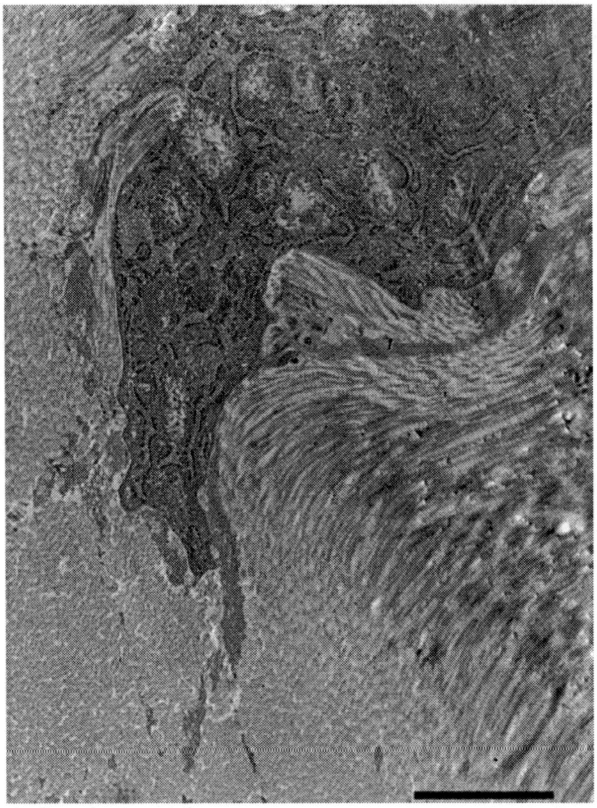

Rat mitral valve; transmission electron microscopy.
Lead citrate and uranyl acetate staining.
Scale bar = 2 μm.

Figure 8. A relatively high magnification image of an active valvar interstitial cell shows the abundant rough endoplasmic reticulum present in the cell; this is indicative of protein synthesis. The cell lies surrounded by the banded collagen of the leaflet – produced by valvar interstitial cells of a synthetic fibroblastic-like phenotype.

In long-term culture of the fibroblastic-like cells of the porcine mitral valve, most likely reflective of the *in vivo* state, these cells present a dual phenotype: an elongated and a cobblestone cell. The former possess reduced rER and Golgi with a prominent cytoskeleton which is suggestive of stress-fibre production and emanates throughout the cell, including into the cytoplasmic processes. The latter contain abundant rER and Golgi with a reduction in the filamentous cytoskeleton and are regarded as being morphologically similar to SMCs in culture [Zacks et al., 1991].

Subendothelial cells of the bovine mitral valve are described as spindle-shaped and on immunostaining were seen to be vWf-negative and α-SMA positive. Morphology conforms to previous reports from other species [Lester et al., 1992].

Cells lying in the subendocardium of the Japanese monkey AV valve are described as being connective tissue cells and are characterised by an abundance of cytoplasmic filaments and numerous cell membrane pits. Located either singly or in rows, each cell extends long slender processes parallel to the overlying endothelium. A few cells were in close association with nerve terminals, which were either ensheathed by a Schwann cell or were naked; the former were within 200 nm of a VIC, the latter were regarded to be in direct contact (20 nm) [Tsumori and Domoto, 1994]

The VICs from the porcine aortic valve *in vitro* exhibit morphology in line with previous reports from other mammals, with a dual phenotype – one being a secretory the other being contractile.

Intercellular junctions included desmosomes and gap junctions. The nuclear profile was round with a high percentage of euchromatin and containing at least one nucleolus. Multinucleate cells are also reported.

The cytoplasm, as has been observed in other species, contained numerous pinocytotic vesicles as well as many caveolae. Lacunae were also noted as was a peppering of glycogen droplets in both cell types. No cells possessed a complete basement membrane. The contractile-type cell had microfilaments dispersed throughout the cytoplasm, electron-dense bodies were generally seen associated with these; the microfilaments were reported as being oriented parallel to the long axis, commonly terminating in submembranous plaques. Some of these contractile cells also contained secretory elements [Messier et al., 1994].

These cells may be termed fibroblast-like, fibroblasts, fibroblast-SMCs, or myofibroblasts. The latter term seems most appropriate in light of their reported ultrastructural morphology as it fits well with the published ultrastructural criteria for the myofibroblast (Figure 9). The characteristics of the myofibroblast are a spindle-shaped cell with fusiform nuclei set in a collagenous matrix, an ill-defined cytoplasm which is less fibrillar than the SMC and contain abundant rER. They stain positively for α-SMA, fibronectin and vimentin; VICs are positive for all of these elements [Lester et al., 1992; Messier et al., 1994; Flanagan et al., 2006a]. They also contain a fibronexus which is defined as intracellular filaments and basement membrane components (chiefly fibronectin) joining to form an anchoring plaque with the ECM [Eyden, 2003].

### *III.II.III. Extracellular matrix (ECM)*

If the cellular components of the valve are regarded as an endothelial sandwich containing a diverse population of synthetic and contractile myofibroblasts, it follows that a description of the ECM components of the valve be addressed prior to the neural elements of the valve. From light microscopic studies [see above), it is clear that the normal structure-function relationship of the valve depends heavily on its connective tissue core.

The zona spongiosa of the chicken mitral valve is composed of small bundles of collagens with a reported diameter of 5 nm and a periodicity of 64 nm along with interspersed smaller fibrils of 1.1-1.3 nm in diameter and an indistinct periodicity. The ground substance in which these elements lie is homogenous and somewhat electron-lucid, although some scattered electron-dense particles were also observed; this is suggestive of mucopolysaccharide proteinaceous material. Heterogeneity of the fibrillar elements is noted, with collagen often not being arranged in discrete bundles, especially directly subendothelially. This superficial layer contains a greater number of fine fibrils and these are again more common on the atrial side. Dense collagen is widespread in the coaptation region.

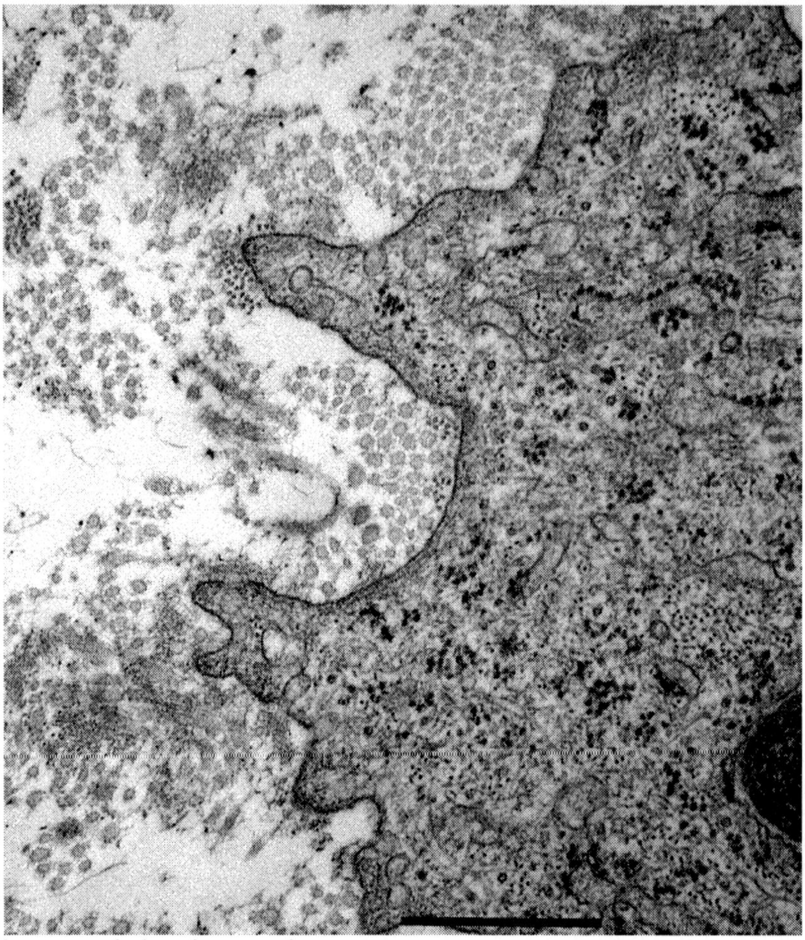

Rat mitral valve; transmission electron microscopy.
Lead citrate and uranyl acetate staining.
Scale bar = 500 nm.

Figure 9. Valvar interstitial cells may also present in a myofibroblast-like phenotype, as indicated by the presence of substantial amounts of cytoplasmic actin filaments and an absence of rough endoplasmic reticulum. The collections of dark spots indicate free ribosomes clumping together to form polyribosomal rosettes.

Elastin fibers are also seen, intermingling with collagen directly subendothelially. These branching fibers are thick yet of low density on the atrial spongiosa, becoming rarer in the spongiosa of the ventricular side presenting as focal electron-dense spots. The atrial-ventricular differences become so indistinct as to disappear nearing the free edge.

The zona fibrosa, as its name suggests, comprises compact collagen bundles which are arranged parallel to the endothelium (Figure 10). The collagen in this region shows an ordered pattern and is periodic [Mitomo et al., 1969].

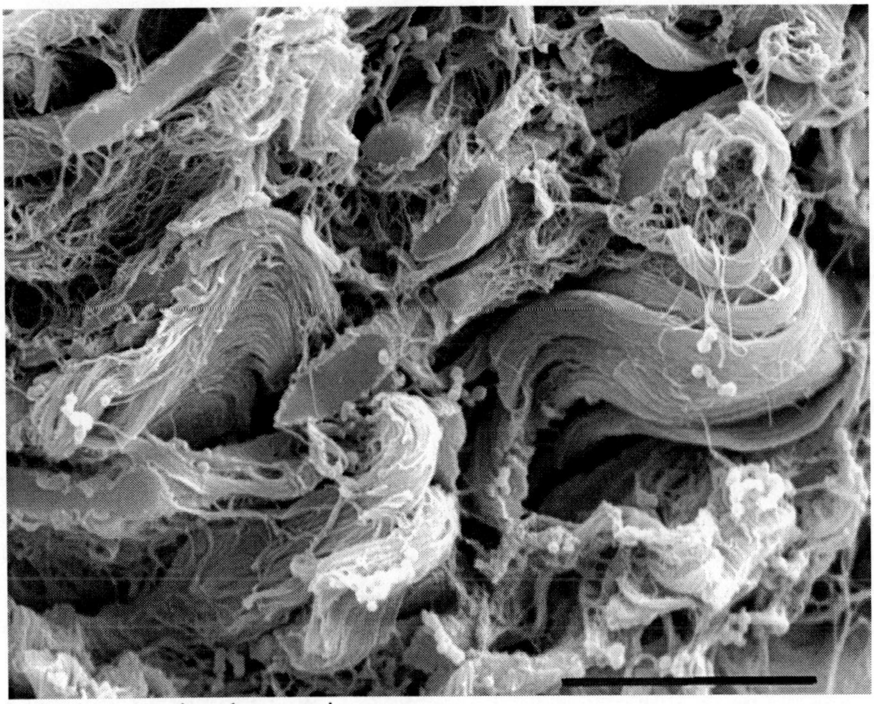

Equine mitral valve; scanning electron microscopy.
Scale bar = 10 μm.

Figure 10. A scanning electron micrograph of the fibrosa of an equine mitral leaflet exhibits large undulating bands of collagen. Interspersed in the collagenous material are bundles of elastin. These structural proteins provide the mechanical strength vital to normal valvar function.

The mouse mitral valve, investigated after endothelial denudement, was revealed to be formed by a fibrous and a spongy layer. The fibrosa being composed of a continuous layer of tightly packed undulating collagen fibers oriented circumferentially from the annular (basal) region. VICs are seen sending processes parallel to these fibers. The spongiosa is a loose network of fine fibrils [Icardo and Colvee, 1995].

The guinea-pig valve demonstrates a large population of banded collagen in the distal portion, especially so near chordal insertion or attachment sites. The stroma of the valve, however, is composed largely of microfibrils of 1-2 nm in diameter; they may be single or grouped in bundles. A 'cottony' material is also noted in this species, and is described as being similar to the material seen composing the incomplete basement membrane of the VIC population. Few elastic fibers are seen with those present lying subendothelially, widely dispersed in an unorganised fashion [Hibbs and Ellison, 1973].

The collagen of the normal porcine mitral leaflet is primarily type I and type III (74% and 24%, respectively) along with 2% of type V. Type I forms tightly packed thick fibers and is generally found in areas of tensile stress. Type III is thought to contribute to the maintenance of morphology. Elastin is capable of extension in a rapid fashion followed by full return to the pre-stressed state with equal rapidity. The ground substance of glycosaminoglycans in which these connective tissue elements are situated thus provides a three-dimensional structural scaffold for structural and functional integrity of the valve. On atrial-ventricular cross-sectional analysis taken parallel to the annulus, the central core or fibrosa made up 68% of leaflet thickness with the atrialis-spongiosa and ventricularis-spongiosa being equal at 16%

each. In base-free edge cross-sectional analysis, the fibrosa was thickest at the base (annular attachment) tapering off distally. In contrast, the atrialis-spongiosa became thicker closer to the free edge, becoming the dominant layer in this area, while the ventricular layer thinned out appreciably as it approached distally [Kunzelman et al., 1993].

The collagen content of human valves was studied by Bashey et al. [1967]. Valve specimens were treated with acetone, chloroform and ether in order to produce a lipid-free dried sample which was then crushed and examined for the presence of collagen and elastin. Mitral valves had an average collagen content of 55% of the total dry weight, with elastin being 10% of dry weight. Collagen varied in a statistically significant manner with age, with dry weight of 70% at age 10 falling to 40% at age 80. Elastin also varied with age, but increased rather than decreased; at age 10 elastin accounted for approximately 8% and at age 80 accounted for approximately 12% [Bashey et al., 1967].

The collagen of denuded human mitral valve chordae was investigated using SEM and revealed a central core of collagen bundles around which were widely spaced fibers. These outer fibers are oriented at a slight angle to the core of the structure, wrapping around it. The central collagen, conversely, is oriented to the long axis of the chorda, some exhibiting a wavy pattern [Shi and Vesely, 2003].

First order chordae from normal human hearts were examined by SEM and light reflectance. Light reflectance studies revealed a consistent pattern of 11 μm periodicity in young subjects along the entire chordal length, although this was not seen in specimens from embalmed cadavers possibly due to the embalming technique. Tangentially sectioned chordae revealed a similar pattern. Several layers of elastin were ascertained, an outer layer which was a subendocardial layer arranged at a slight angle to the chordal surface and an inner layer which was longitudinally arranged in the deep subendocardial region, passing deep into the core collagen where it diminished substantially. A schema for the ECM of the chorda was produced which is as follows from endocardium to the mid-centre: EE, first layer of elastin (slightly angled), second layer of elastin (longitudinally arranged), planar collagen with a 11um repeat pattern, longitudinal collagen with scattered elastin fibers interspersed in the first few superficial layers [Millington-Sanders et al., 1998].

### *III.II.IV. Neural elements*

The presence of nerves in the feline AV, aortic and pulmonary valves was demonstrated by the use of methylene blue staining. Stained fibres were located near the base of the AV valves with diminution of fibre number as they traversed the valve toward the chordae tendineae where they arborised. Simple dot endings were also seen [Nettleship, 1936]. This therefore is the first paper suggesting a function for the neural elements found in AV valves.

The innervation of the AV valves of guinea-pig, rabbit, cat and hedgehog was investigated using cholinesterase staining; a rich pattern of innervation was found in each species. In older animals the appearance of degenerating nerve fibres is noted [Williams, 1964a]. The description of fine beaded nerves agrees with that of Nettleship [1936]. Large myelinated nerve fibres are also noted traversing the valve leaflets in all species studied a sensory role is put forward for the neural elements in the AV valves. Following vagotomy, degeneration was observed among a nerve population in the guinea-pig mitral valve, although no degeneration was observed following either surgical sellatectomy or sympathectomy. It is concluded that these fibres may be proprioceptive [Williams, 1964b].

The afferent innervation of the valve in cat and rabbit revealed two nerve plexuses; these are divided into endocardial and muscular, the endocardial plexus being described as more pronounced on the atrial aspect of the valve in both species. Fine nerve trunks interconnect forming loops which are small and elongated at the valve base. The free edge has larger and more circular loops which may run into the chordae tendineae and from there into the muscular plexus of the ventricular wall via the papillary muscles. Receptors in the valve are free brush endings with numerous afferent endings being found in the connective tissue substance of the valve. Thick medullated fibres of the valve originate from the muscular plexus, rise into thc chordac via thc papillary muscles, loose their myelin ensheathment and afterwards divide in a dichotomous fashion. Some filaments are seen to follow the valve free edge and descend down another chorda tendinea re-entering the muscular plexus. These neural structures are regarded as a type of stretch receptor during the cardiac cycle [Voloschenko, 1964].

Cooper et al. [1966] report the first observations of the AV valves following cardiac transplantation. Canine valves were investigated for the presence of adrenergic nerves. These were found in control animals associated with cardiac muscle bundles in the basal zone, in the aurotransplanted heart, however no adrenergic elements could be found. Silver and cholinesterase staining procedures revealed the presence of nerves throughout the leaflets in both experimental and control animals.

Ehinger et al. [1969] studied the hearts of mice, rats, rabbits, cats and Cynomolgous monkeys. Their fluorescence studies demonstrated the presence of a well developed adrenergic ground plexus on the atrial side of the valve in all of their experimental species, and identified adrenergic fibres.

A series of experiments on canine valve not only reiterated the presence of Schwann cells containing c-fibres, but strengthened the case that there is in fact a neurally mediated contraction in the mitral valve due to the fact that tyramine (which releases endogenous catecholamines from adrenergic nerves) was shown to intensify valvar contraction [Sonnenblick et al., 1967]. Licata [1967] had demonstrated a diverse staining in all cardiac valves for catecholamines, stating that the nerves found should not be seen as mere continuations of the atrial plexus, but a discrete valvar plexus which is present throughout the valve.

Chordal innervation is regarded as being of two sources, one descending from the valve leaflet, the other ascending from the papillary muscle. Bilateral cervical vagotomies on young adult sheep were attempted although this procedure proved to have a high mortality rate so unilateral vagotomies were adopted as the procedure of choice. Neural degeneration was observed on the homolateral side, though minimal adrenergic fibre alteration was noted [Licata, 1967].

1968 saw one valve innervation paper, with Novi as the author. She used TEM to study the papillary muscles with the rat as a model.

A rich terminal innervation pattern was demonstrated in the rat papillary muscle, with a mixture of both granular and agranular vesicles in axons suggesting the presence of adrenergic nerves. Vesiculated granules suggest the presence of catecholamines. Neuro-muscular relationships are distinguished in two ways; the first is the true myo-neuronal junction while the second is loose contact demonstrated by bare axons located at a varied distance from effector cells [Novi, 1968].

There is some mention of innervation in the chicken mitral valve, the majority of the neural elements being located in the zona spongiosa, with only rare elements seen in the zona [Mitomo et al., 1969].

A rich basal and free edge network of cholinergic nerves has been demonstrated in the guinea-pig valve. The connective tissue of the valve is reported as hosting a separate adrenergic plexus, associated with neither muscle nor blood vessel [Anderson 1971]. Smith [1971] investigated the innervation of the AV valves in rabbits, cats, dogs and guinea-pigs. He presented species-specific findings; in the dog, the atrial muscle ring of both AV valves is closely associated with a network transmitting fine fibres into the fibromuscular area of the valve. Large nerve fibres are seen extending from the atrium into the valve, branching as they do so to form a leaflet-wide web. The web is seen to become denser as it approaches the free edge and the chordal attachment sites. The chordae themselves are innervated by a lattice-like plexus; at the papillary muscle attachment area the network enters the ventricular network. The feline heart is more densely innervated, though the leaflet-wide image seen in the dog seems to dissipate in the midzone, although there are fine fibres opposite the chordae. Fibres are beaded, with some terminating in fine points. The rabbit heart is richer in nerves than either the canine or feline, with thick nerves traversing the basal third until they terminate with fine fibre branches. Chordal innervation is similar to that of cat and dog. The guinea-pig is reported to have a similar, though sparser, innervation than the rabbit, though the relation between guinea-pig, cat and dog is not stated. Chordal nerves were infrequently found in this species. The statement that the tricuspid valve is more densely innervated than the mitral contradicts all previous literature.

Fenoglio et al. [1972] briefly mention the occurrence of small nerves scattered between the muscle of the basal leaflet of the mitral valve in dogs. The pattern of adrenergic innervation reported in the mitral valve of the guinea-pig is in concordance with previous studies on this species with the exception of the description of a zone which, extending around the entire leaflet area, is ‘essentially free of adrenergic elements’ [Ellison and Hibbs, 1973].

Human AV valve innervation has been reported as extending through the valve in all directions. Composed of two separate types of nerve, large meshworks of myelinated fibres and non-myelinated fibres arranged in smaller meshes; these webs were wider near the free edge, with chordae possessing both types of nerve. The possible functional significance of the presence of these nerves is reiterated [Ferreira and Rossi, 1974].

The study by the Russian scholars presented the findings gleaned following silver nitrate impregnation into 50 specimens of bovine and 30 specimens of human AV valves revealed the presence myelinated and non-myelinated fibres in the valve which branch into progressively finer fibres [Sokolov and Goriun, 1976], and supports the earlier literature. Neural elements in the human valve are associated with the musculature which is reported to extend into the base of the valve; there is no such distinction observed in bovine heart [Sokolov and Goriun, 1976].

Substance-P-immunoreactive nerves were found in both the AV valves of guinea-pigs travelling through the connective tissue and near the free edge [Wharton et al., 1986].

Porcine valve innervation was studied by silver staining, acetylcholinesterase staining and fluorescence histochemistry. This revealed nerve fibres in all specimens examined with preferential location on the atrial subendocardial surface. The plexus is similar to that previously reported in human valves [De Biasi et al., 1984]. The presence of calcitonin gene-related peptide (CGRP) immunoreactivity was demonstrated in guinea-pig heart including the valves; it was revealed as punctate varicosities [Gerstheimer and Metz, 1986].

The innervation of the human AV valves was demonstrated as having both primary sensory and autonomic components. Neural elements immunoreactive to the pan-neuronal marker protein gene peptide 9.5 (PGP 9.5) were localised to the atrial region of valve leaflets, with branches arising from the basal area. These then branched within the leaflet to form a network of varicose and non-varicose fibres. Neural elements were not seen in the distal one third of the leaflet tissue. Some nerve terminals were closely related to valvar EE cells [Marron et al., 1996]. These data support the report of Oki et al. [1995].

PGP 9.5, tyrosine hydroxylase (TH), neuropeptide Y (NPY), substance P (SP) and CGRP immunoreactivity was found to exist in the valve leaflets of the Dunkin-Hartley guinea-pig and Sprague-Dawley rat. The valve is described in terms of three zones - a basal- (near the annulus) a mid- (the middle third of the leaflet) and a distal-zone (the distal third). The guinea-pig exhibited a denser innervation than the rat throughout. The mitral and tricuspid valve was seen to have similar innervation patterns which consisted of two major plexuses separated by a lozenge-shaped ‘nearly nerve-free’ zone; this was most conspicuous on the anterior mitral leaflet. The first plexus extends through the valve ramifying as it does so, to terminate at the free edge of the distal zone; the second plexus was seen to run from the papillary muscles into the chordae and run parallel to the free edge before either running along the free edge or into adjacent chordae. A few nerves were observed running from one papillary muscle up an attached chorda along the free edge down another attached chorda and terminate in the contralateral papillary muscle. Not all chordae contained nerves [Ahmed et al., 1997]. SP-containing nerves were again demonstrated in the AV valves of the guinea-pig, and revealed a leaflet-wide network of positive fibres, a finding which is not in line with previous studies [Miklosova et al., 1999].

# IV. Myxomatous Mitral Valve Disease (Canine Model)

This section of the chapter will deal with mitral valve disease in the dog and only make occasional reference to the comparative disease in humans, MVP. The section will draw on published information, but also unpublished data where available and data presented at scientific conferences. There will be limited discussion on the clinical aspects of the disease.

Canine myxomatous mitral valve disease (MMD), also know as mitral valve endocardiosis and often referred to as chronic mitral valve degeneration, is the single most common cardiac diseases of the dog. In veterinary clinical practice it will account for 75% of all types of cardiac diseases seen in the dog, and is a significant cause of morbidity and mortality in this species. The clinical aspects of the disease have been clearly outlined over the last 20 years, but there is still limited information on the aetiopathogenesis. The earliest clear reference to MMVD in the dog are from the mid 1960s and early 1970s, and at the same time possible similarities with mitral valve prolapse in humans were first commented on [Detweiler and Patterson, 1965; Pomerance, 1969; Pomerance and Whitney, 1970]. Subsequently, most studies of MMVD in the dog have concentrated on clinical characterisation, diagnosis and treatment, and with the increased use of echocardiography in veterinary cardiology, the haemodynamic consequences of MMVD have been studied in great detail and therapy protocols have been optimised.

## IV.I. Clinical Features and Natural Disease Progression

MMVD is recognised to be an age-associated condition and is particularly prevalent in middle to old-aged dogs (9 years and above), with some evidence of the disease likely to be present in all geriatric dogs [Beardow and Buchanan, 1993]. However, the presence of valve pathology does not necessarily equate with clinical disease and many dogs can remain free of clinical signs throughout their life. The only indicator that they have MMVD would be a pansystolic murmur audible over the left heart apex (mitral valve). The factors that determine which dogs become clinically affected and which do not has not been determined yet. Dogs that are clinically affected show signs of left-sided congestive heart failure, which typically include coughing, tachypnoea, dyspnoea, exercise intolerance and in some cases, syncope [Beardow and Buchanan, 1993; Buchanan, 1977; Darke, 1987]. Once clinical signs of congestive heart failure appear the survival with therapy is poor, with a median survival of only 150 days and most dogs are dead within 12 months [Smith et al., 2005]. Survival beyond that is possible in a minority of cases.

In addition to a close association with age, MMVD has a strong breed association, and is typically associated with small breed dogs. A sub-type of the disease might be present in large breed dogs, where there is mitral valve prolapse but less appreciable valve leaflet distortion on 2-D echocardiography compared to small breed dogs. The disease is particularly prevalent in the cavalier King Charles spaniel world wide, but is also noted to be prevalent in several other breeds [Darke, 1987; Haggstrom et al., 1995; Hamlin, 2005; Olsen et al., 1999; Thrusfield et al., 1985]. There does not appear to be gender association and by inference that any inheritance of the condition is sex linked [Olsen et al., 1999; Thrusfield et al., 1985], although it may be more prevalent in male miniature pinschers and the whippet [Thrusfield et al., 1985]. However, there is a greater tendency among males to develop severe form of the disease compared to females, and for the disease to progress more rapidly in males [Olsen et al., 1999; Swenson et al., 1996]. Taking the cavalier King Charles spaniel (CKCS) as a best example of breed association and the breed that has been most closely studied, there is no gender association nor is there any association with coat colour [Beardow and Buchanan, 1993]. All CKCS dogs above the age of 10 will have evidence of the disease (although this probably has changed in recent years with breeding programmes attempting to eliminate the disease from the breed), and disease can be apparent as young as 1 year of age. In comparison to all other dogs breeds in which the disease is particularly prevalent tend to show evidence of the disease earlier in life [Beardow and Buchanan, 1993; Olsen et al., 1999; Pedersen et al., 1999a]. The close association with breed points toward an inherited basis for the disease in some pedigree breeds, but the high prevalence of the disease in all dogs irrespective of breed and including mixed breeds complicates this issue. Nevertheless, for some pedigree breeds the disease appears to be a multi-factorial, polygenic threshold trait [Olsen et al., 1999; Swenson et al., 1996], in that there is a very clear link between parental status and the appearance of disease in off-spring.

## IV.II. Pathology of Myxomatous Mitral Valve Disease

The gross and histopathological changes of MMVD have been described previously, but this description has not been significantly updated recently [Ernst et al., 1973; Kogure, 1980; Pomerance and Whitney, 1970; Whitney, 1974]. Grossly MMVD primarily affects the edge of the anterior and posterior leaflet and can extend to involve the chordae tendineae. The gross changes to the leaflets are described according to the Whitney classification, and are grade 0 to 4 with 0 being normal and 4 the most advanced form of the disease [Pomerance and Whitney, 1970; Whitney, 1974]. Typically, the disease starts as small numbers of discrete nodules on the leaflet free edge with intervening areas of translucent leaflet (Grade 1), progressing through the development of larger nodules, coalescence of these nodules, involvement of the chordae and finally gross distortion and ballooning of the leaflets with marked chordal thickening and eventually chordal rupture (Grade 4). This system of classification is reasonably robust and follows the time course of development of the disease such that most Grade 3 and 4 dogs are greater than 9 years of age [Han et al., submitted]. Unlike in human MVP, the incidence of endocarditis in affected leaflets is very low or absent [Pomerance and Whitney, 1970; Whitney, 1967]. The valve thickening is most prominent in the distal third of the leaflet, extends to the mid zone in the more severe forms of the disease, but the valve base and mitral annulus are unaffected. The appearance of grade 4 leaflets suggest they are contracted, but morphological analysis in our laboratory show that in fact they are elongated [Han et al., in preparation]. Additionally, the leaflets ends are significantly thickened in severe disease and the posterior leaflet is consistently thicker than the anterior leaflet [Han et al., in preparation].

On histopathology the most striking changes are expansion of the spongiosa and loss of the fibrosa [Buchanan, 1977; Kogure, 1980; Pomerance and Whitney, 1970]. This is best characterised as expansion of the loose connective tissue of the spongiosa and an increase in amorphous metachromatically stained mucoid material (myxomatous degeneration). The remnants of the fibrosa can be appreciated even in advanced disease with Masson trichome staining, but is markedly disorganised [Han et al., in preparation]. Previously these changes had been described as fibro-elastic proliferation, but this does not appear to be the case, and it is connective tissue disorganisation that is the main change. In the myxomatous areas, using image analysis techniques on Masson's trichrome stained sections, there is a measurable reduction in connective tissue density, and this reduction equates with disease severity [Han et al., in preparation]. Usually, the change observed is presumed to represent an increase in the spongiosa and a loss of the fibrosa. However, this gives the impression of two separate ongoing parallel events, while the true change might be destruction of the fibrosa such that it becomes indistinguishable from the adjacent loose connective tissue of the spongiosa. Data from our laboratory would tend to support this description.

Qualitative and quantitative differences in total collagen content have also been demonstrated between lesional and non-lesional areas of the same valve in dogs using Synchotron x-ray diffraction, with a reduction in diseased areas [Hadian et al., 2007]. Furthermore, there is distinct alteration in collagen bundle orientation and fibril alignment in diseased areas, where the fibrils become haphazard, compared to the normal tissue where the fibrils are aligned in a predictable fashion and at the leaflet edge are continuous with the fibrils in the neighbouring chordae tendinae [Hadian et al., 2007]. Overall, there is a reduction in total tissue content (collagenous and non-collagenous) in myxomatous areas, but there is no information on changes in the content of non-collagenous ECM products such as, acid-mucopolysaccarides in affected dog valves. Nevertheless, using quantitative methods we have shown there is 20% decrease in collagen fibrils but only a 10% decrease in total collagen content (Hadian et al., submitted]. Coupled with this change is an increase in reducible covalent cross-link bonds in collagen in affected areas, as determined by neutron diffraction [Hadian et al., in preparation]. This implies there is failure to produce immature fibrillar collagen to replace normal collagen turnover and that the remaining collagen in diseased areas has less tensile strength. This in turn would contribute to poor mechanical performance of the leaflet and the billowing and prolapse seen with this disease. Similar changes in chordal collagen would have a similar effect. The production of reducible cross-links requires lysyl oxidase, which is know to become depleted in old age, and therefore the change seen might be part of the normal aging process. However, the increased deposition of proteoglycans, which is known to occur with MMVD, is speculated to interfere with cross-links in collagen and this might contribute to the change seen in canine leaflets [Scott and Orford, 1981]. The involvement of activated myofibroblasts in this process in both the human and canine forms of the disease is of major interest [Black et al., 2005; Rabkin et al., 2001].

Cellular changes are also noted in the stroma of diseased canine valves. These include phenotypic alteration of the VICs from quiescent vimentin-positive fibroblast-like cells to more activated α-SMA-positive (activated myofibroblasts) [Black et al., 2005; Han et al., 2008]. Such activated myofibroblasts are found to lie in areas of loose collagen bundles and many can be seen to exude fibrillar collagen on electron microscopy, but are also localised away from the myxomatous areas close to the valve edge. This change in cell phenotype and localisation coincides with disease progression and demonstrable temporal and spatial alteration in valve cellularity [Han et al., submitted]. In the more advanced stages of the disease such cells appear more smooth muscle-like, form synchytia and anchor to collagen bundles [Black et al., 2005], and we have speculated this might compensate for the reduction in tensile strength. Coupled with this regionalisation of stromal cells there is a reduction in cell numbers in overtly myxomatous areas compared to normal spongiosa, but no further change in cell numbers as the disease progresses [Han et al., in preparation]. The exact identity of the cells present in myxomatous areas is not know as they are both vimentin and α-SMA negative. However, they retain a spindle shape suggestive of an interstitial phenotype [Han et al., in preparation]. Some of these cells are CD34 and CD117 positive, suggesting a circulating fibrocyte, mast cell and/or stem cell lineage, but further work is ongoing in or laboratory to clarify these issues. There is evidence of a marginal increase in mast cell numbers with advancing disease [O'Connell et al, 2006]. While the role of mast cell chymase in cardiac remodelling has been hypothesised, the potential role in mitral valve disease is worth considering [Dell'Italia et al., 1995]. There is no evidence of involvement of the resident macrophage population in disease pathogenesis [O'Connell et al., 2006] and while it is generally understood that inflammatory cells are also not involved, this has not been proved conclusively. It is still necessary to determine if there is any lymphocyte involvement.

Changes to the endothelium are also noted with MMVD. SEM demonstrates areas of endothelial de-nuding, cell pleomorphism, and increased numbers of surface microappendages [Corcoran et al., 2004]. These changes are indicative of basement membrane abnormalities and, endothelial cell death and reactive changes in the endothelium in response to insult. Similar changes can be identified on TEM and additionally, VIC migration to the sub-endothelial layer is apparent [Black et al., 2005]. This localisation to the periphery matches that seen with α-SMA positive cells on immunostained sections [Han et al., submitted]. It has been speculated that repeated damage to the leaflet edge is likely to play a role in the aetiopathogenesis of MMVD in the dog and the fact the lesions are located to the valve edge and that there is demonstrable changes to the endothelium would support that assertion. But how exactly endothelial damage impacts on the ECM in the valve stroma has not been determined. Functional changes in canine valve endothelium have been identified and even as far back as 1973, Ernst and co-workers noted increased NADH and NADPH-reductase activity in the endothelium of diseased valves [Ernst et al., 1973]. An association between an increase in NADPH diaphorase, as a measure of nitric oxide synthase (NOS) activity, and severity of MMVD, sub-endothelial collagen degeneration and deposition of mucopolysaccarides has been demonstrated in the dog [Olsen et al., 2003]. Furthermore, there is evidence of increased endothelin activity in MMVD, with a close association between increased expression of endothelin receptors on the valve surface and the development of disease [Mow and Pedersen, 1999a]. This suggests nitric oxide (NO) and endothelin (ET) might contribute to the development of MMVD. There is a regulatory balance between NO and endothelin, with NO inhibiting the synthesis of ET, but both also have an effect on ECM production [Olsen et al., 2003]. The migration and localisation of activated myofibroblasts towards the endothelium in MMVD may be a part of this process [Black et al., 2005].

Lastly, there is some information available on canine mitral valve innervation and changes with disease. It is recognised that the mammalian mitral valve is innervated but the extent of innervation in the dog mitral valve has not been previously reported [Ahmed et al., 1997]. Innervation localisation appears to be consistent when comparing normal dogs and dogs with varying severity of MMVD [Culshaw et al., in preparation]. The majority of nerve fibres are found in close association with the myocardial base of the leaflet. Occasional nerve fibre fragments are seen in the mid part of the leaflet, but are absent from the distal portion of the leaflet, the free edge and the chordae tendinae. To date, these nerve fibres have been shown to express PGP 9.5 and TH, suggesting the majority of the innervation is adrenergic. Statistically significant differences in the density of innervation are found with advancing age, but there is no association with the degree of myxomatous degeneration. The reduction in innervation in older dogs coincides with a reduction in the amount to myocardium at the valve base, as a proportion of total leaflet length and it would be interesting to speculate that this loss of muscle might affect themechanical function of the valves.

## IV.III. Pathogenesis and Pathophysiology of Myxomatous Mitral Valve Disease

The exact cause of MMVD in the dog is unknown, but we do have a lot of information on associated risk factors, although these associations are difficult to explain. The effect of age, breed and gender has been mentioned previously, but in addition close association between MMVD has been identified in some dogs and some breeds with platelet dysfunction [Olsen et al., 2001; Tanaka et al., 2002; Tanaka and Yamane, 2000; Tarnow et al., 2005; Tarnow et al., 2003], insulin-like growth factor-1 [Pedersen et al., 2005], low magnesium status [Pedersen and Mow, 1998] and low plasma vWf high molecular weight multimers [Tarnow et al., 2004]. Some of these associations might have very close breed associations, particularly with the CKCS breed, making interpretation of their potential role in MMVD aetiopathogenesis difficult [Cowan et al., 2004]. Furthermore, there is a lot of information on the neuroendocrine changes in response to the haemodynamic consequences of MMVD, and studies have attempted to match such changes in circulating and tissue neuroendocrine factors. This is particularly important considering the potential role of angiotensin II, chymases, ET and other products in the process of myocardial remodelling through effects on myocardial interstitial cells, and how such systems might have a similar effect on VICs [Campbell and Katwa, 1997; Dell'Italia, 2002; Dell'Italia et al., 1995]. Significant changes in the expression of rennin, aldosterone, NO metabolites and the naturetic peptides ANP and BNP and the cardiac troponins have been demonstrated in dogs with MMVD [Oyama and Sisson, 2004; Pedersen et al., 2005; Pedersen et al., 1995a; Pedersen et al., 1995b; Pedersen et al., 1999b; Pedersen et al., 2003], but there is no evidence for up-regulation of angiotensin II receptors in either canine or human diseased valves [Mow and Pedersen, 1999b; Mow et al., 1999].

The biochemical functional consequences of MMVD in the dog have been partially examined and include genomic expression patterns and parallel qualitative protein expression (proteomics) [Oyama and Chittur, 2006; Han et al., in preparation]. This work has only been carried out in a small number of dogs and those with the most advanced form of the disease (Grade 4). Genomic expression profiles show changes in a large number of transcripts involving genes associated with cell signalling, ECM, immune function, cell defence and metabolism [Oyama and Chittur, 2006]. Of particular interest has been the identification of the potential involvement of inflammatory cytokines and the 5-HT-TGF-β pathway. The involvement of inflammatory pathways is contrary to the belief that MMVD is not an inflammatory disease, but the increase in expression of the genes encoding for IL-6, IL-1 and IL-10, as well as the adhesion molecules VCAM-1 and ICAM-1, may represent a response to the endothelial damage associated with MMVD. However, in our laboratory we have detected an increase in immunoglobulin fractions in diseased valves and while this may originate from the blood pool, the potential role of immune mechanisms and inflammation cannot be discounted without further study. The identification of increased expression of NOS and ET-1 matches that reported in previous immunohistochemical studies [Mow and Pedersen, 1999a; Olsen et al., 2003]. Up-regulation of the 5-HT2B receptor (serotonin) is an interesting finding as it brings to mind the valve pathology consequent on the use of the appetite suppressant phentermine-fenfluramine and various anti-Parkinsonian drugs [Roy et al., 2000]. Furthermore, the platelet abnormalities reported in the CKCS [Cowan et al., 2004], platelets being the main store for serotonin, suggests 5-HT might be implicated in the aetiology of MMVD as it is involved in the TGF-β signalling pathway which is important in ECM production, including collagen and fibronectin, and in the transformation of fibroblasts to activated myofibroblasts; all identifiable facets of MMVD.

Protemic data from canine MMVD provides additional information regarding the post-translational protein expression, but data is only available from the severe end-stage form of the disease and changes in protein expression, as well as genomic expression, for the earlier less severe forms of the disease are unknown. Proteomics can be used to complement genomic data, but can also be a better measure of the biological activity in a tissue at a particular time point. However, canine protein databases are somewhat limited and application of proteomic technology will rely on more reliable canine databases being available in the future. 2-D SDS-PAGE & MALDI-TOF, combined with Dymension software, has detected 1880 protein spots in normal leaflets, 1705 spots in moderately affected leaflet and 1687 spots in severely affected leaflets [Han et al., in preparation]. On closer analysis of the normal and severely affected dogs, 41 proteins from normal and 19 proteins from diseased valves have been found to be significantly altered. Of these, 16 proteins are common between the normal and diseased states and 3 proteins are found only in the diseased dogs. The most striking change in Grade 4 disease is the complete loss of expression of tropomyosin and myosin regulatory light chain 2, which regulate contractile function. Both of these proteins are important in general cell function and have a role in normal VIC function through interaction with actin. It is interesting to note this change in conjunction with the interstitial phenotypic change that occurs with progression of canine MMVD. Furthermore, there is an increase in expression of IgG in diseased valves and this is associated with change in disease severity. Comparing this with the suggestion of changes in expression of genes associated with immune function and inflammatory suggests the possible role of inflammation in this disease needs to be evaluated [Oyama and Chittur, 2006].

MMVD is recognised as the single most important cardiovascular disease of the dog and shares enough similarities with human MVP for both to be considered natural models of each other. There is a large amount of information on the clinical features, diagnosis and treatment of this disease, and in recent years there has been a significant expansion of our understanding of the ultrastructural and cellular changes that occur with this disease, and through genomic and proteomic studies we have information on the functional consequences of these changes. The challenge for the future is to determine the reason for these changes and possibly develop therapeutic strategies to arrest or reverse these changes.

## V. Mitral Valve Regeneration & Tissue Engineering

Although mitral valve repair is the preferred initial treatment method to address severe mitral valve disease, valve repair is not feasible in a large number of patients with end-stage valve disease, and replacement of the mitral valve with a biological or mechanical prosthesis is necessary. However, conventional prosthetic mitral valves carry with them a number of limitations, including thromboembolism, life-threatening haemorrhagic complications, limited durability, rejection and transmission of infection. Currently available prosthetic mitral valves also lack the capacity to grow and remodel, which presents a particular disadvantage in paediatric patients as multiple re-operations are required. Bioprosthetic valves are also prone to tissue calcification in younger patients. To overcome these limitations, the focus of prosthetic valve research has shifted to the development of tissue-engineered living valves capable of growth and remodelling; many animal studies have demonstrated the feasibility of the tissue engineering approach [for detailed reviews, see Flanagan and Pandit, 2003; Vesely, 2005].

While a number of different strategies for heart valve tissue engineering are being pursued, most studies have addressed the construction of a tricuspid/trileaflet valved conduit, designed specifically for the most frequently transplanted aortic valve, and the pulmonary valve in paediatric patients. In comparison to aortic and pulmonary valve conduits, the narrow field of research in mitral valve tissue engineering must address the significantly more complicated structure of the entire mitral valve apparatus. Despite this, the basic design principles for tissue-engineered aortic valves are equally applicable to mitral valve tissue engineering. Strategies are typically based on the seeding of scaffold materials (biological, synthetic, or a composite of both) with a suitable source of VICs and EE cells in an appropriate three-dimensional configuration, followed by physical conditioning of the valve construct in a bioreactor system to develop a living, functional implant. Each of the three essential components of the technique have important, specific functions: the cells, or viable component of the valve, will ultimately construct the new tissue and endow the valve with remodelling capabilities, and should also form a thromboresistant coating on the valve surface. The scaffold is designed to maintain the cells in a suitable anatomic configuration at the implantation site, and bio-reactor conditioning guides optimal cellular and physical properties via controlled gene expression, tissue development and remodelling.

## V.I. Cell Sourcing for Mitral Valve Tissue Engineering

The search for a reliable cell source for a tissue-engineered mitral valve has generated intense research over the last decade. Both *in vitro* and *ex vivo* studies of valve cell phenotype and behaviour can provide useful information to aid the selection of suitable cell sources for tissue-engineered valves [Flanagan et al., 2006a; Mulholland and Gotlieb, 1996]. A variety of sources for both VICs and EE cells has been identified thus far, and include those from vascular tissue (Figure 11), skin, bone marrow, umbilical cord, placenta, and even valve tissue itself [Flanagan et al., 2006b; Kadner et al., 2002a, 2002b; Maish et al., 2003; Schmidt et al., 2006; Shinoka et al., 1996, 1997; Sutherland et al., 2005]. The most attractive sources for clinical applications of a tissue-engineered mitral valve are autologous cells harvested from patients themselves, which can be acquired through minimally-invasive surgery, and would present no risk for immune rejection following re-implantation. Arterial or venous sources may also be isolated using minimally-invasive techniques, but patients with an underlying pathological vascular disease may not have suitable cells. While these and other autologous sources may not be suitable for the geriatric population due to reduced proliferative capacities, promising cell sources for the paediatric population have been highlighted in recent reports, and include bone marrow mesenchymal stem cells (isolated by routine bone marrow puncture), umbilical cord-derived cells or chorionic villi-derived cells [Kadner et al., 2002a, 2002b; Schmidt et al., 2006; Sutherland et al., 2005]. Despite such advances, there is no evidence to date that these cell populations, or indeed any other stem cell populations, will adapt and behave as required *in vivo*. Sutherland et al. [2005] reported the presence of differentiated endothelial cells lining the surface of implanted tissue-engineered pulmonary valves after 4 months *in vivo*, following the seeding of synthetic biodegradable constructs with bone marrow-derived mesenchymal stem cells. However, as the seeded cells were not labelled prior to implantation, the origin of the endothelium is unclear, as it is known that structures implanted in the ovine vasculature can rapidly become endothelialised by host cells [Hoffman et al., 1992]. Therefore, a clearer understanding of the factors involved in the differentiation of these stem cells, as well as preservation of gene expression and phenotypic function *in vivo*, will be critical in maintaining the function of a tissue-engineered mitral valve replacement.

## V.II. Scaffold Development for Mitral Valve Tissue Engineering

The ideal scaffold material for development of a successful tissue-engineered heart valve continues to be a matter of intense debate. Bio-degradable scaffolds are designed to immobilise the appropriate cell populations at the implantation site of a tissue-engineered structure, and also to provide appropriate mechanical stability until new tissue has been synthesised, organised and cross-linked into a stable tissue. Traditionally, two principal scaffold types have been applied in the field of heart valve tissue engineering: natural, biological scaffold materials and synthetic scaffold materials. Biological scaffolds have included decellularised native tissue (homograft or xenograft valve tissue, small intestinal submucosa, gall bladder tissue), collagen, glycosaminoglycans (GAGs) and fibrin scaffolds [Brody et al., 2007; Flanagan et al., 2006b, 2007; Jockenhoeval et al., 2001; Matheny et al., 2000; O'Brien et al., 1999; Ramamurthi and Vesely, 2005; Taylor et al., 2002; Wilson et al., 1995]. Proponents of the use of biological scaffolds argue that the natural structure of these protein materials provides a more suitable template for cell growth owing to the presence of natural cell attachment sites, in contrast to synthetic scaffolds, and that biological scaffolds are therefore more suitable for the regulation of gene expression, cell organisation, proliferation and tissue remodeling.

Arguably, the most utilised biological scaffold to date has been decellularised valve tissue itself, designed to be devoid of antigenic foreign cell material and to be either re-seeded with appropriate autologous cells *in vitro*, or to attract endogenous cells from the blood or surrounding host tissue after implantation. The methods of removing the resident foreign cells from such scaffolds (homograft or xenograft) generally entail detergent treatment, enzymatic decellularisation or sonication, resulting in a ready-made natural matrix scaffold for reseeding with patient-derived cells. The concept has been applied and developed by a number of groups worldwide, particularly in Europe, but to date has proven to be relatively unsuccessful. In fact, the first clinical application of these valves was disastrous, with one study reporting the deaths of three out of four children receiving implants due to severe inflammation, degeneration, rupture and stenosis [Simon et al., 2003].

A second, and more technical, approach using biological scaffolds involves the *in vitro* reconstitution of biological proteins and cells into valve-shaped conduits. These proteins, including collagen, elastin and fibrin, as well as GAGs (mucopolysaccharides), have been formulated into sponge, film, mesh and hydrogel structures that allow excellent cell attachment and proliferation, and support the synthesis of ECM proteins by seeded cells [Flanagan et al., 2006b, 2007; Jockenhoevel et al., 2001; Ramamurthi et al., 2005; Taylor et al., 2002]. Cell-mediated contraction of hydrogel scaffolds can result in enhanced, tissue-like matrix densities within these structures, while aligned ECMs can also be achieved by constraining the mechanical forces elicited by the resident cells. This phenomenon has been cleverly manipulated by the groups of Tranquillo and Vesely to develop a highly-aligned ECM for the construction of tissue-engineered vascular grafts and mitral valve chordae, respectively [Barocas et al., 1998; Shi and Vesely, 2003].

Fibrin, a major structural protein involved in the wound healing process, represents a potentially ideal cell delivery vehicle for the rapid synthesis of completely autologous cell-seeded structures due to its routine isolation from patients' blood. Fibrin gel scaffolds have been developed in our group as a matrix for the construction of autologous vascular grafts and heart valves (Figure 12) [Flanagan et al., 2007; Jockenhoevel et al., 2001; Tschoeke et al.,

2008a, 2008b; Ye et al., 2000]. The concept is relatively straightforward: fibrin, the major structural protein of a blood clot, is formed by the enzymatic polymerisation of fibrinogen monomers by thrombin in the presence of calcium ions, and when this process is performed *in vitro*, a gel structure is formed. If cells are added to the mixture during the gelation process, a high cell seeding efficiency and uniform cell distribution is achieved – ideal parameters for the formation of tissue-engineered structures. Further advantages of a fibrin scaffold include biodegradation that can be controlled by supplementing the structure with protease inhibitors (e.g. aprotinin) [Ye et al., 2000], as well as enhanced ECM synthesis by seeded cells within fibrin scaffolds in comparison to other reconstituted proteins (e.g. type I collagen) [Grassl et al., 2002; Long and Tranquillo, 2003]. We have demonstrated the formation of autologous tissue-engineered heart valves using fibrin-based scaffolds which show excellent tissue remodelling by seeded vascular-derived cells (Figure 13) [Flanagan et al., 2007; Jockenhoevel et al, 2001]. A limitation of using hydrogel scaffolds for heart valve tissue engineering is the potential for valve insufficiency caused by cell-mediated shrinkage of the tissue structure; despite this, a multi-factorial approach is being pursued effectively to eliminate potential insufficiency, using both biomechanical and biochemical conditioning techniques [Diamantouros et al., 2007; Flanagan et al., 2007]. Preliminary results of implanted fibrin-based tissue engineered heart valves are encouraging, with excellent tissue remodelling and mechanical stability after 3 months *in vivo* [Flanagan et al., 2008]. The concept demonstrates real potential for the creation of truly "autologous" tissue-engineered mitral or aortic valves - a term which should be reserved for those implanted structures that consist entirely of components isolated initially from the patient in question, and not, as many groups claim, for those structures containing implanted synthetic materials, biodegradable or otherwise.

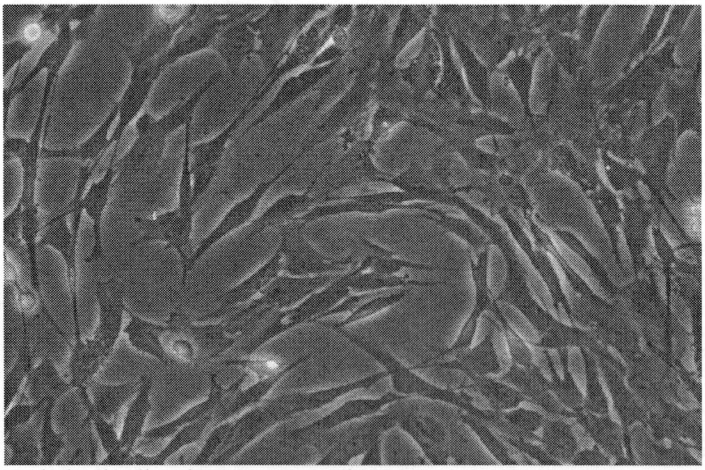

Ovine carotid artery-derived cells; phase contrast microscopy.

Figure 11. A phase contrast micrograph of a culture of cells derived from the ovine carotid artery. Vascular-derived cells could potentially be used to develop living, autologous tissue-engineered mitral valve replacements.

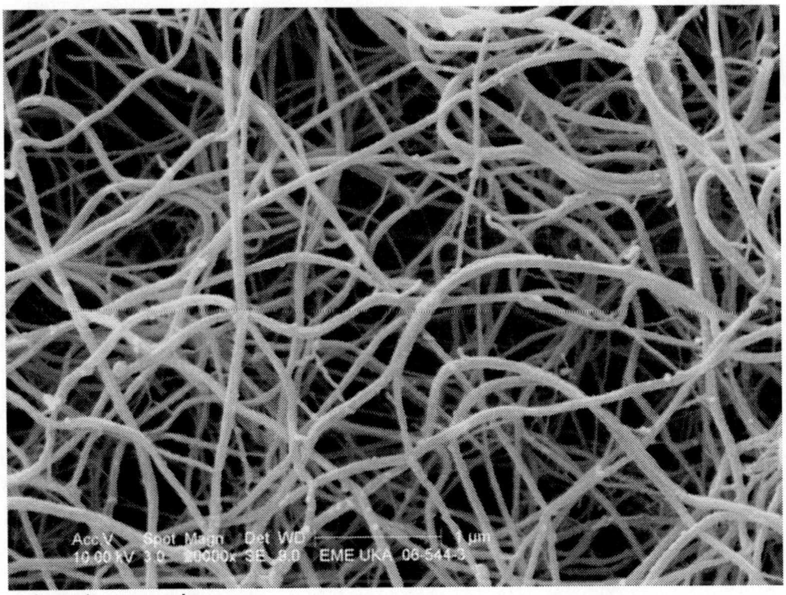


Fibrin gel; scanning electron microscopy.
Scale bar = 1 µm.

Figure 12. A scanning electron micrograph of a the mesh-like internal structure of a fibrin scaffold developed from human blood. Fibrin has excellent potential as an autologous patient-derived scafold material for the construction of mitral valve replacements.

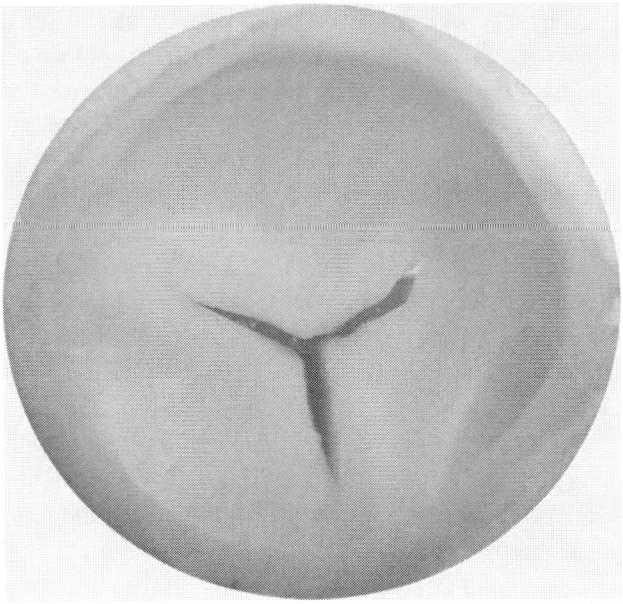

Figure 13. A tissue-engineered hart valve developed from autologous, patient-derived cells, fibrin scaffold material, and rendering implantable through physical conditioning in a bioreactor system.

A variety of synthetic biodegradable polymer materials have also been used as scaffolds for heart valve regeneration, and are favoured by investigators in this area due to their potential for modification, reproducibility and bulk synthesis. Initial attempts by the Boston-based Mayer group at heart valve regeneration based on synthetic biodegradable scaffolds involved the FDA-approved materials, polyglycolic acid (PGA), polylactic acid (PLA), and co-polymers thereof [Shinoka et al., 1996, 1997]. These scaffold materials initially proved to be too stiff for suitable leaflet function in earlier studies, but with subsequent modifications, the group eventually demonstrated functional valves in a sheep model for up to 4 months using mesenchymal stem cells seeded on a co-polymer PGA/PLLA scaffold [Sutherland et al., 2005]. The mechanical properties of these scaffold materials were further altered by dip-coating the scaffolds in polyhydroxyalkanoates (e.g. poly-4-hydroxybutyrate; P4HB), which apparently results in a more flexible structure for improved valve leaflet function [Hoerstrup et al., 2000a]. These valves, seeded with autologous carotid artery-derived cells, have been shown to function in an ovine model for up to five months *in vivo*, and demonstrated histological and mechanical similarities to native valve tissue following explanation [Hoerstrup et al., 2000a]. However, the gradual production of toxic degradation products from synthetic, biodegradable materials can have potentially adverse effects on the surrounding host tissue [van der Giessen et al., 1996; Athanasiou et al., 1996], and it is too early to suggest that such constructs are ready for the clinical setting in either the mitral or aortic position.

## V.III. Bioreactor Development for Mitral Valve Tissue Engineering

The final component of the triad for a tissue-engineered mitral valve is an appropriate method of signaling to enhance or control tissue development and preserve the phenotypic properties of seeded cells. Each heart valve is subjected to a variety of flow, pressure and strain conditions throughout the cardiac cycle *in vivo*, including shear stress, cyclic loading and dynamic flexure. The heart valve "bioreactor" aims to closely mimic such conditions in order to stimulate tissue development and remodelling within the structures, making them suitably safe for implantation [for bioreactor reviews, see Barron et al., 2002; Martin et al., 2004]. It is unclear, however, if identical environmental conditions would condition either mitral and aortic valves adequately, as the mechanical forces experienced by both during the cardiac cycle differ significantly. The human mitral valve, for example, closes against pressures of up to 150 mmHg during systole, whereas the aortic valve closes against diastolic pressures of up to 20 mmHg [Yoganathan et al., 2004]. It is likely that cyclic loading is variable across individual mitral valve leaflets during systole, as the chordae, which are continuous with the leaflet architecture, are restrained by the papillary muscles during ventricular contraction. Surface shear stress, an important parameter for cell adhesion and biosynthetic activity, is also likely to vary considerably between the mitral and aortic valves, owing to the significantly more complex flow patterns through the mitral valve apparatus. Therefore, any tissue-engineered device that functions well in the aortic position may not necessarily perform equally in the mitral position. Despite the differences in the biomechanical environments of these valves, however, bioreactor conditioning *in vitro* has at least been shown to enhance cell proliferation within tissue-engineered heart valves, and to improve ECM synthesis and organisation. Several bioreactors have been developed for routine testing and to subject pre-implantation valves to numerous mechanical conditions, including tension, compression, flexure, shear stress and pulsatile flow of cell culture medium [Engelmayr et al., 2003; Hoerstrup et al., 2000b; Jockenhoevel et al., 2002; Mol et al., 2005].

This results in strengthening of the tissue and confers suitable mechanical properties for *in vivo* animal trials in the low pressure pulmonary system. Whether or not these conditioning techniques can be extended adequately to the variable, high pressure environment of the high pressure mitral and aortic positions remains to be elucidated.

## V.IV. Challenges in the Field of Mitral Valve Tissue Engineering

In a recent controversial review article published in Circulation Research [Vesely, 2005], the author delivers an honest appraisal of the current state of the heart valve tissue engineering field: unfortunately, while many researchers in the field seem to promise much, the reality is that we remain far from being able to credibly apply tissue-engineered mitral or aortic valves in a clinical setting. The challenges that need to be overcome in this field are numerous, with particular regard to the narrower field of mitral valve tissue engineering. In order to improve mechanical properties for an implantable tissue-engineered mitral valve, a greater knowledge of the relationship between normal mitral valve mechanics and intrinsic mitral valve structure and remodelling will prove extremely beneficial. Advances in the understanding of mitral valve embryology and development will aid in the design of suitable bioreactors and signalling tools to improve *in vitro* engineered mitral valves. The design and validation of reliable markers of tissue development and remodelling, both *in vitro* and *in vivo*, will also allow significant advances in the field. Ultimately, however, successful pre-clinical studies remain of paramount importance prior to a responsible transition into the clinical setting. To date, tissue-engineered valves have not been implanted in the high pressure systemic circulation (aortic, mitral position) in pre-clinical studies, and only sparse evidence exists that these valves can function adequately in the low pressure pulmonary circulation. Strict validation methods will need to be developed and implemented, in order to avoid a repetition of such results as those of the Synergraft$^{TM}$ trial [Simon et al., 2003]. Despite the challenges ahead, significant advances have been made in this exciting and promising area of research. The approaches described, in combination with the creativity of researchers in the field, hold great potential for the development of mitral valve prostheses with the ability to grow, remodel and repair their structure following implantation.

# References

Ahmed, A; Johansson, O; Folan-Curran, J. Distribution of PGP 9.5, TH, NPY, SP and CGRP immunoreactive nerves in the rat and guinea pig atrioventricular valves and chordae tendineae. *Journal of Anatomy*, 1997, 191, 547-60.

Anderson, RH. Fluorescing valvular nerves in the guinea-pig heart. *Experentia*, 1971, 27(9), 1063-4.

Anderson, RH; Webb, S; Brown, NA; Lamers, W; Moorman A. Development of the heart: (2) Septation of the atriums and ventricles. *Heart*, 2003a, 89(8), 949-58.

Anderson, RH; Webb, S; Brown, NA; Lamers, W; Moorman A. Development of the heart: (3) formation of the ventricular outflow tracts, arterial valves, and intrapericardial arterial trunks. *Heart*, 2003b, 89(9), 1110-8.

Andries, LJ. *Endocardial endothelium: functional morphology.* 1st ed.- Austin, Texas: Landes; 1994.

Andries, LJ; Brustsaert DL. Differences between endocardial and vascular endothelium. *Journal of Cardiovascular Pharmacology*, 1991, 17(S3), 243-6.

Athanasiou, KA; Niederauer, GG; Agrawal, CM. Sterilization, toxicity, biocompatibility and clinical applications of polylactic acid/polyglycolic acid copolymers. *Biomaterials*, 1996, 17(2), 93-102.

Barocas, VH; Girton, TS; Tranquillo, RT. Engineered alignment in media equivalents: magnetic prealignment and mandrel compaction. *Journal of Biomechanical Engineering*, 1998, 120(5), 660-6.

Barron, V; Lyons, E; Stenson-Cox, C; McHugh, PE; Pandit, A. Bioreactors for cardiovascular cell and tissue growth: a review. *Annals of Biomedical Engineering*, 2002, 31(9), 1017-30.

Bashey, RI; Torii, S; Angrist, A. Age-related collagen and elastin content of human heart valves. *Journal of Gerontology*, 1967, 22, 203-8.

Beardow, AW; Buchanan, JW. Chronic mitral valve disease in cavalier King Charles spaniels: 95 cases (1987-1991). *Journal of the American Veterinary Medical Association*, 1993, 203(7), 1023-9.

Black, A; French, AT; Dukes-McEwan, J; Corcoran, BM. Ultrastructural morphologic evaluation of the phenotype of valvular interstitial cells in dogs with myxomatous degeneration of the mitral valve. *American Journal of Veterinary Research*, 2005, 66(8), 1408-14.

Brody, S; McMahon, J; Yao, L; O'Brien, M; Dockery, P; Pandit, A. The effect of cholecyst-derived extracellular matrix on the phenotypic behaviour of valvular endothelial and valvular interstitial cells. *Biomaterials*, 2007, 28(8), 1461-9.

Buchanan, JW. Chronic valvular disease (endocardiosis) in dogs. *Advances in Veterinary Science & Comparative Medicine*, 1977, 21, 75-106.

Campbell, SE; Katwa, LC. Angiotensin II stimulated expression of transforming growth factor-beta1 in cardiac fibroblasts and myofibroblasts. *Journal of Molecular and Cellular Cardiology*, 1997, 29(7), 1947-58.

Cooper, T; Napolitano, LM; Fitzgerald, MJT; Moore, KE; Daggett, WM; Willman, VL; Sonnenblick, EH; Hanlon CR. Structural basis of cardiac valvar function. *Archives of Surgery*, 1966, 93, 767-71.

Corcoran, BM; Black, A; Anderson, H; McEwan, JD; French, A; Smith, P; Devine, C. Identification of surface morphologic changes in the mitral valve leaflets and chordae tendineae of dogs with myxomatous degeneration. *American Journal of Veterinary Research*, 2004, 65(2), 198-206.

Cowan, SM; Bartges, JW; Gompf, RE; Hayes, JR; Moyers, TD; Snider, CC; Gerard, DA; Craft, RM; Muenchen, RA; Carroll, RC. Giant platelet disorder in the Cavalier King Charles Spaniel. *Experimental Hematology*, 2004, 32(4), 344-50.

Culshaw, G; French, A; Han, R; Black, A; Pearson, G; Corcoran BM. *Innervation of the canine mitral valve and the effects of myxomatous degeneration*. 2008 (submitted).

Darke, PG. Valvular incompetence in cavalier King Charles spaniels. *Veterinary Record*, 1987, 120(15), 365-6.

De Biasi, S; Vitellaro-Zuccarello, L; Blum, I. Histochemical and ultrastructural study on the innervation of human and porcine atrio-ventricular valves. *Anatomy and Embryology*, 1984, 169(2), 159-65.

De la Cruz, MV; Giménez-Ribotta, M ; Saravalli, O; Cayré, R. The contribution of the inferior endocardial cushion of the atrioventricular canal to cardiac septation and to the development of the atrioventricular valves: study in the chick embryo. *American Journal of Anatomy*, 1983, 166(1), 63-72.

Deck, JD. Endothelial cell orientation on aortic valve leaflets *Cardiovascular Research*, 1986, 20(10), 760-7.

Dell'Italia, LJ. The renin-angiotensin system in mitral regurgitation: a typical example of tissue activation. *Current Cardiology Reports*, 2002, 4(2), 97-103.

Dell'Italia, LJ; Meng, QC; Balcells, E; Straeter-Knowlen, IM; Hankes, GH; Dillon, R; Cartee, RE; Orr, R; Bishop, SP; Oparil, S. Increased ACE and chymase-like activity in cardiac tissue of dogs with chronic mitral regurgitation. *American Journal of Physiology*, 1995, 269(6[2]), H2065-73.

Detweiler, DK; Patterson, DF. The prevalence and types of cardiovascular disease in dogs. *Annals of the New York Academy of Sciences*, 1965, 127(1), 481-516.

Diamantouros, S; Flanagan, TC; Sachweh, JS; Schmitz-Rode, T; Jockenhoevel, S. Vasoactive drugs reduce smooth muscle cell-mediated contraction of fibrin gel in culture: implications for fibrin-based heart valve tissue engineering. *Tissue Engineering*, 2007, 13(7), 1775.

Ehinger, B; Falck, B; Steveni, U. Adrenergic and non-adrenergic valvular nerves of the heart. *Experientia*, 1969, 25(7), 742-3.

Ellison, JP; Hibbs, RG. The atrioventricular valves of the guinea-pig I. A light microscope study. *American Journal of Anatomy*, 1973, 138, 331-46.

Engelmayr, GC Jr; Hildebrand, DK; Sutherland, FW; Mayer, JE Jr; Sacks, MS. A novel bioreactor for the dynamic flexural stimulation of tissue engineered heart valve biomaterials. *Biomaterials*, 2003, 24(14), 2523-32.

Ernst, E; Schneider, P; Trautwein, G. Etiology and pathogenesis of the endocardiosis and endocarditis in dogs. II. Anatomicopathological findings. *Deutsche Tierarztliche Wochenschrifte*, 1973, 80(14), 322-8.

Eyden, B. Electron microscopy in the study of myofibroblastic lesions. *Seminars in Diagnostic Pathology*, 2003, 20(1), 13-24.

Fenoglio, JJ; Pham, TD; Wit, AL; Bassett, AL; Wagner, BM. Canine mitral complex: ultrastructure and electromechanical properties. *Circulation Research*, 1972 31, 417-30.

Ferreira, AL; Rossi, MA. Innervation of human atrioventricular valves. *Acta Anatomica*, 1974, 87, 57-65.

Filip, DA; Radu, A; Simionescu, M. Interstitial cells of the heart valves possess characteristics similar to smooth muscle cells. *Circulation Research*, 1986, 59, 310-20.

Flanagan, TC; Black, A; O'Brien, M; Smith, TJ; Pandit, A. Reference models for mitral valve tissue engineering based on valve cell phenotype and extracellular matrix analysis. *Cells Tissues and Organs*, 2006a, 183, 12-23.

Flanagan, TC; Cornelissen, C; Koch, S; Tschoeke, B; Sachweh, JS; Schmitz-Rode, T; Jockenhoevel, S. The in vitro development of autologous fibrin-based tissue-engineered heart valves through optimised dynamic conditioning. *Biomaterials*, 2007, 28(23), 3388-97.

Flanagan, TC; Frese, J; Sachweh, JS; Bernstein, N; Schmitz-Rode, T; Jockenhoevel, S. In vivo evaluation of fibrin-based tissue-engineered heart valves in a sheep model. *Tissue Engineering Part A*, 2008, 14(5), 746-7.

Flanagan, TC; Pandit, A. Living artificial heart valve alternatives: a review. *European Cells and Materials*, 2003, 6, 28-45.

Flanagan, TC; Wilkins, B; Black, A; Jockenhoevel, S; Smith, TJ; Pandit AS. A collagen-glycosaminoglycan co-culture model for heart valve tissue engineering applications. *Biomaterials*, 2006b, 27(10), 2233-46.

Gerstheimer, FP; Metz, J. Distribution of calcitonin gene-related peptide-like immunoreactivity in the guinea pig heart. *Anatomy and Embryology*, 1986, 175, 255-60.

Grassl, ED; Oegema, TR; Tranquillo, RT. Fibrin as an alternative biopolymer to type-I collagen for the fabrication of a media equivalent. *Journal of Biomedical Materials Research*, 2002, 60(4), 607-12.

Gross, L; Kugel, MA. Topographic anatomy and histology of the valves in the human heart. *American Journal of Pathology*, 1931, **7**, 445-95.

Hadian, M; Corcoran, BM; Bradshaw, JP. Molecular changes in fibrillar collagen in myxomatous mitral valve disease. 2008 (submitted, *Biophysical Journal*).

Hadian, M; Corcoran, BM; Han, RI; Grossmann, JG; Bradshaw, JP. Collagen organisation in canine myxomatous mitral valve disease, an x-ray diffraction study. *Biophysical Journal*, 2007, 93(7), 2472-6.

Haggstrom, J; Kvart, C; Hansson, K. Heart sounds and murmurs: changes related to severity of chronic valvular disease in the Cavalier King Charles spaniel. *Journal of Veterinary Internal Medicine*, 1995, 9(2), 75-85.

Hamlin, RL. Geriatric heart diseases in dogs. *Veterinary Clinics of North America Small Animal Practice*, 2005, 35(3), 597-615.

Han, RI; Black, A; Corcoran, BM. *Structural and cellular changes in myxomatous mitral valve disease: an image analysis study*. 2008 (submitted).

Han, RI; Black, A; Culshaw, G; French, AT; Else, RW; Corcoran, BM. The distribution of myofibroblasts, smooth muscle-like cells, macrophages and mast cells in canine myxomatous mitral valve disease. *American Journal of Veterinary Research*, 2008, 69(6), 763-9.

Harasaki, H; Hanano, H; Tanaka, J; Tokunaga, K; Torisu, M. Surface structure of the human cardiac valve. A comparative study of normal and diseased valves. *Journal of Cardiovascular Surgery*, 1978, 19(3), 281-90.

Harasaki, H; Suzuki, I; Tanaka, J; Hanano, H; Torisu, M. Ultrastructural research of the endocardial endothelium of monkeys. *Archives Histologica Japonica*, 1975, 38(1), 71-84.

Hibbs, RG; Ellison, JP. The atrio-ventricular valves of the guinea-pig II. An ultrastructural study. *American Journal of Anatomy*, 1973, 138, 347-70.

Hill, ADK; Folan-Curran J. Microappendages on the atrioventricular valves of the guinea pig. *Journal of Anatomy*, 1993, 182, 425-8.

Hoerstrup, SP; Sodian, R; Daebritz, S; Wang, J; Bacha, EA; Martin, DP; Moran, AM; Guleserian, KJ; Sperling, JS; Kaushal, S; Vacanti, JP; Schoen, FJ; Mayer, JE Jr. Functional living trileaflet heart valves grown in vitro. *Circulation*, 2000a, 102(19 suppl 3), II144-9.

Hoerstrup, SP; Sodian, R; Sperling, JS; Vacanti, JP; Mayer, JE Jr. New pulsatile bioreactor for in vitro formation of tissue engineered heart valves. *Tissue Engineering*, 2000b, 6(1), 75-9.

Hoffmann, D; Gong, G; Liao, K; Macaluso, F; Nikolic, SD; Frater, RWM. Spontaneous host endothelial growth on bioprostheses. *Circulation*, 1992, 89(Suppl II), II75-9.

Icardo, JM; Arrechedera, H; Colvee, E. The atrioventricular valves of the mouse: I. A scanning electron microscope study. *Journal of Anatomy*, 1993, 182, 87-94.

Icardo, JM; Colvee, E. Atrioventricular valves of the mouse: II. Light and transmission electron microscopy. *The Anatomical Record*, 1995, 241, 391-400.

Iemoto, Y; Kondo, Y. Endocardial lesions in acute serum sickness in the rabbit. A scanning electron microscopic study. *Virchows Archive B, Cell Pathology Including Molecular Pathology*, 1982, 40(2), 191-200.

Jockenhoevel, S; Chalabi, K; Sachweh, JS; Groesdonk, HV; Demircan, L; Grossmann, M; Zund, G; Messmer, BJ. Tissue engineering: complete autologous valve conduit - a new moulding technique. *Thoracic and Cardiovascular Surgery*, 2001, 49(5), 287-90.

Jockenhoevel, S; Zund, G; Hoerstrup, SP; Schnell, A; Turina, M. Cardiovascular tissue engineering: a new laminar flow chamber for in vitro improvement of mechanical tissue properties. *ASAIO Journal*, 2002, 48(1), 8-11.

Kadner, A; Hoerstrup, SP; Tracy, J; Breymann, C; Maurus, CF; Melnitchouk, S; Kadner, G; Zund, G; Turina, M. Human umbilical cord cells: a new cell source for cardiovascular tissue engineering. *Annals of Thoracic Surgery*, 2002a, 74(4), S1422-8.

Kadner, A; Hoerstrup, SP; Zund, G; Eid, K; Maurus, C; Melnitchouk, S; Grunenfelder, J; Turina, MI. A new source for cardiovascular tissue engineering: human bone marrow stromal cells. *European Journal of Cardiothoracic Surgery*, 2002b, 21(6), 1055-60.

Kanani, M; Moorman, AF; Cook, AC; Webb, S; Brown, NA; Lamers, WH; Anderson, RH. Development of the atrioventricular valves: clinicomorphological correlations. *Annals of Thoracic Surgery*, 2005, 79(5), 1797-804.

Kim, JS; Virágh, S; Moorman, AF; Anderson, RH; Lamers, WH. Development of the myocardium of the atrioventricular canal and the vestibular spine in the human heart. *Circulation Research*, 2001, 88(4), 395-402.

Kogure, K. Pathology of chronic mitral valvular disease in the dog. *Nippon Juigaku Zasshi*, 1980, 42(3), 323-35.

Koprla, EC; Nemeseri, L. Essential features of endocardial and myocardial morphology: SEM and TEM studies. *Acta Physiologica Hungarica*, 1984, 64(1), 65-79.

Kunzelman, KS; Cochran, RP; Murphree, SS; Ring, WS; Verrier, ED; Eberhart, RC. Differential collagen distribution in the mitral valve and its influence on biomechanical behaviour. *Journal of Heart Valve Disease*, 1993, 2, 236-44.

Lamers, WH; Moorman, AF. Cardiac septation: a late contribution of the embryonic primary myocardium to heart morphogenesis. *Circulation Research*, 2002, 91(2), 93-103.

Lamers, WH; Virágh, S; Wessels, A; Moorman, AF; Anderson, RH. Formation of the tricuspid valve in the human heart. *Circulation*, 1995, 91(1), 111-21.

Lester, WM; Damji, AA; Tanaka, M; Gedeon, I. Bovine mitral valve organ culture: role of interstitial cells in repair of valvular injury. *Journal of Molecular and Cellular Cardiology*, 1992, 24, 43-5.

Licata, RH. Possible reflexogenic mechanisms regulating heart valve function. *Rocky Mountain Medical Journal*, 1967, 64(3), 65-8.

Lim, KO; Boughner, DR. Scanning electron microscopical study of human mitral valve chordae tendineae. *Archives of Pathology and Laboratory Medicine*, 1977, 101(5), 236-8.

Long, JL; Tranquillo, RT. Elastic fiber production in cardiovascular tissue equivalents. *Matrix Biology*, 2003, 22(4), 339-50.

Lupu, F; Simionescu, M. Organization of the intercellular junctions in the endothelium of cardiac valves. *Journal of Submicroscopic Cytology*, 1985, 17(2), 119-32.

Maish, MS; Hoffman-Kim, D; Krueger, PM; Souza, JM; Harper, JJ 3rd; Hopkins, RA. Tricuspid valve biopsy: a potential source of cardiac myofibroblast cells for tissue-engineered cardiac valves. *Journal of Heart Valve Disease*, 2003, 12(2), 264-9.

Marron, K; Yacoub, MH; Polak, J; Sheppard, MN; Fagan, D; Whitehead, BF; De Leval, MR; Anderson, RH; Wharton, J. Innervation of human atrioventricular and arterial valves. *Circulation*, 1996, 94, 368-75.

Martin, I; Wendt, D; Heberer, M. The role of bioreactors in tissue engineering. *Trends in Biotechnology*, 2004, 22, 80-8.

Matheny, RG; Hutchison, ML; Dryden, PE; Hiles, MD; Shaar, CJ. Porcine small intestine submucosa as a pulmonary valve leaflet substitute. *Journal of Heart Valve Disease*, 2000, 9(6), 769-74.

Melax, H; Leeson, TS. Fine structure of the endocardium in adult rats. *Cardiovascular Research*, 1967, 1(4), 349-55.

Messier, RH; Bass, BL; Aly, HM; Jones, JL; Domkowski, PW; Wallace, RB; Hopkins, RA. Dual structural and functional phenotypes of the porcine aortic valve interstitial population: characteristics of the leaflet myofibroblast. *Journal of Surgical Research*, 1994, 57, 1-21.

Miklosova, M; Sivrev, D; Kocisova, M; Schmidtova, K; Rybarova, S; Kluchova, D; Lovasova, K; Dorko, F. The distribution of substance P-like immunoreactive nerves in the atrioventricular valves of the guinea pig. *Biologia, Bratislava*, 1999, 54(Supp 6), 233-8.

Millington-Sanders, C; Meir, A; Lawrence, L; Stolinski, C. Structure of chordae tendineae in the left ventricle of the human heart. *Journal of Anatomy*, 1998, 192, 573-81.

Mitomo, Y; Nakao, K; Angrist, A. The fine structure of the heart valves in the chicken I. Mitral valve. *American Journal of Anatomy*, 1969, 125, 147-68.

Mol, A; Driessen, NJ; Rutten, MC; Hoerstrup, SP; Bouten, CV; Baaijens, FP. Tissue engineering of human heart valve leaflets: a novel bioreactor for a strain-based conditioning approach. *Annals of Biomedical Engineering*, 2005, 33(12), 1778-88.

Moorman, A; Webb, S; Brown, NA; Lamers, W; Anderson, RH. Development of the heart: (1) formation of the cardiac chambers and arterial trunks. *Heart*, 2003, 89(7), 806-14.

Morse, DE; Hamlett, WC; Noble, CW Jr. Morphogenesis of chordae tendineae. I: Scanning electron microscopy. *Anatomical Record*, 1984, 210(4), 629-38.

Mow, T; Pedersen, HD. Increased endothelin-receptor density in myxomatous canine mitral valve leaflets. *Journal of Cardiovascular Pharmacology*, 1999a, 34(2), 254-60.

Mow, T; Pedersen, HD. No expression of angiotensin II receptors angiotensin-converting enzyme in myxomatous canine mitral valve leaflets. An autoradiographic study. *Journal of Veterinary Medicine Series A*, 1999b, 46(8), 465-72.

Mow, T; Poulsen, K; Nielsen, AH; Baandrup, U; Hansen, BF; Pedersen, HD. Species differences in expression of angiotensin II receptors and angiotensin-converting enzyme in human, canine and rat mitral valve leaflets. *Comparative Biochemistry and Physiology. Part C, Pharmacology, Toxicology & Endocrinology*, 1999, 124(1), 11-7.

Mulholland, DL; Gotlieb, AI. Cell biology of valvular interstitial cells. *The Canadian Journal of Cardiology*, 1996, 12(3), 231-6.

Nettleship, AW. Experimental Studies on the afferent innervation of the cat's heart. *Journal of Comparative Neurology*, 1936, 64(1), 115-31.

Novi, AM. An electron microscopic study of the innervation of papillary muscles in the rat. *Anatomical Record*, 1968, 160(1), 123-41.

O'Brien, MF; Goldstein, S; Walsh, S; Black, KS; Elkins, R; Clarke, D. The SynerGraft valve: a new acellular (nonglutaraldehyde-fixed) tissue heart valve for autologous recellularization first experimental studies before clinical implantation. *Seminars in Thoracic and Cardiovascular Surgery*, 1999, 11(4 suppl 1), 194-200.

O'Connell, P; Han, RI; Black, A; French, AT; Else, RW; Corcoran, BM. Distribution of macrophages and mast cells in the leaflets of dogs with myxomatous mitral valve disease. *European College of Veterinary Internal Medicine Congress*, 2006.

Oki, T; Fukuda, N; Kawano, T; Iuchi, A; Tabata, T; Manabe, K; Kageji, Y; Sasaki, M; Yamada, H; Ito, S. Histopathologic studies of innervation of normal and prolapsed human mitral valves. *Journal of Heart Valve Disease*, 1995, 4, 496-502.

Olsen, LH; Fredholm, M; Pedersen, HD. Epidemiology and inheritance of mitral valve prolapse in Dachshunds. *Journal of Veterinary Internal Medicine*, 1999, 13(5), 448-56.

Olsen, LH; Kristensen, AT; Häggström, J; Jensen, AL; Klitgaard, B; Hansson, H; Pedersen, HD. Increased platelet aggregation response in Cavalier King Charles Spaniels with mitral valve prolapse. *Journal of Veterinary Internal Medicine*, 2001, 15(3), 209-16.

Olsen, LH; Mortensen, K; Martinussen, T; Larsson, LI; Baandrup, U; Pedersen, HD. Increased NADPH-diaphorase activity in canine myxomatous mitral valve leaflets. *Journal of Comparative Pathology*, 2003, 129(2-3), 120-30.

Oosthoek, PW; Wenink, AC; Vrolijk, BC; Wisse, LJ; DeRuiter, MC; Poelmann, RE; Gittenberger-de Groot, AC. Development of the atrioventricular valve tension apparatus in the human heart. *Anatomy and Embryology*, 1998a, 198(4), 317-29.

Oosthoek, PW; Wenink, AC; Wisse, LJ; Gittenberger-de Groot, AC. Development of the papillary muscles of the mitral valve: morphogenetic background of parachute-like asymmetric mitral valves and other mitral valve anomalies. *Journal of Thoracic and Cardiovascular Surgery*, 1998b, 116(1), 36-46.

Oyama, MA; Chittur, SV. Genomic expression patterns of mitral valve tissues from dogs with degenerative mitral valve disease. *American Journal of Veterinary Research*, 2006, 67(8), 1307-18.

Oyama, MA; Sisson, DD. Cardiac troponin-I concentration in dogs with cardiac disease. *Journal of Veterinary Internal Medicine*, 2004, 18(6), 831-9.

Pedersen, HD; Falk, T; Haggstrom, J; Tarnow, I; Olsen, LH; Kvart, C; Nielsen, MO. Circulating concentrations of insulin-like growth factor-1 in dogs with naturally occurring mitral regurgitation. *Journal of Veterinary Internal Medicine*, 2005, 19(4), 528-32.

Pedersen, HD; Koch, J; Poulsen, K; Jensen, AL; Flagstad, A. Activation of the renin-angiotensin system in dogs with asymptomatic and mildly symptomatic mitral valvular insufficiency. *Journal of Veterinary Internal Medicine*, 1995a, 9(5), 328-31.

Pedersen, HD; Lorentzen, KA; Kristensen, BO. Echocardiographic mitral valve prolapse in cavalier King Charles spaniels: epidemiology and prognostic significance for regurgitation. *Veterinary Record*, 1999a, 144(12), 315-20.

Pedersen, HD; Mow, T. Hypomagnesemia and mitral valve prolapse in Cavalier King Charles spaniels. *Zentralbl Veterinarmed A*, 1998, 45(10), 607-14.

Pedersen, HD; Olsen, LH; Arnorsdottir, H. Breed differences in the plasma renin activity and plasma aldosterone concentration of dogs. *Zentralbl Veterinarmed A*, 1995b, 42(7), 435-41.

Pedersen, HD; Olsen, LH; Mow, T; Christensen, NJ. Neuroendocrine changes in Dachshunds with mitral valve prolapse examined under different study conditions. *Research in Veterinary Science*, 1999b, 66(1), 11-7.

Pedersen, HD; Schutt, T; Sondergaard, R; Qvortrup, K; Olsen, LH; Kristensen, AT. Decreased plasma concentration of nitric oxide metabolites in dogs with untreated mitral regurgitation. *Journal of Veterinary Internal Medicine*, 2003, 17(2), 178-84.

Peine, CJ; Low, FN. Scanning electron microscopy of cardiac endothelium of the dog. *American Journal of Anatomy*, 1975, 142, 137-58.

Pomerance, A. Ballooning deformity (mucoid degeneration) of atrioventricular valves. *British Heart Journal*, 1969, 31(3), 343-51.

Pomerance, A; Whitney, JC. Heart valve changes common to man and dog: a comparative study. *Cardiovascular Research*, 1970, 4(1), 61-6.

Puff, A. Functional anatomy of the heart valve apparatus. *Verhandlungen der Deutschen Gesellschaft fur Kreislaufforschung*, 1965, 31, 1-15.

Rabkin, E; Aikawa, M; Stone, JR; Fukumoto, Y; Libby, P; Schoen, FJ. Activated interstitial myofibroblasts express catabolic enzymes and mediate matrix remodeling in myxomatous heart valves. *Circulation*, 2001, 104(21), 2525-32.

Ramamurthi, A; Vesely, I. Evaluation of the matrix-synthesis potential of crosslinked hyaluronan gels for tissue engineering of aortic heart valves. *Biomaterials*, 2005, 26(9), 999-1010.

Riddle, JM; Wang, CH; Magilligan, DJ; Stein, PD. Scanning electron microscopy of surgically excised human mitral valves in patients over 45 years of age. *American Journal of Cardiology*, 1989, 63, 471-7.

Roy, A; Brand, NJ; Yacoub, MH. Expression of 5-hydroxytryptamine receptor subtype messenger RNA in interstitial cells from human heart valves. *Journal of Heart Valve Disease*, 2000, 9(2), 256-60.

Sarphie, TG. Pleomorphic surface features of mammalian endocardium: fine structure of canine bicuspid valves. *Journal of Molecular and Cellular Cardiology*, 1980, 12, 241-55.

Sarphie, TG. Surface topography of mitral valve endothelium from diet-induced, hypercholesterolemic rabbits. *Atherosclerosis*, 1982, 45, 203-20.

Sarphie, TG; Allen, DJ. Scanning and transmission electron microscopy of normal and methotrexate treated endocardial cell populations in dogs. *Journal of Submicroscopic Cytology*, 1978, 10(1), 15-25.

Schmidt, D; Mol, A; Breymann, C; Achermann, J; Odermatt, B; Gössi, M; Neuenschwander, S; Pretre, R; Genoni, M; Zund, G; Hoerstrup, SP. Living autologous heart valves engineered from human prenatally harvested progenitors. *Circulation*, 2006, 114(1 suppl), I125-31.

Scott, JE; Orford, CR. Dermatan sulphate-rich proteoglycan associates with rat tail-tendon collagen at the d band in the gap region. *Biochemical Journal*, 1981, 197(1), 213-6.

Shi, Y; Vesely, I. Fabrication of mitral valve chordae by directed collagen gel shrinkage. *Tissue Engineering*, 2003, 9(6), 1233-42.

Shinoka, T; Ma, PX; Shum-Tim, D; Breuer, CK; Cusick, RA; Zund, G; Langer, R; Vacanti, JP; Mayer, JE Jr. Tissue-engineered heart valves: autologous valve leaflet replacement study in a lamb model. *Circulation*, 1996, 94(9 suppl), II164-8.

Shinoka, T; Shum-Tim, D; Ma, PX; Tanel, RE; Langer, R; Vacanti, JP; Mayer, JE Jr. Tissue-engineered heart valve leaflets: does cell origin affect outcome? *Circulation*, 1997, 96(9 suppl), II102-7.

Simon, P; Kasimir, MT; Seebacher, G; Weigel, G; Ullrich, R; Salzer-Muhar, U; Rieder, E; Wolner, E. Early failure of the tissue engineered porcine heart valve SYNERGRAFT in pediatric patients. *European Journal of Cardiothoracic Surgery*, 2003, 23(6), 1002-6.

Smith, PJ; French, AT; Van Israël, N; Smith, SG; Swift, ST; Lee, AJ; Corcoran, BM; Dukes-McEwan, J. Efficacy and safety of pimobendan in canine heart failure caused by myxomatous mitral valve disease. *Journal of Small Animal Practice*, 2005, 46(3), 121-30.

Smith, RB. Intrinsic innervation of the atrioventricular and semilunar valves in various mammals. *Journal of Anatomy*, 1971, 108(1), 115-21.

Sokolov, VV; Goriun, GG. Vascular-nervous relationships in the valves of the heart *Arkhiv Anatomii, Gistologii I Embriologii*, 1976, 70(4), 103-6.

Somi, S; Buffing, AA; Moorman, AF; Van Den Hoff, MJ. Dynamic patterns of expression of BMP isoforms 2, 4, 5, 6, and 7 during chicken heart development. *Anatomical Record Part A: Discoveries in Molecular, Cellular and Evolutionary Biology*, 2004, 279(1), 636-51.

Song, SH. Endocardial surface structures of the feline heart observed with a scanning electron microscope. *Acta Anatomica*, 1977, 99, 67-75.

Sonnenblick, EH; Napolitano, LM; Daggett, WM; Cooper, T. An intrinsic neuromuscular basis for mitral valve motion in the dog. *Circulation Research*, 1967, 21, 9-15.

Stein, PD; Wang, CH; Riddle, JM; Sabbah, HN; Magilligan, DJ Jr; Hawkins, ET. Scanning electron microscopy of operatively excised severely regurgitant floppy mitral valves. *American Journal of Cardiology*, 1989, 64(5), 392-4.

Sutherland, FW; Perry, TE; Yu, Y; Sherwood, MC; Rabkin, E; Masuda, Y; Garcia, GA; McLellan, DL; Engelmayr, GC Jr; Sacks, MS; Schoen, FJ; Mayer, JE Jr. From stem cells to viable autologous semilunar heart valve. *Circulation*, 2005, 111(21), 2783-91.

Swenson, L; Haggstrom, J; Kvart, C; Juneja, RK. Relationship between parental cardiac status in Cavalier King Charles spaniels and prevalence and severity of chronic valvular disease in offspring. *Journal of the American Veterinary Medical Association*, 1996, 208(12), 2009-12.

Tanaka, R; Murota, A; Nagashima, Y; Yamane, Y. Changes in platelet life span in dogs with mitral valve regurgitation. *Journal of Veterinary Internal Medicine*, 2002, 16(4), 446-51.

Tanaka, R; Yamane, Y. Platelet aggregation in dogs with mitral valve regurgitation. *American Journal of Veterinary Research*, 2000, 61(10), 1248-51.

Tarnow, I; Kristensen, AT; Olsen, LH; Falk, T; Haubro, L; Pedersen, LG; Pedersen, HD. Dogs with heart diseases causing turbulent high-velocity blood flow have changes in platelet function and von Willebrand factor multimer distribution. *Journal of Veterinary Internal Medicine*, 2005, 19(4), 515-22.

Tarnow, I; Kristensen, AT; Olsen, LH; Pedersen, HD. Assessment of changes in hemostatic markers in Cavalier King Charles Spaniels with myxomatous mitral valve disease. *American Journal of Veterinary Research*, 2004, 65(12), 1644-52.

Tarnow, I; Kristensen, AT; Texel, H; Olsen, LH; Pedersen, HD. Decreased platelet function in Cavalier King Charles Spaniels with mitral valve regurgitation. *Journal of Veterinary Internal Medicine*, 2003, 17(5), 680-6.

Taylor, PM; Allen, SP; Dreger, SA; Yacoub, MH. Human cardiac valve interstitial cells in collagen sponge: a biological three-dimensional matrix for tissue engineering. *Journal of Heart Valve Disease*, 2002, 11(3), 298-307.

Thrusfield, MV; Aitken, CGG; Darke, PGG. Observations on breed and sex in relation to canine heart valve incompetence. *Journal of Small Animal Practice*, 1985, 26, 709-17.

Tschoeke, B; Flanagan, TC; Cornelissen, A; Koch, S; Roehl, A; Sri Harwoko, M; Sachweh, JS; Gries, T; Schmitz-Rode, T; Jockenhoevel, S. Development of a composite degradable/nondegradable tissue-engineered vascular graft. *Artificial Organs*, 2008a, 32(10), 800-9.

Tschoeke, B; Flanagan, TC; Koch S; Sri Harwoko, M; Deichmann, T; Ellä, V; Sachweh, JS; Kellomäki, M; Gries, T; Schmitz-Rode, T; Gries, T; Jockenhoevel, S. Tissue-engineered small-calibre vascular graft based on a novel biodegradable composite fibrin-polylactide scaffold. *Tissue Engineering*, 2008b (in press).

Tsumori, T; Domoto, T. Ultrastructural evidence for innervation of the endothelium and interstitial cells in the atrioventricular valves of the Japanese monkey. *Anatomical Record*, 1994, 240, 157-66.

van der Giessen, WJ; Lincoff, AM; Schwartz, RS; van Beusekom, HM; Serruys, PW; Holmes, DRJr; Ellis, SG; Topol, EJ. Marked inflammatory sequelae to implantation of biodegradable and nonbiodegradable polymers in porcine coronary arteries. *Circulation*, 1996, 94(7), 1690-7.

Vesely, I. Heart valve tissue engineering. *Circulation Research*, 2005, 97(8), 743-55.

Voloschchenko, AA. Afferent innervation of atrioventricular valve. *Arkhiv Anatomii, Histologii i Embriologii*, 1964, 47(8), 81-4.

Webb, S; Anderson, RH; Lamers, WH; Brown, NA. Formation of the atrioventricular septal structures in the normal mouse. *Circulation Research*, 1998, 82(6), 645-56.

Webb, S; Qayyum, SR; Anderson, RH; Lamers, WH; Richardson, MK. Septation and separation within the outflow tract of the developing heart. *Journal of Anatomy*, 2003, 202(4), 327-42.

Weibel, ER; Palade, GE. New cytoplasmic components in arterial endothelia. *Journal of Cell Biology*, 1964, 23, 101-12.

Wenink, AC. Quantitative morphology of the embryonic heart: an approach to development of the atrioventricular valves. *Anatomical Record*, 1992, 234(1), 129-35.

Wenink, AC; Gittenberger-de Groot, AC. Embryology of the mitral valve. *International Journal of Cardiology*, 1986, 11(1), 75-84.

Wenink, AC; Gittenberger-de Groot, AC; Brom, AG. Developmental considerations of mitral valve anomalies. *International Journal of Cardiology*, 1986, 11(1), 85-101.

Wharton, J; Gulbenkian, S; Mulderry, PK; Ghatei, MA; McGregor, GP; Boom, SR; Polak, JM. Capsaicin induces a depletion of CGRP-immunoreactive nerves in the cardiovascular system of the guinea-pig and rat. *Journal of the Autonomic Nervous System*, 1986, 6, 289-309.

Whitney, JC. Cardiovascular pathology. *Journal of Small Animal Practice*, 1967, 8(8), 459-65.

Whitney, JC. Observations on the effect of age on the severity of heart valve lesions in the dog. *Journal of Small Animal Practice*, 1974, 15(8), 511-22.

Williams, PL; Bannister, LH; Berry, MM; Collins, P; Dyson, M; Dussek, JE; Ferguson, MWJ (Eds.), *Gray's Anatomy. The Anatomical Basis of Medicine and Surgery*. 38th edition. London: Churchill Livingstone; 1995.

Williams, TH. Fast-conducting fibres in the mitral valve. *British Heart Journal*, 1964b, 26(4), 554-7.

Williams, TH. Mitral and tricuspid valve innervation. *British Heart Journal*, 1964a, 26(1), 105-15.

Wilson, GJ; Courtman, DW; Klement, P; Lee, JM; Yeger, H. Acellular matrix: a biomaterials approach for coronary artery bypass and heart valve replacement. *Annals of Thoracic Surgery*, 1995, 60(2 suppl), S353-8.

Ye, Q; Zund, G; Benedikt, P; Jockenhovel, S; Hoerstrup, SP; Sakyama, S; Hubbell, JA; Turina, M. Fibrin gel as a three dimensional matrix in cardiovascular tissue engineering. *European Journal of Cardiothoracic Surgery*, 2000, 17(5), 587-91.

Yoganathan, AP; He, Z; Casey Jones, S. Fluid mechanics of heart valves. *Annual Review of Biomedical Engineering*, 2004, 6, 331-62.

Zacks, S; Rosenthal, A; Granton, B; Havenith, M; Opas, M; Gotlieb, AI. Characterization of cobblestone mitral valve interstitial cells. *Archives of Pathology and Laboratory Medicine*, 1991, 115, 774-9.

In: Advances in Cardiovascular Research, Volume 1
Editors: L. Schmitt, T. Konig, pp. 47-83
ISBN: 978-1-60741-720-0


*Chapter II*

# Review of Treatment of Ventricular Fibrillation

***Rajiv Sankaranarayanan[1*], Hanney Gonna[2**] and Michael James[3***]***
[1]Cardiology Specialty Registrar, Manchester Heart Centre,
Manchester Royal Infirmary, Oxford Road, Manchester M13 9WL, UK
[2]Cardiology Specialty Registrar, London Deanery, UK
[3]Consultant Cardiologist, Taunton Hospital,
Musgrove Park, Taunton TA1 5DA, UK

## Abstract

The annual incidence of sudden cardiac deaths in the United States is about 300,000 cases. Ventricular fibrillation (VF) remains an important cause of sudden death both in hospitals and in the community contributing to about half of these cases, although in monitored setting with rapid response times, VF is the presenting rhythm in almost three quarters of these patients. Despite an overall declining trend in the incidence of VF, the management of the arrhythmia remains challenging due to the fact that the event is usually unexpected and almost certainly lethal in the absence of resuscitation within the first few minutes. There has been a dramatic improvement in survival from VF due to the introduction of defibrillation as a part of resuscitation but in a significant proportion of patients, the process of resuscitation proves futile due to lack of return of spontaneous circulation or significant neurological disability caused by cerebral anoxia.

This review article traces the historical evolution in the management of VF from the era when the term cardiopulmonary resuscitation or CPR was coined less than 50 years ago to represent the series of concerted steps to provide life support and thereby minimize tissue hypoxia by maintaining airway, breathing and circulatory systems through airway patency maneuvers and adjuncts, artificial breathing and delivery of oxygen, chest

* Corresponding authors: Tel.: 044 161 276 1234, 044 7525826672 E-mail: rajiv-s@doctors.org.uk
** E-mail: hanney@doctors.org.uk
*** Tel: 01823 333444, E-mail: michael.james@tst.nhs.uk

compressions and defibrillation, to the modern era of "cardio-cerebral resuscitation". There have been significant changes both in the sequence and methodology of these steps and the persons delivering resuscitation. For instance, there were a series of studies in the 1970s demonstrating the importance of early initiation of resuscitation and therefore the concept of "first responder" or "bystander" CPR leading to improved survival and neurological recovery.

There has been a paucity of high level evidence for many of the resuscitation therapies due to the restrictions on human research created by consent legislation and therefore most of the traditional recommendations such as epinephrine, atropine and strength or type of current delivered by defibrillators, are based on animal research or observational studies. Despite this, there have been many radical developments such as the introduction of automated external defibrillators(AEDs), biphasic defibrillation and re-emphasis on chest compressions preceding defibrillation especially in out of hospital arrests, leading to frequent changes in resuscitation guidelines. The importance of the neurological outcome has also led to the 21st century term cardio-cerebral resuscitation. We hope that by charting the evolution of the treatment of VF, this review article can help to discern the progress made and also to foment further novel ideas in this field.

## Cardiopulmonary Resuscitation

CPR along with prompt defibrillation forms the core component of the management of VF. The various components of CPR and drugs delivered have been devised over the centuries through a combination of chance discovery and trials. While there have been descriptions of airway maintenance and mouth to mouth resuscitation many hundred years back [1], the first cardiac compressions were performed by Moritz Schiff in 1874 in an open canine thorax [2, 3] and by Friedrich Maass in 1892 in a closed chest [4]. The 1st successful human defibrillation is credited to Claude Beck in 1947 and Paul Zoll performed this externally 8 years later [5,6]. Direct current was shown to be superior to alternating current defibrillation by Bernard Lown in 1962 [7]. The first portable automatic external defibrillator was developed in 1979 [1] and 2 years later Michel Mirowski described for the 1st time the use of an implantable automatic defibrillator in humans [8]. While Åsmund Laerdal had devised a mannequin calling it "Resusci Anne" to facilitate CPR education [9], the use of mannequins for CPR practice were first advocated in guidelines in 1966 [10]. Dissemination of information and educating the public regarding resuscitation was first given importance by Dr Beck in the 1950s [1] but this was developed to a much larger scale in Seattle in 1970 [11]. Paramedics were then approved to administer medications during resuscitation in the field and in 1991 the "chain of survival" with 4 links: early access (alerting emergency medical services), early CPR, early defibrillation, and early adult cardiac life support was devised [12]. Data has shown that with each passing minute of untreated VF, the likelihood of survival is reduced by 8 to 10% thereby reiterating the need for early access to defibrillation [12]. This has led to a widespread expansion in public access to AEDs especially in busy public areas such as airports, train stations and shopping centres. A study of resuscitation in casinos reported up to three quarters of patients survive to hospital discharge if defibrillated within 3 minutes [13]. The 2005 American Heart Association guidelines advise that the goal is rapid delivery of a shock within 3 minutes of victim collapse [14]. However chest compressions prior to defibrillation have also been shown to facilitate return of spontaneous circulation with defibrillation [15, 16].It is therefore recommended that CPR should be initiated during AED retrieval and setup if more than 1 rescuer is present, but early defibrillation should be the priority if the defibrillator is available [14]. Hypothermia has been shown to facilitate resuscitation from VF both in animal studies as well as in humans and has therefore become a standard part of post-resuscitation care [17, 18, 19]. Over the last 5 years, the emphasis has been shifted to trying to ensure continuous chest compressions or "minimally-interrupted chest compressions" even if this is to deliver ventilation. This concept is substantiated by studies which have shown that continuous chest compressions alone were associated with a better survival and neurological outcome than that achieved with standard CPR [20, 21]. These opinions by some authors have given rise to the concept of "cardio-cerebral resuscitation" instead of the widely used term "cardiopulmonary resuscitation" [22,23].

# Drug Therapy of Ventricular Fibrillation

## Introduction

Early pharmacological attempts to improve the prognosis of patients at risk of sudden cardiac death centered upon the 'Premature Ventricular Complex Hypothesis' [24]. The hypothesis is simple; the frequency of ventricular ectopy is related to the risk of developing malignant ventricular arrhythmias therefore the suppression of ventricular ectopy should in turn reduce the risk of SCD.

In the 1980s, this hypothesis was so widely held to be self evident that drugs known to reduce ventricular premature complexes, such as the type I anti-arrhythmics, were routinely prescribed in the post infarct period. However it has since transpired that not only is such a strategy ineffective but is actually associated with excess mortality.

The IMPACT [25, 26] and CAST trials [27] were early demonstrations of the deleterious effects of class I anti-arrhythmic agents in this scenario. IMPACT compared mexiletine with placebo in 630 patients who had sustained recent MI. A non-significant trend towards increased mortality in the treatment group was observed. However as IMPACT did not specifically assess the effect of the agent on the frequency of ambient arrhythmias, the premature ventricular complex hypothesis was left still plausible. A pilot study was therefore performed [28] using encainide, flecainide, imipramine and moricizine to examine the efficacy of these agents on reducing the frequency of premature ventricular complexes in post MI patients, with only imipramine shown to be ineffective. Therefore the CAST study was designed to use encainide, flecainide and moricizine or placebo in almost 1500 post MI patients with mild left ventricular dysfunction who had demonstrated either increased premature ventricular complexes or asymptomatic VT on holter monitoring. After just 10 months of follow up the study was terminated due to significant threefold increases in rates of all cause mortality and sudden death in the treatment arms. The moricizine subgroup appeared not suffer quite as significant deleterious effects and were recruited into a larger follow-on study CAST II [29] which again terminated early following an observed fivefold increase in deaths. Combined analysis of both trials revealed a 5% increase in absolute risk of one year all cause mortality [30]. In the light of the CAST trials and other discouraging meta-analysis of type I anti-arrhythmics [31] attention quickly turned away from this class of electrophysiologically active drugs to other potentially more mechanistically attractive agents, most notably the class III drugs amiodarone and sotalol.

## Amiodarone

Over 30 trials of amiodarone in patients at risk of sudden cardiac death have been conducted, with variable results. The most notable early trials, CAMIAT [32] and EMIAT [33] showed reductions in rates of sudden death in the region of 35-40%. Those reductions however did not translate into a statistically significant impact on overall mortality. Interestingly, a positive drug interaction transpired on pooled analysis of the two trials. Patients with a prior myocardial infarction receiving the combination of beta blockade and amiodarone appeared to fare better than those on one agent or neither with respects to both all cause mortality and arrhythmic death at a statistically significant level. As the majority of the amiodarone trials were underpowered to detect moderate reductions in mortality, subsequent meta-analysis have been performed.

A recent meta-analysis of amiodarone for the prevention of SCD by Piccini et al. [34] incorporating data from over 8500 patients in 15 trials including ScD-HeFT found significant reductions in rates of cardiovascular mortality and sudden death of 18% ($p=0.004$) and 29%($p<0.001$) respectively. However, once more these reductions did not translate into a statistically significant reduction in the rates of overall mortality (1.5% absolute risk reduction, $p=0.093$) and was associated with increased rates of pulmonary and thyroid toxicity with almost 10% of randomised patients discontinuing therapy. Interestingly there also appears to be a trend towards an increased incidence of cancer related deaths and this could be postulated to be due to a reduced cardiac death rate.

Thus it appears that amiodarone may have a place in the treatment of high risk post MI or heart failure patients to reduce SCD in those not eligible for ICD therapy and also in adjunct to ICD to reduce device therapy.

## Sotalol

Sotalol, in its commercially marketed preparation, is a racemic mixture of two enantiomers; d-sotalol provides the drug's class III properties and l-sotalol has non-cardioselective ß-blocking activity. Potentially protective effects of the drug in lowering the incidence of ventricular arrhythmias post simulated myocardial infarction were found over 30 years ago in a number of animal studies, such as following the ligation of canine coronary arteries [35]. Early human trials of post myocardial infarction prophylactic use of sotalol displayed promising trends towards reduced mortality, albeit non significant [36]. Unfortunately, despite being a mechanistically plausible therapy with positive initial animal and human study data, sotalol like many other anti-arrhythmics did not fare well when scrutinized in a large properly conducted randomised controlled trial environment. The largest such study, the SWORD [37] trial, examined the efficacy of d-Sotalol in patients with either a recent myocardial infarction associated left ventricular dysfunction (LVEF<40%) or a remote

MI with symptomatic left ventricular dysfunction. The trial was terminated early due to an increase in mortality rates, primarily driven by an increase in arrhythmic deaths (relative risk 1·77, p=0·008).

### *Non anti-arrhythmic drugs that reduce risk of SCD*

Following the largely disappointing experience with anti-arrhythmic agents, attention has turned away from the use of directly electrophysiologically active agents to drugs that may prevent the development of pro-arrhythmic substrates and triggers for VT/VF and/or modulate their interaction. Many of these agents prevent adverse electrical and mechanical remodeling by reducing pathophysiological processes such as myocardial fibrosis, hypertrophy and inflammation. Such drugs include angiotensin converting enzyme inhibitors, aldosterone antagonists, statins and most notably beta-blockers. These agents are discussed below.

### *Angiotensin Converting Enzyme (ACE) Inhibitors*

The reduction in rates of SCD by ACE inhibitors have been postulated to occur by a variety of mechanisms such as positive impact on electrical and mechanical remodeling and neuro-hormonal modulation [38]. A number of clinical trials have demonstrated significant reductions in major adverse cardiovascular events in a variety of study populations and in particular the post myocardial infarct group. However, individually the majority of trials were underpowered to specifically comment on the impact of ACEIs on the rates of sudden cardiac death. However a meta-analysis of 15 randomised controlled trials incorporating over 15000 patients enrolled into studies examining the use of ACE inhibitors vs placebo within 14 days of a MI, has been performed [39]. The results strongly indicate that ACE inhibitors not only reduce all cause mortality but also significantly reduce the risk of SCD by approximately 20% in this post-myocardial infarct population. In patients with chronic heart failure, trial data supports a reduction in cardiovascular mortality with ACE inhibitors however the effect on sudden cardiac death on balance appears not to be significant but rather the conferred mortality advantage arises from reductions in rates of progressive heart failure [40].

### *Aldosterone antagonists*

It appears that after an initial period of reduced aldosterone levels with the commencement of ACEI therapy there is a subsequent rebound effect whereby levels rise once more. Therefore direct aldosterone receptor antagonists mechanistically are an attractive potential therapy and their use has been justified through two major trials. The aldosterone antagonists, spironolactone and eplerenone, have been demonstrated to significantly reduce all cause mortality and sudden death in patients with left ventricular dysfunction in the RALES [41] and EPHESUS [42] trials respectively. EPHESUS was a large scale trial of 6632 post myocardial infarction patients with LVEF < 40%, clinical or radiographic signs of heart failure or diabetes. The primary endpoint of relative risk of all cause mortality was reduced by a factor of 0.85 (p=0.008) as was the secondary endpoint of SCD (RR 0.85, p=0.03). It is important to note that this effect was with the use of aldosterone antagonists in addition to standard ACE inhibition in the majority of the study populations.

**Statins**

The pivotal role of statin therapy in the management of patients with coronary artery disease is unequivocal. A number of trials have demonstrated significant reductions in all cause mortality with the use of these agents, however closer scrutiny indicates that statins may also exhibit anti-arrhythmic effects that are likely independent of their lipid lowering effect. Hypotheses explaining this effect are myriad and include; anti-inflammatory, anti-oxidant, vulnerable plaque stabilisation, endothelial function improvement, reduced ischaemia induced myocyte hypertrophy, improvement in autonomic function, anti-thrombotic and direct effects on ion channel function [43, 44].

Two large scale randomised trials of statins in secondary prevention have reported SCD rates as secondary endpoints. The Long-Term Intervention with Pravastatin in Ischaemic Disease Study (LIPID) randomised 9014 patients with a history of ischemic heart disease to pravastatin or placebo [45].With a mean follow up of over 6 years, overall mortality was significantly reduced by 22%. Rates of sudden cardiac death also appeared to be modestly reduced from 4.7% in the placebo group to 4% in the pravastatin group. The Scandinavian Simvastatin Survival Study [46] had a similar design but used simvastatin in a study population of 4444 patients. Again SCD rates appear to have been reduced from 3.9% to 2.3%.

The protective effects of statins appear to be stronger in the immediate post myocardial infarction period than in secondary prevention studies, perhaps because of the higher baseline risk in this population. Retrospective analysis of national registry data [47] of acute myocardial infarction patients indicates significant substantial reductions in rates of in-hospital mortality with early (within 24 hours) use of statins from 15.4% to 5.3% ($p<0.001$). This benefit is obviously too early to be attributed to plaque regression and strongly points towards a mechanism unrelated to lipid lowering in reducing the rates of sudden death. Further evidence for a non atherosclerotic modifying process comes from the post hoc analysis [48] of statin use in patients with non-ischemic dilated cardiomyopathy (the DEFINITE ICD Trial).. Intriguingly, there was one arrhythmic sudden death in the statin therapy group (0.9%) versus 18 arrhythmic sudden deaths in the 348 patients not receiving statin therapy (5.2%; $p = 0.04$). It is important to note however that these effects have not been directly assessed with arrhythmic death as a pre-defined primary end-point.

**Fish Oils**

Epidemiological indications of a cardio-protective effect of fish oil fatty acids were first noted in the 1970s, when it was observed that Inuit Eskimos with a high intake of dietary fish oils displayed lower rates of fatal coronary heart disease [49].

Major inroads have since been made in the understanding of potential protective mechanisms and which active compounds are responsible for this effect. The eicosapentaenoic acid (EPA) and docosahexenoic acid (DHA) subgroups appear to be particularly relevant and are contained, in varying proportions, in currently commercially available supplements. Given the attractiveness of replicating a 'healthy diet' and perceived low likelihood of significant side effects, many studies of n3-polyunsaturated fatty acids have been conducted in a number of clinical contexts including the post MI context. One of the most notable of these trials being the GISSI-P trial [50] conducted in the 1990s which indicated significant reductions in the primary endpoints of death, non-fatal myocardial infarction and stroke when 2836 post recent MI patients were supplemented with n-3 polyunsaturated fatty acids. Of particular interest was the observation that this maybe primarily driven by a reduction in sudden cardiac death rates, thus generating the hypothesis that PUFA maybe anti-arrhythmic. A recent systematic review [51] of 12 studies encompassing over 32000 patients yields a less convincing argument for a significant anti-arrhythmic effect with a non-significant risk reduction on sudden cardiac death being found. A significant reduction in deaths from cardiac causes (RR 0.80, 95% CI 0.69 to 0.92) but not on all cause mortality was also found. There is however a number of difficulties associated with such an analysis. Notably, there was significant variation in the formulations and dosages employed in the trials, at present there is little consensus on the optimal preparation and or dosage. Furthermore funnel plot analysis indicates a high likelihood of significant publication bias with survival neutral or negative studies being excluded. Finally the examined study populations vary significantly ranging from elective Percutaneous Coronary Intervention patients to patients in their first week post myocardial infarction.

Currently the AHA nutrition committee [52] advocates, in the context of secondary prevention management of IHD, the consumption of approximately 1 g of eicosapentaenoic acid and docosahexenoic acid per day, preferably from oily fish. However they also concede that this maybe difficult to attain and that eicosapentaenoic acid and docosahexenoic acid supplements could be considered at physician discretion.

**Beta blockers**

Of all the drugs with direct electrophysiological activity, only beta-blockers have consistently demonstrated benefit in the reduction of SCD events. This has led to their recommendation as the only anti-arrhythmics that have a primary role in the prevention of SCD in the recent consensus guidelines for the management of ventricular arrhythmias and the prevention of SCD [53].

Their effectiveness predominantly derives from their capacity to modulate cardiac sympathetic tone. Cardiac autonomic imbalance favouring excessive sympathetic drive is clearly implicated in the genesis of lethal ventricular arrhythmias. Sympathetic effects on the heart are mediated through the action of norepinephrine on β1 and β2 adrenergic receptors which are inhibited by the β blocking class of drugs to varying extents depending on the specific agent. β-blockade is associated with decreased ischaemia, fibrosis, hypertrophy, LV dilatation and dispersion of refractory periods, all of which predispose to ventricular arrhythmogenesis [54].

β blockers have been used predominantly in two groups of patients who are at high risk of SCD; those who have sustained a myocardial infarction and in patients with heart failure.

## Use of β blockers post myocardial infarction

The beneficial effects of beta blockade in patients with prior myocardial infarction were reported initially over 40 years ago. From a sudden cardiac death perspective, this group of patients represent an important at risk group.

The Norwegian Multicentric Study Group Trial [55] in the early 1980s was the first large trial to demonstrate a significant reduction (44%, p=0.0001) in rates of SCD in patients assigned to beta blocker therapy (timolol) post myocardial infarction. The benefits were demonstrated to persist for at least six years post index event [56]. A number of other beta blockers were also demonstrated to have a similar beneficial effect in the 1980s. The Beta-

Blocker Heart Attack Trial (BHAT) [57] showed significant improvements in both all cause mortality (7.2% vs 9.8%) and SCD (3.3% vs 4.6%) with propranolol use. Metoprolol [58, 59] and atenolol [60] were also demonstrated to reduce rates of sudden death.

With the advent of routine reperfusion therapy with thrombolysis or percutaneous coronary intervention and therapies such as ACE inhibition, a need arose for more contemporary appraisal of the value of beta blockade post myocardial infarct. The CAPRICORN study [61] sought to clarify the role of carvedilol in the new so called 'reperfusion era'. The trial enrolled almost 2000 patients with proven acute MI and left ventricular dysfunction (LVEF<40%) who were randomised to either carvedilol or placebo. Of note almost all patients were receiving ACE inhibitors and half had received reperfusion therapy. All cause mortality was reduced by 23% (p=0.03) and a trend towards reduction of SCD, but not reaching statistical significance, 5% vs 7% (HR 0·74, p=0.09) was displayed. However, a subsequent post hoc blinded analysis of arrhythmias in the CAPRICORN study population [62] yields some more dramatic reductions in the rates in ventricular malignant arrhythmias with carvedilol therapy by 70% (from 3.9% to 0.9%, HR 0.24, p<0.0001). It is also interesting to note the magnitude of the reduction of all cause mortality is similar to that of trials in the pre-reperfusion era. The limitations of a post hoc analysis notwithstanding, beta-blockade therefore appears to have significant incremental benefit in the management of post myocardial infarct patients in the present era. However, even today, beta-blockade remains underutilized in patients at risk of malignant ventricular arrhythmias.

### Use of β blockers in heart failure

The first documented use of β blockade in heart failure in 1973 by Dr. Finn Waagstein was met with stiff criticism. At that time and for decades subsequent to that, the practice of giving a negative inotrope to a failing heart seemed counterintuitive. However, many trials since have demonstrated convincing reductions in the rates of SCD and all cause mortality in this important patient population.

### CIBIS I

The Cardiac Insufficiency Bisoprolol Study (CIBIS) [63] was the first large prospective analysis of the mortality impact of beta-blockade in patients with chronic heart failure. The study randomised 641 patients with class III and IV heart failure with an LVEF<40% receiving optimal medical therapy to either bisoprolol or placebo. Although demonstrating significant improvements in functional class and reduced hospital admissions the bisprolol arm showed only a non-significant trend towards reduction of all cause mortality and no appreciable impact on SCD rates. The study was underpowered due to a lower than expected background mortality rate. In part this may have been a reflection of the fact that less than 5% of patients were in class IV NYHA heart failure.

### CIBIS II

In 1999, two important trials elevated the status of beta-blockers to standard therapy for patients with chronic LV systolic dysfunction heart failure. CIBIS II [64] attempted to rectify some of the failings of the first trial through recruitment of a much larger sample size with more severe HF. 2647 patients with severe symptomatic heart failure (83% with Class III NYHA symptoms and the remainder class IV)) and LV systolic dysfunction (LVEF<35%)

receiving standard therapy with diuretics and ACE inhibitors were randomized to receive placebo or bisoprolol.

The trial was terminated following the second interim analysis, which demonstrated a significant mortality benefit in the bisoprolol arm. On an intention to treat analysis, there were significant reductions in both all-cause mortality (11·8% vs. 17·3%, RR 34%, p<0·0001) and rates of SCD (3·6% vs 6·3%, RR 44%, p=0·0011) in the bisoprolol treatment arm. Treatment effects were independent of the severity or cause of heart failure.

## MERIT HF

Later in the same year, the MERIT-HF study group announced similar findings but this time with sustained release metoprolol used in a broader group of patients [65]. The trial enrolled 3991 patients with NYHA class II–IV symptoms with LVEF<40% on optimum standard therapy. Randomisation was preceded by a 2 week run in phase. 1990 patients were randomised to metoprolol CR/XL 12·5 mg (NYHA III–IV) or 25·0 mg once daily (NYHA II) and 2001 were assigned to placebo. MERIT-HF was also terminated early due to the demonstration of a significant survival advantage with beta-blockade. Treatment with long-acting metoprolol was associated with a statistically significant 34% reduction in all-cause mortality, being reduced from 11·0% to 7·2%. There also were significantly fewer sudden deaths in the metoprolol group than those receiving the placebo. As in CIBIS-II, for those in class III-IV failure a risk reduction of 41% was demonstrated (44% in CIBIS-II).

Both metoprolol and bisoprolol are lipophilic and highly selective for beta1-receptors. Carvedilol on the other hand is a non-cardioselective, non-lipid soluble beta-antagonist that also exhibits β2 and α1 adrenergic blockade, additionally it has also been reported to have anti-oxidant actions, anti-endothelin and anti-proliferative actions. As such, it has been postulated that this may confer incremental benefits. Three trials have reported on sudden cardiac death in patients with heart failure on carvedilol.

### US Carvedilol Heart Failure Study

The US carvedilol heart failure study [66] enrolled 1094 patients with symptomatic heart failure and a LVEF<35% to carvedilol or placebo. Although the trial demonstrated a significant reduction in mortality from 7.8% in the placebo group to 3.2% with carvedilol therapy which in part arose from reduction in rates of sudden death (from 3.8% to 1.7%), the trial design was such that non-fatal endpoints were the primary outcomes and mortality was only specified a priori to assess safety and potential benefit. This is unusual for a trial that is designed to examine the mortality impact of a drug therapy. This design somewhat limited the conclusions that could be drawn about to what degree carvedilol exhibited mortality benefit and for what duration this effect persisted.

### COPERNICUS

These limitations were addressed by members of the study group in the subsequent trial COPERNICUS [67], which examined 2289 patients with severe symptomatic (dyspnoea on minimal exertion or at rest) and echocardiographic heart failure (LVEF <25%). Patients were randomised to carvedilol or placebo and were assessed for an average of 10.4 months. The trial was prematurely terminated following the demonstration of a significant positive treatment effect with carvedilol, most notably a 35% reduction in the risk of death (p=0.00013) and reduction in sudden death from 6.1% to 3.9%.

**COMET (& BEST) Trial**

Thus it has been demonstrated that cardioselective (metoprolol and bisoprolol) and non-cardioselective beta-Blockers (carvedilol) reduce both all cause and sudden death mortality in patients with chronic heart failure. However beta-Blockers are heterogeneous in their pharmacological action and it should not be assumed that this is a class effect. The BEST trial [68] which studied the use of bucindolol, a non-selective beta-blocker, in patients with class III and IV heart failure with significant left ventricular dysfunction yielded only non-significant trends towards improved mortality, albeit with some overlap of confidence intervals with the previous trials. This may in part be explained by study population differences as the BEST trial recruited a higher proportion of black patients. There are documented racial differences in the polymorphisms of the β1-adrenergic receptor, which is the predominant beta-adrenergic receptor expressed on cardiac myocytes [69].

Specifically black patients are more likely to express a hypoactive β1AR polymorphism thereby potentially reducing the relative efficacy of beta blockade. However previous trials have reported no significant differences in the benefit of beta-blockade in black and non-black heart failure patients [66]. This therefore still leaves the possibility that different beta-blockers may be more or less efficacious in reducing the rates of sudden cardiac death and all-cause mortality. It is in this light that the COMET trial was conceived. This was a head to head superiority comparison of metoprolol and carvedilol in over 3000 symptomatic heart failure patients with a LVEF <35% [70]. On first glance of the reported results it would appear that carvedilol displayed a survival advantage over metoprolol, all-cause mortality was 34% in the carvedilol group and 40% in those treated with metoprolol with a relative risk reduction of 17% (p=0.0017). However a number of mechanistic and trial design issues have been raised which cast into doubt the clinical validity of the findings [71], the most salient being that equipotent dosing regimens may not have been used. The degree of β1 blockade exhibited in the metoprolol group being less that shown in MERIT-HF. Unfortunately there was insufficient data collated to truly compare the degree of β1 blockade in the metoprolol and carvedilol arms.

An analysis of 13 beta-blocker trials that report SCD rates show that the average incidence of sudden death in the placebo treated group was 51% as apposed to 43% in those treated with a beta-blocker [72]. Although the rates of SCD are higher than reported elsewhere in the more contemporary literature, they nonetheless illustrate the positive impact of this class of drug. Current ESC guidelines advocate the use of beta blockers in ischaemic heart failure and during or post MI for the prevention of sudden cardiac death as a class I recommendation [73].

# Automated External Defibrillators & Public Access Defibrillation

## Introduction

The key determinant of successful defibrillation from ventricular arrhythmias is the time elapsed between the onset of VT/VF and the delivery of the first defibrillation shock. It has been estimated that for every minute of delay in delivering defibrillation the probability of survival decreases by approximately 5-10% [74]. This has been illustrated by the very high rates of successful defibrillation attained in closely monitored environments that have rapid, almost immediate, defibrillation capacity at hand such in cardiac rehabilitation programmes and electrophysiological study laboratories in contrast with the poor outcomes seen in out of hospital cardiac arrests. As such, access to early defibrillation is considered to be one of the four interdependent links that constitute the "chain of survival" [75].

Despite a number of well planned initiatives providing early defibrillation has proved problematic for many communities. Both urban and rural environments have presented specific challenges that prevent consistently short delays in delivering trained personnel with appropriate equipment to victims of out an of hospital sudden cardiac arrest, these include problems such as high traffic density and remote locations. In an attempt to circumvent the inherent delay involved in delivering trained healthcare professionals with standard defibrillator equipment to the site of a cardiac arrest the concept of an automated external defibrillator has gathered much attention. This allows persons with no formal training in cardiac rhythm recognition to successfully and rapidly defibrillate a patient.

The automated external defibrillator was developed in the late 1970s and its first reported use was in 1979 [76]. First clinical reports of the use of fully transthoracic defibrillator paddle electrodes arrived in the mid 1980s [77]. It is important to note the distinction between an automated and automatic external defibrillator. The former only advises the need for defibrillation and requires an operator to activate the discharge whereas the latter would perform this automatically. For reasons of safety the currently described AED is automated.

## The Modern AED

The modern AED as we know it is in part a response by industry to the American Heart Association's Public Access Defibrillation Task force's 1994 recommendations as to what would constitute an ideal device. Specifically the task force requested the medical manufacturing industry to produce AEDs that were small, light, easy to use, durable, maintenance free, and voice prompted. The American Heart Association even went so far to recommend strategies for cost reduction. It can be said that most modern AEDs fulfill these specifications. The AED microprocessor must be able to determine, from a surface electrocardiogram whether a rhythm is shockable or non-shockable. This is achieved through analysis algorithms that incorporate data such as wave morphology, amplitude and slope. Noise artifacts must also be filtered to avoid degrading the specificity and sensitivity of the algorithm. In 1997, the American Heart Association AED task force recommended developmental and validation performance goals regarding the accuracy of the arrhythmia analysis algorithms incorporated into AEDs.

The current sensitivity and specificity for shockable rhythm detection by AEDs now approaches 100%. Testament to this fact is the absence of reported inappropriately delivered shocks in field trials of public access defibrillation. The few cases of failure to defibrillate have been in cases of fine VF where misinterpretation as asystole has occurred. This is probably of limited clinical significance. The use of biphasic waveforms has had an advantageous impact on AED design. As biphasic shocks require reduced energy levels most AEDs now utilise a lithium battery instead of older nickel or lead cadmium. Lithium batteries are energy dense and have predictable life spans resulting in smaller devices that require less maintenance. Although modern AEDs have been on the whole reliable, there has been a recent class I recall issued by the Food and Drug Administration for a specific model which failed to deliver shocks following the inability of the device's battery-monitoring software to detect battery failure.

The operation of most modern AEDs follows a four step principle; power on, attach pads, analyze rhythm, shock advisory. In order to illustrate the ease of use of the devices, Gundry et al [78] compared the performance of 15 sixth grade children with no previous training in operating an AED with that of 22 paramedics in a mock cardiac arrest scenario. The primary outcome measure was time from entry on scene to delivery of the shock into simulated ventricular fibrillation. Mean time to defibrillation was 90 seconds for the children and 67 seconds for the paramedics. Electrode pad placement was appropriate for all subjects. All remained clear during shock delivery.

## Public Access Defibrillation (PAD)

Unfortunately most cardiac arrests occur outside a healthcare facility with the vast majority taking place in the home. It follows that non-healthcare professionals in the immediate vicinity or relatively close proximity to a victim of cardiac arrest could attain significantly decreased defibrillation times if they had the capacity to defibrillate when compared to paramedics who are remote to the location. The AED allows lay persons with minimal, or even potentially no training, to achieve exactly this. The strategy of equipping lay persons or high risk environments with AEDs has come to be known as 'Public Access Defibrillation.'

Probably the first attempt in implementing a PAD was performed by Chamberlain et al. in the late 1980s [79].Five patients were successfully defibrillated by British Transport Police officers at a busy London railway station, following basic resuscitation training [80].However the concept dates back to even before the development of AEDs. In 1972 Charles Freidberg in an introduction to a symposium on myocardial infarction hypothesized "Possibly every home with a person at risk should have a portable defibrillator next to the television set."

### *Forms of PAD*

PAD strategies broadly fall into one of three strategies:

1. Site Specific: High risk locations, such as sports arenas, where a large number of people are present have their own AED.
2. Community Based: Lay persons, which maybe members of other emergency services, respond with a mobile AED to the site of an arrest.
3. Home Based: High risk persons have a device placed in their residences.

Certain hybrid strategies have also been proposed which combine site specific and community based programmes.

A significant amount of data documenting the experiences with public access defibrillation has recently become available and salient studies are described below.

**Site Specific**

### Airline studies

Two reports from the late 1990s document experience with the use of AED onboard commercial aircraft [81, 82]. It has been estimated that up to 1000 annual deaths occur onboard commercial flights [81]. The unique aspects of that environment both likely precipitate and contribute to increased mortality from SCD. Of particular concern is that even under optimal conditions, a minimum of 20 minutes would be required to reach conventional medical assistance on the ground. This is both virtually futile and of significant cost to the airline. American Airlines reported their use of AEDs in 200 patients, 14 of which had electrocardiographically documented VF. All of the 13 patients in whom defibrillation was attempted successfully cardioverted on the first shock and an overall rate of survival to discharge from the hospital after shock with the automated external defibrillator was 40%.

### Airport studies

Large airports represent an attractive location for AED placement, by virtue of the sheer volume of people who maybe exposed to the devices. In 2002, Caffrey et al. reported their experience over a 2 year period with the placement of AEDs 90 seconds walking distance apart throughout 3 airports in the Chicago area with an estimated annual passenger volume of 100 million people [83]. Although the incidence rate of arrests was not particularly high (18 cases of VF arrest), the overall long-term survival rate was 56 percent and 67 percent among the 12 patients who underwent defibrillation within five minutes. What is most interesting about this report however is that in half the successfully defibrillated cases, the defibrillator users had no prior training or experience with AEDs. Awareness of the defibrillators was promoted by public service videos in waiting areas and pamphlets only. This is testament to the intuitive AED user interface and suggests good feasibility of public use of defibrillators with minimal costs and training periods.

### Casino studies

Casinos also pose an instructional environment due to their high SCD event rate and unique level of video tape surveillance which allows for very precise time course analysis. In the late 1990s a series of 105 VF arrests (86% witnessed) occurring in 10 casinos with on site AEDs was reported [84]. In witnessed arrests, a mean (±SD) of 4.4±2.9 minutes from collapse to the delivery of the first defibrillation shock and 9.8± 4.3 minutes from collapse to the arrival of the paramedics was achieved. A survival rate of 74% for those who received defibrillation less than three minutes after a witnessed collapse and 49% for those who received defibrillation after more than three minutes provided a glimpse of what an early defibrillation with an effective PAD system can achieve.

**Community Based**

In many areas emergency services such as the police force and firefighters arrive at the scene of an arrest many minutes prior to the arrival of the ambulance service. A number of studies have illustrated the potential impact that trained personnel from these services can have if equipped with AEDs. Weaver et al [80] and Mosesso et al [85] have showed that both firefighters and police provide faster response times with an associated mortality benefit.

### Public Access Defibrillation Trial

To determine the real world effect of public access defibrillation programmes the National Heart, Lung and Blood Institute, American Heart Association and other stakeholders funded a large North American multi-center prospective trial of public access defibrillation [86]. This involved almost a thousand centres, 20,000 volunteers were trained and reported on 239 out of hospital SCDs. It found in comparison with CPR only sites those with AEDs had a shorter interval from collapse to first rhythm assessment (6 vs 8.7 minutes) and a higher incidence of VF (57% vs 47%). Importantly, there were more survivors to hospital discharge in the units assigned to have volunteers trained in CPR plus the use of AEDs than there were in the units assigned to have volunteers trained only in CPR. Residential sites represented 16% of the study sites and accounted for 28% of the cardiac arrests but <5% of the survivors. The study lacked statistical power to detect whether lay rescuer AED programs increase survival from SCA in residential settings.

### Hybrid approaches

A hybrid approach combining both static and dynamically deployed AEDs has also been evaluated particularly by Italian investigators in Piacenza [87] and Brescia [88]. This strategy used AEDs at high risk locations and devices used by lay staffed ambulances and police cars. AED training was only given in addition to traditional CPR training. Response times were reduced by almost 2 minutes and were associated with up to threefold increases of survival in witnessed arrests. However there are some methodological concerns particularly as historical controls were used. Recently the United Kingdom has established a national defibrillator programme, the first programme of its type in the world [89]. The programme uses a combination of on-site and mobile AEDs. Early results from the prospective audit of this national initiative have recently been published [90] showing significant promise. In particular on-site AEDs appear to be particularly effective with 39% of patients having a return of spontaneous circulation and 26% surviving to hospital discharge. These results are favorable when compared to contemporary rates of successful resuscitation with paramedic crew only attended cardiac arrests. The mobile devices were associated understandably with longer response times and higher mortality rates but have the advantage that each device can potentially reach a larger population.

### Recent CPR vs CPR & AED Meta-analysis

A recent meta-analysis [91] comparing CPR only to CPR and mobile AED use by lay-rescuers provides some foundation for the further development of community based public access defibrillation programmes. Remarkably given the relatively widespread uptake of public access defibrillation, on the basis of Jadad scoring for randomized control trial quality, only three trials were deemed suitable for the meta-analysis [ 92-94]. Of these selected trials , although displaying a trend towards AED benefit, none were powered sufficiently to show statistically significant confidence intervals except one which only demonstrated increased survival to hospital admission [93]. However on pooled analysis of the individual trials, amounting to 1583 cases of out of hospital cardiac arrests, a statistically significant survival benefit with CPR + AED as compared with CPR only was demonstrated. This translates into number needed to treat of 17 and 24 for survival to hospital admission and discharge respectively. However, as the authors acknowledge, this analysis does not take into account the potential impact of continuous cardiac compression algorithms described elsewhere as the component trials utilized standard CPR treatment recommendations.

There are some inherent difficulties in comparing the results of community based public access defibrillation studies. Local topography and response times are very different and as such the European Society of Cardiology guidelines take this into account by recommending that local conditions be taken into account when establishing a public access defibrillation programme. Factors such as physical and social isolation due to community structure, physical location and accessibility will significantly impact on attainable defibrillation times.

### Cost effectiveness of public access defibrillation in public places

One of the very legitimate concerns raised by public access defibrillation programmes is the significant cost associated with employing such a strategy. Cost effectiveness analyses vary widely depending on population and exact strategy used for reasons detailed above. In the previously described cohort of VF arrests in casinos a cost analysis has been performed yielding a cost of $56700 per quality-adjusted life year which is comparable with other interventions deemed to be cost-effective [95]. However, it must been borne in mind that this environment specifically lends itself well to rapid defibrillation times and is not representative of the majority of public access defibrillation times attained. The cost-effectiveness of AEDs is quite sensitive to the number of people the device is exposed to. In a cost analysis of AEDs on US aircraft incorporating costs to airline industries and healthcare organisations cost per quality-adjust life year of $94700 with AEDs placed on all aircraft reduces to $35300 if restricted to use only on larger aircraft with capacity for over 200 passengers. A prime difficulty is in the accurate prediction of where public arrests will occur in all except the highest incidence areas. The Public Access Defibrillation trial showed an average interval between arrests per site of 3.5 years or 9.1 years per AED. This money could be used to decrease paramedic response times and for primary and secondary prevention measures instead and as such it is imperative that the cost effectiveness of such a strategy is clearly elucidated before its widespread implementation.

**Home Programmes**

Perhaps one of the greatest challenges in resuscitation medicine is how to reach the locus of the vast majority of cardiac arrests, the home. It is currently estimated that 80% of all SCD occurs at home, which is associated with a dismal 2% survival rate [96]. It is therefore by logical extension that researchers have hypothesized that the placement of AEDs in the home has the potential to significantly impact on the overall mortality associated with sudden cardiac arrest.

### Early AED at Home trials

Early attempts at the use of AEDs deployed in high risk patients in their homes, date back to the late 1980s. Eisenberg et al. enrolled 97 survivors of out-of-hospital VF arrests to a study, with 59 receiving home AEDs [97]. There were a total of 14 out of hospital arrests, of which 10 were in the AED group. Only 6 of the AED group arrests actually had the device applied, 2 patients were in VF and 1 of those survived but with significant neurological dysfunction and died several months later. The authors concluded that there was small potential for in-home AED use in high risk patients. Although this study and other small series had demonstrated, at best, a minor impact on the problem there have been continued efforts along this front for a number of reasons. These studies used earlier generation devices with a user interface not fully optimized for lay person use, the cost of devices has reduced and most importantly even a modest treatment effect when multiplied by the vast number of arrests that occur at home would have a potentially significant impact on this public health problem. It is in this light that the strategy of in-home AED deployment has been conceived. However, given the huge potential cost implications of such a project, validation of the efficacy of such a strategy must occur prior to widespread implementation.

## Home AED Trial (HAT)

The recently reported HAT study specifically sought to provide such validation in patients with a previous anterior myocardial infarct and no ICD in situ, a population perceived to be at high risk for SCD [98]. This large international trial randomised 7001 patients to either conventional resuscitation (CPR and triggering of emergency medical services) or conventional resuscitation and the use of a home AED. The primary outcome measure was all cause mortality with a median follow up period of over 3 years.

The trial found no significant reduction in all cause mortality with the strategy of home AED placement. This finding although disconcerting for proponents of home AEDs has some salient messages. Firstly, the overall event rate of both all cause mortality and SCD was lower than previously assumed. Historical data from the GUSTO I trial in the early 1990s was used to determine an expected annual rate of death of 4% in power calculations. In fact the HAT results demonstrated a annual mortality of 2%. Secondly, patients were equally likely to die from non-cardiac causes as from SCD. The rate of SCD was less than 1% per year which was lower than anticipated prior to the study commencing. Furthermore less than half of SCD events were witnessed and, as with early home AED trials, not all had AEDs applied. Both study population characteristics and improvements in standard care go some way in explaining these findings. Both control and intervention groups had high rates of previous revascularisation (72%) and use of modern drug therapy. The resultant median ejection fraction was 45% (approximately 80% of the intervention and control groups had a documented EF). Finally, it is of note that the overall survival rate from cardiac arrest in the home of 12% is another significant improvement from previously reported figures. On the basis of this trial it has been argued that future funding should be diverted away from home public access defibrillation programmes to directions like minimizing the global burden of SCD such as primary prevention of heart disease [99].

### Summary of public access defibrillation

On balance it appears there is a direct proportional relationship between the efficacy of public access defibrillation programmes and the percentage burden of out-of-hospital cardiac arrests it is designed to target. A major problem is the majority of arrests occur in locations that are not defined as high incidence locations. And as such AEDs placed even in high incidence locations still will not reach the majority of out-of-hospital cardiac arrests. Conversely the placement of AEDs where the majority of arrests occur will only be able to reach limited numbers of patients per AED. At present the American Heart Association recommends that AEDs be placed where at least one arrest will occur every two years. It is likely that prospective audit data from national programmes, such as that instituted in the UK, will shed further light on an optimal strategy when developing public access defibrillation programmes.

# The Implantable Cardioverter-Defibrillator

## Introduction

Early electrical defibrillation is the primary treatment for VF. The primary determinant of successful defibrillation is the time elapsed from the onset of the arrhythmia to the administration of a defibrillatory electrical charge. Even with ubiquitous deployment of external defibrillators there is an inherent time delay between the recognition of the patient with a potentially lethal arrhythmia and defibrillation. This time delay is frequently fatal. To overcome this time delay, in the mid 1960s Michel Mirowski started to develop the implantable cardioverter-defibrillator [100]. However it was not until 1980 that the first internal defibrillator was implanted in a human [101]. Since then multiple technological advances and trial data have established the device as being the treatment of choice for a substantial number of patients with over 100,000 devices being implanted annually.

In essence, the device functions primarily to sense atrial and ventricular electrocardiogram signals, classifies those signals, provide an electrical shock if deemed appropriate and finally provides pacing for bradycardia if needed. Indications for ICD implantation fall into two broad categories; as secondary prevention in patients who have previously sustained a potentially lethal ventricular arrhythmia and as primary prevention for those who are at high risk but as yet have not suffered a ventricular arrhythmia.

## Primary Prevention

Frequently, the first episode of VF is lethal. Often this first fatal presentation occurs in patients who were to some degree at predictably higher risk of developing ventricular arrhythmias due to a history of predisposing conditions such as coronary artery disease or left ventricular dysfunction. The role of the ICD as primary prevention in such patients has been extensively studied in a number of trials.

### *MADIT I*

The Multicenter Automatic Defibrillator Implantation Trial (subsequently renamed MADIT-I) [102], reported in 1996, was the first study to examine the effect of ICDs in patients with prior myocardial infarctions. A total of 196 NYHA class I-III patients with a prior MI, LVEF <35%, a documented episode of asymptomatic non-sustained VT and inducible, non suppressible (by intravenous administration of procainamide) VT/VF on electrophysiological studies (EPS) were randomly assigned to receive an ICD or conventional medical therapy (most commonly amiodarone).At 32 months, there was a statistically significant mortality relative risk reduction of 59% (16% in ICD group vs 39% control group).Being an early trial in the so called ‘epicardial era’, almost half of all device implantations were via the thoracotomy route. Despite the impressive mortality advantage demonstrated, a number of issues regarding the trial’s methodology and generalizability limited its impact on clinical practice. The inclusion only of patients who have non-pharmacologically suppressible VT may have inherently introduced bias as these patients could also have had VT which was difficult to treat by ICD therapy. There was also higher proportion of patients receiving beta-blockers in the ICD arm which in itself is associated with improved mortality. Importantly the actual number of real world patients who would be eligible by MADIT I criteria for an ICD, although difficult to accurately estimate, is likely to be low.

### *MUSTT*

The Multicenter Unsustained Tachycardia Trial (MUSTT) [103], although not designed as a ICD primary prevention trial, provided some important early insights regarding the use of ICDs. The trial enrolled 704 prior MI patients with LVEF<40% and inducible VT to no anti-arrhythmics or to EPS guided therapy with either an anti-arrhythmic or, if one such agent was ineffective, to implantation of an ICD. As such it primarily examined the value of an EPS guided management strategy. The decision to implant an ICD was not randomised. The primary endpoint was arrhythmic death or resuscitated SCA as opposed to all cause mortality which was a secondary endpoint. A non-randomised analysis of patients in the EP guided arm demonstrated trends towards reduction of all cause mortality with ICD implantation when compared to anti-arrhythmic therapy at five years (24% in ICD group vs 55% in anti-arrhythmic group, p=0.06). There was no significant mortality difference between those in the control group or those receiving anti-arrhythmics and as such the authors concluded that the survival benefit associated with electrophysiologically guided therapy was due solely to the use of defibrillators, not to anti-arrhythmic drugs.

### *MADIT II*

Following the limitations of their first study, the MADIT investigators designed MADIT-II [104], a significantly larger trial with more simplified and inclusive entry criteria. MADIT II recruited 1232 patients with a history of remote MI (>30 days or greater than 3 months if surgical revascularisation was performed) and significant LV dysfunction (LVEF<30%). In contrast to MADIT-I, no further risk stratification was performed; neither EPS nor ambulatory electrocardiography to demonstrate ventricular arrhythmias was required for inclusion. With a mean follow up of 20 months the trial was terminated prematurely, after an interim data and safety monitoring board analysis demonstrated a significant mortality difference between the two groups that had reached the pre-specified efficacy boundary. Due entirely to reduced rates of SCD, treatment with an ICD reduced all cause mortality from 19.8% with standard therapy to 14.2%. This is the smallest mortality advantage demonstrated in a positive ICD trial. Some commentators have remarked that this in part maybe due to the high rate of beta blocker use in both the control and intervention arms, which may have attenuated the benefit gained from ICD therapy [105]. Further scrutiny of the MADIT-II results reveals a number of unexpected findings. Firstly, ICD therapy appeared not only to confer a mortality advantage but more disconcertingly an increased trend towards new or worsened heart failure; 14.9% of the conventional-therapy group and 19.9% the defibrillator group were hospitalized with heart failure (p=0.09). There are multiple potential mechanisms explaining this finding; RV pacing is known to induce ventricular dyssynchrony and has been associated with worsening heart failure previously, the ICD by treating potentially fatal ventricular arrhythmias reduces SCD but does not modify the underlying disease process which ultimately progresses to more severe heart failure, finally the ICD shocks themselves may injure myocardium leading to further impaired ventricular function. Secondly, when compared with MADIT I, the beneficial effects of ICD appear later after implantation and the survival curve separated after a few months in MADIT-I but only after a year in MADIT-II. Also, the magnitude of survival benefit appears to be more modest then demonstrated previously.

*DINAMIT*

All of the primary prevention ICD trials, with the exception of the MUSTT trial which was not primarily designed to study the role of ICDs specifically, have excluded patients with a recent myocardial infarction. The risk of SCD following a myocardial infarction exhibits marked time dependence starting with the highest risk immediately post infarct and decreasing as the event becomes more remote [106]. The Defibrillator in Acute Myocardial Infarction Trial (DINAMIT) [107] was designed to test whether the prophylactic implantation of an ICD in the early post myocardial infarction period could prevent these early events and reduce mortality. The study enrolled 674 patients who had sustained a myocardial infarction in the preceding 6-40 days and followed up patients for a mean of 30 months. Entry criteria were impaired LV systolic function (EF<35%) and cardiac autonomic dysfunction (reduced heart rate variability or elevated resting heart rate). While patients known to surgical revascularisation or 3 vessel PCI were excluded, coronary angiography itself was not a mandatory requirement and therefore in a proportion of the trial population, the nature of their coronary artery disease was unknown. While a large number of the trial population did undergo angiography, the ones with severe coronary disease requiring revascularization were ultimately excluded and the ones without severe disease were a poor target population because they would have had a low event rate (as the trial did find and commented upon) and therefore predictably had a low likelihood of benefit from the ICD. Even worse mortality in those who did not undergo angiography would have increased the mortality rate in the ICD patients and reduced the survival benefit. Furthermore as we do not know the coronary anatomy they could not have been equally randomised and may have skewed the results if they were not evenly split between the groups. Due to these methodological deficiencies, the trial did not exclude a survival advantage for patients who underwent adequate re-vascularisation combined with an ICD implant (as this group excluded from DINAMIT).Also of note, patients with VT/VF greater than 48 hours after the index event were excluded. While the current ICD guidelines advocate a longer "cooling off" period before assessment for ICD implant, this was another drawback of the trial as these were the very patients who were likely to have needed ICD therapy. The majority of patients had anterior myocardial infarcts and two thirds received reperfusion therapy. Despite a significant reduction in deaths due to arrhythmia (hazard ratio in the ICD group, 0.42, p=0.009) by a magnitude similar to that seen in previous trials, this did not translate into an all cause mortality advantage. It appears that the SCD reduction was offset by other cardiac causes of death. It is largely on the basis of the results in this trial that the current joint ACC/AHA/ESC Guidelines for the Management of Patients with Ventricular Arrhythmias and the Prevention of Sudden Cardiac Death [108] recommend the deferral of ICD implantation post infarct for at least 40 days. There a number of other possible explanations as to why DINAMIT failed to demonstrate benefits shown in other trials. The exclusion of patients with significant ventricular arrhythmias and relatively low rate of revascularisation may have selected a population that were at lower risk of SCD but who had higher risk of death from further ischemic events and heart failure. The marker of impaired autonomic function may in itself have selected a group of patients who are at risk of non-arrhythmic cardiac death. In summary, however, there are several major criticisms of the DINAMIT trial. There was no requirement to undertake angiography prior to randomisation, which meant that a large proportion of the trial population had undisclosed CAD, which will have reduced the survival benefit from ICD. Patients who did undergo angiography tended to be excluded from the trial because of their need for revascularisation, and yet this was an important target population, because patients with the most severe disease have the most to gain from ICD therapy. Finally as a result of a failure to routinely revascularise patients recruited into the study, no account has been taken of the beneficial effect of CABG on prevention of non-sudden cardiac death, from prevention of progression of LV dysfunction or recurrent infarction. This probably accounts for why the trial failed to demonstrate the significant reduction in all cause mortality rates that would have been expected from the reduction in sudden death rates, which were comparable with other ICD trials. Thus, the significant reduction in sudden death from ICD implants was unfortunately counterbalanced by an equivalent increase in non-sudden cardiac death. The important and unanswered question is whether ICD implantation would provide a survival advantage when combined with adequate revascularisation. Thus whilst the DINAMIT study has provided some useful insights, for instance it demonstrates that early post-MI patients are at higher risk of acute non-sudden cardiac deaths than other, more stable, ICD eligible patients, it has not answered the important question as to whether ICD implantation in adequately revascularised patients is a worthwhile strategy early post infarction.

#### *CABG-PATCH*

Another trial that examined patients specifically with a known ischemic substrate was the CABG-PATCH trial [109]. This trial randomised 1055 patients scheduled for elective coronary artery bypass grafting with a LVEF <36% and a positive signal averaged electrocardiogram (a proposed marker of increased arrhythmic death risk) to an epicardial sited ICD and CABG or CABG alone. The trial found no survival benefit from the prophylactic implantation of an ICD at the time of bypass grafting. A likely explanation for this finding is a strong anti-arrhythmic effect of revascularisation in itself. However there are some unclear aspects that potentially confound this conclusion. The discharge rates observed were similar to that in MADIT-I. Unfortunately the majority of the ICDs placed did not have the capacity to store electrocardiograms as these were only marketed in the late phases of the trial. Also, unlike modern ICDs, the devices were committed. That is once a shockable rhythm has been detected the device will deliver a therapy without a pre-shock reanalysis. This makes it difficult to ascertain what proportion of shocks were appropriate. Regardless, even using appropriate shocks as a surrogate marker of averted SCD events is problematic due to the possible pro-arrhythmic effect of the ICD system itself.

#### *DEFINITE*

Patients with non-ischemic dilated cardiomyopathy are also at risk of fatal ventricular arrhythmias [110]. The CAT [111], AMIOVIRT [112] and DEFINITE [113] trials have specifically examined primary prevention with an ICD in this important sub-population. Both CAT and AMIOVIRT were small trials of approximately one hundred patients that terminated early and failed to demonstrate a mortality benefit of ICD therapy. They were underpowered to detect a significant treatment effect. The DEFINITE trial, although larger with 458 patients, also was underpowered due to a lower than expected all cause mortality rate in medical therapy arm. Inclusion criteria were a non-ischemic dilated cardiomyopathy

LVEF< 36% resulting in symptomatic heart failure and the presence of ambient arrhythmias on Holter monitoring. Ambient arrhythmias were defined as an episode of non-sustained VT on Holter or an average of at least 10 premature ventricular complexes per hour. At two years, the trial did however show a trend towards all-cause mortality reduction with an ICD (7.9% vs 14.1%, RRR 35%, p=0.08). Subset analysis of patients with class III heart failure symptoms did show a significant survival advantage. An interesting prospective sub-study [114] from DEFINITE followed 274 participants from the trial who underwent 24-hour Holter recording for analysis of heart rate variability at study onset. It found that those patients identified as having preserved heart rate variability appeared to be at very low risk of death.

### *ScD-HeFT*

The largest and most contemporary primary prevention study the ScD-HeFT trial [115] also enrolled a substantial proportion of patients with non-ischemic cardiomyopathy (48%). Overall the study recruited 2521 patients with class II (70%) and III (30%) symptomatic heart failure and LVEF<35% with median follow-up of 45.5 months. Somewhat differently to previous trials, ScD-HeFT used a common control design as opposed to a separate control design resulting in three treatment groups; placebo control, amiodarone or ICD therapy. This design can improve the power of a trial resulting in fewer patients needing to be recruited. The amiodarone and placebo groups fared equally with no significant mortality difference between them. ICD therapy was associated with a significant reduction in all cause mortality with hazard ratio of 0.77 (p=0.007). Patients with non-ischemic cardiomyopathy derived a similar statistically significant mortality benefit to those with an underlying ischemic etiology, thereby expanding on the findings of the previous DEFINITE trial. In comparison to DEFINITE, the magnitude of this benefit was reduced in ScD-HeFT (35% vs 27% relative mortality reduction). However in contradiction to DEFINITE's finding of greater benefit in those with class III failure and MADIT-II's finding of equal benefit across class I-III patients, ScD-HeFT actually appeared to show that class III NYHA patients had no benefit from ICD implantation. This has become known as the 'ScD-HeFT paradox.' It is unlikely that this is a true effect, but more plausibly is an aberration resultant from using a common control design. A number of subsequent analyses have arisen from the ScD-HeFT trial, providing insight on a number of relevant factors. It has become apparent the single most important and clinically utilizable risk-stratifier is the presence of LV dysfunction. However it is also generally accepted that intra-observer and inter-observer reliability in estimating EF is poor. A further confounder is that estimation by other modalities may not be any more or less accurate. Thus, although the trial methodology did not dictate a standardised means of measuring EF, post hoc sub-group analysis did not show that there was any difference between the groups of EF's established by different means in terms of risks or outcomes, suggesting that the groups identified by different methods were broadly similar despite the known inaccuracies of measurement [116]. AF is common in patients with heart failure and LV dysfunction who are suitable for ICD therapy. On occasion, atrial fibrillation with a fast ventricular response rate maybe misinterpreted by an ICD as a ventricular tachyarrhythmia, resulting in inappropriate therapies being delivered. It is also possible that AF may predispose to true ventricular tachyarrhythmias through initiation of short-long-short stimulation sequences. Singh et al. [117] indeed demonstrated an increase in the rates of both appropriate and inappropriate shocks in ScD-HeFT patients with baseline AF. Interestingly despite similar mortality rates for patients in AF or sinus rhythm, ICD's did not appear to improve mortality in the patients with AF. Poole et al. [118] examined the prognostic significance of defibrillator shocks in ScD-HeFT patients. They found that both inappropriate and appropriate shocks as compared with no shocks conferred a significantly higher risk of death and the most common cause of this was progressive heart failure. It is important to consider that both the findings of Poole and Singh et al. are in the context that the ScD-HeFT utilised primarily single lead ICDs and no anti-tachycardia pacing (ATP), although at present there is no prognostically favourable data on the use of dual chamber systems or ATP is plausible that these both may reduce the number of appropriate and inappropriate shocks delivered.

#### *META-ANALYSIS*

A meta-analysis of primary prevention with ICD therapy incorporating 10 trials indicates that regardless of etiology and QRS duration ICD therapy is significantly associated with a 26% reduction in all cause mortality [119]. This amounts to an almost 8% absolute risk reduction in all cause death in the intermediate term and equates to a number needed to treat of 13. The authors place this data in context with other currently available therapies such as ACE inhibitors and beta-blockers (6.1% and 4.4% absolute risk reduction respectively). It should however also be noted that this mortality advantage is additive.

### Summary

At present the indications for the implantation of an ICD as primary prevention with the strongest levels of evidence is for those with an LVEF of less than 35% who are at least 40 days post MI and display NYHA class II or III symptoms or for those with a remote MI and have a LVEF less than 30%. A number of other patient groups also derive benefit from ICD therapy as recommended by the recently updated ACC/AHA/HRS guidelines for device based therapy [120].

## Secondary Prevention

### Introduction

Survivors of sudden cardiac arrests (SCA) are at high risk of further events. In the late 1980s a number of series demonstrated significant reductions in the rate of SCD [121-123] with the implantation of an ICD. However, a legitimate concern regarding these studies is that the ICD may merely change the modality of death rather than actually confer a true overall mortality advantage. As such four prospective trials addressing the use of ICDs in secondary prevention have been conducted. All these trials compared the use of an ICD with drug therapy using all cause mortality as the primary endpoint. The trials differ in the populations recruited and the pharmacological agents utilized.

## Early and DUTCH Trials

The first trial examining the use of ICDs in secondary prevention was the relatively small DUTCH trial [124] which commenced in the early 1980s but did not report until 1995. Sixty patients with prior SCD, MI (>4 weeks prior) and inducible ventricular arrhythmia on EPS were randomised to either drug therapy (class Ia/c or III anti-arrhythmics) with subsequent evaluation of response on EPS or early ICD implantation. Patients randomised to the drug therapy arm who were deemed non-responders (60%) underwent either map-guided VT surgery or late ICD implantation. On intention-to-treat analysis, a 63% mortality reduction was demonstrated with ICD implantation.

### *CASH*

The CASH trial [125] initially randomized patients previously resuscitated from SCD secondary to documented sustained ventricular arrhythmias to an ICD, amiodarone, propafenone, or metoprolol. Subsequently the propafenone arm was discontinued after an interim analysis found a significantly raised all cause mortality rate. The CASH trial has the longest follow up duration of all the secondary prevention trials, with some patients being followed up for 10 years. In an intention-to-treat analysis of 390 patients, at a mean follow up of 57 months there was a non-significant trend towards reduction in all cause mortality of 23% (p=0.08). The secondary end point of SCD showed a significant reduction of 61%. A notable feature of the intervention arm of the CASH trial was its high proportion of ICDs implanted via the thoracotomy route (44%).

### *CIDS*

Although follow up duration was shorter than the CASH trial and the total number of patients recruited was fewer that in AVID, the Canadian Implantable Defibrillator Study (CIDS) [126] has contributed the greatest number of total patient years to subsequent meta-analyses of secondary prevention of SCD using ICDs. The trial enrolled 659 patients with resuscitated VF or VT or unmonitored syncope (not due to recent MI or electrolyte imbalance) to either amiodarone or ICD implantation. A 20% relative risk reduction occurred in all-cause mortality and a 33% reduction occurred in arrhythmic mortality with ICD therapy compared with amiodarone, however these reductions did not reach statistical significance. Subsequent multivariate analysis [127] of the CIDS dataset identified age, poor functional NYHA status (class III/IV) and LV dysfunction (LVEF<35%) as independent predictors of high risk. When these risk factors are constructed into quartiles a significant interaction between quartiles and the ICD treatment effect was demonstrated. Specifically those patients in the highest risk quartile (greater than 2 risk factors) derived a statistically significant 50% relative risk reduction of death with an ICD. Patients in the 3 lower quartiles appear to gain no statistically significant benefit with ICD therapy over standard medical therapy.

### *AVID*

The largest of the secondary prevention trials, the multi-center AVID study [128] randomised 1016 patients who were resuscitated from with near-fatal VF, sustained VT with syncope, or sustained VT with an LVEF <40% and symptoms suggesting severe haemodynamic compromise to ICD or drug therapy (predominantly amiodarone). The trial was terminated early due to an interim analysis by the Data and Safety Monitoring board, showing a significant survival advantage with ICD therapy of reduction in death rates of 39, 27 and 31 percent at one, two and three years respectively. Relatively few patients were followed up for more than two years. The average unadjusted length of additional life associated with ICD therapy was 2.7 months. Despite similar design, patients and treatments the observed risk reduction in the AVID was greater than that in the CIDS trial. Owing to the premature cessation of the trial, the AVID study has the shortest follow up duration of the secondary prevention ICD trials.

#### *META-ANALYSIS*

To date, only one prospective RCT has demonstrated a statistically significant all cause mortality advantage with implantation of an ICD for the secondary prevention of SCD when compared with anti-arrhythmic therapy. In general the reported trials did not allow for accurate sub-group analysis to determine which patients benefit the most from the implantation of an ICD. In response to this, a meta-analysis of pooled data from the three largest randomized controlled trials has been performed with the goal of comparing the relative effects of amiodarone and ICD treatment [129]. Planning for this analysis commenced prior to completion of any of the three major trials. Raw patient level data was pooled into a master database which was subsequently analysed to reveal overall statistically significant reductions in all cause mortality (Hazard Ratio 0.73, $p<0.001$) and SCD (HR 0.49, $p<0.001$) with ICD implantation. The survival advantage of 2.1 months at 3 years of follow up was also found to be statistically significant. Two statistically significant subgroup interactions were found. As with the CIDS subgroup analysis, patients with a LVEF of $>35\%$ had significantly less benefit from implantation than those with a lower ejection fraction. The second key subgroup effect not immediately apparent from the individual trial analyses, was that patients who required a thoracotomy for device implantation appeared to gain no benefit from ICD therapy, likely in part due to increased peri-operative mortality.

### Summary

Present consensus guidelines consider the ICD to be the treatment of choice for survivors of SCA who have no completely reversible causes [120]. Although encouraging for many, it must be bourn in mind that this group of patients represents only a small fraction of the global burden of disease caused by ventricular arrhythmias.

## Cost effectiveness of ICDs

The ICD presents a significant economic challenge for finite-resource organisations overseeing healthcare provision. It is a costly device with a large potentially eligible patient population. Multiple health economic analyses have been performed to assess the value of ICD implantation. These have taken the forms of trial based studies [130-132], disease-simulation models and hybrid studies [133]. In one such hybrid study [133], sensitivity analysis revealed five key factors that affected incremental cost-effectiveness: device efficacy in mortality reduction, device implantation cost, device replacement frequency, quality of life impact and time horizon used for analysis. Corollaries of these findings are that ICD implantation is most cost effective when the device is cheap to purchase, implant and has a significant positive impact on mortality and quality of life.

With all economic analyses, there are a number of potential pitfalls that policy makers and clinicians should be aware of. For instance the time period over which economic analyses are performed can be a substantial source of bias in economic studies leading to both under- and over-estimation of the cost-effectiveness of high up-front cost interventions such as ICDs. Short time-frames may be insufficient to demonstrate the cumulative benefit of ICDs and the ongoing costs of drug therapy. Conversely if the analysis period does not encompass device generator changes due to battery depletion, the bias will be towards over-estimation of the cost-effectiveness of ICDs. Unfortunately a number of ICD trials have been terminated prior to the predicted trial duration. The significant impact of the time horizon of analysis has been particularly apparent in the MADIT-II & ScD-HeFT trials [132]. The incremental cost-effectiveness of $235000 per year of life saved derived from the actual 3.5 year actual study period reduces substantially to between $79000 and $114000 when the analysis is extrapolated to a 12 year projection. Similarly the ScD-HeFT cost-effectiveness data shows a similar trend with a cost-effectiveness ratio of $127500 per year of life saved based on the 5 year actual study period time horizon dropping to $58500 when a 12 year extrapolation is used.

It has been previously suggested that interventions that impact on mortality should have their cost-effectiveness analysed based on a patients life time [134]. Such projections can be problematic as they inherently carry a number of assumptions, all of which have a degree of uncertainty associated with them. There is also uncertainty linked to any expressed trial based cost effectiveness ratio. In an attempt to account for this, the ScD-HeFT investigators performed bootstrap re-sampling yielding a cost-effectiveness ratio of < $100,000 in 99% of their repetitions. There are further dynamic considerations that may not be immediately apparent from currently available trial data. Market forces will likely result in more competitive pricing strategies and technology enhancements may both increase and decrease device manufacturing costs. It is currently uncertain what impact remote monitoring will have on device follow up expenditure. Another consideration is that although the majority of trial data examines the use of single lead systems a substantial proportion of currently implanted devices also employ an atrial lead. It is not clear what overall impact this has on incremental initial and aftercare costs.

## Summing up and Future Directions

Overall the outcomes of both trial and disease model based analyses, their limitations withstanding, have suggested cost-effectiveness ratios for ICDs that comparable to other accepted therapies in developed economies. However it still remains that the total budgetary impact of the intervention is substantial. It is likely therefore that the determination of optimal methods for accurate risk prediction, and therefore who will benefit the most from device implantation, will continue to receive the considerable attention that is apparent from the perusal of contemporary published studies in electrophysiological therapy. Costs are only part of any cost effectiveness analysis. Clinical effectiveness is a major determinant of whether a therapeutic strategy will be economically favorable and this in turn depends on the population who receive the intervention. Lower risk patients will derive lower absolute benefit from device implantation. This further underpins the importance of robust methods for risk stratification. Conversely patients who are at high risk from non-SCD related death may not survive for duration long enough to accrue benefits in comparison to their healthier counterparts.

### *VF ABLATION*

While ICD therapy significantly enhances survival due to VF, frequent use of the device can lead to significant morbidity in patients with "electrical storms". There have been reports of clinically significant anxiety and depression in more than half of ICD patients [135-137] ICD storm can occur in up to 25 % of patients. [138,139]Even in patients with ICDs, the incidence of sudden cardiac death due to unresponsiveness of ICDs can be as high as 5% and therefore ICDs do not offer absolute protection against sudden cardiac death [140].VF ablation is postulated to reduce device therapy and therefore improve quality of life of ICD patients in addition to improving longevity of the device.

There have been many reports of the use of radiofrequency catheter ablation to treat idiopathic VF. PVCs from the Purkinje system or the right ventricular outflow tract have been shown to be culprits in initiating idiopathic VF [141-143]. Some of these authors [144-147] have ablated foci responsible for initiating "culprit" premature ventricular complexes which trigger VF [144]. The premature beats had morphology identical or similar to that initiating VF thereby allowing mapping of their common origin. The authors postulate that ablation potentially eliminates not only the trigger for VF but also modifies the substrate for the same [144].

There has been a suggestion of the involvement of Purkinje system and PVCs in some cases of post-MI electrical storm. A study of 29 ischaemic cardiomyopathy patients with documented VF initiation showed that monomorphic PVCs from the scar border zone always initiated VF and that these PVCs were preceded by a Purkinje-like potential (PLP) [148]. Ablation eliminating these PVCs also prevented further VF storms in this study over a mean follow-up of about a year. A case series of 4 patients with repetitive VF and VT post-MI reported similar successful results with ablation and the authors also suggest that the mechanism of initiation of the VPCs is triggered activity [149].

Advanced mapping systems nowadays have allowed identification of foci and triggers for VF. There was a recent case report of post –MI VF where the focus was in the right ventricular myocardium (not from the Purkinje network) [150]. With ablation of this focus, there was no recurrence over a 4 month follow-up.

Studies have also looked at the role of prophylactic ablation in ICD patients with a history of MI to prevent defibrillator therapy and have shown a 73% reduction of subsequent shocks through "prophylactic ablation" [151]. While ablation for VF in day-to day practice has been generally reserved for patients with ICDs and electrical storms or with poor quality of life due to frequent appropriate firing of ICD despite anti-arrhythmic drugs, encouraging results such as these and with rapid progress in advanced mapping systems could envision an age when ablation could widen the indications for VF ablation.

# Abbreviations

VF – Ventricular Fibrillation
MI – Myocardial infarction
CPR – Cardiopulmonary Resuscitation
AED – Automated External Defibrillator
PVC – Premature Ventricular Complex
SCD – Sudden Cardiac Death
ICD – Internal Cardioverter Defibrillator
ACEI – Angiotensin Converting Inhibitor
RCT – Randomised Controlled Trial
LVEF – Left Ventricular Ejection fraction
IHD – Ischaemic Heart Disease
AHA – American Heart Association

# References


2005 American Heart Association Guidelines for Cardiopulmonary Resuscitation and Emergency Cardiovascular Care. *Circulation.*, 2005, 112 (suppl IV), 1-211

A comparison of antiarrhythmic-drug therapy with implantable defibrillators in patients resuscitated from near-fatal ventricular arrhythmias. The antiarrhythmics versus implantable defibrillators (AVID) investigators. *N Engl J Med*, 1997, Nov 27, 337(22), 1576-83.

A randomized trial of beta-blockade in heart failure. The cardiac insufficiency bisoprolol study (CIBIS). CIBIS investigators and committees. *Circulation*, 1994, Oct, 90(4), 1765-73.

A randomized trial of propranolol in patients with acute myocardial infarction. I. Mortality results. *JAMA*, 1982, Mar 26, 247(12), 1707-14.

Ad Hoc Committee on Cardiopulmonary Resuscitation of the Division of Medical Sciences, National Academy of Sciences–National Research Council. Cardiopulmonary resuscitation. *JAMA.*, 1966, 198, 138-145

Adamson, PB; Gilbert, EM. Reducing the risk of sudden death in heart failure with beta-blockers. *J Card Fail*, 2006, Dec, 12(9), 734-46.

Anderson, KP. Sudden cardiac death unresponsive to implantable defibrillator therapy: an urgent target for clinicians, industry and government. *J Interv Card Electrophysiol.*, 2005, 14, 71-8.

Arshad, A; Mandava, A; Kamath, G; Musat, D. Sudden cardiac death and the role of medical therapy. *Prog Cardiovasc Dis*, 2008, 50(6), 420-38.

Bardy, GH; Lee, KL; Mark, DB; Poole, JE; Packer, DL; Boineau, R; et al. Sudden cardiac death in heart failure trial (scd-heft) investigators. Amiodarone or an implantable cardioverter-defibrillator for congestive heart failure. *N Engl J Med*, 2005, 352(3), 225-37.

Bardy, GH; Lee, KL; Mark, DB; Poole, JE; Toff, WD; Tonkin, AM; et al. Home use of automated external defibrillators for sudden cardiac arrest. *New England Journal of Medicine*, 2008.

Beck, CS; Pritchard, WH; Feil, HS. Ventricular fibrillation of long duration abolished by electric shock. *JAMA.*, 1947, 135, 985.

Bernard, SA; Gray, TW; Buist, MD; Jones, BM; Silvester, W; Gutteridge, G; Smith, K. Treatment of comatose survivors of out-of-hospital cardiac arrest with induced hypothermia. *N Engl J Med*

Beta-Blocker Evaluation of Survival Trial Investigators. A trial of the beta-blocker bucindolol in patients with advanced chronic heart failure. *N Engl J Med*, 2001, May 31, 344(22), 1659-67.

Bigger, JT. Prophylactic use of implanted cardiac defibrillators in patients at high risk for ventricular arrhythmias after coronary-artery bypass graft surgery. Coronary artery bypass graft (CABG) patch trial investigators. *N Engl J Med*, 1997, Nov 27, 337(22), 1569-75.

Bilge, AK; Ozben, B; Demircan, S; Cinar, M; Yilmaz, E; Adalet, K. Depression and anxiety status of patients with implantable cardioverter defibrillator and precipitating factors. *Pacing Clin Electrophysiol.*, 2006, 29, 619-26

Bristow, MR; Adams, KF Jr.; Bauman, JL; Feldman, AM; Giles, TD; Goldstein, S; Mann, DL; Talbert, RL. The COMET Trial. *Congest Heart Fail*, 2005 Jan-Feb, 11910, 39-47

Bristow, MR; Feldman, AM; Adams, KF; Goldstein, S. Selective versus nonselective β-blockade for heart failure therapy: Are there lessons to be learned from the COMET trial? *J Card Fail*, 2003, 9(6), 444-53.

Buxton, A; Lee, K; Fisher, JD; Josephson, ME; Prystowsky, EN; Hafley, G. For the multicenter unsustained tachycardia trial investigators. A randomized study of the prevention of sudden death in patients with coronary artery disease. *N Engl J Med*, 1999, 341(25), 1882-90.

Bänsch, D; Antz, M; Boczor, S; Volkmer, M; Tebbenjohanns, J; Seidl, K; et al. Primary prevention of sudden cardiac death in idiopathic dilated cardiomyopathy: The cardiomyopathy trial (CAT). *Circulation*, 2002, Mar 26, 105(12), 1453-8.

Bänsch, D; Oyang, f; Antz, M; Arentz, T; Weber, R; Val-Mejias, JE; Ernst, S; Kuck, KH. Successful Catheter Ablation of Electrical Storm After Myocardial Infarction. *Circulation.*, 2003, 108, 3011

Caffrey, SL; Willoughby, PJ; Pepe, PE; Becker, LB. Public use of automated external defibrillators. *N Engl J Med.*, 2002 Oct 17, 347(16), 1242-7.

Cairns, JA; Connolly, SJ; Roberts, R; Gent, M. Randomised trial of outcome after myocardial infarction in patients with frequent or repetitive ventricular premature depolarisations: CAMIAT. Canadian amiodarone myocardial infarction arrhythmia trial investigators. *Lancet*, 1997, Mar 8, 349(9053), 675-82.

Callans, DJ. Can home aeds improve survival? *New England Journal of Medicine*, 2008, 358(17), 1853.

Cappato, R; Curnis, A; Marzollo, P; Mascioli, G; Bordonali, T; Beretti, S; et al. Prospective assessment of integrating the existing emergency medical system with automated external defibrillators fully operated by volunteers and laypersons for out-of-hospital cardiac arrest: The brescia early defibrillation study (BEDS). *Eur Heart J*, 2006, Mar, 27(5), 553-61.

Capucci, A; Aschieri, D; Piepoli, MF; Bardy, GH; Iconomu, E; Arvedi, M. Tripling survival from sudden cardiac arrest via early defibrillation without traditional education in cardiopulmonary resuscitation. *Circulation*, 2002, Aug 27, 106(9), 1065-70.

Carson, PA; O'Connor, CM; Miller, AB; Anderson, S; Belkin, R; Neuberg, GW; et al. Circadian rhythm and sudden death in heart failure: Results from prospective randomized amlodipine survival trial. *J Am Coll Cardiol*, 2000, Aug, 36(2), 541-6.

Cobb, LA; Alvarez, H; Kopass, MK. A rapid response system for out-of-hospital cardiac emergencies. *Med Clin North Am.*, 1976, 60, 283-290.

Cobb, LA; Fahrenbruch, CE; Walsh, TR; Copass, MK; Olsufka, M; Breskin, M; Hallstrom, AP. Influence of cardiopulmonary resuscitation prior to defibrillation in patients with out-of-hospital ventricular fibrillation. *JAMA.*, 1999, 281, 1182-1188.

Cohen, DJ; Reynolds, MR. Interpreting the results of cost-effectiveness studies. *J Am Coll Cardiol*, 2008, Dec 16, 52(25), 2119-26.

Colquhoun, MC; Chamberlain, DA; Newcombe, RG; Harris, R; Harris, S; Peel, K; et al. A national scheme for public access defibrillation in england and wales: Early results. *Resuscitation*, 2008, Sep, 78(3), 275-80.

Connolly, SJ; Gent, M; Roberts, RS; Dorian, P; Roy, D; Sheldon, RS; et al. Canadian implantable defibrillator study (CIDS) : A randomized trial of the implantable cardioverter defibrillator against amiodarone. *Circulation*, 2000, Mar 21, 101(11), 1297-302.

Connolly, SJ; Hallstrom, AP; Cappato, R; Schron, EB; Kuck, KH; Zipes, DP; Greene, HL; Boczor, S; Domanski, M; Follmann, D; Gent, M; Roberts, RS. Meta-analysis of the implantable cardioverter defibrillator secondary prevention trials. AVID, CASH and CIDS studies. Antiarrhythmics vs Implantable Defibrillator study. Cardiac Arrest Study Hamburg . Canadian Implantable Defibrillator Study. *Eur Heart J.*, 2000 Dec, 21(24), 2071-8

Copper, JA; Copper, JD; Cooper, JM. Cardiopulmonary Resuscitation -History, Current Practice, and Future Direction. *Circulation.*, 2006, 114, 2839-2849

Credner, SC; Klingenheben, T; Mauss, O; Sticherling, C; Hohnloser, SH. Electrical storm in patients with transvenous implantable cardioverter-defibrillators: incidence, management and prognostic implications. *J Am Coll Cardiol.*, 1998, 32, 1909-15]

Cummins, RO; Ornato, JP; Thies, WH; Pepe, PE. Improving survival from sudden cardiac arrest: the 'chain of survival' concept. *Circulation.*, 1991, 83, 1833-1847

Dargie, HJ. Effect of carvedilol on outcome after myocardial infarction in patients with left-ventricular dysfunction: The CAPRICORN randomised trial. *Lancet*, 2001, May 5, 357(9266), 1385-90.

Davies, CS; Colquhoun, MC; Boyle, R; Chamberlain, DA. A national programme for on-site defibrillation by lay people in selected high risk areas: Initial results. *Heart*, 2005, Oct, 91(10), 1299-302.

Diack, AW; Welborn, WS; Rullman, RG; Walter, CW; Wayne, MA. An automatic cardiac resuscitator for emergency treatment of cardiac arrest. *Med Instrum*, 1979, 13(2), 78-83.

Dietary supplementation with n-3 polyunsaturated fatty acids and vitamin E after myocardial infarction: Results of the gissi-prevenzione trial. Gruppo italiano per lo studio della sopravvivenza nell'infarto miocardico. *Lancet*, 1999, Aug 7, 354(9177), 447-55.

Domanski, MJ; Exner, DV; Borkowf, CB; Geller, NL; Rosenberg, Y; Pfeffer, MA. Effect of angiotensin converting enzyme inhibition on sudden cardiac death in patients following acute myocardial infarction. A meta-analysis of randomized clinical trials. *J Am Coll Cardiol*, 1999, Mar, 33(3), 598-604.

Dyerberg, J; Bang, HO; Hjorne, N. Fatty acid composition of the plasma lipids in Greenland Eskimos. *American Journal of Clinical Nutrition*, 1975, 28, 958-966.

Echt, DS; Liebson, PR; Mitchell, LB; Peters, RW; Obias-Manno, D; Barker, AH; et al. Mortality and morbidity in patients receiving encainide, flecainide, or placebo. The cardiac arrhythmia suppression trial. *N Engl J Med*, 1991, Mar 21, 324(12), 781-8.

Effect of the antiarrhythmic agent moricizine on survival after myocardial infarction. The cardiac arrhythmia suppression trial II investigators. *N Engl J Med*, 1992, Jul 23, 327(4), 227-33.

Effects of encainide, flecainide, imipramine and moricizine on ventricular arrhythmias during the year after acute myocardial infarction: The CAPS. The cardiac arrhythmia pilot study (CAPS) investigators. *Am J Cardiol*, 1988, Mar 1, 61(8), 501-9.

Eisenberg, MS; Moore, J; Cummins, RO; Andresen, E; Litwin, PE; Hallstrom, AP; Hearne, T. Use of the automatic external defibrillator in homes of survivors of out-of-hospital ventricular fibrillation. *Am J Cardiol*, 1989, Feb 15, 63(7), 443-6.

Epstein, AE; DiMarco, JP; Ellenbogen, KA; Estes, NA; Freedman, RA; Gettes, LS; et al. ACC/AHA/HRS 2008 guidelines for device-based therapy of cardiac rhythm abnormalities: A report of the american college of cardiology/american heart association task force on practice guidelines (writing committee to revise the ACC/AHA/NASPE 2002 guideline update for implantation of cardiac pacemakers and antiarrhythmia devices) developed in collaboration with the american association for thoracic surgery and society of thoracic surgeons. *J Am Coll Cardiol*, 2008, May 27, 51(21), e1-62.

Epstein, AE; Hallstrom, AP; Rogers, WJ; Liebson, PR; Seals, AA; Anderson, JL; et al. Mortality following ventricular arrhythmia suppression by encainide, flecainide, and moricizine after myocardial infarction. The original design concept of the cardiac arrhythmia suppression trial (CAST). *JAMA*, 1993, Nov 24, 270(20), 2451-5.

European Heart Rhythm Association, Heart Rhythm Society, Zipes, DP; Camm, AJ; Borggrefe, M; Buxton, AE; et al. ACC/AHA/ESC 2006 guidelines for management of patients with ventricular arrhythmias and the prevention of sudden cardiac death: A report of the american college of cardiology/american heart association task force and the european society of cardiology committee for practice guidelines (writing committee to develop guidelines for management of patients with ventricular arrhythmias and the prevention of sudden cardiac death). *J Am Coll Cardiol*, 2006, Sep 5, 48(5), e247-346.

Ewy, GA. Cardiocerebral Resuscitation-The New Cardiopulmonary Resuscitation. *Circulation.*, 2005, 111, 2134-2142.

Ewy, GA; Kern, KB. Recent Advances in Cardiopulmonary Resuscitation- Cardiocerebral Resuscitation. *J Am Coll Cardiol*, 2009, 53, 149-157.

Fonarow, GC; Wright, RS; Spencer, FA; Fredrick, PD; Dong, W; Every, N; et al. Effect of statin use within the first 24 hours of admission for acute myocardial infarction on early morbidity and mortality. *Am J Cardiol*, 2005, Sep 1, 96(5), 611-6.

Garg, R; Yusuf, S. Overview of randomized trials of angiotensin-converting enzyme inhibitors on mortality and morbidity in patients with heart failure. Collaborative group on ACE inhibitor trials. *JAMA*, 1995, May 10, 273(18), 1450-6.

Goldberger, JJ; Subacius, H; Schaechter, A; Howard, A; Berger, R; Shalaby, A; et al. Effects of statin therapy on arrhythmic events and survival in patients with nonischemic dilated cardiomyopathy. *J Am Coll Cardiol*, 2006, Sep 19, 48(6), 1228-33.

Guidelines 2000 for cardiopulmonary resuscitation and emergency cardiovascular care. Part 12: From science to survival: Strengthening the chain of survival in every community. The american heart association in collaboration with the international liaison committee on resuscitation. *Circulation*, 2000, Aug 22, 102(8 Suppl), I358-70.

Gula, LJ; Klein, GJ; Hellkamp, AS; Massel, D; Krahn, AD; Skanes, AC; et al. Ejection fraction assessment and survival: An analysis of the sudden cardiac death in heart failure trial (scd-heft). *Am Heart J*, 2008, Dec, 156(6), 1196-200.

Gundry, JW; Comess, KA; DeRook, FA; Jorgenson, D; Bardy, GH. Comparison of naive sixth-grade children with trained professionals in the use of an automated external defibrillator. *Circulation*, 1999, Oct 19, 100(16), 1703-7.

Haissaguerre, M; Extramiana, F; Hocini, M; et al. Mapping and ablation of ventricular fibrillation associated with long-QT and Brugada syndromes, *Circulation*, 108 (2003), pp. 925-928.

Haissaguerre, M; Shah, DC; Jais, P; et al. Role of Purkinje conducting system in triggering of idiopathic ventricular fibrillation, *Lancet*, 359 (2002), pp. 677-678.

Haissaguerre, M; Shoda, M; Jais, P; et al. Mapping and ablation of idiopathic ventricular fibrillation, *Circulation*, 106 (2002), 962-967

Haïssaguerre, M; Shoda, M; Jaïs, P; Nogami, A; Shah, DC; Kautzner, J; Arentz, T; Dietrich Kalushe, MD; Dominique Lamaison, MD; Mike Griffith, MD; Fernando Cruz, MD; Angelo de Paola, MD; Fiorenzo Gaïta, MD; Mélèze Hocini, MD; Stéphane Garrigue, MD; Laurent Macle, MD; Rukshen Weerasooriya, MD; Jacques Clémenty, MD. Mapping and Ablation of Idiopathic Ventricular Fibrillation. *Circulation.*, 2002, 106, 962

Hake, TG. Studies on ether and chloroform from Professor Schiff's physiological laboratory. *Practitioner.*, 1874, 12, 241.

Hallstrom, AP; Ornato, JP; Weisfeldt, M; Travers, A; Christenson, J; McBurnie, MA, et al. Public-Access defibrillation and survival after out-of-hospital cardiac arrest. *N Engl J Med*, 2004, 351(7), 637.

Hallstrom, AP; Ornato, JP; Weisfeldt, M; Travers, A; Christenson, J; McBurnie, MA; et al. Public-Access defibrillation and survival after out-of-hospital cardiac arrest. *N Engl J Med*, 2004, Aug 12, 351(7), 637-46.

Heidenreich, PA; Keeffe, B; McDonald, KM; Hlatky, MA. Overview of randomized trials of antiarrhythmic drugs and devices for the prevention of sudden cardiac death. *Am Heart J*, 2002, Sep, 144(3), 422-30.

Hjalmarson, A; Herlitz, J; Holmberg, S; Rydén, L; Swedberg, K; Vedin, A; et al. The göteborg metoprolol trial. Effects on mortality and morbidity in acute myocardial infarction. *Circulation*, 1983, Jun, 67(6 Pt 2), I26-32.

Hohnloser, SH; Kuck, KH; Dorian, P; Roberts, RS; Hampton, JR; Hatala, R; et al. Prophylactic use of an implantable cardioverter-defibrillator after acute myocardial infarction. *N Engl J Med*, 2004, Dec 9, 351(24), 2481-8.

Holzer, M. For the Hypothermia after Cardiac Arrest Study Group. Mild therapeutic hypothermia to improve the neurologic outcome after cardiac arrest. *N Engl J Med.*, 2002, 346, 549-556.

International mexiletine and placebo antiarrhythmic coronary trial (IMPACT): II. Results from 24-hour electrocardiograms. IMPACT research group. *Eur Heart J*, 1986, Sep, 7(9), 749-59.

International mexiletine and placebo antiarrhythmic coronary trial: I. Report on arrhythmia and other findings. Impact research group. *J Am Coll Cardiol*, 1984, Dec, 4(6), 1148-63.

Julian, DG; Camm, AJ; Frangin, G; Janse, MJ; Munoz, A; Schwartz, PJ; Simon, P. Randomised trial of effect of amiodarone on mortality in patients with left-ventricular dysfunction after recent myocardial infarction: EMIAT. European myocardial infarct amiodarone trial investigators. *Lancet*, 1997, Mar 8, 349(9053), 667-74.

Julian, DG; Prescott, RJ; Jackson, FS; Szekely, P. Controlled trial of sotalol for one year after myocardial infarction. *Lancet*, 1982, May 22, 1(8282), 1142-7.

Kadish, A; Dyer, A; Daubert, JP; Quigg, R; Estes, NA; Anderson, KP; et al. Prophylactic defibrillator implantation in patients with nonischemic dilated cardiomyopathy. *N Engl J Med*, 2004, May 20, 350(21), 2151-8.

Kamphuis, HCM; de Leeuw, RJ; Derksen, R; Hauer, RN; Winnubst, JA. Implantable cardioverter defibrillator recipients: quality of life in recipients with and without ICD shock delivery: a prospective study. *Europace.*, 2003, 5, 381-9.

Kaumann, AJ; Aramendía, P. Prevention of ventricular fibrillation induced by coronary ligation. *J Pharmacol Exp Ther*, 1968, Dec, 164(2), 326-32.

Kellermann, AL; Hackman, BB; Somes, G; Kreth, TK; Nail, L; Dobyns, P. Impact of first-responder defibrillation in an urban emergency medical services system. *JAMA*, 1993, Oct 13, 270(14), 1708-13.

Kern, KB; Hilwig, RW; Berg, RA; Sanders, AB; Ewy, GA. Importance of continuous chest compression during cardiopulmonary resuscitation: improved outcome during a simulated single lay-rescuer scenario. *Circulation.*, 2002, 105, 645-649

Kohsaka, S; Razavi, M; Massumi, A. Idiopathic ventricular fibrillation successfully terminated by radiofrequency ablation of the distal Purkinje fibers. *Pacing Clin Electrophysiol.*, 2007 May, 30(5), 701-4.

Kostapanos, MS; Liberopoulos, EN; Goudevenos, JA; Mikhailidis, DP; Elisaf, MS. Do statins have an antiarrhythmic activity? *Cardiovasc Res*, 2007, Jul 1, 75(1), 10-20.

Kris-Etherton, PM; Harris, WS; Appel, LJ. American Heart Association. Nutrition Committee. Fish consumption, fish oil, omega-3 fatty acids, and cardiovascular disease. *Circulation*, 2002, Nov 19, 106(21), 2747-57.

Kuck, KH; Cappato, R; Siebels, J; Rüppel, R. Randomized comparison of antiarrhythmic drug therapy with implantable defibrillators in patients resuscitated from cardiac arrest: The cardiac arrest study hamburg (CASH). *Circulation*, 2000, Aug 15, 102(7), 748-54.

Larsen, MP; Eisenberg, MS; Cummins, RO; Hallstrom, AP. Predicting survival from out-of-hospital cardiac arrest: A graphic model. *Ann Emerg Med*, 1993, Nov, 22(11), 1652-8.

Lechat, P; Brunhuber, KW; Hofmann, R; Osterziel, AL. The cardiac insufficiency bisoprolol study II (CIBIS-II): A randomised trial. *Lancet*, 1999, 353, 9-13.

León, H; Shibata, MC; Sivakumaran, S; Dorgan, M; Chatterley, T; Tsuyuki, RT. Effect of fish oil on arrhythmias and mortality: Systematic review. *BMJ*, 2008, 337, a2931.

Lown, B; Neuman, J; Amarasingham, R; Berkovits, BV. Comparison of alternating current with direct current electroshock across the closed chest. *Am J Cardiol.*, 1962, 10, 223.

Majmudar, MD; Tompkins, C; Bachmann, JM; Blumenthal, RS; Marine, JE. Effects of lipid-altering therapies on ventricular arrhythmias and sudden cardiac death. *Cardiol Rev*, 2009, 17(2), 60-9.

Mark, DB; Nelson, CL; Anstrom, KJ; Al-Khatib, SM; Tsiatis, AA; Cowper, PA; et al. Cost-Effectiveness of defibrillator therapy or amiodarone in chronic stable heart failure: Results from the sudden cardiac death in heart failure trial (scd-heft). *Circulation*, 2006, Jul 11, 114(2), 135-42.

Marsden, AK; Chamberlain, D; Tunsdall-Pedoe, H. United Kingdom resuscitation outcome study. *Resuscitation*, 1989, 17(suppl), S157-S159

McMurray, J; Køber, L; Robertson, M; Dargie, H; Colucci, W; Lopez-Sendon, J; et al. Antiarrhythmic effect of carvedilol after acute myocardial infarction: Results of the carvedilol post-infarct survival control in left ventricular dysfunction (CAPRICORN) trial. *J Am Coll Cardiol*, 2005, Feb 15, 45(4), 525-30.

Metoprolol in acute myocardial infarction (MIAMI). A randomised placebo-controlled international trial. The MIAMI trial research group. *Eur Heart J*, 1985, Mar, 6(3), 199-226.

Mirowski, M; Mower, MM; Reid, PR. Treatment of malignant ventricular arrhythmias in man with an implanted automatic defibrillator. *Crit Care Med.*, 1981, 9, 388-389

Mirowski, M; Mower, MM; Staewen, WS; Tabatznik, B; Mendeloff, AI. Standby automatic defibrillator. An approach to prevention of sudden coronary death. *Arch Intern Med*, 1970, Jul, 126(1), 158-61.

Mirowski, M; Reid, PR; Mower, MM; Watkins, L; Gott, VL; Schauble, JF; et al. Termination of malignant ventricular arrhythmias with an implanted automatic defibrillator in human beings. *N Engl J Med*, 1980, Aug 7, 303(6), 322-4.

Moore, JD; Mason, DA; Green, SA; Hsu, J; Liggett, SB. Racial differences in the frequencies of cardiac beta(1)-adrenergic receptor polymorphisms: Analysis of c145a>G and c1165g>C. *Hum Mutat*, 1999, Sep 19, 14(3), 271.

Mosesso, VN; Davis, EA; Auble, TE; Paris, PM; Yealy, DM. Use of automated external defibrillators by police officers for treatment of out-of-hospital cardiac arrest. *Ann Emerg Med*, 1998, Aug, 32(2), 200-7.

Moss, AJ; Hall, WJ; Cannom, DS; Daubert, JP; Higgins, SL; Klein, H; et al. Improved survival with an implanted defibrillator in patients with coronary disease at high risk for ventricular arrhythmia (multicenter automatic defibrillator implantation trial investigators). *N Engl J Med*, 1996, 335(26), 1933-40.

Moss, AJ; Zareba, W; Hall, WJ; Klein, H; Wilber, DJ; Cannom, DS; et al. Prophylactic implantation of a defibrillator in patients with myocardial infarction and reduced ejection fraction. *N Engl J Med*, 2002, Mar 21, 346(12), 877-83.

Mushlin, AI; Hall, WJ; Zwanziger, J; Gajary, E; Andrews, M; Marron, R; et al. The cost-effectiveness of automatic implantable cardiac defibrillators: Results from MADIT. Multicenter automatic defibrillator implantation trial. *Circulation*, 1998, Jun 2, 97(21), 2129-35.

Myerburg, RJ; Kessler, KM; Castellanos, A. Sudden cardiac death: Epidemiology, transient risk, and intervention assessment. *Ann Intern Med*, 1993, Dec 15, 119(12), 1187-97.

Myerburg, RJ; Luceri, RM; Thurer, R; Cooper, DK; Zaman, L; Interian, A; et al. Time to first shock and clinical outcome in patients receiving an automatic implantable cardioverter-defibrillator. *J Am Coll Cardiol*, 1989, Aug, 14(2), 508-14.

Nagao, K; Kanmatsuse, K; Kikushima, K; Sakamoto, T; Igarashi, M; Saito, A; Hori, S; Kanesaka, S; Hamabe, Y; Hayashi, N. The effect of chest compression alone during bystander-initiated cardiopulmonary resuscitation. *Circulation.*, 2004, 110 (suppl III), III-455. Abstract.

Nanthakumar, K; Epstein, AE; Kay, GN; Plumb, VJ; Lee, DS. Prophylactic implantable cardioverter-defibrillator therapy in patients with left ventricular systolic dysfunction: A pooled analysis of 10 primary prevention trials. *J Am Coll Cardiol*, 2004, Dec 7, 44(11), 2166-72.

Nassir, F; Marrouche, MD*; Atul Verma, MD*; Oussama Wazni, MD*; Robert Schweikert, MD*; David, O; Martin, MD*; Walid Saliba, MD*; Fethi Kilicaslan, MD*; Jennifer Cummings, MD*; David Burkhardt, J; MD*; Mandeep Bhargava, MD*; Dianna Bash, RN*; Johannes Brachmann, MD*; Jens Guenther, MD*; Steven Hao, MD*; Salwa Beheiry, RN*; Antonio Rossillo, MD*; Antonio Raviele, MD*; Sakis Themistoclakis, MD*; Andrea Natale, MD. Mode of initiation and ablation of ventricular fibrillation storms in patients with ischemic cardiomyopathy. *Journal of the American College of Cardiology*, Volume 43, Issue 9, 5 May 2004, Pages 1715-1720

Nichol, G; Valenzuela, T; Roe, D; Clark, L; Huszti, E; Wells, GA. Cost effectiveness of defibrillation by targeted responders in public settings. *Circulation*, 2003, Aug 12, 108(6), 697-703.

Norris, RM. UK Heart Attack Study Collaborative Group. Circumstances of out of hospital cardiac arrest in patients with ischaemic heart disease. *Heart*, 2005, Dec, 91(12), 1537-40.

Nuttall, SL; Toescu, V; Kendall, MJ. B blockade after myocardial infarction: B blockers have key role in reducing morbidity and mortality after infarction. *BMJ: British Medical Journal*, 2000, 320(7234), 581

O'Rourke, MF; Donaldson, E; Geddes, JS. An airline cardiac arrest program. *Circulation*, 1997, Nov 4, 96(9), 2849-53.

Packer, M; Bristow, MR; Cohn, JN; Colucci, WS; Fowler, MB; Gilbert, EM; Shusterman, NH. The effect of carvedilol on morbidity and mortality in patients with chronic heart failure. US carvedilol heart failure study group. *N Engl J Med*, 1996, 334(21), 1349-55.

Packer, M; Fowler, MB; Roecker, EB; Coats, AJ; Katus, HA; Krum, H; et al. Effect of carvedilol on the morbidity of patients with severe chronic heart failure: Results of the carvedilol prospective randomized cumulative survival (COPERNICUS) study. *Circulation*, 2002, Oct 22, 106(17), 2194-9.

Page, RL; Joglar, JA; Kowal, RC; Zagrodzky, JD; Nelson, LL; Ramaswamy, K; et al. Use of automated external defibrillators by a U.S. Airline. *N Engl J Med*, 2000, Oct 26, 343(17), 1210-6.

Pedersen, TR. Six-Year follow-up of the norwegian multicenter study on timolol after acute myocardial infarction. *N Engl J Med*, 1985, Oct 24, 313(17), 1055-8.

Piccini, JP; Berger, JS; O'Connor, CM. Amiodarone for the prevention of sudden cardiac death: A meta-analysis of randomized controlled trials. *Eur Heart J*, 2009, Mar 31.

Pitt, B; Pierard, LA; Bilge, A; Bourassa, G; White, M; Lepage, S; et al. Effectiveness of spironolactone added to an angiotensin-converting enzyme inhibitor and a loop diuretic for severe chronic congestive heart failure (the randomized aldactone evaluation study [RALES]). *Am J Cardiol*, 1996, 78, 902-7.

Pitt, B; Remme, W; Zannad, F; Neaton, J; Martinez, F; Roniker, B; et al. Eplerenone post-acute myocardial infarction heart failure efficacy and survival study investigators. Eplerenone, a selective aldosterone blocker, in patients with left ventricular dysfunction after myocardial infarction. *N Engl J Med*, 2003, 348(14), 1309-21.

Poole, JE; Johnson, GW; Hellkamp, AS; Anderson, J; Callans, DJ; Raitt, MH; et al. Prognostic importance of defibrillator shocks in patients with heart failure. *N Engl J Med*, 2008, Sep 4, 359(10), 1009-17.

Prevention of cardiovascular events and death with pravastatin in patients with coronary heart disease and a broad range of initial cholesterol levels. The Long-Term Intervention with Pravastatin in Ischaemic Disease (LIPID) Study Group. *N Engl J Med.*, 1998 Nov 5, 339(19), 1349-57.

Priori, SG; Aliot, E; Blomstrom-Lundqvist, C; Bossaert, L; Breithardt, G; Brugada, P; et al. Task force on sudden cardiac death of the european society of cardiology. *Eur Heart J*, 2001, Aug 22, 22(16), 1374-450.

Randomised trial of cholesterol lowering in 4444 patients with coronary heart disease: The scandinavian simvastatin survival study (4S). *Lancet*, 1994, Nov 19, 344(8934), 1383-9.

Randomised trial of intravenous atenolol among 16 027 cases of suspected acute myocardial infarction: ISIS-1. First international study of infarct survival collaborative group. *Lancet*, 1986, Jul 12, 2(8498), 57-66.

Rashba, EJ; Estes, NA; Wang, P; Schaechter, A; Howard, A; Zareba, W; et al. Preserved heart rate variability identifies low-risk patients with nonischemic dilated cardiomyopathy: Results from the DEFINITE trial. *Heart Rhythm*, 2006, Mar, 3(3), 281-6.

Safar, P. Resuscitation from clinical death: pathophysiologic limits and therapeutic potentials. *Crit Care Med.*, 1988, 16, 923-941.

Saliba, W; Abul Karim, A; Tchou, P; Natale, A. Ventricular fibrillation: ablation of a trigger? *J Cardiovasc Electrophysiol.*, 2002 Dec, 13(12), 1296-9.

Sanders, GD; Hlatky, MA; Owens, DK. Cost-Effectiveness of Implantable cardioverter-defibrillators. *N Engl J Med*, 2005, Oct 6, 353(14), 1471-80.

Sanna, T; La Torre, G; de Waure, C; Scapigliati, A; Ricciardi, W; Dello Russo, A; et al. Cardiopulmonary resuscitation alone vs. Cardiopulmonary resuscitation plus automated external defibrillator use by non-healthcare professionals: A meta-analysis on 1583 cases of out-of-hospital cardiac arrest. *Resuscitation*, 2008, Feb, 76(2), 226-32.

Schiff, M. Ueber direkte reizung der herzoberflaeche. *Arch Ges Physiol.*, 1882, 28, 200.

Sears, SE Jr.; Conti, JB. Understanding implantable cardioverter defibrillator shocks and storms: medical and psychosocial considerations for research and clinical care. *Clin Cardiol.*, 2003, 26, 107-11.

Sheldon, R; Connolly, S; Krahn, A; Roberts, R; Gent, M; Gardner, M. Identification of patients most likely to benefit from implantable cardioverter-defibrillator therapy: The canadian implantable defibrillator study. *Circulation*, 2000, Apr 11, 101(14), 1660-4.

Singh, SN; Poole, J; Anderson, J; Hellkamp, AS; Karasik, P; Mark, DB; et al. Role of amiodarone or implantable cardioverter/defibrillator in patients with atrial fibrillation and heart failure. *Am Heart J*, 2006, Nov, 152(5), 974.e7-11.

Strickberger, SA; Hummel, JD; Bartlett, TG; Frumin, HI; Schuger, CD; Beau, SL; et al. Amiodarone versus implantable cardioverter-defibrillator:Randomized trial in patients with nonischemic dilated cardiomyopathy and asymptomatic nonsustained ventricular tachycardia--amiovirt. *J Am Coll Cardiol*, 2003, May 21, 41(10), 1707-12.

Takahashi, Y; et al. Ventricular fibrillation initiated by premature beats from the ventricular myocardium not associated with the Purkinje system after myocardial infarction. *Heart Rhythm.*, 2008, 5, 1458-1460

Takatsuki, S; Mitamura, H; Ogawa, S. Catheter ablation of a monofocal prematureventricular complex triggering idiopathic ventricular fibrillation. *Heart*, 2001, 86, e3

Taw, RL. Dr. Friedrich Maass: 100th anniversary of "new" CPR. *Clin Cardiol.*, 1991, 14, 1000-1002.

Tchou, PJ; Kadri, N; Anderson, J; Caceres, JA; Jazayeri, M; Akhtar, M. Automatic implantable cardioverter defibrillators and survival of patients with left ventricular dysfunction and malignant ventricular arrhythmias. *Ann Intern Med*, 1988, Oct 1, 109(7), 529-34.

Teo, KK; Yusuf, S; Furberg, CD. Effects of prophylactic antiarrhythmic drug therapy in acute myocardial infarction. An overview of results from randomized controlled trials. *JAMA*, 1993, Oct 6, 270(13), 1589-95.

The MERIT-HF Study Group. Effects of Controlled-Release Metoprololon Total Mortality, Hospitalizations, and Well-being in Patients With Heart FailureThe Metoprolol CR/XL Randomized Intervention Trialin Congestive Heart Failure (MERIT-HF). *JAMA*, March 8, 2000—Vol 283, No. 10 1295

Timolol-Induced reduction in mortality and reinfarction in patients surviving acute myocardial infarction. *N Engl J Med*, 1981, Apr 2, 304(14), 801-7.

Tjomsland, N; Baskett, P; Laerdal, ÅS. *Resuscitation.*, 2002, 53, 115-119.

Tung, R; Zimetbaum, P; Josephson, ME. A critical appraisal of implantable cardioverter-defibrillator therapy for the prevention of sudden cardiac death. *J Am Coll Cardiol*, 2008, Sep 30, 52(14), 1111-21.

Waldo, AL; Camm, AJ; deRuyter, H; Friedman, PL; MacNeil, DJ; Pauls, JF; et al. Effect of d-sotalol on mortality in patients with left ventricular dysfunction after recent and remote myocardial infarction. The SWORD investigators. Survival with oral d-sotalol. *Lancet*, 1996, Jul 6, 348(9019), 7-12.

Valenzuela, TD; Roe, DJ; Nichol, G; Clark, LL; Spaite, DW; Hardman, RG. Outcomes of rapid defibrillation by security officers after cardiac arrest in casinos. *N Engl J Med.*, 2000, 343, 1206-1209

Valenzuela, TD; Roe, DJ; Nichol, G; Clark, LL; Spaite, DW; Hardman, RG. Outcomes of rapid defibrillation by security officers after cardiac arrest in casinos. *N Engl J Med*, 2000, Oct 26, 343(17), 1206-9.

van Alem, AP; Vrenken, RH; de Vos, R; Tijssen, JG; Koster, RW. Use of automated external defibrillator by first responders in out of hospital cardiac arrest: Prospective controlled trial. *BMJ*, 2003, Dec 6, 327(7427), 1312.

Weaver, WD; Copass, MK; Hill, DL; Fahrenbruch, C; Hallstrom, AP; Cobb, LA. Cardiac arrest treated with a new automatic external defibrillator by out-of-hospital first responders. *Am J Cardiol*, 1986, 57(13), 1017.

Weaver, WD; Hill, D; Fahrenbruch, CE; Copass, MK; Martin, JS; Cobb, LA; Hallstrom, AP. Use of the automatic external defibrillator in the management of out-of-hospital cardiac arrest. *N Engl J Med*, 1988, Sep 15, 319(11), 661-6.

Wever, EF; Hauer, RN; van Capelle, FL; Tijssen, JG; Crijns, HJ; Algra, A; et al. Randomized study of implantable defibrillator as first-choice therapy versus conventional strategy in postinfarct sudden death survivors. *Circulation*, 1995, Apr 15, 91(8), 2195-203.

Wik, L; Hansen, TB; Fylling, F; Steen, T; Vaagenes, P; Auestad, BH; Steen, PA. *Delaying defibrillation to give basic cardiopulmonary resuscitation to patients with out-of-hospital ventricular fibrillation.*

Villacastín, J; Almendral, J; Arenal, A; et al. Incidence and clinical significance of multiple consecutive, appropriate, high-energy discharges in patients with implanted cardioverter-defibrillators. *Circulation.*, 1996, 93, 753-62.

Winkle, RA; Mead, RH; Ruder, MA; Gaudiani, VA; Smith, NA; Buch, WS; et al. Long-Term outcome with the automatic implantable cardioverter-defibrillator. *J Am Coll Cardiol*, 1989, May, 13(6), 1353-61.

Vivek Y. Reddy, MD; Matthew R. Reynolds, MD; Petr Neuzil, MD, Ph.D.; Allison W. Richardson MD; Milos Taborsky, MD, PhD; Krit Jongnarangsin, MD; Stepan Kralovec, Lucie Sediva, MD; Jeremy N. Ruskin, MD; Mark E. Josephson, MD. Prophylactic Catheter Ablation for the Prevention of Defibrillator Therapy. *N Engl J Med.*, 2007 December 27, 357(26), 2657-2665.

Zipes, DP; Camm, AJ; Borggrefe, M; Buxton, AE; Chaitman, B; Fromer, M; et al. ACC/AHA/ESC 2006 guidelines for management of patients with ventricular arrhythmias and the prevention of sudden cardiac death: A report of the american college of cardiology/american heart association task force and the european society of cardiology committee for practice guidelines (writing committee to develop guidelines for management of patients with ventricular arrhythmias and the prevention of sudden cardiac death): Developed in collaboration with the european heart rhythm association and the heart rhythm society. *Circulation*, 2006, Sep 5, 114(10), e385-484.

Zoll, PM; Linenthal, AJ; Gibson, W; Paul, MH; Norman, LR. Termination of ventricular fibrillation in man by externally applied electric countershock. *N Engl J Med.*, 1956, 254, 727

Zwanziger, J; Hall, WJ; Dick, AW; Zhao, H; Mushlin, AI; Hahn, RM, et al. The cost effectiveness of implantable cardioverter-defibrillators: Results from the multicenter automatic defibrillator implantation trial (MADIT)-II. *J Am Coll Cardiol*, 2006, Jun 6, 47(11), 2310-8.

In: Advances in Cardiovascular Research, Volume 1
Editors: L. Schmitt, T. Konig, pp. 85-119
ISBN: 978-1-60741-720-0


*Chapter III*

# A Historical View of Advances in the Resuscitation of Patients in Ventricular Fibrillation from the Perspective of Emergency Medical Services

***Paul W. Baker and Hugh J.M. Grantham***
South Australian Ambulance Service, Australia

## Abstract

Since the first use of basic life support (BLS) and defibrillation in the pre-hospital setting in Belfast in 1966, few would argue that there have been major improvements in the rate of survival for out-of-hospital cardiac arrests. Indeed, until the widespread introduction of BLS and defibrillators to emergency medical service (EMS) vehicles, an out-of-hospital cardiac arrest would mean certain death.

The initial rhythm of a patient in cardiac arrest is predictive of their chances of survival. In this regard, the rhythms with the highest rate of survival to hospital discharge are ventricular fibrillation (VF) and ventricular tachycardia (VT). In the past century we have learnt much about VF and VT, with this knowledge forming the bedrock of present day resuscitation guidelines. In the last decade there has been a truly international effort, headed by the International Liaison Committee on Resuscitation (ILCOR), aimed at reducing the mortality from cardiac arrest. This effort has resulted in the publication of the 2005 guidelines for resuscitation. While there is still much to learn, the 2005 guidelines appear to have reduced mortality from VF/VT arrests more than any before.

The concept of providing cardiopulmonary resuscitation (CPR), defibrillation, and advanced cardiac life support, in a timely fashion to reduce mortality from cardiac arrests evolved in the late 1980's. It was formalised in 1991 by Cummings as the *"Chain of Survival"*. It is the role of EMS, with regards to cardiac arrest, to provide the final critical links in the chain of survival. Aside from this vital function, EMS have been invaluable in enabling an assessment of the impact of the many changes to resuscitation protocols over the years on the mortality rate from cardiac arrest by facilitating research in the pre-hospital domain.

As VF is a more common presenting rhythm in out-of-hospital cardiac arrest and much of our knowledge of VF is relevant to VT, this chapter will focus primarily on VF cardiac arrest. It will begin by examining the birth of modern CPR and the mechanism and epidemiology of cardiac arrest and sudden cardiac death. It will then touch on the evolution of EMS, equipping them to deal with out-of-hospital cardiac arrests like never before and to make a significant contribution to research in this area. This chapter will also examine some of the issues surrounding the research that has lead to our current guidelines for VF cardiac arrests and how these guidelines have been shaped by a concerted international effort headed by ILCOR.

## Introduction

Those who work in the Emergency Medical Services (EMS) are all too aware of the grief and devastation that befalls a family following the death of a loved one. For some, death is premature, occurring in apparently healthy individuals in the most unexpected of settings, such as dinner at the kitchen table with family, in the fruit and vegetable aisle at the local supermarket or while playing sport with friends. Such events remind us of our own mortality, a fact that is perhaps cemented into place by the familiarity of the context in which they occur.

Each of us has a vested interest in research into sudden cardiac death (SCD) and the management of cardiac arrest as given the right conditions, any one of us, at any time, may experience one. Dr Myron Weisfeldt highlights this fact in his recollection of a successful resuscitation he attended in 1967, where they used the newly described procedure of closed-chest cardiac massage [1]. The patient, a well-dressed gentleman, went into cardiac arrest in a lift. He happened to be the newly appointed Chairman of the Department of Medicine on his first day in that position. This chapter will begin by examining, in brief, the development of closed-chest cardiac massage and the external cardiac defibrillator, both of which form the bedrock of modern day resuscitation.

In the recent past, which can be defined as 20 to 40 years ago for most places in the developed world, a sudden cardiac arrest out-of-hospital would have meant certain death. Nowadays the overall survival rate for an out-of-hospital cardiac arrest is around 7.5%, with figures ranging from 3 to 17%. Undoubtedly, things have improved, but a rate of 7.5% is still low - especially if you are one of the 92.5% with an unsuccessful outcome. This figure is even more significant when considering the fact that under optimal conditions survival rates approaching 70% are possible for out-of-hospital cardiac arrest [2-4]. Having said this, it is important to remember, that due to the unexpected nature of cardiac arrest and the unavoidable systemic and geographic constraints there is naturally an upper limit to the maximal survival that can be attained. Some of these issues will be discussed in this chapter.

Much work has and is still being done to improve the chances of survival from a cardiac arrest. In Australia, and in most developed countries, the majority of cardiac arrests occur in the community - 86% according to the Australian Institute of Health and Welfare [5]. Accordingly, EMS play a key role in the management of out-of-hospital cardiac arrests, as well as being highly active in both initiating and participating in resuscitation research. EMS are commonly the testing ground for many of the guideline changes in resuscitation protocols that are now coordinated at an international level by the International Liaison Committee on Resuscitation (ILCOR), and in Australia at a national level by the Australian Resuscitation

Council (ARC). In this chapter we will also discuss the evolution of EMS and their pivotal role in out-of-hospital cardiac arrest resuscitation, as well as their role in testing past and present resuscitation protocols and treatments, determining what has and hasn't worked. This chapter will also discuss the framework that is now in place thanks to ILCOR and the recent progress that has been made in resuscitation as well as some of the current controversies.

Finally, and most importantly, as ventricular fibrillation (VF) is the most commonly encountered cardiac rhythm on arrival of EMS crews at a cardiac arrest, and the rhythm with the highest rate of survival to hospital discharge, this chapter will give a brief account of the mechanism of VF to enable an understanding of the results of recent studies. Moreover, all of the above will be discussed with specific reference to VF cardiac arrests.

## A Brief History of the Development of Modern Day Cardiopulmonary Resuscitation and Defibrillation

The King James version of the Holy Bible [6] contains a reference to what is widely cited as the first recorded resuscitation, circa 896 BC [7-10]. It is as follows;

> *"And Gehazi passed on before them, and laid the staff upon the face of the child; but there was neither voice, nor hearing. Wherefore he went again to meet him, and told him, saying, The child is not awaked.*
>
> *And when Elisha was come into the house, behold, the child was dead, and laid upon his bed.*
>
> *And he went up, and lay upon the child, and put his mouth upon his mouth, and his eyes upon his eyes, and his hands upon his hands: and he stretched himself upon the child; and the flesh of the child waxed warm.*
>
> *Then he returned, and walked in the house to and fro; and went up, and stretched himself upon him: and the child sneezed seven times, and the child opened his eyes."*

Since biblical times the face of resuscitation has changed markedly, with many of the significant advances occurring in the last 50 to 60 years – reviewed in [8-14]. Undoubtedly, one of the pivotal developments occurred in 1960 when Kouwenhoven, Jude and Knickerbocker, from Johns Hopkins Hospital, published a manuscript entitled "Closed-Chest Cardiac Massage" [15]. In this paper they described a technique, employed in their hospital over the preceding 10 months, which yielded an unprecedented 70% survival from cardiac arrest with good neurological recovery. This method now forms the backbone of modern cardiopulmonary resuscitation strategies. The history of the findings of the Johns Hopkins team has been reviewed at length and is discussed in brief below [16-19].

In the 1920's and 30's many electricity company linesman died from VF secondary to electrocution – it had been known since around 1850's that an electric current across the heart caused fibrillation ([20] in [21] and [22] in [10]). In 1925, in response to these deaths, the electricity companies began searching for teams suitably positioned to research solutions to this problem. In 1926, Johns Hopkins (both the School of Medicine and the School of

Hygiene and Public Health) received funding from Consolidated Edison of New York for this purpose. Three other sites were also selected: Colombia University, Harvard Engineering Committee and the Rockefeller Institute.

In 1928 when the official work started at Johns Hopkins, William Kouwenhoven now aged 42, was a Professor of electrical engineering and the Dean of the Hopkins' Whiting School of Engineering. Although he had little medical experience he had a very creative mind and a keen interest in the ability of electricity to induce VF, stemming from his previous research on high-tension wire transmission of electricity.

History shows that Kouwenhoven was an excellent choice and by the mid 1930's he led the investigations in Baltimore. Based on work by Prevost and Battelli published in 1899, in the late 1920's to early 30's Kouwenhovens' team rediscovered that application of a counter-shock to an already fibrillating heart could restore a perfusing rhythm [23-25]. These finding sparked the development of the first cardiac defibrillators for application in a clinical setting. It wasn't until 1947 that Dr Claude Beck performed the first successful open-chest defibrillation of a patient with VF ([26] as reprinted in [27]). The patient was a 14 year-old boy having surgery to correct a funnel chest (pectus excavatum). On closing the patient's chest he arrested into VF. His chest was re-opened and cardiac massage was performed until termination of his VF some 45 minutes later following two defibrillations. The patient made a full neurological recovery.

The team at Johns Hopkins developed three defibrillators between 1928 and the mid 1950's [28]. The early defibrillators were open-chest defibrillators, requiring direct application of the electrodes to the heart. This was in keeping with the resuscitation techniques of the time where direct cardiac massage was used to provide cardiac output, as with the 14 year old boy above. As open-chest cardiac massage and defibrillation were impractical in the community setting, and electricity company lines men were still dying from fibrillation, there was a need to develop techniques for both external cardiac compression and closed-chest defibrillation. In 1950 Kouwenhoven began developing a closed-chest defibrillator [17]. In 1956 however, Paul Zoll, working at Harvard University, reported not only the development of an external defibrillator for use in humans but also the first successful external defibrillation of a human [28].

It was in 1958 that Guy Knickerbocker, an electrical engineer who joined Kouwenhovens team in 1954, discovered quite fortuitously that when the heavy electrodes of their external defibrillator were applied to the chest of a dog in cardiac arrest there was a transitory rise in blood pressure [17]. The technique of external cardiac compression was born. The team at Johns Hopkins spent the next year optimising this technique and incorporating the newly developed method of mouth-to-mouth ventilation. From mid 1959 to early 1960, they set about collecting clinical data on the efficacy of the combination of external cardiac compression, mouth-to-mouth ventilation and closed-chest defibrillation. Their results were published in July 1960 [15]. The combination of external cardiac compression and mouth-to-mouth ventilation as reported in the 1960 publication would later be referred to as cardiopulmonary resuscitation or CPR.

It should be recognised that the history of the findings of the Johns Hopkins team is just a small part of the development of modern day resuscitation. Their findings were based on the work of many that came before them over the preceding centuries (reviewed in depth in [8,10,14]). For example, in the late 1800's, there was experimental and clinical evidence that coronary artery obstruction caused ventricular fibrillation and SCD, and that an electric shock could terminate the fibrillation [29]. The work of Kouwenhoven et al. was chosen as they were the first to publish in the peer review literature a complete method for resuscitation, including CPR and defibrillation, and its clinical efficacy over a period of observation.

## Cardiovascular Disease and Sudden Cardiac Death: The Demographics and Survival Rates of Patient in VF

Cardiovascular Disease (CVD) is a broad term encompassing a spectrum of diseases of the heart and blood vessels [30]. Of particular relevance to this discussion however, are CVD's due to coronary artery disease which manifest as myocardial ischemia and infarction, resulting in arrhythmias, heart failure and SCD.

In Australia, as in other industrialised countries, the mortality rate from CVD has been declining for many years, with some evidence that it is now beginning to plateau [31,32]. Interestingly, in countries that are becoming westernised the mortality rate for CVD is said to be increasing [33]. Despite the decline in CVD mortality in Australia, in 2006, ischemic heart disease was the leading cause of mortality, accounting for around 18% of all deaths and claiming the life of some 22,983 people [31]. Given the number of hospital admissions in the 2003 to 2004 period for patients with coronary artery disease (~ 166,000), arrhythmias (~ 63,000) and heart failure (~ 40,000) there is also a significant economic burden associated with CVD [30].

SCD, defined as "natural death from cardiac causes, heralded by abrupt loss of consciousness within 1 hour of the onset of an acute change in cardiovascular status" [34], is one of the most dramatic presentations of coronary artery disease. SCD is important to any discussion on VF, as primary arrhythmias are believed to be the cause of arrest in more than 90% of cases (see below) [35,36].

It is important to consider when reviewing data on the incidence of cardiac arrests that not all arrests are due to cardiac causes – unless specified, the data usually includes arrests due to trauma, drug overdoses, cerebrovascular accidents, respiratory failure, etc. The incidence of cardiac arrest, from all causes, is higher in-hospital than it is out-of-hospital (100 to 500 per 100,000 admission-years versus between 33 and 190 per 100,000 person-years). However the vast majority of SCD actually occur out-of-hospital [37-43]. Indeed, in Australia between 2001 and 2002, 86% of cardiac related deaths occurred out-of-hospital [5] – over 90% of SCD are attended by EMS [38,44]. The incidence of SCD in the community is reported to be in the range of 37 to 100 per 100,000 person-years (reviewed in [45]). Around 20 to 25% of these deaths are said to be the first clinical manifestation of previously silent or unrecognised coronary artery disease [46,47].

Patients in cardiac arrest are most commonly found to be in VF, asystole or pulse-less electrical activity (PEA) on arrival of EMS or hospital staff (see Table 1) [38,40,42,43,48-63]. Primary ventricular tachycardia (VT) is a relatively uncommon rhythm out-of-hospital [30], occurring more commonly in the hospital setting (1% vs. 8%) [60,64-66]. For this reason VF and VT are often grouped together in many studies. The lower occurrence of VT as an initial rhythm for out-of-hospital cardiac arrests is thought to be a function of the longer response time for EMS compared to hospital resuscitations – EMS takes on average 5 to 10 minutes from initial call to arrival on scene [43,49-51,56,67-69,70-74]. During this time VT is presumed to deteriorate into VF (discussed below). The approximate rates of VF/VT, asystole and PEA as the presenting rhythm for in-hospital compare to out-of-hospital arrests are as follows; 31 vs. 34%, 30 v. 47% and 34 vs. 19% (see Table 1). The higher rate of asystole as the first presenting rhythm for out-of-hospital cardiac arrest, again, is most likely a function of response time [69,72]. The remaining rhythms are most commonly bradyarrhythmias. The incidence of the VF as a presenting rhythm to EMS has changed with time and is now less prevalent. The explanation of this change is subject to speculation and may include changes in cardiac care in the pre-arrest stage.

**Table 1. Rhythm on arrival of EMS or hospital staff in out-of-hospital or in-hospital* cardiac arrest.**

| Reference | VF | VT/VF | VT | PEA | Asystole |
|---|---|---|---|---|---|
| [38] | - | 27 | - | 5 | 68 |
| [43] | - | 52 | - | 18 | 30 |
| [50] | 33.3 | - | - | 7.1 | 59.6 |
| [60] | 32 | - | 1 | 20 | 47 |
| [64] | 15.0 | - | 1.2 | 16.9 | 63.7 |
| [65] | 34.7 | - | .6 | 24.7 | 38.2 |
| [66] | 46.7 | - | 0.5 | 27.4 | 25.4 |
| [71] | - | 23.6 | - | 21.8 | 54.6 |
| [122] | 34.2 | - | - | 18.1 | 44.6 |
| [128] | - | 33.4 | - | 25.4 | 41.2 |
| [199] | - | 37.5 | - | 20.3 | 40.0 |
| [200] | - | 36.1 | - | 20.9 | 40.8 |
| [201] | 43 | - | - | 18 | 39 |
| [52]* | 24.7 | - | 8.5 | 41.3 | 25.4 |
| [53]* | - | 31.4 | - | 37.1 | 24.8 |
| [54]* | - | 23 | - | 32 | 35 |
| [202]* | - | 41 | - | 29 | 30 |
| [203]* | - | 25 | - | 30 | 36 |

Of all the rhythms that patients in out-of-hospital cardiac arrests are found to be in on arrival of the EMS, VF has the highest rate of survival to hospital discharge with an average of 19% (~ 84,000 arrests) (see Table 2) [38,40,48-51,56,58-62]. Occurrence of VF cardiac arrests in-hospital has a much higher rate of survival at an average of 39% (~38,000 arrests) (see Table 2) [53,54]. Again, in part this is most probably a reflection of the shorter response time for hospital resuscitation, including the ready availability of trained staff to provide CPR before arrival of medical emergency teams [69,72,75,76]. In studies of out-of-hospital arrests with much shorter response times [2-4], survival rates for VF arrest of up to 70% have been reported. Interestingly, the value of 70% survival to hospital discharge equates well with the 67% predicted by Larsen when defibrillation, CPR and advanced life support (ALS) occur without delay [77]. It is also identical to that reported by Kouwenhoven, Jude and Knickerbocker in their landmark paper on CPR in 1960 [15]. One might assume this to be the maximal attainable survival rate, bounded by not only practical constraints but more importantly perhaps the heterogeneity of aetiologies of cardiac arrest, some of which are irreversible no matter how hard one tries.

**Table 2. Survival for out-of-hospital or in-hospital* cardiac arrest with respect to rhythm on arrival of EMS or hospital staff.**

| Reference | Overall | VF | VT/VF | PEA | Asystole |
|---|---|---|---|---|---|
| [38] | 7.2 | 41.7 | - | - | - |
| [40] | 10.7 | 21.2 | - | - | - |
| [42] | 8 | - | - | - | - |
| [43] | 6.8 | 10.6 | - | - | - |
| [48] | - | - | 4.6 | - | - |
| [49] | - | 26.6 | - | - | - |
| [50] | - | 18.5 | - | - | - |
| [51] | - | 13.9 | - | - | - |
| [55] | - | - | - | - | 0.5 |
| [56] | - | 9-17 | - | - | - |
| [57] | 3.8 | - | - | - | - |
| [58] | - | 9.5 | - | - | 1.6 |
| [59] | 4.6 | 22 | - | - | - |
| [60] | 11.5 | 18.3 | - | 7.6 | 3.4 |
| [61] | 8.4 | 17.7 | - | - | - |
| [62] | - | 9 | - | - | - |
| [62] | - | 22 | - | - | - |
| [62] | 17 | - | - | - | - |
| [62] | 5 | - | - | - | - |
| [62] | 3 | - | - | - | - |
| [62] | - | 18 | - | - | - |
| [62] | - | 21 | - | - | - |
| [65] | 3.8 | | - | - | - |
| [52]* | 21.9 | - | - | - | - |
| [53]* | 17.6 | - | 42.2 | - | - |
| [54]* | 18 | 36.0 | - | 11.2 | 10.6 |
| [63]* | 20 | - | - | - | - |

There is great heterogeneity in survival rates for cardiac arrest as seen in Table 2. Bystander CPR and a shorter response time have been repeatedly shown to correlate with improved survival for out-of-hospital cardiac arrest [43,65,76], hence these factors are integral in the chain of survival. Consistent with this, the overall survival for all rhythms for in-hospital cardiac arrests is also greater than that observed out-of-hospital, 18% (~40,000 arrests) [38,40,42,48-51,55-62] vs. 7.5% (~ 86,000 arrests) [52-54,63].

In Australia, the pre-hospital VF presentation rate is between 7 and 16 per 100,000 person-years [43,51,60,66]. This translates roughly to between 1400 and 3400 arrests presenting in VF across Australia per year. This is consistent with the results of a large retrospective review (~ 36,000 arrests) of the peer-reviewed literature form the United States

– incidence of arrest with the first rhythm observed by EMS providers being VF was 21 per 100,000 person-years [61].

## Mechanism of Sudden Cardiac Death and Ventricular Fibrillation: The Arrhythmogenicity of Myocardial Ischaemia

Not only do the vast majority of SCD's occur out-of-hospital but ventricular arrhythmias triggered by ischaemia are know to be the cause of many of these deaths. Any analysis of recent advances in modern day resuscitation strategies should be preceded by a discussion on factors responsible for the initiation of ventricular arrhythmias in patients with ischaemic heart disease.

In 1840 Erichsen, experimenting with the ligation of coronary arteries in dogs, established a causal relationship between myocardial ischaemia and ventricular arrhythmia, described at the time as 'a slight tremulous motion alone continuing' ([78] in [29]). It was not until 1849 however, that Hoffa and Ludwig formally described VF after induction of cardiac arrest in a dog following an electrical stimulus ([20] in [21]). In 1889, McWilliam was the first to hypothesise a causal link between atherosclerotic coronary artery disease, myocardial ischemia, ventricular fibrillation and SCD. He wrote, '…sudden syncope from plugging or obstructing some portion of the coronary system is very probably determined or ensued by the occurrence of fibrillar contractions in the ventricles. The cardiac pump is thrown out of gear, and the last of its vital energy is dissipated in a violent and prolonged turmoil of fruitless activity in the ventricular walls' ([79] in [29]).

In the majority of cases ventricular arrhythmias, such as VF, result from a complex series of interactions between metabolic and ionic factors in ischemic myocardium leading to spatial and temporal aberrations in impulse conduction [36,47,80]. Today, myocardial ischemia is known to be the precipitating factor in 75 to 80% of SCD [47] with greater than 80% of patients having significant coronary artery disease [38,45].

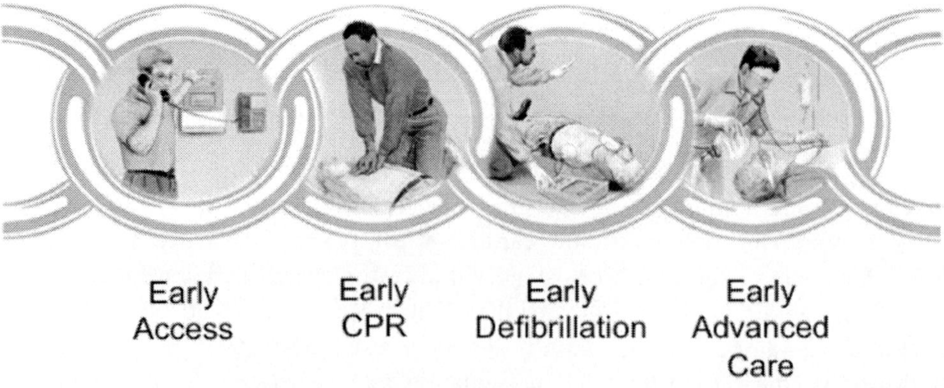


Figure 1. The Chain of Survival for Cardiac Arrest as described by Collins [198].

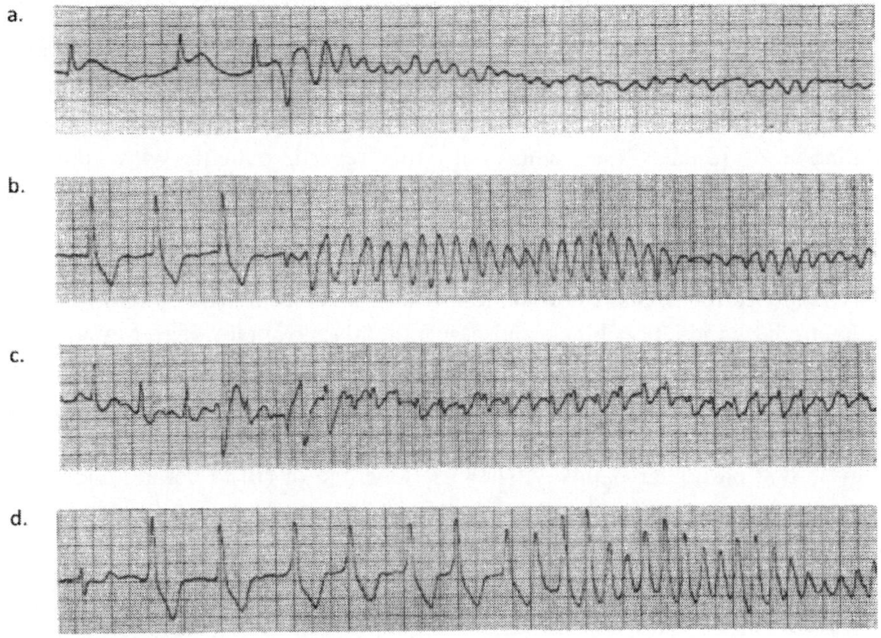


Figure 2. Initiation of ventricular fibrillation: R on T extrasystole (panel a), late cycle extrasystole (panel b), ventricular tachycardia/ventricular flutter which degenerated into ventricular fibrillation (panel c), idioventricular rhythm with rapid acceleration into ventricular fibrillation (panel d) (reproduced from [81] with permission from the British Medical Journal).

Premature ventricular contractions, or PVC's, originating from the margins of ischemic myocardium, have been identified as triggers of VF [47,81-84]. Indeed, they are the most common ECG anomaly preceding witnessed out-of-hospital ischemic VF arrest [81]. In 1982 Adgey et al. published the findings from 48 consecutive cases of patients with acute ischemic heart disease [81]. These patients arrested into VF, while undergoing cardiac monitoring, following arrival of the mobile coronary care team. Specifically they looked at events in the ECG preceding the initiation of VF. They report that in the majority of cases (69%) it was a PVC occurring on the T-wave of a normal beat, referred to as R-on-T, that preceded VF. The next most common (19%) was primary VT that degenerated into VF, with the least common (12%) being a late cycle ectopic beat or an idioventricular rhythm with rapid acceleration into VF [81]. Examples of these can be seen in Figure 2.

In 1989 Bayes de Luna published the results of a similar study of 157 patients with a stable health status who died from cardiac arrhythmia whilst wearing a Holter monitor [35]. Although these deaths were not due to any significant acute ischemic event such as a myocardial infarction they are still of interest as the majority of them occurred out-of-hospital and would have been attended by EMS. They found that 83% of the arrests were due to ventricular arrhythmia with the remaining 17% being due to bradyarrhythmia. Specifically, of the ventricular arrhythmias, a short run of VT with degeneration into VF was the most common (62%), followed by torsades-de-pointes (13%) and then primary VF (8%). Both of these studies highlight the role of ventricular arrhythmias as a primary cause of SCD and also demonstrate the role of PVC's in triggering VF.

Myocardial tissue is known to produce PVC's through three mechanisms, they are, triggered activity, re-entry and enhanced automaticity [85] – for reviews see [86,87]. While experimental studies have shown re-entry to be a significant factor in the initiation of many ventricular arrhythmias, they have also shown that it is solely responsible for the propagation and maintenance of VF [87,88]. This is supported by the increased risk of SCD in individuals with structural and conductive anomalies in cardiac tissue, as these anomalies provide a nidus for the initiation of re-entry (see below). In this regard, patients with cardiomyopathy, fibrosis, or myocardial scar tissue, secondary to previous infarction, are particular vulnerable [35,47,89].

Structural re-entry is enabled by a small focal abnormality in myocardial tissue providing two distinct pathways for impulse conduction. It can only occur when one of these pathways has a unidirectional conduction block and a sufficiently slow rate of retrograde conduction. Well-written, comprehensive reviews can be found elsewhere [86,87]. The conduction block can be permanent or temporary and is usually caused by either, (i) a structural anomaly in the myocardial syncytium, (ii) a derangement in the rate of depolarisation or repolarisation, due to pathology in that particular pathway, such as ischemia, or (iii) a combination of both. For example, a wave of depolarisation, originating from the sino-atial (SA) node, approaches the proximal ends of such a dual pathway, contained in the ventricular tissue (Figure 3, panel a). In one pathway (the right-hand side), the impulse meets a unidirectional block, due to ischaemia, resulting in the delayed conduction of the preceding impulse and subsequent repolarisation of this pathway [82]. The block, caused by this pathway being temporarily refractory to conduction, results in the impulse being extinguished (Figure 3, panel c). In the other pathway however, the impulse is conducted as usual (Figure 3, panel b to e). At the distal end of the pathway, the normal impulse exits and continues through the myocardial syncytium resulting in a normal beat (Figure 3, panel e). As the first pathway has now had time to repolarise it is no longer refractory, and so the normal impulse is conducted in a retrograde manner up this pathway resulting in a premature beat, or PVC (Figure 3, panels e to h) [85]. Re-entry can produce single ectopic beats, such as a PVC, or it can trigger ventricular tachycardia if the conditions are right and the impulse continues to travel in a circular motion around the dual pathway (Figure 3, cycling from panel e to j continually).

In a non-diseased, non-ischemic, structurally normal heart PVC's do not normally result in arrhythmias [88]. In the presence of structural and electrophysiological abnormalities however, the wavefront of depolarisation of a PVC, can collide with the normal wave of depolarisation propagating through the ventricles. This collision, termed a wave-wave interaction, can produce functional re-entry due to spatial heterogeneity in refractoriness in tissue surrounding the wave fronts. Such a re-entry may produce VT which can rapidly deteriorates into VF [47,90]. An example of this can be seen in the phenomena known as R-on-T (Figure 2, panel a). The wavefront of depolarisation of a PVC may also spontaneously break, referred to as wave break or wave splitting, producing two daughter wavelets that also lead to functional re-entry in a manner similar to wave-wave interaction [90].

In the setting of acute myocardial ischemia, with hypoxic myocytes and increased sympathetic tone, both re-entry and enhanced automaticity are significant contributors to the generation of PVC's [47,87,91]. Automaticity is a term used to describe the intrinsic ability of myocytes to spontaneously depolarise. While most myocytes have this capability, under normal conditions only specialised myocardial cells in the conduction system function as pacemakers. The level of automaticity present in myocardial cells varies. The SA node has a higher intrinsic rate (60–100/minute) and is usually the dominant pacemaker [92]. The atrio-ventricular node has a slower rate (40-60/minute) while ventricular tissue tends to have an even slower rate (<40/minute). In times of stress increased sympathetic tone can lead to spontaneous depolarisation of normal ventricular myocytes producing PVC's. In a patient experiencing cardiac chest pain, PVC's are indicative of irritable and hypoxic ventricular myocytes, as such they should be considered a warning sign. Other factors may affect the stability of the myocardial resting membrane potential, lowering its threshold for activation, increasing myocardial automaticity and the generation of PVCs. These include acidosis, electrolyte imbalances and drugs.

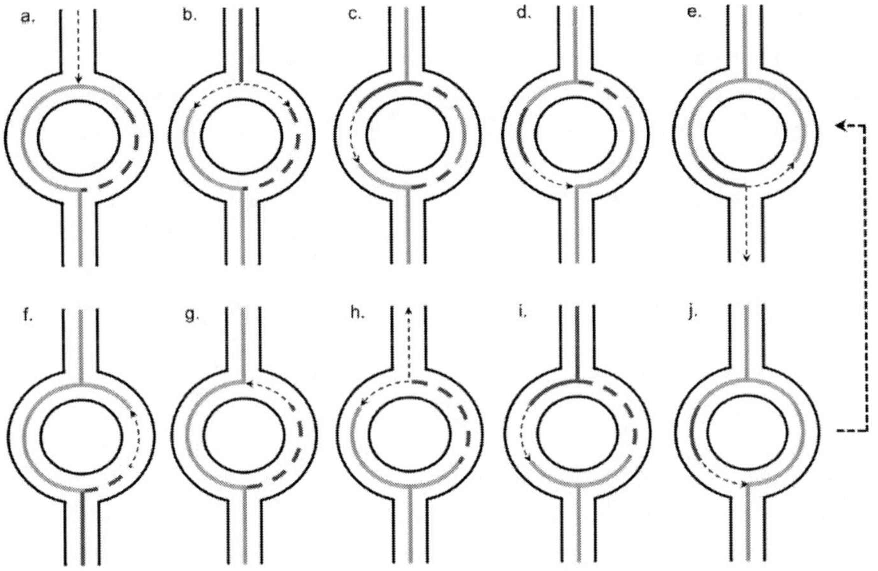


Figure 3. A simplified pictorial representation of a commonly accepted mechanism of ventricular re-entry. A wave of depolarisation approaches the proximal ends of a dual pathway in the ventricle (panel a). In the right-hand pathway, the impulse meets a temporary unidirectional block (panel b), extinguishing it (panel c). In the left-hand pathway the impulse is conducted as usual (panels b to e) resulting in a normal beat as it exits the distal end (panel e). As the unidirectional block has now had time to repolarise it is no longer refractory, and so the normal impulse is conducted in a retrograde manner up this pathway (panels e to h) resulting in a premature beat, or PVC, as it exits the proximal end of the dual pathway (panel h). Re-entry can produce a single ectopic beats, such as a PVC, or it can trigger ventricular tachycardia if the conditions are right and the impulse continues to travel in a circular motion around the dual pathway (cycling from panels e to j continually).

Interestingly, many studies have reported circadian variation in the incidence of out-of-hospital SCD, with the highest rates being observed between 6am and midday [43,93-96]. Increases in sympathetic nervous system activity in the morning, due to postural changes and stressors, with subsequent changes in vascular tone and myocardial excitability have been hypothesised as one reason for this circadian variation [47,91,95,97,98].

The studies by Adgey and Bayes de Luna (described above) highlight the importance of ventricular arrhythmias, particularly VF, as a major cause of out-of-hospital SCD. Of course these studies refer to the rhythm at the time of collapse. As noted in the section above, the most commonly found rhythm on arrival of EMS post witnessed arrests is asystole (47%), followed by VT/VF (34%) and then PEA (19%). This difference is thought to be due to the 5 to 10 minute response time of most EMS, enabling VT/VF to degenerate into asystole [69]. Without bystander CPR before arrival of EMS, VT degenerates into course VF as the myocardium becomes more hypoxic [35], which further degenerates into fine VF and eventually asystole [69]. Effective bystander CPR has been shown to slow the rate of deterioration of VT/VF into asystole [43,64,65,69,70,75,99].

As seen above, VF is the result of chaotic uncoordinated, cyclic electrical discharge within the myocardial syncitium. As evidenced by the high rates of return of spontaneous circulation observed with implantable cardioverter-defibrillator (ICD), or in patients fortunate enough to have early manual external defibrillation, there is no doubt that for witnessed cardiac arrest with VT or VF as the first presenting rhythm, defibrillation is definitive treatment [100]. The delivery of a small electric current to the heart, a process known as defibrillation, is believed to work by depolarising a critical mass of myocardial tissue, thereby terminating the aberrant electrical activity in the ventricles and enabling a dominant pacemaker such as the SA node to re-establish coordinated control. In recent years, there has been some discussion as to whether defibrillation of a patient with an out-of-hospital VF arrest should take precedence or whether EMS personnel should provide a period of CPR before defibrillation in an effort to combat the effects of prolonged myocardial hypoxia (this is discussed below).

## The Management of Out-of-Hospital Cardiac Arrest: Evolution of Emergency Medical Services

In the very early years following publication of the 1960 paper by Kouwenhoven, CPR and defibrillation were confined to the realms of the hospital. It was not until the mid 1960 that CPR and to a lesser extent defibrillators began to filter out into the community [101]. In January 1966 in Belfast, a revolutionary Irish cardiologist named Dr Frank Pantridge, put into practice his idea of taking the defibrillator to patients with early myocardial infarction [102]. The results of an 18-month trial of this mobile cardiac intensive care unit were published in 1967 [103]. In this time they treated 312 patients en-route to hospital and performed the first successful out-of-hospital defibrillation. In the United States, the first successful out-of-hospital defibrillation with good neurological recovery did not occur until 1969 [104]. In closing, Pantridge et al. stated, "it has been shown perhaps for the first time that the correction of cardiac arrest outside of hospital is a practical proposition."

Following the success in Belfast, the idea of bringing cardiac care to patients spread rapidly. Defibrillators started appearing on ambulances and ambulance drivers or attendants, as they were referred to at the time, began to be trained in BLS, including modern CPR [101,104]. So began a revolutionary change in the service delivery model of EMS [104]. The "load and go" mentality, where patient's received little intervention en-route to hospital, was replaced by a model in which patient's received life saving medical interventions at the scene and en-route [105]. Education of ambulance drivers, to a higher level, made it possible for them to take on a greater level of clinical responsibility with less risk to the community. It was from this increased level of training and clinical responsibility that the emergency medical technician (EMT) and paramedic were born.

In 1993 Cummins published an extensive review on the role of EMS in increasing survival from out-of-hospital cardiac arrests by improving links in the Chain of Survival [44]. He noted that while some communities had approached what was considered at the time to be a practical limit for survivability from SCD (15-20% for all rhythms and 25-30%for VF), it was clear that many communities operated with defects in their EMS chain of survival resulting in poor outcomes. In this regard, Cummins concluded that "people are more likely to survive out-of-hospital cardiac arrest when the following sequence of events occurs as rapidly as possible: recognition of early warning signs, activation of the emergency medical system, basic CPR, defibrillation, intubation, and intravenous medications." This view was consistent with the results of many studies showing that survival from VF arrest is improved through early bystander CPR [65,74,100,106-108], a rapid EMS response time, enabling early defibrillation and BLS [43,65,74,106,107,109], and the implementation of ALS [55,100,107,110-114]. Indeed, one large-scale study (1,667 arrests) has even quantified the relationship between these determinants and survival to discharge in patients with underlying heart disease, who had witnessed arrests and were found to be in VF upon arrival of EMS; Survival Rate = 67% - 2.3% per minute to CPR - 1.1% per minute to defibrillation - 2.1% per minute to ALS [77]. In the early 90's although it was clear that much progress had been made by EMS in some countries, many still had not yet achieved the optimum performance.

Although defibrillators were first used in the pre-hospital setting in the mid 1960's their widespread appearance on ambulances was a slow process, continuing through the 1970's and right up until the early 1990's in some countries [49,104,115,116] - there are many countries throughout the world where the desirable standard of a defibrillator on every ambulance has yet to be achieved. Certainly in Australia in the late 1980's to early 1990's only selected ambulances carried defibrillators, they were an expensive scant resource. The use of a defibrillator was initially seen as the preserve of a senior paramedic or a medical officer. Over time defibrillators have moved from this elite group to being standard paramedic equipment and are now considered part of the basic life support pathway. In the very early years, the lack of portability of the units impeded their widespread use out-of-hospital. Over the ensuing decades this was solved. Indeed, while the first defibrillators weighed around 90kg in the early 1950's, refinements made the next generation around 45kg in the late 50's, with the early portable versions weighing only 35kg in the mid 60's [18,101]! In the late 60's the weight was down to around 20kg with it reaching current day levels of around 10kg in the mid 70's [101,117]. Modern fully optioned manual defibrillators weigh around 5 to 10kg with automatic external defibrillators, or AEDs, weighing around 3kg. Such technological advances have made it practical for all first line emergency ambulances to be equipped with defibrillators, taking definitive care to the patient's side.

Today, all emergency ambulances in Australia are equipped with defibrillators, many having 12-lead capability, capnography and non-invasive blood pressure monitoring. One of the catalysts for the introduction of defibrillators to all ambulances in Australia occurred in October 1990. Whilst at a Polo match in Warwick Farm, Sydney, Kerry Packer, one of Australia's wealthiest men went into cardiac arrest. He was in arrests for 6 to 8 minutes before being resuscitated by paramedics. Fortunately, for Mr Packer, an ambulance, complete with defibrillator, was in the area. After recovering, Mr Packer donated millions of dollars to the New South Wales Ambulance Service, in a 1:1 deal with the government, to equip all ambulances with defibrillators [118-120]. The addition of defibrillators to every front line ambulance and single response vehicle in Australia has no doubt improved survival for cardiac arrests by strengthening the early defibrillation link in the chain of survival.

In Australia ambulance services have strengthened the early advanced care link in the chain of survival by training Paramedics in ALS. There is a degree of variation between states, but generally this includes the use of cardiac specific drugs such as adrenaline, amiodarone, lignocaine, adenosine and atropine as well as cardiac pacing and endotracheal intubation. In most states Paramedics, are referred to as Intensive Care Paramedics. The New South Wales (level 5 officers) and Victorian ambulance services (MICA officers) introduced ALS and Intensive Care Paramedics in the mid to late 1970's, other services followed. Indeed, within Australian ambulance services there is now clear evidence that attendance of an Intensive Care Paramedic at a cardiac arrest significant improves the odds of survival to hospital discharge over that seen with attendance of Paramedics alone [66,110,111]. There is a great deal of variation in terms of training, experience and equipment between paramedics across the world. This makes it difficult to interpret much of the evidence purporting to evaluate the impact of paramedics upon cardiac arrest survival. In EMS systems where physicians provide ALS (the Franco-German model), the survival rate for VF arrests is comparable to those where well-trained paramedics provide ALS (the Anglo-American model) [2,49-51,121].

Undoubtedly early defibrillation and early advanced care are two crucial elements in the chain of survival. There is little point however, in having ambulances equipped with defibrillators and manned by staff trained in ALS if they cannot respond to a cardiac arrest within a critical window [100]. Unfortunately, due to increasing demand on EMS in many communities there is a constant struggle for ambulance services to maintain response times within acceptable criteria. The current criteria are by necessity a pragmatic balance between the need for a rapid response and economic factors. Baring an ambulance on every street corner, something that is prohibited by finite health resources, there will always be a practical limit to EMS response times. This is especially true in rural and remote communities where other strategies, such as an increased reliance on dispatcher initiated bystander CPR and community AED programs for early defibrillation, may be of benefit [66]. In this regard, dispatcher initiated CPR, in both rural and remote communities, has been shown to be beneficial in increasing bystander CPR rates, which in turn increase survival [65,74,106-108,123-125].

## The Evolution of Advanced Life Support

Since the advent of modern CPR and the introduction of community-based defibrillation and ALS programs, the goal has always been to improve the survival rate from cardiac arrest. In some EMS, the early implementation of resuscitation efforts was characterised by rapidly increasing survival rates. In this regard, the rate observed in the King County region of Washington State set a particularly high benchmark of around 30% [2]. From this time onwards survival rates have not risen nearly as dramatically despite significant advances in technology and our understanding of the aetiology of cardiac arrest. In some regions most of the subsequent advances in survival from out-of-hospital cardiac arrests appear to be related to the introduction of ALS to EMS [66,110,111]. Primarily, ALS involves the use of advanced airway techniques and cardiac specific pharmacology.

Starting with simple oropharyngeal airways a variety of airway devices have been used to improve airway patency and facilitate adequate ventilation. While the endotracheal tube remains the gold standard for definitive airway management, providing both a means of ventilation and a secured airway, it requires a level of skill and currency above that which is needed for other airway management techniques. According to a 2008 Cochrane review, "the efficacy of emergency intubation as currently practiced has not been rigorously studies"

[126]. This review concluded that there was no strong evidence to support the use of intubation, as opposed to other airway management techniques, for acutely ill or injured patients. This is in stark contrast to the results of a more recent study from Japan, published in 2009, of 42,873 out-of-hospital cardiac arrests [127]. This study demonstrated a small but clear benefit of early intubation with regards to the neurological outcome of survivors [127]. A similar result was also found in an Australian study of 1,790 out-of-hospital arrests published in 2006. In this study endotracheal intubation was associated with a significant improvement in survival to hospital discharge [66]. Other studies, such as the OPALS study, have found no changes in survival to hospital discharge following introduction of ALS [128]. Again, the difficulty in comparing the results of such studies stems from the heterogeneity of EMS systems around the world, particularly the level of education, training and skill of the paramedics concerned. The issues include not only the success rate of intubation but also the expediency of the procedure and the judgment as to when to carry out the procedure and when not to.

Although other devices such as the laryngeal mask airway and Combi-tube have been used successfully in the management of cardiac arrest to produce an effective airway [129], there is again insufficient data regarding the effect of their use as a specific intervention on survival post cardiac arrest.

Various pharmacological interventions, such as calcium and sodium bicarbonate, have been used in the clinical setting from time to time in an attempt to improve survival. Their use, primarily based on the empirical extrapolation of their actions in non-arrested patient and laboratory animals, was common practice. They have now for the most part disappeared from practice, being brought out under only very specific circumstances. This is consistent with the 2005 ILCOR guidelines where no significant evidence was found to support their use [130].

The use of adrenaline in cardiac arrest is one pharmacological intervention that has stood the test of time, despite a lack of evidence that it significantly impacts on survival. The dose used today is still very much the same as the empirical dose first suggested [131]. If adrenaline provides any benefit, it is though to be due to its ability to cause peripheral vasoconstriction, thereby increasing central venous pressure and venous return to the heart, in turn increasing aortic root pressure and both cerebral and coronary perfusion. In the late 80's and early 90's enthusiasm for high-dose adrenaline, which in theory produced superior perfusion pressures, failed to produce a significant improvement in survival [132-137]. Other vasoconstrictors such as vasopressin (a.k.a. antidiuretic hormone or arginine vasopressin) have been considered and tried. When compared with the results from adrenaline however, the majority of studies also failed to demonstrate a significant improvement in survival (reviewed in [138]).

Various devices have been constructed and tested with the aim of improving myocardial perfusion by improving the efficiency of chest compressions with regard to rate and depth. In the early 70's a pneumatically driven piston device, powered by compressed oxygen, was described in the literature [139]. In more recent times there have been a number of pilot trials investigating a device that enables rescuers to perform "minimally invasive cardiac massage". This involves the insertion of the device into the thoracic cavity though a small incision in the chest wall. This enables direct contact with the heart and compression of the ventricles [140]. Load distributing band compression devices, which squeeze the thorax in a cyclical manner, have also been trialled. While many of these devices undoubtedly produce higher perfusion pressures and improve the choreography of compression, conclusive evidence that they improve survival is still elusive [130].

With regard to ventricular arrhythmias a myriad of anti-arrhythmics, such as lignocaine, procainamide, bretylium, magnesium sulfate and amiodarone have seen clinical use - some have maintained a place in practice, others have not. Clinically many of these agents were first used to suppress myocardial irritability in patient following infarction or who were experiencing ventricular arrhythmias but were haemodynamically stable. It was the success of some of these agents in this context that led to their use in cardiac arrest due to VT and VF [141]. For many years lignocaine has been the anti-arrhythmic of choice in this setting. In recent times however it has fallen from favour, being replaced by amiodarone. Primarily, this seems to relate to the fact that amiodarone, when compared to lignocaine, results in a higher rate of ROSC and survival to hospital admission [142]. Again however, there is a lack of significant clinical evidence that amiodarone promotes survival to hospital discharge and beyond – this is also the case for most other anti-arrhythmics [130,143].

Undoubtedly both lignocaine and amiodarone are effective in stabilising myocardial electrical activity. If however, they are successful in reverting a ventricular arrhythmia to a perfusing rhythm that is more conducive to life, it may come at the expense of a significant reduction in myocardial contractility and hence cardiac output [141,143,144]. The growing awareness of the negative impact of these anti-arrhythmics on contractility, coupled with the lack of dramatic improvements in survival to hospital discharge probably accounts for the recent change in attitude towards anti-arrhythmics in cardiac arrest. There has been a move away from the routine use of these drugs to a position where they are now used with discretion and careful consideration depending upon the circumstance.

Advances in defibrillator technology have seen changes in the wave-form of the defibrillating current from monophasic to biphasic. The evidence of their effectiveness when compared with monophasic shocks of similar energy has been one of the drivers of this change [145-148]. It is now well recognised that defibrillation causes reversible myocardial dysfunction, such as reduced contractility. This dysfunction is associated with reversible ST-segment changes on the ECG, such as elevation or depression indicative of injury and ischaemia [147]. Biphasic shocks that are effective at a lower energy appeared to be associated with less myocardial impact following a defibrillation [146,148]. Once again the extrapolation of this theory into practice, whilst making good clinical sense, does not seem to be associated with a dramatic improvement in long-term survival [149,150].

Post cardiac arrest management, which for a long time was largely supportive and expectant, has now been modified to include the benefits of hypothermia, supported by two independent studies [151,152]. These studies have been backed up at both the national and international level by guidelines recommending hypothermia for a period of time in the post arrest phase [130,153]. The evidence suggest that a period of hypothermia for 12 to 24-hours at a temperature of approximately 32 to 34° C is beneficial. Interestingly enough, although the evidence has been widely available for some time the uptake of routine hypothermia for cardiac arrest survivors has been patchy. This is possibly explained by the technical difficulties associated with achieving and maintaining hypothermia under these circumstances. The greater accessibility of angiography and angioplasty/stenting for the post arrest victim is another trend that will not only improve mortality but also impact significantly upon morbidity.

Despite the significant improvements in ALS and post resuscitation care as described above, one of the most dramatic improvement in survival rates seen in the recent decades (discussed below) appears to have been associated with the introduction of the revised ILCOR CPR guidelines in 2005 [2,51,122]. This observation supports a very fundamental line of though. That is, without the basics being done, and being done well, there is little benefit to be gained from the advanced techniques. In this regard much is to be gained from improving both the quality and quantity of bystander CPR. Reviews of cardiac arrest victims reveal that bystander CPR rates vary considerably from 60% in some countries [51] to around 15% in others [154]. As bystander CPR has been shown unequivocally to be a determinant of survival, hence its place in the chain of survival, such variation is surprising. To some extent these differences can be explained by cultural differences as well as the local EMS-dispatcher protocols with regards to persuading bystanders to perform CPR. The issue of compression only CPR [155], to overcome reluctance to carry out full CPR has been studied and current phone advice guidelines support compression only CPR if the rescuer is at all reluctant to do full CPR [156]. It is important to recognise that compression only CPR should not necessarily be considered as CPR without ventilation, as if the airway is open a degree of gas exchange does occur with the changes in intra-thoracic pressure. If compression only CPR is performed simple airway manoeuvre, or devices, would be advantageous.

## Establishment of the International Liason Committee on Resuscitation to Develop a Concerted International Approach

Historically, guidelines for the management of cardiac arrest were extrapolated from the observations of smaller observational studies and expert opinion. The field has now progressed to a stage where current guidelines are based on evidence from large-scale clinical trials, with expert opinion playing an integral part in interpreting the evidence and developing the guidelines. In the late 80's, due to the complexity of the field of resuscitation research and the many disciplines involved, the need for uniformity in the reporting of data from out-of-hospital cardiac arrests was recognised. In June 1990, a meeting was held in the Utstein Abbey, on the remote Norwegian Island of Mosteroy, for the purpose of developing a standardised data set [157]. Present at the meeting were representatives for the American Heart Association (AHA), European Resuscitation Council (ERC), Heart and Stroke Foundation of Canada (HSFC), and the Australian Resuscitation Council (ARC). It was from this meeting that the Utstein style was born [158]. It describes a standardised set of data required of any study investigating out-of-hospital cardiac arrest. It has become such an important tool that without compliance and reporting of studies in the Utstein style many journals will not consider a manuscript for publication. The Utstein style enables one to compare 'apples to apples' and evaluate the lessons learnt from different systems.

In 1996, the AHA, ERC, HSFC and ARC, in collaboration with other resuscitation committees were pivotal in the formation of an international body, termed the International Liason Committee on Resuscitation or ILCOR. The name ILCOR, or "ill cor", was a deliberate play on words referring to "sick heart" [157]. For many years, the individual resuscitation organisations had been providing a local framework for considering appropriate management recommendations for resuscitation, based mostly on empirical evidence from experts in the field. In Australia, the ARC has been in existence since the early days of modern resuscitation. With the development of ILCOR, local organisations were now working in a close international collaboration, reviewing peer reviewed literature on a regular basis and providing recommendations that were now grounded in evidence base medicine wherever possible.

In November 2005, ILCOR published it's second round of recommendations for emergency cardiac care and cardiopulmonary resuscitation [130,159-161] - it's first round came in 2000. The recommendations were the result of a critical analysis of the peer review literature containing the best available evidence at the time of review. They were adopted by all local resuscitation councils - only minor relevant local changes were made. The third iteration of this process, for release in 2010, will take into account evidence obtained since the last international recommendations were released.

There are still considerable areas of resuscitation that remained the preserve of expert opinion in the absence of a firm evidence base. Where recommendations are based purely on expert opinion, this is now clearly recognised and acknowledged by ILCOR.

## The 2005 ILCOR Guidelines for Resuscitation: CPR before Defirbillation in VF Cardiac Arrest

As discussed above, in November 2005 ILCOR published its most recent recommendations for emergency cardiac care and cardiopulmonary resuscitation [130,159-161]. With regards to resuscitation of out-of-hospital VF arrests by EMS the major changes in the 2005 resuscitation guidelines, as summarised by the Australian Resuscitation Council (ARC) [162], were, (i) more emphasis on chest compression, with a compression to ventilation ratio of 30:2, compared to the earlier 15:2, (ii) a single shock for unwitnessed VF arrests, compared to the earlier stack of 3, (iii) 2 minutes of CPR post defibrillation without a rhythm or pulse check, compared to the earlier pause for a rhythm check post defibrillation and only 1 minute of CPR.

It is now apparent that the coordinated efforts of ILCOR have paid off. A handful of independent studies, published recently in the peer review literature, from Denmark, the United States and Australia, have report significant increases in the survival rate for out-of-hospital VF arrests following introduction of the 2005 guidelines [2,51,122].

When the ILCOR recommendations were published a list of controversial topics from the 2005 International Consensus Conference was identified [163]. A degree of resolution was reached in most cases, due to the availability of appropriate data. With regards to the question of whether it is best, upon arrival at a patient in VF arrest, to, (i) stop and provide an extended period of CPR before defibrillation or (ii) defibrillate immediately, controversy remained. In the 2005 Guidelines the statement made by ILCOR [164] with respect to this issue was rightly, a cautious one, 'a 1.5- to 3-minute period of CPR before attempting defibrillation may be considered in adults with out-of-hospital VF or pulseless VT and EMS response (call to arrival) intervals of 4 to 5 minutes'.

The hesitancy of ILCOR to commit either way to an extended period of CPR before the first defibrillation was due to a lack of appropriate evidence at the time. Indeed, there were 2 studies [49,50] showing a significant improvement in survival following an extended period of CPR before not just the first, but all defibrillations. Unfortunately, these studies could not be used to confirm outright the effectiveness of CPR before the first defibrillation only (see below). Especially, in light of a study, that had been published at that time, by Jacobs et al. showing no significant increase in survival following 90 seconds of CPR before the first defibrillation only [48]. The caution exercised by ILCOR in 2005 was justified when in 2008 the results of a study by Baker et al. could not demonstrate an increase in survival following 3 minutes of CPR before the first defibrillation only [51] – in fact there was a strong trend, that did not reach significance, implying that CPR before defibrillation may be detrimental to survival. The relevance of these studies in the debate over CPR before the first defibrillation is discussed below.

The idea of providing an extended period of CPR before all defibrillation in out-of-hospital VF arrest gained significant clinical momentum following the publication of a paper by Cobb et al. in 1999 [49]. In brief, this study showed an increase in the overall survival to hospital discharge of 25% following a change in resuscitation guideline from immediate defibrillation to providing 90 seconds of CPR before not just the first, but all defibrillations. The increase in overall survival was due largely to a 58% increase in survival of patients who had an EMS response time of ≥4 minutes. Although this study was not a randomised control trial, it was an observational, prospectively defined study with pre- and post-intervention analysis, yielding a result that could not be ignored. It is important to note, in light of studies by Jacobs and Baker [48,51], that there is no way of determining from the Cobb study the relative magnitude of the effect of 90 seconds of CPR before the first or subsequent defibrillations on survival. It may be that the improvement in survival was gained solely from the 90 seconds of CPR before subsequent defibrillations with no additional benefit being gained by delaying defibrillation in the first instance to provide 90 seconds of CPR.

The idea of an extended period of CPR before defibrillation gained even more momentum in 2002 when Weisfeldt and Becker hypothesised that VF cardiac arrest, if left to run its natural course, progresses through three phases. This hypothesis, referred to as the 3-phase time-sensitive model, was the culmination of 2 decades of studies into VF cardiac arrest [165]. Of particular interest was the second postulated phase, 4 to 8 minutes post-arrest, termed the circulatory phase. The hallmark of this phase is increased myocardial ischaemia and acidosis with a reduction in the likelihood of a successful resuscitation [166-169]. Attempts at defibrillation in this phase can result in refractory VF, pulse-less electrical activity (PEA) and even asystole [170,171]. The importance of this phase lies in the fact that a significant number of patient in VF arrest are reached by EMS within this window [43,49-51,56,67-74]. More importantly, evidence, predominantly from studies with laboratory animals, suggested that a period of CPR before defibrillation within this phase improved survival. The hypothesis is that CPR reverses ischaemia sufficiently to alter the dynamics of the VF waveform enabling a successful defibrillation [172-174], that is, a ROSC. In this regard, it seems reasonable to expect that an extended period of CPR by EMS, before the first defibrillation, would yield the greatest results as, (i) the average patient had been in arrest for some 6 to 10 minutes upon arrival of EMS and (ii) post defibrillation, in most arrests, there are always periods of CPR, so the expected benefit post the first defibrillation from any additional duration of CPR may be minimal.

Briefly, the first phase postulated by Weisfeldt and Becker, 0 to 4 minutes post-arrest, was termed the electrical phase. There is little doubt that immediate defibrillation is the treatment of choice during the electrical phase. This is evidenced by not only the success of

ICD's, with regards to long term patient survival [175-177], but also the very high rates of survival to hospital discharge (70%) of patient experiencing VF cardiac arrest in public venues with AED's on hand and short collapse to defibrillation times [3,4]. Additionally, in patients experiencing out of hospital VF arrest and call to first shock times of around 5 minutes, the rate of success of the first, second and third defibrillations, with respect to obtaining ROSC, have been shown to be around 90, 98 and 99% respectively [178]. Whether CPR is performed or not during the electrical phase appears to have little effect on the rate of survival to hospital discharge [49,50,167,166] - the myocardium is still energy replete and benefits mostly from defibrillation. Historically it is the effectiveness of defibrillation during this phase that led to the widespread acceptance of immediate defibrillation as definitive therapy for VF arrest, irrespective of call-to-defibrillation time. The third postulated phase, 8 minutes post-arrest, has been called the metabolic phase. This phase is characterised by systemic ischemia and a very low probability of establishing a ROSC.

There is no doubt that in the studies of laboratory animals, as reported by Weisfeldt and Becker [165], an extended period of CPR before all defibrillations in the second, or circulatory, phase improves survival [179-184]. Again, from these studies however, it is not possible to determine the relative contribution of CPR before the first or subsequent defibrillations on survival as all of these animals required more than one defibrillation to achieve ROSC. More importantly perhaps, in all of these studies VF was induced through the delivery of a small current to the right ventricular endocardium by a pacing catheter, advanced from a peripheral venous site. The results of a recent study by Niemann et al. questions the relevance of VF induced in this manner to the human condition, namely, VF arrest secondary to myocardial ischemia [185]. Specifically, they compared the ease of resuscitation from VF that had been induced through either electrical stimulation, as described for the studies above, or ischaemia brought about through balloon occlusion of the mid-left anterior descending coronary artery. In comparison to the group with electrically induced VF, those animals with ischemia induced VF required more defibrillations to achieve ROSC (9.4 vs. 2.7 defibrillation), took a longer time to achieve ROSC (7.2 vs. 2.5 minutes) and had a much lower rate of survival (40 vs. 90% survival). The authors concluded that, 'Ischemically induced ventricular fibrillation is a more clinically relevant model for the evaluation of resuscitation interventions.'

In 2003 Wik et al. published the results of a well-constructed randomised control trial, comparing, in patients with out-of-hospital VF cardiac arrest, 3 minutes of CPR before all defibrillations versus immediate defibrillation, followed by 1 minute of CPR before subsequent defibrillations [50]. This again fuelled interest in the concept of CPR before defibrillation. In contrast to the observations of Cobb [49], there was no significant difference in overall survival between the groups in the Wik study. Consistent with the observations of Cobb though, a 16%, or 5 fold, increase in survival to discharge was observed for patients with an ambulance response time of > 5 minutes who received 3 minutes of CPR before all defibrillations. Again, while this is a fantastic observation it cannot be interpreted solely as justification for the use of an extended period of CPR before the first defibrillation, especially in light of the studies by Jacobs and Baker [48,51] based on the logic discussed above. In 2004, Pepe et al. published a clinical review [186] entitled, "Reappraising the concept of immediate defibrillatory attempts for out-of-hospital ventricular fibrillation.' In this review the studies by Wik and Cobb were again used to justify CPR before the first defibrillation, following the same error in logic as others in the interpretation of the results of these studies.

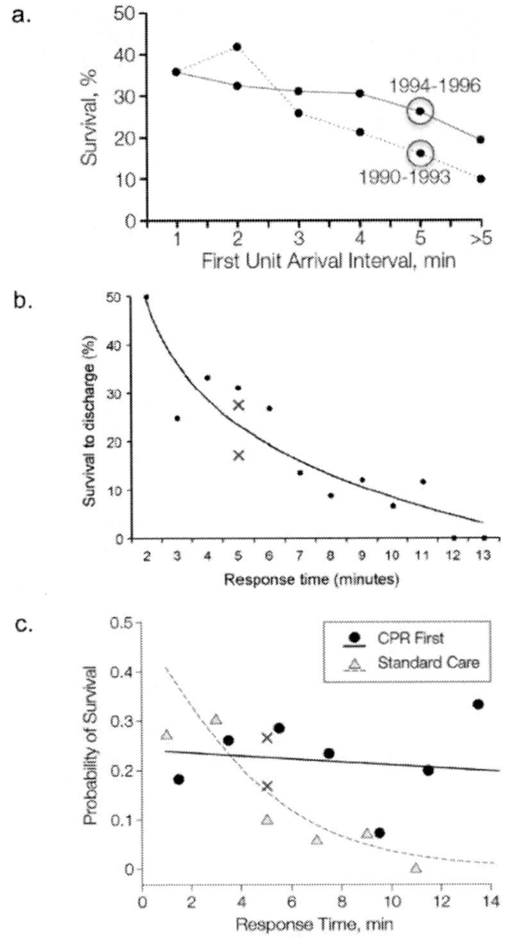


Figure 4. Survival curves for patients receiving immediate defibrillation or CPR before defibrillation in the studies of Cobb (panel a), Baker (panel b) and Wik (panel c) (reproduced with permission from the Journal of the American Medical Association [49,51] and Resuscitation [50] respectively). In panel b and c, the X placed on the graph represents the approximate position of the 5 minute first unit arrival interval in the Cobb study (the points contained in the circles). In panel b, the study by Baker et al., the curves for the immediate defibrillation and CPR before defibrillation groups were combined as there were no significant differences with regard to survival.

The observation of Wik and Cobb [49,50], on one hand, and Baker and Jacobs [48,51] on the other, are not mutually exclusive. Rather, they are consistent with the following hypothesis; an extended period of CPR before the first defibrillation is futile, defibrillation should occur immediately, it is the extended period of CPR before subsequent defibrillations that significant improves survival. This view is supported by the remarkably similar 2-fold increases (8.8 vs. 18% [51] and 8.3 vs. 16% [122] respectively) in overall survival for VF cardiac arrests observed in Australia by Baker et al. and in Denmark by Steinmetz et al., following introduction of the 2005 ILCOR guidelines for resuscitation, with minor regional modifications. The most significant change in the new guideline was an increase in the duration of CPR following all defibrillations from 1 to 2 minutes, similar to that used by WIk and Cobb in the intervention arms of their studies. The significant increase in survival, in the group receiving 3 minutes of CPR before defibrillation, following introduction of the 2006 ARC guideline in the study by Baker [51], suggests that failure to observe any significant effect of CPR before the first defibrillation was not due to poor resuscitation efforts or techniques by the EMS personnel involved, rather, it strongly suggests that CPR before the first defibrillation is a flawed treatment regime.

It is important to recognise that part of the increase in survival, following introduction of the new guidelines, may also relates to replacement of the 3 stacked defibrillation policy with a single defibrillation strategy. The change in the compression to ventilation ratio from 15:2 to 30:2 may have also played a part. Unless specific studies are performed the extent of each of these changes to the overall increase in survival will never be known.

If the above hypothesis is correct then why should delaying defibrillation to provide CPR have little effect on survival, and may even be detrimental. Certainly, in large population studies the sooner both bystander CPR [113,168,187-189] and defibrillation [94,187-191] occur the higher the rate of survival. As mentioned previously, a study by Larsen et al. even went as far as to quantitate this relationship showing that, survival = 67% - 2.3% per minute to CPR - 1.1% per minute to defibrillation - 2.1% per minute to ALS [77]. While the rate of survival is influenced by all factors in this equation, only one of the factors, defibrillation, is a corrective treatment, having the ability to terminate fibrillation enabling a ROSC. Perhaps immediate defibrillation is simply an immutable fact of life.

Even with bystander CPR, the probability of survival still declines over time, although at a much slower rate than that seen in patients who do not receive bystander CPR [166,167]. Perhaps this is also true when the first defibrillation is delayed by professional rescuers, such as EMS, to perform CPR, in the hope of improving oxygenation and the VF waveform. Evidence for this can be seen quite clearly in the survival curves in the studies by Cobb et al. [49] (Figure 4, panel a) and to a lesser extend in the one by Wik et al. [50] (Figure 4, panel c). This may relate to the fact that while fibrillating the heart uses up at least the amount of energy of the resting heart, if not more, depleting cellular ATP stores and increasing lactate levels [192-194]. Effective CPR has only been shown to provide around 30% [195,196] of the normal cardiac output. Hence, as the duration of the arrests extends there will always be a widening deficit in the energy required by the heart to fibrillate and what can be provided by CPR. Defibrillation, if effective, terminates fibrillation and lessens myocardial energy requirements, it does however cause temporary and reversible myocardial dysfunction [197], essentially stunning the heart. The provision of 2 minutes of CPR in this post defibrillation period of stunning, as in the new guideline, provides an opportunity for the heart to rest, enabling a dominant pacemaker to gain control and some reversal of the metabolic catastrophe that has occurred. Perhaps this is why immediate defibrillation should be the treatment of choice.

## Conclusion: A Look to the Future

Our understanding of the science of resuscitation has improved over the years with anecdote and opinion being replaced slowly by evidence based approaches. The future may well hold some significant advances in technology but these must be supported with system advances enabling rapid community responses and shorter delays to definitive resuscitation efforts. While technological advances can improve survival rates, the results of recent studies have highlighted that greater improvement in survival can be achieved by optimising the basics of resuscitation. Specifically, these changes have focused on the importance of reducing interruptions to CPR achieved by removing the pulse and rhythm check following defibrillation and doubling the duration of CPR from 1 to 2 minutes as well as increasing the compression to ventilation ratio from 15:2 to 30:2. It is a lesson to us all, we must never forget the basics.

Looking to the future one can envisage community CPR rates at higher level, enabled by dispatcher initiated CPR and greater community awareness of the need for timely CPR. This would be supported by perhaps a higher community availability of defibrillators and possibly a simple community airway device to ensure that compression only CPR is occurring in the presence of an open airway.

The ALS component could be driven by the analysis of the VF waveform to provide a tailored response. There may well be a variation in ideal shock characteristics in terms of waveform duration and power, dependent upon the presenting rhythm, and associated with the duration of the arrest. Similarly, vasopressor regimes may well be delivered in a more tailored format, again depending on the duration of the arrest and the presenting rhythm, all of which could be driven from the rhythm analysis software in the defibrillator.

Lastly, rapid EMS access and response would ensure early commencement of ALS, including routine cooling and greater access to angiography suites, as well as strategies to reduce the post arrest inflammatory response. Certainly, we have come far, but undoubtedly there is more to do.

## References

[1] Weisfeldt, ML; Ornato, JP. Closed-chest cardiac massage: progress measured by the exceptions. *JAMA.*, 2008 Oct 1, 300(13), 1582-4.

[2] Becker, L; Gold, LS; Eisenberg, M; White, L; Hearne, T; Rea, T. Ventricular fibrillation in King County, Washington: a 30-year perspective. *Resuscitation.*, 2008 Oct, 79(1), 22-7.

[3] Wassertheil, J; Keane, G; Fisher, N; Leditschke, JF. Cardiac arrest outcomes at the Melbourne Cricket Ground and shrine of remembrance using a tiered response strategy-a forerunner to public access defibrillation. *Resuscitation.*, 2000 Apr, 44(2), 97-104.

[4] Valenzuela, TD; Roe, DJ; Nichol, G; Clark, LL; Spaite, DW; Hardman, RG. Outcomes of rapid defibrillation by security officers after cardiac arrest in casinos. *N Engl J Med.*, 2000 Oct 26, 343(17), 1206-9.

[5] Australia AIoHaWatNHFo. Heart, Stroke and Vascular Diseases. *Australian Facts 2004.* 2004 May 2004.

[6] American Bible Society. *The Holy Bible*, King James Version. 2000 [07/01/2009]. URL: www.bartelby.com/108/.

[7] Rogers, MC. New developments in cardiopulmonary resuscitation. *Pediatrics.*, 1983 Apr, 71(4), 655-8.

[8] Eisenberg, MS; Baskett, P; Chamberlain, D. *Cardiac Arrest: The Science and Practice of Resuscitation Medicine*. Second Edition, In N. A. Paradi, H. R. Halperin, K. B. Kern, V. Wenzel, & D. A. Chamberlain (Eds.), Cambridge University Press, 2008.

[9] Divers, U. History of CPR: Fascinating insight into early attempts to resuscitate people. 2007. URL:http://www.ukdivers.net/history/cpr.htm.

[10] Cooper, JA; Cooper, JD; Cooper, JM. Cardiopulmonary resuscitation: history, current practice, and future direction. *Circulation.*, 2006 Dec 19, 114(25), 2839-49.

[11] Ardagh, M. A brief history of resuscitation. *Journal of the New Zealand Medical Association.*, 2004, 117(1193), 868.

[12] Foundation, AH. *History of CPR: Highlights of the History of Cardiopulmonary Resuscitation (CPR).* 2008. URL:http://www.americanheart.org/presenter.jhtml?identifier=3012990.

[13] The lifesaver known as CPR - cardiopulmonary resuscitation. 1986. URL: http://findarticles.com/p/articles/mi_m1370/is_/ai_4119043.

[14] Safar, P. On the history of modern resuscitation. *Crit Care Med.*, 1996 Feb, 24(2 Suppl), S3-11.

[15] Kouwenhoven, WB; Jude, JR; Knickerbocker, GG. Closed-chest cardiac massage. *JAMA.*, 1960 Jul 9, 173, 1064-7.

[16] Cavagnaro, L; Kiviat, BJ. Simply CPR. *Johns Hopkins School of Medicine.*, 2000. URL: http://www.jhu.edu/~jhumag/0400web/12.html.

[17] Acosta, P; Varon, J; Sternbach, GL; Baskett, P. Resuscitation great. Kouwenhoven, Jude and Knickerbocker: The introduction of defibrillation and external chest compressions into modern resuscitation. *Resuscitation.*, 2005 Feb, 64(2), 139-43.

[18] Worthington, J. The engineer who could. Baltimore: Johns Hopkins School of Medicine. 1998. URL:http://www.hopkinsmedicine.org/hmn/W98/engr.html.

[19] Fye, WB. Ventricular fibrillation and defibrillation: historical perspectives with emphasis on the contributions of John MacWilliam, Carl Wiggers, and William Kouwenhoven. *Circulation.*, 1985, 71, 858-65.

[20] Hoffa, M; Ludwig, C. Einige neue Versuche uber Herzbewegung. *Zeitschrift Rationelle Medizin.*, 1850, 9, 107-44.

[21] Efimov, IR. *History of fibrillation and defibrillation.* 2004. URL: http://efimov.wustl.edu/defibrillation/history/defibrillation_history.htm.

[22] Hoffa, M; Ludwig, C. Einige neue versuche uber herzbewegung. *Zeitschrift Rationelle Medizin*, 1850, 9, 107-44.

[23] Hooker, DR. On the recovery of the heart in electric shock. *American Journal of Physiology.*, 1929, 91, 305-28.

[24] Hooker, DR; Kouwenhoven, WB; Langworthy, O. The effect of alternating electric current on the heart. *American Journal of Physiology.*, 1933, 103, 444-54.

[25] Kouwenhoven, WB; Hooker, DR. Resuscitation by countershock. *Electrical Engineering.*, 1933, 52, 475-7.

[26] Beck, CS; Pritchard, WH; Feil, HS. Ventricular fibrillation of long duration abolished by electric shock. *JAMA.*, 1947 December 13, 135(15), 985-6.

[27] Moss, AJ. History of Electrocardiology. *Ann Noninvasive Electrocardiol.*, 1998 July, 3(3), 281-3.

[28] Romanowski, P. External defibrillator. 2007. URL:http://www.madehow.com/Volume-7/External-Defibrillator.html.

[29] Janse, MJ. A brief history of sudden cardiac death and its therapy. *Pharmacol Ther.*, 2003 Oct, 100(1), 89-99.

[30] Cardiovascular Disease in Australia: A Snapshot, 2004-05. *Australian Bureau of Statistics*. 2006. URL:http://www.abs.gov.au/ausstats/abs@.nsf/mf/4821.0.55.001.

[31] Causes of Death, Australia, 2006. *Australian Bureau of Statistics*. 2006. URL:http://www.abs.gov.au/ausstats/abs@.nsf/mf/3303.0.

[32] Wilson, A; Siskind, V. Coronary heart disease mortality in Australia: is mortality starting to increase among young men? *Int J Epidemiol.*, 1995 Aug, 24(4), 678-84.

[33] Epstein, FH. Recent international changes in coronary heart disease mortality. *Nutr Metab.*, 1980, 24 Suppl 1, 45-9.

[34] Myerburg, RJ; Castellanos, A. Chapter 36. Cardiac Arrest and Sudden Cardiac Death. In: P. Libby, R. O. Bonow, D. L. Mann, & D. P. Zipes (Eds.), Libby: Braunwald's *Heart Disease: A Textbook of Cardiovascular Medicine*. Philadelphia: Saunders Elsevier, 2008. 933-71.

[35] Bayes de Luna, A; Coumel, P; Leclercq, JF. Ambulatory sudden cardiac death: mechanisms of production of fatal arrhythmia on the basis of data from 157 cases. *Am Heart J.*, 1989 Jan, 117(1), 151-9.

[36] Martinez-Rubio, A; Bayes-Genis, A; Guindo, J; Bayes de Luna, A. Sudden cardiac death. *Contributions to Science.*, 1999, 1(2), 147-57.

[37] Foundation, AH. Out-of-Hospital Cardiac Arrest. Statistical Fact Sheet. 2008 Update. In: A. H. Foundation (Edr.), *American Heart Foundation*, 2008, 3.

[38] Moore, MJ; Glover, BM; McCann, CJ; Cromie, NA; Ferguson, P; Catney, DC; et al. Demographic and temporal trends in out of hospital sudden cardiac death in Belfast. *Heart.*, 2006 Mar, 92(3), 311-5.

[39] Yasuyuki, H; Atsushi, H; Hiroshi, M; Hirotsugu, A; Isao, N; Hitoshi, Y. Incidence and Characteristics of Out-of-Hospital Cardiac Arrest in 5 International Regions. A Comparison of Prospective Studies. *Journal of Japanese Association for Acute Medicine.*, 2000, 11(1), 8-15.

[40] Atwood, C; Eisenberg, MS; Herlitz, J; Rea, TD. Incidence of EMS-treated out-of-hospital cardiac arrest in Europe. *Resuscitation.*, 2005 Oct, 67(1), 75-80.

[41] Capewell, S; O'Flaherty, M. What explains declining coronary mortality? Lessons and warnings. *Heart.*, 2008 Sep, 94(9), 1105-8.

[42] Chugh, SS; Jui, J; Gunson, K; Stecker, EC; John, BT; Thompson, B; et al. Current burden of sudden cardiac death: multiple source surveillance versus retrospective death certificate-based review in a large U.S. community. *J Am Coll Cardiol.*, 2004 Sep 15, 44(6), 1268-75.

[43] Finn, JC; Jacobs, IG; Holman, CD; Oxer, HF. Outcomes of out-of-hospital cardiac arrest patients in Perth, Western Australia, 1996-1999. *Resuscitation.*, 2001 Dec, 51(3), 247-55.

[44] Cummins, RO. Emergency medical services and sudden cardiac arrest: the "chain of survival" concept. *Annu Rev Public Health.*, 1993, 14, 313-33.

[45] Chugh, SS; Reinier, K; Teodorescu, C; Evanado, A; Kehr, E; Al Samara, M; et al. Epidemiology of sudden cardiac death: clinical and research implications. *Prog Cardiovasc Dis.*, 2008 Nov-Dec, 51(3), 213-28.

[46] Myerburg, RJ; Kessler, KM; Castellanos, A. Sudden cardiac death: epidemiology, transient risk, and intervention assessment. *Ann Intern Med.*, 1993 Dec 15, 119(12), 1187-97.

[47] Luqman, N; Sung, RJ; Wang, CL; Kuo, CT. Myocardial ischemia and ventricular fibrillation: pathophysiology and clinical implications. *Int J Cardiol.*, 2007 Jul 31, 119(3), 283-90.

[48] Jacobs, IG; Finn, JC; Oxer, HF; Jelinek, GA. CPR before defibrillation in out-of-hospital cardiac arrest: a randomized trial. *Emerg Med Australas.*, 2005 Feb, 17(1), 39-45.

[49] Cobb, LA; Fahrenbruch, CE; Walsh, TR; Copass, MK; Olsufka, M; Breskin, M; et al. Influence of cardiopulmonary resuscitation prior to defibrillation in patients with out-of-hospital ventricular fibrillation. *JAMA.*, 1999 Apr 7, 281(13), 1182-8.

[50] Wik, L; Hansen, TB; Fylling, F; Steen, T; Vaagenes, P; Auestad, BH; et al. Delaying defibrillation to give basic cardiopulmonary resuscitation to patients with out-of-hospital ventricular fibrillation: a randomized trial. *JAMA.*, 2003 Mar 19, 289(11), 1389-95.

[51] Baker, PW; Conway, J; Cotton, C; Ashby, DT; Smyth, J; Woodman, RJ; et al. Defibrillation or cardiopulmonary resuscitation first for patients with out-of-hospital cardiac arrests found by paramedics to be in ventricular fibrillation? A randomised control trial. *Resuscitation.*, 2008 Dec, 79(3), 424-31.

[52] Cooper, S; Cade, J. Predicting survival, in-hospital cardiac arrests: resuscitation survival variables and training effectiveness. *Resuscitation.*, 1997 Aug, 35(1), 17-22.

[53] Gwinnutt, CL; Columb, M; Harris, R. Outcome after cardiac arrest in adults in UK hospitals: effect of the 1997 guidelines. *Resuscitation.*, 2000 Oct, 47(2), 125-35.

[54] Nadkarni, VM; Larkin, GL; Peberdy, MA; Carey, SM; Kaye, W; Mancini, ME; et al. First documented rhythm and clinical outcome from in-hospital cardiac arrest among children and adults. *JAMA.*, 2006 Jan 4, 295(1), 50-7.

[55] Vayrynen, T; Kuisma, M; Maatta, T; Boyd, J. Medical futility in asystolic out-of-hospital cardiac arrest. *Acta Anaesthesiol Scand.*, 2008 Jan, 52(1), 81-7.

[56] Myerburg, RJ; Fenster, J; Velez, M; Rosenberg, D; Lai, S; Kurlansky, P; et al. Impact of community-wide police car deployment of automated external defibrillators on survival from out-of-hospital cardiac arrest. *Circulation.*, 2002 Aug 27, 106(9), 1058-64.

[57] Byrne, R; Constant, O; Smyth, Y; Callagy, G; Nash, P; Daly, K; et al. Multiple source surveillance incidence and aetiology of out-of-hospital sudden cardiac death in a rural population in the West of Ireland. *Eur Heart J.*, 2008 Jun, 29(11), 1418-23.

[58] Holmberg, M; Holmberg, S; Herlitz, J. Incidence, duration and survival of ventricular fibrillation in out-of-hospital cardiac arrest patients in sweden. *Resuscitation.*, 2000 Mar, 44(1), 7-17.

[59] Nichol, G; Thomas, E; Callaway, CW; Hedges, J; Powell, JL; Aufderheide, TP; et al. Regional variation in out-of-hospital cardiac arrest incidence and outcome. *JAMA.*, 2008 Sep 24, 300(12), 1423-31.

[60] Cheung, W; Flynn, M; Thanakrishnan, G; Milliss, DM; Fugaccia, E. Survival after out-of-hospital cardiac arrest in Sydney, Australia. *Crit Care Resusc.*, 2006 Dec, 8(4), 321-7.

[61] Rea, TD; Eisenberg, MS; Sinibaldi, G; White, RD. Incidence of EMS-treated out-of-hospital cardiac arrest in the United States. *Resuscitation.*, 2004 Oct, 63(1), 17-24.

[62] McR. Meyer, AD; Cameron, PA; Smith, KL; McNeil, JJ. Out-of-hospital cardiac arrest. *Med J Aust.*, 2000 Jan 17, 172(2), 73-6.

[63] de Vos, R; de Haes, HC; Koster, RW; de Haan, RJ. Quality of survival after cardiopulmonary resuscitation. *Arch Intern Med.*, 1999 Feb 8, 159(3), 249-54.

[64] SOS-KANTO. Incidence of ventricular fibrillation in patients with out-of-hospital cardiac arrest in Japan: survey of survivors after out-of-hospital cardiac arrest in Kanto area (SOS-KANTO). *Circ J.*, 2005 Oct, 69(10), 1157-62.

[65] Fridman, M; Barnes, V; Whyman, A; Currell, A; Bernard, S; Walker, T; et al. A model of survival following pre-hospital cardiac arrest based on the Victorian Ambulance Cardiac Arrest Register. *Resuscitation.*, 2007 Nov, 75(2), 311-22.

[66] Jennings, PA; Cameron, P; Walker, T; Bernard, S; Smith, K. Out-of-hospital cardiac arrest in Victoria: rural and urban outcomes. *Med J Aust.*, 2006 Aug 7, 185(3), 135-9.

[67] Callaham, M; Madsen, CD. Relationship of timeliness of paramedic advanced life support interventions to outcome in out-of-hospital cardiac arrest treated by first responders with defibrillators. *Ann Emerg Med.*, 1996 May, 27(5), 638-48.

[68] De Maio, VJ; Stiell, IG; Wells, GA; Spaite, DW. Cardiac arrest witnessed by emergency medical services personnel: descriptive epidemiology, prodromal symptoms, and predictors of survival. OPALS study group. *Ann Emerg Med.*, 2000 Feb, 35(2), 138-46.

[69] Waalewijn, RA; Nijpels, MA; Tijssen, JG; Koster, RW. Prevention of deterioration of ventricular fibrillation by basic life support during out-of-hospital cardiac arrest. *Resuscitation.*, 2002 Jul, 54(1), 31-6.

[70] Dowie, R; Campbell, H; Donohoe, R; Clarke, P. 'Event tree' analysis of out-of-hospital cardiac arrest data: confirming the importance of bystander CPR. *Resuscitation.*, 2003 Feb, 56(2), 173-81.

[71] Polentini, MS; Pirrallo, RG; McGill, W. The changing incidence of ventricular fibrillation in Milwaukee, Wisconsin (1992-2002). *Prehosp Emerg Care.*, 2006 Jan-Mar, 10(1), 52-60.

[72] Pell, JP; Sirel, JM; Marsden, AK; Ford, I; Cobbe, SM. Effect of reducing ambulance response times on deaths from out of hospital cardiac arrest: cohort study. *BMJ.*, 2001 Jun 9, 322(7299), 1385-8.

[73] Fredriksson, M; Herlitz, J; Engdahl, J. Nineteen years' experience of out-of-hospital cardiac arrest in Gothenburg--reported in Utstein style. *Resuscitation.*, 2003 Jul, 58(1), 37-47.

[74] Stiell, IG; Wells, GA; DeMaio, VJ; Spaite, DW; Field, BJ 3rd; Munkley, DP; et al. Modifiable factors associated with improved cardiac arrest survival in a multicenter basic life support/defibrillation system: OPALS Study Phase I results. Ontario Prehospital Advanced Life Support. *Ann Emerg Med.*, 1999 Jan, 33(1), 44-50.

[75] Swor, RA; Boji, B; Cynar, M; Sadler, E; Basse, E; Dalbec, DL; et al. Bystander vs EMS first-responder CPR: initial rhythm and outcome in witnessed nonmonitored out-of-hospital cardiac arrest. *Acad Emerg Med.*, 1995 Jun, 2(6), 494-8.

[76] Swor, RA; Jackson, RE; Cynar, M; Sadler, E; Basse, E; Boji, B; et al. Bystander CPR, ventricular fibrillation, and survival in witnessed, unmonitored out-of-hospital cardiac arrest. *Ann Emerg Med.*, 1995 Jun, 25(6), 780-4.

[77] Larsen, MP; Eisenberg, MS; Cummins, RO; Hallstrom, AP. Predicting survival from out-of-hospital cardiac arrest: a graphic model. *Ann Emerg Med.*, 1993 Nov, 22(11), 1652-8.
[78] Erichsen, JE. On the influence of the coronary circulation on the action of the heart. *Lond Med Gaz.*, 1841-1842, 2, 561-5.
[79] McWilliam, JA. Cardiac failure and sudden death. *Br Med J.*, 1989, 1, 6-7.
[80] Cascio, WE. Myocardial ischemia: what factors determine arrhythmogenesis? *J Cardiovasc Electrophysiol.*, 2001 Jun, 12(6), 726-9.
[81] Adgey, AA; Devlin, JE; Webb, SW; Mulholland, HC. Initiation of ventricular fibrillation outside hospital in patients with acute ischaemic heart disease. *Br Heart J.*, 1982 Jan, 47(1), 55-61.
[82] De Groot, JR; Coronel, R. Acute ischemia-induced gap junctional uncoupling and arrhythmogenesis. *Cardiovasc Res.*, 2004 May 1, 62(2), 323-34.
[83] Enjoji, Y; Mizobuchi, M; Shibata, K; Yokouchi, I; Funatsu, A; Kanbayashi, D; et al. Catheter ablation for an incessant form of antiarrhythmic drug-resistant ventricular fibrillation after acute coronary syndrome. *Pacing Clin Electrophysiol.*, 2006 Jan, 29(1), 102-5.
[84] Varma, N. Onset of ventricular fibrillation: opportunities for paced prevention. *Pacing Clin Electrophysiol.*, 2008 Feb, 31(2), 141-3.
[85] Keany, JE; Desai, AD. Premature Ventricular Contraction. e-Medicine. 2008. URL:http://emedicine.medscape.com/article/761148-overview.
[86] Grant, AO; Durrani, S. Chapter 57. Mechanisms of Cardiac Arrhythmias. In: E. J. Topol (Ed.), *Textbook of Cardiovascular Medicine*. 3rd ed. Philadelphia: Lippincott Williams and Wilkins, 2007.
[87] Rubart, M; Zipes, DP. Chapter 31 - Genesis of Cardiac Arrhythmias: Electrophysiological Considerations. In: P. Libby, R. O. Bonow, D. L. Mann, & D. . Zipes (Eds.), *Libby: Braunwald's Heart Disease: A Textbook of Cardiovascular Medicine*. Philadelphia: Sanders Elsevier, 2008. 727-61.
[88] Rho, RW; Page, RL. Chapter 39. Ventricular Arrhythmias. In: V. Fuster, R. Walsh, R. A. O'Rourke, & P. Poole-Wilson (Eds.), *Hurst's the Heart*. 12th ed. New York: McGraw Hill Medical, 2008.
[89] Okada, T; Yamada, T; Murakami, Y; Yoshida, N; Ninomiya, Y; Toyama, J. Mapping and ablation of trigger premature ventricular contractions in a case of electrical storm associated with ischemic cardiomyopathy. *Pacing Clin Electrophysiol.*, 2007 Mar, 30(3), 440-3.
[90] Kim, YH; Yashima, M; Wu, TJ; Doshi, R; Chen, PS; Karagueuzian, HS. Mechanism of procainamide-induced prevention of spontaneous wave break during ventricular fibrillation. Insight into the maintenance of fibrillation wave fronts. *Circulation.*, 1999 Aug 10, 100(6), 666-74.
[91] Ulucan, C; Cetintas, V; Tetik, A; Eroglu, Z; Kayikcioglu, M; Can, LH; et al. Beta1 and beta2-adrenergic receptor polymorphisms and idiopathic ventricular arrhythmias. *J Cardiovasc Electrophysiol.*, 2008 Oct, 19(10), 1053-8.
[92] Huszar, RJ. *Basic Dysrhythmias*. A. Allen (Eds.), St Louis: Mosby, 2002.
[93] Jones-Crawford, JL; Parish, DC; Smith, BE; Dane, FC. Resuscitation in the hospital: circadian variation of cardiopulmonary arrest. *Am J Med.*, 2007 Feb, 120(2), 158-64.

[94] Martens, PR; Calle, P; Van den Poel, B; Lewi, P. Further prospective evidence of a circadian variation in the frequency of call for sudden cardiac death. Belgian Cardiopulmonary Cerebral Resuscitation Study Group. *Intensive Care Med.*, 1995 Jan, 21(1), 45-9.

[95] Lateef, F; Ong, ME; Alfred, T; Leong, BS; Ong, VY; Tiah, L; et al. Circadian rhythm in cardiac arrest: the Singapore experience. *Singapore Med J.*, 2008 Sep, 49(9), 719-23.

[96] Savopoulos, C; Ziakas, A; Hatzitolios, A; Delivoria, C; Kounanis, A; Mylonas, S; et al. Circadian rhythm in sudden cardiac death: a retrospective study of 2,665 cases. *Angiology.*, 2006 Mar-Apr, 57(2), 197-204.

[97] Samuels, MA. The brain-heart connection. *Circulation.*, 2007 Jul 3, 116(1), 77-84.

[98] Lerman, BB; Stein, K; Engelstein, ED; Battleman, DS; Lippman, N; Bei, D; et al. Mechanism of repetitive monomorphic ventricular tachycardia. *Circulation.*, 1995 Aug 1, 92(3), 421-9.

[99] Tovar, OH; Jones, JL. Electrophysiological deterioration during long-duration ventricular fibrillation. *Circulation.*, 2000 Dec 5, 102(23), 2886-91.

[100] Valenzuela, TD; Roe, DJ; Cretin, S; Spaite, DW; Larsen, MP. Estimating effectiveness of cardiac arrest interventions: a logistic regression survival model. *Circulation.*, 1997 Nov 18, 96(10):3308-13.

[101] Beonadonna, P. *The History of Paramedics*. Rochester, New York: Public Safety Training Centre, Monroe Community College. 2003. URL:http://www.monroecc.edu/depts/pstc/backup/parashis.htm.

[102] Shurlock, B. *Pioneers in cardiology: Frank Pantridge*, CBE, MC, MD, FRCP, FACC. *Circulation.*, 2007 Dec 18, 116(25), f145-8.

[103] Pantridge, JF; Geddes, JS. A mobile intensive-care unit in the management of myocardial infarction. *Lancet.*, 1967 Aug 5, 2(7510), 271-3.

[104] *A little history*. URL:http://www.angelfire.com/co/fantasyfigures/710history.html.

[105] *Ambulance*. Wikipedia. 2008. URL:http://en.wikipedia.org/wiki/Ambulance.

[106] Herlitz, J; Svensson, L; Engdahl, J; Silfverstolpe, J. Characteristics and outcome in out-of-hospital cardiac arrest when patients are found in a non-shockable rhythm. *Resuscitation.*, 2008 Jan, 76(1), 31-6.

[107] Nichol, G; Stiell, IG; Laupacis, A; Pham, B; De Maio, VJ; Wells, GA. A cumulative meta-analysis of the effectiveness of defibrillator-capable emergency medical services for victims of out-of-hospital cardiac arrest. *Ann Emerg Med.*, 1999 Oct, 34(4 Pt 1), 517-25.

[108] Spaite, DW; Hanlon, T; Criss, EA; Valenzuela, TD; Wright, AL; Keeley, KT; et al. Prehospital cardiac arrest: the impact of witnessed collapse and bystander CPR in a metropolitan EMS system with short response times. *Ann Emerg Med.*, 1990 Nov, 19(11), 1264-9.

[109] Estner, HL; Gunzel, C; Ndrepepa, G; William, F; Blaumeiser, D; Rupprecht, B; et al. Outcome after out-of-hospital cardiac arrest in a physician-staffed emergency medical system according to the Utstein style. *Am Heart J.*, 2007 May, 153(5), 792-9.

[110] Woodall, J; McCarthy, M; Johnston, T; Tippett, V; Bonham, R. Impact of advanced cardiac life support-skilled paramedics on survival from out-of-hospital cardiac arrest in a statewide emergency medical service. *Emerg Med J.*, 2007 Feb, 24(2), 134-8.

[111] Grantham, HJ. New Paradigm paramedic., 1997.

[112] Kette, F; Pellis, T. Increased survival despite a reduction in out-of-hospital ventricular fibrillation in north-east Italy. *Resuscitation.*, 2007 Jan, 72(1), 52-8.

[113] Weston, CF; Wilson, RJ; Jones, SD. Predicting survival from out-of-hospital cardiac arrest: a multivariate analysis. *Resuscitation.*, 1997 Feb, 34(1), 27-34.

[114] Dickinson, ET; Schneider, RM; Verdile, VP. The impact of prehospital physicians on out-of-hospital nonasystolic cardiac arrest. *Prehosp Emerg Care.*, 1997 Jul-Sep, 1(3), 132-5.

[115] *Early Defibrillation.* Rochester Police EMS History. 2007. URL: http://www.rochestermn.gov/departments/police/defibrillation/EDP%20History.asp.

[116] Scott, IA; Fitzgerald, GJ. Early defibrillation in out-of-hospital sudden cardiac death: an Australian experience. *Arch Emerg Med.*, 1993 Mar, 10(1), 1-7.

[117] Physio-Control International Corp. History of Life-Pak and other commercial defibrillators. 1997. URL:http://www.fundinguniverse.com/company-histories/PhysioControl-International-Corp-Company-History.html.

[118] Davies, O. Defibrillation. Wikipedia. 2008. URL:http://en.wikipedia.org/wiki/User:Owain.davies/Defibrillation.

[119] Kerry Packer. *Wikipedia.* 2009. URL:http://en.wikipedia.org/wiki/Kerry_Packer.

[120] Obituary: Kerry Packer. *The Times On-line.* 2005. URL: http://www.timesonline.co.uk/tol/comment/obituaries/article782808.ece.

[121] Fleischmann, T; Fulde, G. Emergency medicine in modern Europe. *Emerg Med Australas.*, 2007 Aug, 19(4), 300-2.

[122] Steinmetz, J; Barnung, S; Nielsen, SL; Risom, M; Rasmussen, LS. Improved survival after an out-of-hospital cardiac arrest using new guidelines. *Acta Anaesthesiol Scand.*, 2008 Aug, 52(7), 908-13.

[123] Hallstrom, AP; Cobb, LA; Johnson, E; Copass, MK. Dispatcher assisted CPR: implementation and potential benefit. A 12-year study. *Resuscitation.*, 2003 May, 57(2), 123-9.

[124] Rea, TD; Eisenberg, MS; Culley, LL; Becker, L. Dispatcher-assisted cardiopulmonary resuscitation and survival in cardiac arrest. *Circulation.*, 2001 Nov 20, 104(21), 2513-6.

[125] Culley, LL; Clark, JJ; Eisenberg, MS; Larsen, MP. Dispatcher-assisted telephone CPR: common delays and time standards for delivery. *Ann Emerg Med.*, 1991 Apr, 20(4), 362-6.

[126] Lecky, F; Bryden, D; Little, R; Tong, N; Moulton, C. Emergency intubation for acutely ill and injured patients2009 Contract No.: 2.

[127] Iwami, T; Nichol, G; Hiraide, A; Hayashi, Y; Nishiuchi, T; Kajino, K; et al. Continuous improvements in "chain of survival" increased survival after out-of-hospital cardiac arrests: a large-scale population-based study. *Circulation.*, 2009 Feb 10, 119(5), 728-34.

[128] Stiell, IG; Wells, GA; Field, B; Spaite, DW; Nesbitt, LP; De Maio, VJ; et al. Advanced cardiac life support in out-of-hospital cardiac arrest. *N Engl J Med.*, 2004 Aug 12, 351(7), 647-56.

[129] Rumball, CJ; MacDonald, D. The PTL, Combitube, laryngeal mask, and oral airway: a randomized prehospital comparative study of ventilatory device effectiveness and cost-effectiveness in 470 cases of cardiorespiratory arrest. *Prehosp Emerg Care.*, 1997 Jan-Mar, 1(1), 1-10.

[130] ILCOR. Part 4: Advanced Life Support. *Circulation.* 2005 November 29, 112(Suppl. 1), III-25 - III-54.

[131] Hubloue, I; Lauwaert, I; Corne, L. Adrenaline dosage during cardiopulmonary resuscitation: a critical review. *Eur J Emerg Med.*, 1994 Sep, 1(3), 149-53.

[132] Marwick, TH; Case, C; Siskind, V; Woodhouse, SP. Adverse effect of early high-dose adrenaline on outcome of ventricular fibrillation. *Lancet.*, 1988 Jul 9, 2(8602), 66-8.

[133] Goetting, MG; Paradis, NA. High-dose epinephrine improves outcome from pediatric cardiac arrest. *Ann Emerg Med.*, 1991 Jan, 20(1), 22-6.

[134] Stiell, IG; Hebert, PC; Weitzman, BN; Wells, GA; Raman, S; Stark, RM; et al. High-dose epinephrine in adult cardiac arrest. *N Engl J Med.*, 1992 Oct 8, 327(15), 1045-50.

[135] Brown, CG; Martin, DR; Pepe, PE; Stueven, H; Cummins, RO; Gonzalez, E; et al. A comparison of standard-dose and high-dose epinephrine in cardiac arrest outside the hospital. The Multicenter High-Dose Epinephrine Study Group. *N Engl J Med.*, 1992 Oct 8, 327(15), 1051-5.

[136] Lipman, J; Wilson, W; Kobilski, S; Scribante, J; Lee, C; Kraus, P; et al. High-dose adrenaline in adult in-hospital asystolic cardiopulmonary resuscitation: a double-blind randomised trial. *Anaesth Intensive Care.*, 1993 Apr, 21(2), 192-6.

[137] Carvolth, RD; Hamilton, AJ. Comparison of high-dose epinephrine versus standard-dose epinephrine in adult cardiac arrest in the prehospital setting. *Prehosp Disaster Med.*, 1996 Jul-Sep, 11(3), 219-22.

[138] Wyer, PC; Perera, P; Jin, Z; Zhou, Q; Cook, DJ; Walter, SD; et al. Vasopressin or epinephrine for out-of-hospital cardiac arrest. *Ann Emerg Med.*, 2006 Jul, 48(1), 86-97.

[139] Little, K; Auchincloss, J; Reaves, C. A mechanical cardiopulmonary life-support system. *Resuscitation.*, 1974, 3, 63-8.

[140] Rozenberg, A; Incagnoli, P; Delpech, P; Spaulding, C; Vivien, B; Kern, KB; et al. Prehospital use of minimally invasive direct cardiac massage (MID-CM): a pilot study. *Resuscitation.*, 2001 Sep, 50(3), 257-62.

[141] Kudenchuk, PJ. Advanced cardiac life support antiarrhythmic drugs. *Cardiol Clin.*, 2002 Feb, 20(1), 79-87.

[142] Dorian, P; Cass, D; Schwartz, B; Cooper, R; Gelaznikas, R; Barr, A. Amiodarone as compared with lidocaine for shock-resistant ventricular fibrillation. *N Engl J Med.*, 2002 Mar 21, 346(12), 884-90.

[143] Lang, E; Raisi, M. Ventricular tachyarrhythmias (out of hospital cardiac arrests). *BMJ Clinical Evidence.*, 2006, 07(216), 1-7.

[144] Marill, KA; deSouza, IS; Nishijima, DK; Stair, TO; Setnik, GS; Ruskin, JN. Amiodarone is poorly effective for the acute termination of ventricular tachycardia. *Ann Emerg Med.*, 2006 Mar, 47(3), 217-24.

[145] Dell'Orfano, JT; Naccarelli, GV. Update on external cardioversion and defibrillation. *Curr Opin Cardiol.*, 2001 Jan, 16(1), 54-7.

[146] Faddy, SC; Powell, J; Craig, JC. Biphasic and monophasic shocks for transthoracic defibrillation: a meta analysis of randomised controlled trials. *Resuscitation.*, 2003 Jul, 58(1), 9-16.

[147] Reddy, RK; Gleva, MJ; Gliner, BE; Dolack, GL; Kudenchuk, PJ; Poole, JE; et al. Biphasic transthoracic defibrillation causes fewer ECG ST-segment changes after shock. *Ann Emerg Med.*, 1997 Aug, 30(2), 127-34.

[148] Ambler, JJ; Deakin, CD. A randomized controlled trial of efficacy and ST change following use of the Welch-Allyn MRL PIC biphasic waveform versus damped sine monophasic waveform for external DC cardioversion. *Resuscitation.*, 2006 Nov, 71(2), 146-51.

[149] Forcina, MS; Farhat, AY; O'Neil, WW; Haines, DE. Cardiac arrest survival after implementation of automated external defibrillator technology in the in-hospital setting. *Crit Care Med.*, 2009 Apr, 37(4), 1229-36.

[150] Freeman, K; Hendey, GW; Shalit, M; Stroh, G. Biphasic defibrillation does not improve outcomes compared to monophasic defibrillation in out-of-hospital cardiac arrest. *Prehosp Emerg Care.*, 2008 Apr-Jun, 12(2), 152-6.

[151] Bernard, SA; Gray, TW; Buist, MD; Jones, BM; Silvester, W; Gutteridge, G; et al. Treatment of comatose survivors of out-of-hospital cardiac arrest with induced hypothermia. *N Engl J Med.*, 2002 Feb 21, 346(8), 557-63.

[152] Mild therapeutic hypothermia to improve the neurologic outcome after cardiac arrest. *N Engl J Med.*, 2002 Feb 21, 346(8), 549-56.

[153] Guideline 11.9: Therapeutic Hypothermia After Cardiac Arrest: Australian Resuscitation Council2006.

[154] Vaillancourt, C; Stiell, IG; Wells, GA. Understanding and improving low bystander CPR rates: a systematic review of the literature. *CJEM.*, 2008 Jan, 10(1), 51-65.

[155] Bohm, K; Rosenqvist, M; Herlitz, J; Hollenberg, J; Svensson, L. Survival is similar after standard treatment and chest compression only in out-of-hospital bystander cardiopulmonary resuscitation. *Circulation.*, 2007 Dec 18, 116(25), 2908-12.

[156] Dias, JA; Brown, TB; Saini, D; Shah, RC; Cofield, SS; Waterbor, JW; et al. Simplified dispatch-assisted CPR instructions outperform standard protocol. *Resuscitation.*, 2007 Jan, 72(1), 108-14.

[157] Chamberlain, D. The International Liaison Committee on Resuscitation (ILCOR)-past and present: compiled by the Founding Members of the International Liaison Committee on Resuscitation. *Resuscitation*. 2005 Nov-Dec, 67(2-3), 157-61.

[158] Cummins, RO; Chamberlain, DA; Abramson, NS; Allen, M; Baskett, PJ; Becker, L; et al. Recommended guidelines for uniform reporting of data from out-of-hospital cardiac arrest: the Utstein Style. A statement for health professionals from a task force of the American Heart Association, the European Resuscitation Council, the Heart and Stroke Foundation of Canada, and the Australian Resuscitation Council. *Circulation.*, 1991 Aug, 84(2), 960-75.

[159] ILCOR. Part 1: Introduction. *Circulation*. 2005 November 29, 112(Suppl. 1), III-1-III-4.

[160] ILCOR. Part 2: Adult Basic Life Support. *Circulation*. 2005 November 29, 112(Suppl. 1), III-5 - III-16.

[161] ILCOR. Part 3: Defibrillation. *Circulation*. 2005 November 29, 112(Suppl. 1), III-17 - III-24.

[162] Jacobs, IG; Morley, P. New Changes to Resuscitation Guidelines2006 March 27.

[163] Hazinski, MF; Nolan, JP; Becker, LB; Steen, PA. Controversial Topics From the 2005 International Consensus Conference on Cardiopulmonary Resuscitation and Emergency Cardiovascular Care Science With Treatment Recommendations. *Circulation.*, 2005 November 29, 112(Suppl. 1), III-133 - III-6.

[164] Kerber, RE; Martins, JB; Kienzle, MG; Constantin, L; Olshansky, B; Hopson, R; et al. Energy, current, and success in defibrillation and cardioversion: clinical studies using an automated impedance-based method of energy adjustment. *Circulation.*, 1988 May, 77(5), 1038-46.

[165] Weisfeldt, ML; Becker, LB. Resuscitation after cardiac arrest: a 3-phase time-sensitive model. *JAMA.*, 2002 Dec 18, 288(23), 3035-8.

[166] Campbell, RL; Hess, EP; Atkinson, EJ; White, RD. Assessment of a three-phase model of out-of-hospital cardiac arrest in patients with ventricular fibrillation. *Resuscitation.*, 2007 May, 73(2), 229-35.

[167] Gilmore, CM; Rea, TD; Becker, LJ; Eisenberg, MS. Three-phase model of cardiac arrest: time-dependent benefit of bystander cardiopulmonary resuscitation. *Am J Cardiol.*, 2006 Aug 15, 98(4), 497-9.

[168] Vilke, GM; Chan, TC; Dunford, JV; Metz, M; Ochs, G; Smith, A; et al. The three-phase model of cardiac arrest as applied to ventricular fibrillation in a large, urban emergency medical services system. *Resuscitation.*, 2005 Mar, 64(3), 341-6.

[169] Ornato, JP; Gonzalez, ER; Coyne, MR; Beck, CL; Collins, MS. Arterial pH in out-of-hospital cardiac arrest: response time as a determinant of acidosis. *Am J Emerg Med.*, 1985 Nov, 3(6), 498-502.

[170] Idris, AH; Becker, LB; Fuerst, RS; Wenzel, V; Rush, WJ; Melker, RJ; et al. Effect of ventilation on resuscitation in an animal model of cardiac arrest. *Circulation.*, 1994 Dec, 90(6), 3063-9.

[171] Kerber, RE; Sarnat, W. Factors influencing the success of ventricular defibrillation in man. *Circulation.*, 1979 Aug, 60(2), 226-30.

[172] Eftestol, T; Wik, L; Sunde, K; Steen, PA. Effects of cardiopulmonary resuscitation on predictors of ventricular fibrillation defibrillation success during out-of-hospital cardiac arrest. *Circulation.*, 2004 Jul 6, 110(1), 10-5.

[173] Reed, MJ; Clegg, GR; Robertson, CE. Analysing the ventricular fibrillation waveform. *Resuscitation.*, 2003 Apr, 57(1), 11-20.

[174] Menegazzi, JJ; Callaway, CW; Sherman, LD; Hostler, DP; Wang, HE; Fertig, KC, et al. Ventricular fibrillation scaling exponent can guide timing of defibrillation and other therapies. *Circulation.*, 2004 Feb 24, 109(7), 926-31.

[175] A comparison of antiarrhythmic-drug therapy with implantable defibrillators in patients resuscitated from near-fatal ventricular arrhythmias. The Antiarrhythmics versus Implantable Defibrillators (AVID) Investigators. *N Engl J Med.*, 1997 Nov 27, 337(22), 1576-83.

[176] Connolly, SJ; Gent, M; Roberts, RS; Dorian, P; Roy, D; Sheldon, RS; et al. Canadian implantable defibrillator study (CIDS) : a randomized trial of the implantable cardioverter defibrillator against amiodarone. *Circulation.*, 2000 Mar 21, 101(11), 1297-302.

[177] Connolly, SJ; Hallstrom, AP; Cappato, R; Schron, EB; Kuck, KH; Zipes, DP; et al. Meta-analysis of the implantable cardioverter defibrillator secondary prevention trials. AVID, CASH and CIDS studies. Antiarrhythmics vs Implantable Defibrillator study. Cardiac Arrest Study Hamburg . Canadian Implantable Defibrillator Study. *Eur Heart J.*, 2000 Dec, 21(24), 2071-8.

[178] White, RD; Blackwell, TH; Russell, JK; Snyder, DE; Jorgenson, DB. Transthoracic impedance does not affect defibrillation, resuscitation or survival in patients with out-

of-hospital cardiac arrest treated with a non-escalating biphasic waveform defibrillator. *Resuscitation.*, 2005 Jan, 64(1), 63-9.

[179] Garcia, LA; Allan, JJ; Kerber, RE. Interactions between CPR and defibrillation waveforms: effect on resumption of a perfusing rhythm after defibrillation. *Resuscitation.*, 2000 Nov, 47(3), 301-5.

[180] Niemann, JT; Cairns, CB; Sharma, J; Lewis, RJ. Treatment of prolonged ventricular fibrillation. Immediate countershock versus high-dose epinephrine and CPR preceding countershock. *Circulation.*, 1992 Jan, 85(1), 281-7.

[181] Niemann, JT; Cruz, B; Garner, D; Lewis, RJ. Immediate countershock versus cardiopulmonary resuscitation before countershock in a 5-minute swine model of ventricular fibrillation arrest. *Ann Emerg Med.*, 2000 Dec, 36(6), 543-6.

[182] Yakaitis, RW; Ewy, GA; Otto, CW; Taren, DL; Moon, TE. Influence of time and therapy on ventricular defibrillation in dogs. *Crit Care Med.*, 1980 Mar, 8(3), 157-63.

[183] Menegazzi, JJ; Davis, EA; Yealy, DM; Molner, RL; Nicklas, KA; Hosack, GM; et al. An experimental algorithm versus standard advanced cardiac life support in a swine model of out-of-hospital cardiac arrest. *Ann Emerg Med.*, 1993 Feb, 22(2), 235-9.

[184] Menegazzi, JJ; Seaberg, DC; Yealy, DM; Davis, EA; MacLeod, BA. Combination pharmacotherapy with delayed countershock vs standard advanced cardiac life support after prolonged ventricular fibrillation. *Prehosp Emerg Care.*, 2000 Jan-Mar, 4(1), 31-7.

[185] Niemann, JT; Rosborough, JP; Youngquist, S; Thomas, J; Lewis, RJ. Is all ventricular fibrillation the same? A comparison of ischemically induced with electrically induced ventricular fibrillation in a porcine cardiac arrest and resuscitation model. *Crit Care Med.*, 2007 May, 35(5), 1356-61.

[186] Pepe, PE; Fowler, RL; Roppolo, LP; Wigginton, JG. Clinical review: Reappraising the concept of immediate defibrillatory attempts for out-of-hospital ventricular fibrillation. *Crit Care.*, 2004 Feb, 8(1), 41-5.

[187] Hallstrom, AP; Ornato, JP; Weisfeldt, M; Travers, A; Christenson, J; McBurnie, MA; et al. Public-access defibrillation and survival after out-of-hospital cardiac arrest. *N Engl J Med.*, 2004 Aug 12, 351(7), 637-46.

[188] Weaver, WD; Cobb, LA; Hallstrom, AP; Fahrenbruch, C; Copass, MK; Ray, R. Factors influencing survival after out-of-hospital cardiac arrest. *J Am Coll Cardiol.*, 1986 Apr, 7(4), 752-7.

[189] Valenzuela, TD; Spaite, DW; Meislin, HW; Clark, LL; Wright, AL; Ewy, GA. Emergency vehicle intervals versus collapse-to-CPR and collapse-to-defibrillation intervals: monitoring emergency medical services system performance in sudden cardiac arrest. *Ann Emerg Med.*, 1993 Nov, 22(11), 1678-83.

[190] Martens, P; Vandekerckhove, Y. Optimal defibrillation strategy and follow-up of out-of-hospital cardiac arrest. The Belgian CPCR Study Group. *Resuscitation.*, 1996 Feb, 31(1), 25-32.

[191] Ladwig, KH; Schoefinius, A; Danner, R; Gurtler, R; Herman, R; Koeppel, A; et al. Effects of early defibrillation by ambulance personnel on short- and long-term outcome of cardiac arrest survival: the Munich experiment. *Chest.*, 1997 Dec, 112(6), 1584-91.

[192] Kern, KB; Garewal, HS; Sanders, AB; Janas, W; Nelson, J; Sloan, D; et al. Depletion of myocardial adenosine triphosphate during prolonged untreated ventricular fibrillation: effect on defibrillation success. *Resuscitation.*, 1990 Dec, 20(3), 221-9.

[193] Ditchey, RV; Horwitz, LD. Metabolic evidence of inadequate coronary blood flow during closed-chest resuscitation in dogs. *Cardiovasc Res.*, 1985 Jul, 19(7), 419-25.

[194] Grover, FL; Fewel, JG; Ghidoni, JJ; Norton, JB; Arom, KV; Trinkle, JK. Effects of ventricular fibrillation on coronary blood flow and myocardial metabolism. *J Thorac Cardiovasc Surg.*, 1977 Apr, 73(4), 616-24.

[195] Babbs, CF. Circulatory adjuncts. Newer methods of cardiopulmonary resuscitation. *Cardiol Clin.*, 2002 Feb, 20(1), 37-59.

[196] Weil, MH; Tang, W. Cardiopulmonary resuscitation: a promise as yet largely unfulfilled. *Dis Mon.*, 1997 Jul, 43(7), 429-501.

[197] Walcott, GP; Killingsworth, CR; Ideker, RE. Do clinically relevant transthoracic defibrillation energies cause myocardial damage and dysfunction? *Resuscitation.*, 2003 Oct, 59(1), 59-70.

[198] Cummins, RO; Ornato, JP; Thies, WH; Pepe, PE. Improving survival from sudden cardiac arrest: the "chain of survival" concept. A statement for health professionals from the Advanced Cardiac Life Support Subcommittee and the Emergency Cardiac Care Committee, American Heart Association. *Circulation.*, 1991 May, 83(5), 1832-47.

[199] Stiell, IG; Wells, GA; Field, BJ; Spaite, DW; De Maio, VJ; Ward, R; et al. Improved out-of-hospital cardiac arrest survival through the inexpensive optimization of an existing defibrillation program: OPALS study phase II. Ontario Prehospital Advanced Life Support. *JAMA.*, 1999 Apr 7, 281(13), 1175-81.

[200] Vaillancourt, C; Lui, A; De Maio, VJ; Wells, GA; Stiell, IG. Socioeconomic status influences bystander CPR and survival rates for out-of-hospital cardiac arrest victims. *Resuscitation.*, 2008 Dec, 79(3), 417-23.

[201] Stecher, FS; Olsen, JA; Stickney, RE; Wik, L. Transthoracic impedance used to evaluate performance of cardiopulmonary resuscitation during out of hospital cardiac arrest. *Resuscitation.*, 2008 Dec, 79(3), 432-7.

[202] Skogvoll, E; Nordseth, T. The early minutes of in-hospital cardiac arrest: Shock or CPR? A population based prospective study. *Scand J Trauma Resusc Emerg Med.*, 2008, 16(1), 11.

[203] Peberdy, MA; Kaye, W; Ornato, JP; Larkin, GL; Nadkarni, V; Mancini, ME; et al. Cardiopulmonary resuscitation of adults in the hospital: a report of 14720 cardiac arrests from the National Registry of Cardiopulmonary Resuscitation. *Resuscitation.*, 2003 Sep, 58(3), 297-308.

In: Advances in Cardiovascular Research, Volume 1
Editors: L. Schmitt, T. Konig, pp. 121-151
ISBN: 978-1-60741-720-0


*Chapter IV*

# The Ambiguous Role of Epinephrine in Ventricular Fibrillation

***Theodoros Xanthos, Konstantinos Stroumpoulis and Lila Papadimitriou***
University of Athens, Medical School, Laboratory of Experimental Surgery and Surgical Research, Greece

## Abstract

Cardiac arrest affects more than 250,000 people per year in the USA. Ventricular Fibrillation (VF) is the rhythm observed in up to 40% of the cases, when help arrives. Current guidelines recommend initiation of immediate bystander cardiopulmonary resuscitation (CPR), electrical defibrillation and epinephrine (adrenaline) administration.

Since the restoration of threshold levels of coronary perfusion pressure (CPP) has been found to be the only independent determinant of return of spontaneous circulation (ROSC), the use of a vasopressor agent has been considered indispensable for successful CPR. Epinephrine holds a predominant role as the drug of choice for more than 100 years. However, recent studies have shown that eventhough the use of epinephrine increases the possibility of ROSC, it does not result in higher hospital discharge rates when compared to placebo in VF cardiac arrest setting.

Epinephrine is an endogenous catecholamine which possesses both alpha and beta adrenergic actions. Its beneficial effects are assumed to be primarily due to its $\alpha_2$ action leading to peripheral arteriolar vasoconstriction, increasing thus the aortic pressure and consequently myocardial and cerebral perfusion.

On the other hand, epinephrine's $\alpha_1$, $\beta_1$ and $\beta_2$ actions have serious arrhythmogenic effects originated from the resulting increase of oxygen demands in an already fasting myocardium, the increase of myocardial lactate levels and the decrease of myocardial ATP reserves, increasing thus the severity of post-resuscitation myocardial dysfunction. Furthermore, epinephrine is very sensitive to the effects of acidosis, which is the case in VF setting. Lastly, in cardiac arrest victims, endogenous catecholamine levels have been found to be in extremely elevated concentrations. Therefore, it is possible that almost all the catecholamine receptors have been already been stimulated and an epinephrine administration will not have the expected impact.

The aforementioned data have oriented CPR research to the quest for alternative pharmacologic agents which will either replace epinephrine or attenuate its undesired effects.

## Introduction

Cardiac arrest affects more than 250.000 people in North America and Europe each year [1,2] with dismal survival and hospital discharge rates [2-5]. In out-of hospital cardiac arrest, overall survival to hospital discharge barely reaches an average of 6% [2,3,5,7-10]. Survival of patients suffering from in-hospital cardiac arrest is slightly better, reaching 16% [11,12,13]. Ventricular fibrillation is the electrocardiographic (ECG) rhythm observed in up to 40% of the cases when help arrives, but it is estimated to be the etiologic factor for more than 70% of cardiac arrests [14-20]. However, VF is potentially the most treatable rhythm in cardiac arrest [1,9,14]. The optimal treatment for VF CA is "immediate bystander cardiopulmonary resuscitation (CPR) plus electrical defibrillation" [1]. It has been found that during CPR, the pressure gradient between the aorta and the right atrium during the decompression phase, the coronary perfusion pressure (CPP), is positively correlated with return of spontaneous circulation (ROSC) and survival [21,22]. However, the blood flow generated during CPR, rarely exceeds 30% of normal cardiac output [23-26].Therefore, a further increase in systemic vascular resistance is necessary for achieving CPP compatible with life. This is the place for vasopressor use as an adjunctive therapy to CPR in order to increase both myocardial and cerebral perfusion pressures [1,25,27].

## Epinephrine in CPR

Epinephrine (Adrenaline) has been the drug of choice in CPR for more than 100 years [28] and it is still the recommended vasopressor agent by the International Liaison Committee on Resuscitation (ILCOR) and by both European Resuscitation Council (ERC) [1] and American Heart Association (AHA) [29]. However, in 2005 guidelines it is stated that "*despite the widespread use of adrenaline (epinephrine)…… during resuscitation, there is no placebo controlled study that shows that the routine use of any vasopressor at any stage during human cardiac arrest increases survival to hospital discharge. Current evidence is insufficient to support or refute the routine use of any particular drug or sequence of drugs. Despite the lack of human data, the use of adrenaline is still recommended, based largely on animal data*" [1,29]. In addition, there is emerging evidence that survival outcomes may not be affected by epinephrine use [5,9,30-33]. Therefore, a large proportion of current CPR research is oriented towards vasopressor use, examining the mode of action of different agents, possible drug combinations and the appropriate timing for their administration during CPR.

Epinephrine has been used experimentally in animals since 1896 [34]. In humans, it has been used in resuscitation since the early 60s as an intracardiac injection initially [28]. Since then, its use is widespread during resuscitation with the first guidelines edited in 1974 [35] and is still recommended by the current guidelines. ERC guidelines state that "if VF persists after two shocks give epinephrine and repeat every 3-5 min during cardiac arrest" [1]. AHA guidelines recommend: "If VF/VT persists after delivery of 1 or 2 shocks plus CPR, give a vasopressor (epinephrine every 3 to 5 minutes...)" [29] (Figure 1). The relatively short intervals between each administration are dictated by epinephrine's short duration of action that does not exceed 5 min [36,37]. The distribution of epinephrine through the circulatory system is achieved by chest compressions.

## Epinephrine in the Human Organism

Epinephrine is an endogenous catecholamine released by the adrenal medulla as a short-term response to stress. The Greek words epi + nephros mean "on the kidney" designating thus the position of adrenal glands. Epinephrine is a potent vasopressor and its release and entry into circulation causes an increase in venous return, arterial and arteriolar constriction. It also has a positive chronotropic and inotropic action, increasing thus cardiac output and blood pressure [22,28,38-42].

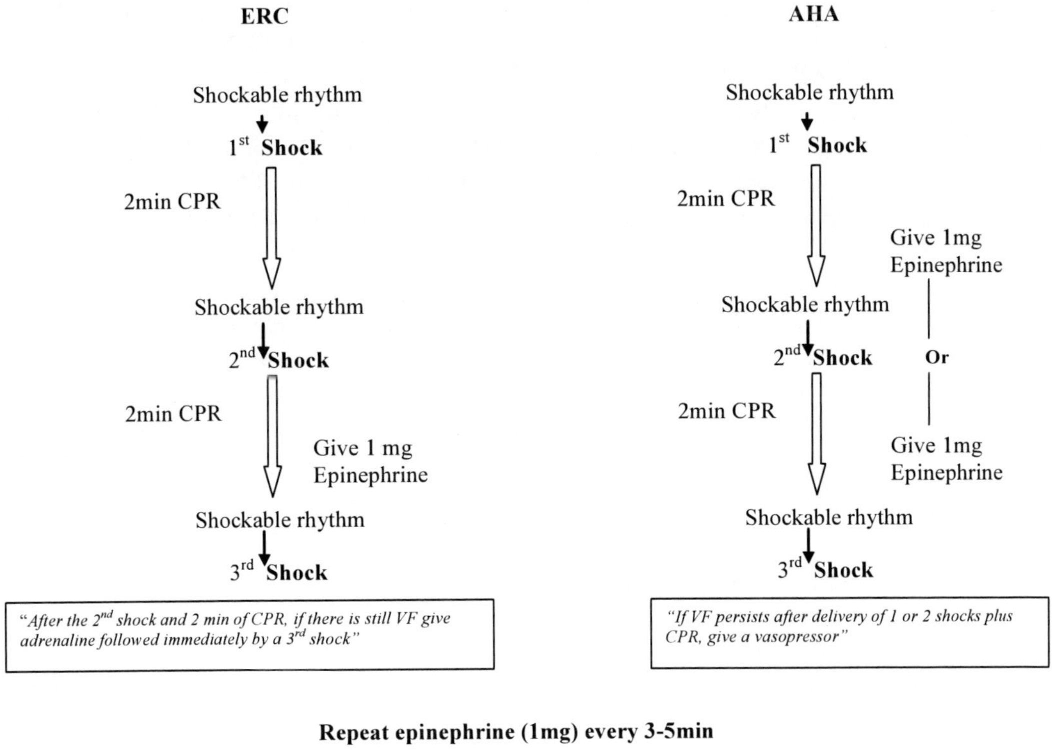


Figure 1. 2005 Guidelines for treatment of VF cardiac arrest. ERC: European Resuscitation Council, AHA: American Heart Association

### Adrenergic Receptor Classification

In 1948 Ahlquist first described the existence of two types of adrenergic receptors and designated them by the initials α and β [28]. In 1960s, Lands et al [43,44] further subdivided the adrenergic receptors into $\alpha_1$, $\alpha_2$, $\beta_1$, $\beta_2$. To date, 9 receptor subtypes have been identified. There are 3 $\alpha_1$-subtypes ($\alpha_{1A}$, $\alpha_{1B}$, $\alpha_{1D}$), 3 $\alpha_2$-subtypes ($\alpha_{2A}$, $\alpha_{2B}$, $\alpha_{2C}$) and 3 β-receptor subtypes ($\beta_1$, $\beta_2$, $\beta_3$) [28].

### Epinephrine's Actions

Epinephrine is a non selective α ($\alpha_1$ and $\alpha_2$) and β-adrenoreceptor ($\beta_1$ and $\beta_2$) agonist. Its beneficial effects are mediated by α-adrenergic receptors causing arterial and arteriolar vasoconstriction in the skin, mucosa and kidney, accompanied by vasoconstriction in veins. Furthermore, epinephrine reverses and prevents arterial collapse which occurs in cardiac arrest setting (loss of vascular tone) and during CPR (the increase of intrathoracic pressure may exceed intraluminal pressure) [26,38,45]. Hence, blood flow is created from peripheral to central circulation protecting the vital organs from ischemia via volume redistribution. This action raises both CPP directly and brain perfusion pressure (BPP) indirectly (as all catecholamines do not penetrate the blood brain barrier, the increase in BPP occurs as a result of volume redistribution) [28,38]. The improvement in cardiac blood supply in general has a double effect. It does not only protect the myocardium from ischemic damage, but may also lower defibrillation energy requirements [46]. On the other hand, epinephrine's $\beta_1$ action causes vasodilation and activation of heart $\beta_1$-receptors mediating for positive inotropic and chronotropic effects, increasing thus myocardial oxygen demands in an already fasting myocardium [25,42,47,48]. $\beta_2$-adrenoreceptor activation causes vasodilation in skeletal muscles and bronchodilation [42,47,49-51]. Eventhough until recently it was thought that there are no $\alpha_2$ adrenoreceptors in the myocardium and a possible role for a selective $\alpha_2$ agonist in CPR was sought [36,46,52], however this is not the case. Both $\alpha_1$ and $\alpha_2$ adrenoreceptors are present in the human coronary circulation with $\alpha_2$ adrenoreceptors predominant in the microcirculation (coronary arterioles) [53-58]. Hence, epinephrine causes extensive vasoconstriction making no discrimination between myocardial and peripheral vessels.

## Pathophysiology of CA

In order to further analyze and understand epinephrine's actions in VF setting, a brief description of what happens to the myocardium under ischemic conditions should be undertaken. Myocardial ischemia plays a double role in cardiac arrest. It can be at the same time both the underlying cause and the result of cardiac arrest giving thus feedback to a never ending circle. Usually a thrombus is formed in a coronary artery leading to ischemic myocardial damage, infarct formation and finally electromechanical dysfunction leading to various spontaneous asynchronized depolarizations (VF) and cessation of blood flow. The stress (if the patient had initially conscience) or the hypovolemia (circulatory arrest) are potent stimuli for catecholamine release from the adrenal glands. In fact adrenaline levels in cardiac arrest victims have been found to be form 170 to 500 times baseline pre VF levels [39,46,59,60]. However, the magnitude of this response is limited and administration of vasopressors is needed [25,46,60].

As ischemia occurs, myocardial oxygen demands raise significantly, all adenosine triphosphate (ATP) levels are depleted, lactate levels are significantly elevated and consequently acidosis develops [22,61,62]. As time progresses, acidosis affects in cellular level the $Na^+$-$K^+$ ATPase pump and the $Na^+$-$Ca^{2+}$ exchanger, resulting in intracellular $Na^+$ and $Ca^{2+}$ overload, finally affecting myocardial cell function and viability [63-66]. Furthermore, the impairment of the $Na^+$-$K^+$ ATPase, prolongs the action potential duration impairing thus the ability of myocytes to repolarize in synchrony [62]. Severe ischemia results into coronary artery endothelial damage and myocardial tissue necrosis. At the same time the phenomenon of ischemic contracture of the heart develops, causing progressive ventricular wall thickening and ventricular cavity size reduction [28,41].

### Reperfusion Injury & Post-Resuscitation Myocardial Dysfunction

If resuscitation attempts are successful and ROSC is achieved, myocardium and many other organs face a second threat, reperfusion injury. Damage in myocytes and endothelial cells occurs not only by ischemia, but also by rapid reperfusion. At that time, the accumulated, during the ischemic period oxygen free radicals, the activated leucocytes and the apoptotic residues, enter the circulation and in association with coronary hypercontracture, further enhance the endothelial damage and cellular necrosis creating thus a very arrhythmogenic substrate sensible to VF recurrence [37,40,59,60,63-66]. The result of these disturbances is a decreased ejection fraction, a decreased peak systolic left ventricular pressure/end-systolic volume ratio and a rightward shift in the pressure-volume relationship [67-70]. This phenomenon, called "post-resuscitation myocardial dysfunction", is so severe and may persist even for up to 14 days [71] that it is probably the major reason why only 1 out of 8 CA victims who achieved ROSC (the majority of them dies within the first 72 hours after ROSC), are finally discharged from hospital [50,72-77]. Ischemia duration has been found to be directly related to the extent of post-resuscitation myocardial dysfunction [78,79]. Eventhough reperfusion injury is difficult to avoid, it is nevertheless amenable to treatment and CPR research is oriented to various agents such as adenosine, opioids, dobutamine, or vasoactive agents that are not β-adrenoreceptor dependent [76,80-89] that could possibly attenuate its effects.

## Three-Phase Ventricular Fibrillation Model

A relatively new (2002) approach of the pathophysiology and therapy of VF has been developed. It is the 3-phase model of VF (Figure 2) proposed by Weisfeldt and Becker [90] which is divided into the following phases: 1) the *electrical* phase (up to 4 min after CA begins), 2) the *circulatory* (or hemodynamic) phase (4-10min post CA) and 3) the *metabolic* phase (after 10 min).

As this model postulates and clinical and research data support, VF response to therapies is time-dependent. In the electrical phase, the fibrillating myocardium has not by that time used up all its energy stores and a rescue countershock has most chances to be successful if attempted as soon as possible without any prior intervention. This is the reason why the benefit of automated external defibrillator (AED) use has been shown in various settings including casinos, airplanes, airports and the community [61,91-99].

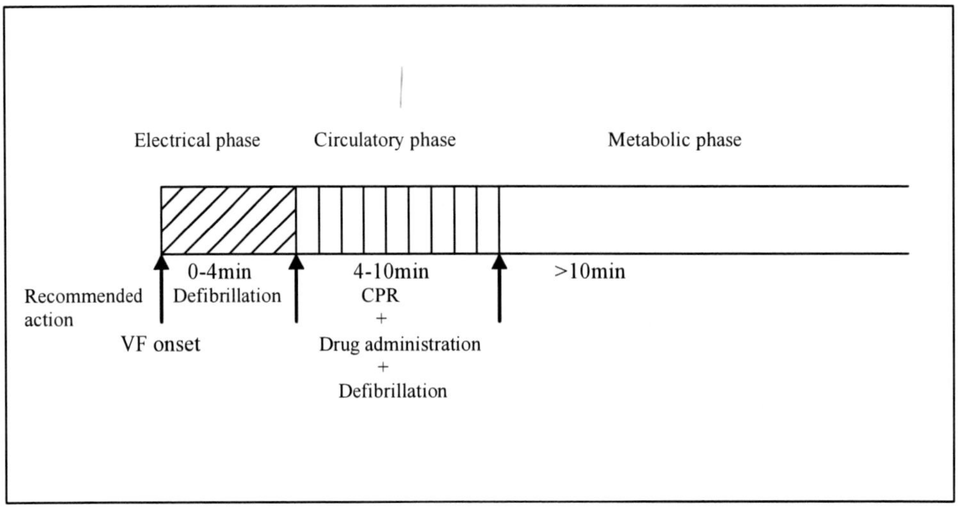


Figure 2. Illustration of the 3-phase VF model.

The second phase of VF arrest, the circulatory phase, lasts approximately from minute 4-5, to minute 10 of cardiac arrest. During this time, immediate electrical defibrillation is typically unsuccessful and reduces the chances of survival [61,96,100-106]. In this period, generation of adequate cerebral and coronary perfusion pressure first, is critical to successful defibrillation and survival without any neurological deficits. During this phase, evidence supports administration of vasopressors with CPR. In fact, even when chest compression are performed by mechanical or high impulse means, vasopressor administration is necessary to elevate CPP higher than the required threshold (20mmHg) to attain ROSC [107-111] and to "coarsen" VF waveform [26,111]. There are indications that this phase can be extended even to 17 min post cardiac arrest with optimal resuscitation techniques (good quality chest compressions, right timing of vasopressor administration), increasing thus the chances of ROSC and meaningful survival [107].

Lastly, the third phase of VF cardiac arrest is the metabolic phase. Prolonged ischemia in association with epinephrine-induced vasoconstriction and endotoxin release in circulation, results in severe organ damage. In this period, resuscitative efforts are rarely successful. This a not thoroughly investigated field of CPR research. Induction of hypothermia [112] or cardiopulmonary bypass [100,113] in these survivors has been shown to improve their outcome.

## Adverse Effects of Epinephrine

After having analyzed the rationale for epinephrine use in CPR and the pathophysiological changes that occur during CA and after ROSC, a further discussion of epinephrine's possible adverse effects in VF setting can be undertaken (Table 1).

**Table 1. Adverse effects of the use of epinephrine in VF cardiac arrest.**

| Adverse effects of Epinephrine |
|---|
| Coronary vasoconstriction |
| Increase in myocardial oxygen consumption |
| Increased ventricular ectopic activity |
| Pulmonary ventilation perfusion defects |
| Increase in defibrillation energy requirements |
| Platelet aggregation |
| Catecholamine oxidation |
| Mast cell degranulation |
| Increase of the severity of post-resuscitation myocardial dysfunction |

## Coronary Vasoconstriction

The indiscriminate α and β-adrenoreceptor activation by epinephrine may result in both vasoconstriction (α-adrenoreceptors) and vasodilation (β-adrenoreceptors). However, in cardiac arrest setting the overwhelming endogenous epinephrine release in association with exogenous epinephrine administration result in intense vasoconstriction and most importantly, in coronary vasoconstriction (induced by both $\alpha_1$ and $\alpha_2$ adrenoreceptor activation), further reducing thus the blood supply to the myocardium [28,53-57,114-117].

## Increase in Myocardial Oxygen Consumption

The aforementioned vasoconstrictive effects lead to a further increase of oxygen demands of an already dramatically fasting myocardium. This situation is further aggravated by the cardiac $a_1$ and $\beta_1$-adrenoreceptor activation that mediate for positive inotropic and chronotropic effects raising even more myocardial oxygen demands and worsening ischemia [42,47,49-51,116].

## Increased Ventricular Ectopic Activity

Epinephrine acts by increasing myocardial oxygen demands leading to myocardial ATP depletion [42,62]. ATP depletion in turn, impairs the function of $Na^+$-$K^+$ ATPase causing a prolongation of the action potential duration and by consequence impairs the ability of myocytes to repolarize in synchrony accentuating thus ventricular ectopic activity [36,42,50,118-120]. Moreover, epinephrine increases myocardiac lactate levels, that can also contribute to arrhythmogenesis [36,42,69]. Furthermore, $\beta_2$-adrenoreceptor activation has been proven to be inducing hypokalaemia [28] which can result to severe arrhythmias. These actions increase the possibility of VF recurrence.

## Pulmonary Ventilation Perfusion Defects

In cardiac arrest, global ischemia results in hypoxia. As a natural response, hypoxic vasoconstriction develops in hypoperfused lung regions in order to redirect blood flow to better ventilated regions of the lung as an attempt to increase oxygen delivery. β-Adrenoreceptor activation by epinephrine causes generalized bronchodilation and vasodilation reversing thus this compensatory mechanism [121]. This effect causes arterial oxygen desaturation and decreases end-tidal $CO_2$ tension [122-126] and may lead to an increase of the intrapulmonary shunting by 30% [127].

## Increase in Defibrillation Energy Requirements

$\beta_1$-Adrenoreceptor activation leads to positive inotropic and chronotropic action, stimulating exhausted myocytes to depolarize, a fact that increases defibrillation energy requirements [25,47,48].

## Platelet Aggregation

It is well known that $\alpha_2$-adrenoreceptor stimulation induces platelet aggregation that in turn initiates the blood clotting cascade [128,129]. Given the fact that VF cardiac arrest usually occurs after a myocardial infarction (MI), it is at least contradictory to administrate an agent with prothrombotic actions in order to save the victim's life. The fact that the majority of MI patients will receive thrombolytic drugs does not justify at any case the use of a vasopressor with even a moderate prothrombotic action.

## Catecholamine Oxidation

Oxidation of catecholamines leads to a further increase of the already high levels of free radicals causing peroxidation of the phospholipids of the myocytes' cell membrane disrupting hence its structure and increasing its permeability leading to cell death [28].

## Mast Cell Degranulation

Mast cells have also $\alpha_1$-adrenoreceptors and their stimulation provokes release of mast cell peroxidase which is cytotoxic. This effect occurs naturally during ischemia and it is further enhanced by exogenous epinephrine administration [130].

### Increase of the Severity of Post-Resuscitation Myocardial Dysfunction

All the aforementioned epinephrine's adverse effects affect not only ROSC, but also meaningful survival because the lead to the previously described post-resuscitation myocardial dysfunction. Both animal and human data directly correlate (as an independent factor) epinephrine administration with that clinical entity and suggest that epinephrine may contribute to its genesis more than reperfusion injury does [42,50,62,79,84,131]. Arrhythmias, VF recurrence, low ejection fraction (epinephrine has been found to be an independent factor) [47,79] are the aspects of this devastating feature which minimizes hospital discharge rates.

## Factors Influencing Epinephrine's Effectiveness

### Epinephrine's Activity in VF Setting

Obviously, human organism's status during VF varies considerably from that during normal circumstances. It is therefore logical that the different conditions may affect epinephrine's activity. Firstly, during cardiac arrest the human organism is under severe (especially if the arrest is prolonged) acidosis [61,62]. Epinephrine is not resistant to the effects of acidosis [62]; hence its effectiveness may be reduced, leading to the false need of multiple repetitive doses when it is established that the cumulative dose of epinephrine is an independent predictor of poor neurological outcome [30,132,133].

### Receptor Desensitization

As mentioned above, catecholamine levels in VF setting are extremely elevated and the adrenoreceptors are possibly already maximally stimulated before vasopressor administration [46]. There is evidence that receptor desensitization [134,135] and/or down regulation [136] occurs under these conditions. Therefore, the real extent of epinephrine's activity is not really known.

### CPR Quality

In cardiac arrest victims, CPR is performed in order to restore critical blood flow [1,137,138]. This is achieved by chest compressions. There are 2 proposed mechanisms as to how chest compressions work. According to the "cardiac pump theory", active compression of the ventricles leads to closure of the atrioventricular valves ejecting thus, blood into the aorta and the pulmonary artery. The "thoracic pump theory" advocates that chest compressions increase intrathoracic pressure which creates a blood flow from the thorax to peripheral circulation and also leads to an increase in venous return by compressing the thoracic vena cava and pulmonary vein [139]. It is to be noted that these 2 theories are not mutually exclusive.

In order for any drug to act during cardiac arrest, a simple injection is not sufficient. Drug circulation and distribution is absolutely dependent upon CPR generated blood flow. Quickly interrupted or inadequate chest compressions severely limit any pharmacologic agent's circulation; hence, efficacy. Recent literature has addressed the issue of chest compressions quality. Evidence indicates that optimal CPR, both in out-of hospital and in-hospital cardiac arrest setting, does not occur often [140-144]. Too often, chest compressions are performed only for a small amount (down to only 50%) of CPR time; they are too shallow and rescue breaths attempts last too long (up to 16seconds) annihilating during this period myocardial and cerebral perfusion [143,145-147]. Furthermore, in experimental conditions simulating clinical CPR it has been found that epinephrine administration did not result in hemodynamic improvement in contrast to when administered under optimal CPR [39]. In addition to the above, it is well established that early bystander CPR significantly improves survival [2,91,148]. However, only 20%-25% [137,148-153] of patients with out-of hospital cardiac arrest receive early bystander CPR, with a further deterioration of acidotic conditions under which epinephrine is supposed to act.

### Time to Drug Administration

Whereas according to the time-dependent 3-phase VF model, epinephrine is supposed to be administered during the circulatory phase of cardiac arrest, meaning between min 4 and min 10 post cardiac arrest; this, according to clinical data almost never occurs. In fact, various clinical trials report average times to first drug administration ranging from 15 to more than 21 minutes after cardiac arrest [2,3,6,7,96,108,154-157]. Even when optimal CPR is performed and the circulatory phase may be extended to 17 min post cardiac arrest [107]; still, in most of the studies, drugs are not administered during this period. In addition to all that, it has to be noted that these intervals do not include the time elapsed between cardiac arrest incidence and emergency medical services (EMS) dispatch. In best-case scenario, with bystander-witnessed cardiac arrest, this interval has been estimated to range from 1 to 4 min [9,158-161]. Of course, when the arrest is un-witnessed, the time to EMS dispatch is probably much longer. If the times of EMS dispatch and time to drug administration are added, it easily occurs that epinephrine is administered well into the metabolic phase where the possibilities of successful resuscitation are minimal.

## Epinephrine's Dose

The recommended dose for epinephrine by both AHA and ERC is 0.014mg/kg (1mg for a 70kg adult) every 3 to 5 min during cardiac arrest [1,29]. In the previous years research was also oriented towards the appropriate epinephrine dosage. Although the accurate dose is not yet known [1,29], it has become evident by both animal [37,162] and clinical data [3,27,103,131,163-166] that high doses of epinephrine (up to 0.2mg/kg) may further increase CPP, but fail to improve long-term survival and neurological outcome. Furthermore, high doses of epinephrine seem to increase in-hospital mortality [3,27] and its cumulative dose is an independent predictor of poor neurological outcome [30,132,133]. Therefore, high doses of epinephrine are no longer recommended [1,29].

# Epinephrine in CPR Research

## Epinephrine vs Placebo

There are no placebo-controlled trials showing that the use of any vasopressor at any stage of cardiac arrest improves the rates of meaningful survival. On the other hand, there is evidence that their use improves ROSC rates [29]. There are however retrospective clinical studies comparing the outcome of patients who received epinephrine, with patients who did not. Two relatively large (1360 and 10.996 patients) studies from Sweden [30,31], failed to prove any change in survival to hospital discharge of patients treated with epinephrine in comparison with patients who had not received epinephrine. Furthermore, in the larger of the 2 studies [31] the use of epinephrine was found to be independently correlated with poor survival. It has to be noted though, that these studies were retrospective and non-randomized. Another study in Australia also found no difference in survival between those treated and those who were not treated with epinephrine [32]. The most close to a placebo-controlled trial, is a recent prospective before-after clinical study involving 1296 non-trauma cardiac arrest patients in Singapore [5]. It examined the results before and after epinephrine introduction in an EMS system that did not previously used medications in pre-hospital CA setting. The researchers found no difference to ROSC, survival to hospital admission or to hospital discharge rates before and after epinephrine introduction. There was however a trend (although not statistically significant due to sample size) in the subgroup analysis to suggest that epinephrine may improve survival in patients with EMS response times up to 8 min and patients presenting with VF. Nevertheless, this study was limited by the fact that it examined only the effect of a single epinephrine dose, as no repetitive dose was permitted until arrival to a hospital.

# Alternative Pharmacologic Agents

CPR research on vasoactive agents is in progress for several years and has explored various possible alternatives (Table 2).

**Table 2. Pharmacologic agents investigated in CPR research.**

| Alternative agents | Alternative combinations |
|---|---|
| Vasopressin | Epinephrine + vasopressin |
| New α2-agonists | Epinephrine + β-blockers |
| A-methylnorepinephrine | Epinephrine + cariporide |
| norepinephrine | Epinephrine + levosimendan |
| | Epinephrine + Vasopressin + Nitroglycerin |

## Vasopressin

Vasopressin is an endogenous peptide; a natural antidiuretic hormone. It is a potent vasopressor, stimulating (via $V_1$ receptors) vascular contraction in skeletal muscles, small bowel, fat tissue skin and kidneys [167-169]. In contrast to epinephrine it is resistant to acidosis [62,170] and has a more sustained action [36,46,171]. Furthermore, endogenous vasopressin levels were significantly higher in successfully resuscitated patients than in patients who died [132]. Research on vasopressin occupies a large part of CPR research, it has provided encouraging, but ambiguous as all vasopressors results, and its use is still under great debate. Vasopressin is the only alternative vasopressor recommended by AHA as a 40IU single dose that can replace the first or second dose of epinephrine during cardiac arrest advanced life support [29]. On the other hand ERC does not recommend vasopressin stating that "there is currently insufficient evidence to support or refute the use of vasopressin as an alternative to, or in combination with adrenaline (epinephrine) in any cardiac arrest rhythm" [1].

## Vasopressin vs Epinephrine in Animal Studies

Early animal studies on this promising agent indicated improvement in hemodynamic variables [172-174], survival [171,175,176] and neurologic outcome, even in models of prolonged cardiac arrest [177]. In a porcine CPR model comparing the effects of repeated vasopressor doses, each vasopressin administration resulted in CPP increase whereas this was observed only after the first of three epinephrine injections [171]. In another laboratory CPR model, no differences were observed in histological brain sections from animals successfully resuscitated with either vasopressin or epinephrine [178]. Lastly, a meta-analysis of human and animal trials comparing vasopressin to epinephrine or placebo, found in 33 animal trials that vasopressin was superior regarding ROSC, to both epinephrine and placebo [179]. However, there is confounding evidence about the full extent of vasopressin's actions. A post-resuscitation two-fold increase in systemic vascular resistance has been found in swine [180] fact that may deteriorate post-resuscitation myocardial dysfunction.

## Vasopressin vs Epinephrine in Clinical Studies

In 1996, based on animal data, 40IU of vasopressin were administered to 8 adults with refractory cardiac arrest. All patients attained ROSC and 3 of them attained neurologically intact hospital discharge [170]. In a later, small out-of hospital VF cardiac arrest randomized trial, both ROSC and 24 hour survival rates were significantly higher for those treated with vasopressin [181]. Two larger randomized studies for in-hospital [182] and out-of hospital cardiac arrest [183] failed to show an overall increase in ROSC or survival rates of patients treated with vasopressin as the initial vasopressor, in comparison with those treated with epinephrine. However, a subgroup analysis in this last study [183] showed that the successive administration of vasopressin and epinephrine in patients with refractory cardiac arrest improved significantly survival rates to hospital discharge. A systematic review and meta-analysis [184] of 1519 patients with cardiac arrest from 5 randomized controlled trials demonstrated that there is no clear advantage of vasopressin over epinephrine for ROSC, death within 24 hours or death before hospital discharge, regardless the rhythm of cardiac arrest (VF, asystole, pulseless electrical activity). Lastly, a review [157] of 3 high-quality well-reported randomized trials and 1 data meta-analysis, did not find any evidence that establish a benefit of vasopressin over epinephrine neither in survival to discharge nor to neurologic outcomes.

### Vasopressin Combined with Epinephrine vs Epinephrine Alone

There is evidence that when ischemia and advance cardiac life support efforts are prolonged, the combination of epinephrine and vasopressin may be beneficial [183,185-189]. Furthermore, the $V_2$ receptor-mediated vasodilatory effect of vasopressin may attenuate the hypoperfusion resulting from multiple doses of epinephrine [46]. Experimental models have shown a more rapid [190] and significant rise in CPP [189] and increased left ventricular myocardial blood flow during CPR [191]. A relatively large single-center clinical study (598 patients) [122] demonstrated an improve in both ROSC, ROSC and hospital admission, and 24 hour survival rates in patients treated with a combination vasopressin and epinephrine in comparison to patients treated with epinephrine alone. However, it did not show any difference in hospital discharge between the 2 groups. In subgroup analysis, there was a difference found in hospital discharge rates only in patients with asystole treated with the 2 drug combination. Finally, the largest up to date multi-center randomized study (1442 patients) found no difference between the vasopressin-epinephrine group and the epinephrine-only group in ROSC, survival to hospital admission, survival to hospital discharge, 1-year survival or good neurologic recovery at hospital discharge [2].

## Adrenergic Agents

### Selective α 2-adrenoreceptor Agonists

The indiscriminate α and β action of epinephrine has some serious adverse effects which are principally mediated by $\alpha_1$ and β adrenoreceptor activation leading to increase of oxygen consumption, increase of defibrillation energy requirements and increase of the severity of post-resuscitation myocardial dysfunction [36,46,62,191,192]. Epinephrine's beneficial effects are though to be $\alpha_2$ mediated (based on the false assumption that there are no $\alpha_2$-adrenoreceptors in the myocardium); therefore the possibility that a vasopressor with only $\alpha_2$ action could be beneficial in CPR was investigated. In fact, an animal CPR study indicated that eventhough combined $\alpha_1$ and β-adrenergic blockade (prazosin plus propranolol plus epinephrine) in comparison to epinephrine administration alone had no difference in ROSC rates, on the other hand improved significantly post-resuscitation cardiac and neurological recovery without however achieving any improvement in 72 hour survival [36]. Moreover, the administration of carvedilol an antagonist of $\alpha_1$, $\beta_1$ and $\beta_2$-adrenoreceptors prior to epinephrine treatment, significantly improved survival and both myocardial and neurological function [28]. On the other hand, there are limitations in their use, as most currently used $\alpha_2$-

adrenoreceptor agonists such as clonidine, cross the blood brain barrier, activate $\alpha_{2A}$ and $\alpha_{2C}$ adrenoreceptors inducing vasodilation that overcomes the vasoconstrictor effect of $\alpha_{2B}$ adrenoreceptors causing thus a paradoxical fall in blood pressure. Furthermore, the existence of $\alpha_2$-adrenoreceptors in coronary arterioles leads to vasoconstriction, which has detrimental effects on ROSC and survival [53-58].

## α-Methylnorepinephrine (α -MNE)

α-MNE, a supposedly selective $\alpha_2$-adrenoreceptor agonist, has given some promising results in animal studies and there are indications that it does not cross the blood brain barrier [193,194]. In an experimental study of VF cardiac arrest, epinephrine and α-MNE were equally effective in restoring ROSC. However, post-resuscitation heart rate increased by 38% for epinephrine and only by 15% for α-MNE respectively. Furthermore, ejection fraction was reduced by 35% and 14% respectively ($p<0.01$) causing thus a lesser myocardial injury [47]. Another animal study comparing α-MNE, epinephrine and vasopressin in VF cardiac arrest demonstrated significantly better post-resuscitation myocardial function and survival in animals treated with α-MNE [195]. There are no clinical trials assessing the role of α-MNE in VF setting. A small clinical trial in healthy adults however demonstrated that no vasoconstrictor effect was evident until β-adrenoreceptor blockade was performed; suggesting thus that α-MNE probably is not a selective $\alpha_2$-adrenoreceptor agonist [196].

## Norepinephrine

There is only one randomized clinical trial comparing norepinephrine with standard-dose and high-dose epinephrine. However, a non-significant trend towards higher rates of ROSC but worse neurological outcome has been shown [197]. Combination therapies aiming to ameliorate epinephrine's adverse effects.

## Epinephrine and β-Blockers

A large part of epinephrine's adverse effects during resuscitation is attributed to β-adrenergic stimulation which increases the severity of post-resuscitation myocardial dysfunction [25,42,48]. It is therefore logical to investigate the effects of epinephrine and β-blocker combination. Several animal studies have shown that addition of a β-blocker (esmolol, propranolol, atenolol) to epinephrine significantly improves ROSC and survival rates and minimizes post-resuscitation myocardial dysfunction [59,198-200]. There are no clinical trials involving β-blocker use in CPR and the fact that a large proportion of patients susceptible to cardiac arrest already is under β-blocker treatment makes these pharmacologic agents warranting further investigation.

### Epinephrine Combined with Vasopressin and Nitroglycerin

Nitroglycerin is a well-known potent vasodilator agent with a pronounced effect on coronary arteries. Thus, it has been used since many years for patients suffering from angina pectoris and/or myocardial infarction [201-204]. Two animal studies have shown that although triple therapy did not significantly improve ROSC rates it did however improve CPP and vital organ blood flow during CPR. A major limitation of these studies was the selection of the appropriate dose for each agent and especially for nitroglycerine, for which relevant data form CPR research is extremely limited [191,204].

### Epinephrine Combined with Cariporide

Cariporide inhibits the sarcolemmal sodium-hydrogen exchanger isoform-1 (NHE-1) [41] fact that may lead to attenuation of the ischemic contracture developing under prolonged ischemia [205,206]. An amelioration of ischemic contracture renders chest compressions more effective. It seems that its effects are not exerted on vascular beds, but only to myocytes [41]. Administration of cariporide in addition to epinephrine in animal trials has resulted in less ectopic activity, improved hemodynamic function and survival rates [41,207-209].

### Epinephrine Combined with Levosimendan

Levosimendan is a nonadrenergic inotropic calcium sensitizer that enhances myocardial contractility without affecting intracellular calcium. It also mediates for activation of the ATP-dependent potassium channels and reduces the accumulated potassium into the myocytes during ischemia, exerting thus a cardioprotective effect [210,211]. The results from laboratory trials indicate that it can improve survival and ameliorate post-resuscitation myocardial dysfunction [212,213]. However, as with all previously mentioned agents, a large amount of data is still missing before its inclusion in clinical CPR trials.

## Causes of Discrepancies between Laboratory and Clinical Trials in CPR

There is still a great amount of research for the aforementioned agents (with the exception of vasopressin) in order to be considered for involvement in clinical trials. However, the number of agents investigated in animal or ex-vivo trials is indicative of the insufficiency of the currently recommended agent, epinephrine. Furthermore, pharmacologic agents or drug combinations that seem promising in experimental settings, more than often prove disappointing in clinical conditions. The reasons for the discrepancies between laboratory and clinical research are so various and interlaid, that the situation caused resembles to a multifactorial disease.

### Laboratory CPR and Manual CPR

An important factor hindering the exclusion of safe conclusions about epinephrine's (and any other drug's) efficacy during CPR, is the inability to compare the quality of chest compressions performed in clinical and laboratory CPR setting. In laboratory CPR chest compressions are highly standardized, performed by mechanical means [45,107,108,189] whereas in clinical setting manual chest compressions are usually of poor quality [143,144] limiting thus the circulation of drugs and their efficacy. Furthermore, poor quality CPR leads to lower CPP leading in turn to decreased chances of survival and further limiting the researcher's ability to estimate the impact of drug administration.

### Time and Route of Epinephrine Administration

Proper timing of drug administration is crucial for resuscitation success. Almost in all laboratory trials drugs are administered in an early phase of VF leading thus to higher chances of ROSC. As a large literature review covering a 17-year period demonstrated, mean time to first drug administration in animal studies was 9.5 min, whereas time reported in clinical trials was significantly higher attaining 19.4 min [108]. Hence, in laboratory conditions drugs are administered in the circulatory VF phase (where they have more chances to be successful) whereas in clinical setting drugs are administered well into the metabolic VF phase, where any intervention has minimal chances of success. Furthermore in animal studies drugs are usually administered via a central vein [22,36,41,191,195] attaining thus circulation easily, whereas in clinical setting drugs are delivered via a peripheral vein under conditions of hypoperfusion.

### Subjects' Health Status

Most of laboratory trials are performed on young healthy animals. On the other side, in clinical setting, human CA victims are older and have various co-morbidities for which they often take several medications that could possibly interact with the drugs administered.

### End Points in CPR Trials

Although it is necessary for laboratory studies to respond to certain mechanistic questions, the percentage of these studies examining neurologically intact (the ultimate aim of resuscitative efforts) survival is very low [28,108].

## Conclusion

Despite the discrepancies between laboratory and clinical CPR research, it is evident that epinephrine is not the ideal vasopressor for CPR. If epinephrine was a newly discovered agent, probably it would not have been incorporated to current resuscitation guidelines. It is an agent resembling to a double-edged sword with potent vasoconstrictive properties essential for ROSC on one side and deleterious adverse effects affecting survival on the other side. However, in clinical trials no other agent has been found to be more effective, leaving epinephrine in the place of drug of choice for more than a century.

Lastly, before addressing the matter of the proper drug for CPR, the issues of chest compression quality and time of drug administration should be primarily resolved in order to produce scientific results that can be translated into clinical practice. Improvements on resuscitation protocols and in EMS response times will have a positive impact on thousands of lives. CPR research has to work simultaneously on 2 directions: new pharmacologic agents and new strategies to face VF cardiac arrest.

## References

[1] Nolan, JP; Deakin, CD; Soar, J; Bottiger, BW; Smith, G. European Resuscitation Council Guidelines for Resuscitation 2005. Section 4. Adult advanced life support. *Resuscitation*, 2005, 67, S39-S86

[2] Gueugniaud, PY; David, JS; Chanzy, E; Hubert, H; Dubien, PY; Mauriaucourt, P; Bragança, C; Billères, X; Clotteau-Lambert, MP; Fuster, P; Thiercelin, D; Debaty, G; Ricard-Hibon, A; Roux, P; Espesson, C; Querellou, E; Ducros, L; Ecollan, P; Halbout, L; Savary, D; Guillaumée, F; Maupoint, R; Capelle, P; Bracq, C; Dreyfus, P; Nouguier, P; Gache, A; Meurisse, C; Boulanger, B; Lae, C; Metzger, J; Raphael, V; Beruben, A; Wenzel, V; Guinhouya, C; Vilhelm, C; Marret, E. Vasopressin and epinephrine vs. epinephrine alone in cardiopulmonary resuscitation. *N Engl J Med.*, 2008, 359, 21-30.

[3] Gueugniaud, PY; Mols, P; Goldstein, P; Pham, E; Dubien, PY; Deweerdt, C; Vergnion, M; Petit, P; Carli, P. A comparison of repeated high doses and repeated standard doses of epinephrine for cardiac arrest outside the hospital. European Epinephrine Study Group. *N Engl J Med.*, 1998, 339, 1595-1601.

[4] Bobrow, BJ; Clark, LL; Ewy, GA; Chikani, V; Sanders, AB; Berg, RA; Richman, PB; Kern, KB. Minimally interrupted cardiac resuscitation by emergency medical services for out-of-hospital cardiac arrest. *JAMA*, 2008, 299, 1158-1165.

[5] Ong, ME; Tan, EH; Ng, FS; Panchalingham, A; Lim, SH; Manning, PG; Ong, VY; Lim, SH; Yap, S; Tham, LP; Ng, KS; Venkataraman, A. Cardiac Arrest and Resuscitation Epidemiology Study Group. Survival outcomes with the introduction of intravenous epinephrine in the management of out-of-hospital cardiac arrest. *Ann Emerg Med.*, 2007, 50, 635-642.

[6] Haukoos, JS; Lewis, RJ; Niemann, JT. Prediction rules for estimating neurologic outcome following out-of-hospital cardiac arrest. *Resuscitation.*, 2004, 63, 145-155.

[7] Stiell, IG; Wells, GA; Field, B; Spaite, DW; Nesbitt, LP; De Maio, VJ; Nichol, G; Cousineau, D; Blackburn, J; Munkley, D; Luinstra-Toohey, L; Campeau, T; Dagnone, E; Lyver, M. Ontario Prehospital Advanced Life Support Study Group. Advanced cardiac life support in out-of-hospital cardiac arrest. *N Engl J Med.*, 2004, 351, 647-656.

[8] Eckstein, M; Stratton, SJ; Chan, LS. Cardiac Arrest Resuscitation Evaluation in Los Angeles: CARE-LA. *Ann Emerg Med.*, 2005, 45, 504-509.

[9] Herlitz, J; Engdahl, J; Svensson, L; Angquist, KA; Young, M; Holmberg, S. Factors associated with an increased chance of survival among patients suffering from an out of-hospital cardiac arrest in a national perspective in Sweden. *Am Heart J.*, 2005, 149, 61-66.

[10] Becker, LB; Ostrander, MP; Barrett, J; Kondos, GT. Outcome of CPR in a large metropolitan area--where are the survivors? *Ann Emerg Med.*, 1991, 20, 355-361.

[11] van Walraven, C; Stiell, IG; Wells, GA; Hébert, PC; Vandemheen, K. Do advanced cardiac life support drugs increase resuscitation rates from in-hospital cardiac arrest? The OTAC Study Group. *Ann Emerg Med.*, 1998, 32, 544-553.

[12] Peberdy, MA; Kaye, W; Ornato, JP; Larkin, GL; Nadkarni, V; Mancini, ME; Berg, RA; Nichol, G; Lane-Trultt, T. Cardiopulmonary resuscitation of adults in the hospital: a report of 14720 cardiac arrests from the National Registry of Cardiopulmonary Resuscitation. *Resuscitation.*, 2003, 58, 297-308

[13] Cooper, S; Janghorbani, M; Cooper, G. A decade of in-hospital resuscitation: outcomes and prediction of survival? *Resuscitation.*, 2006 Feb, 68, 231-237.

[14] Faddy, SC; Powell, J; Craig, JC. Biphasic and monophasic shocks for transthoracic defibrillation: a meta analysis of randomised controlled trials. *Resuscitation.*, 2003, 58, 9-16.

[15] Cobb, LA; Fahrenbruch, CE; Olsufka, M; Copass, MK. Changing incidence of out-of-hospital ventricular fibrillation 1980-2000. *JAMA*, 2002, 288, 3008-3013

[16] Rea, TD; Eisenberg, MS; Sinibaldi, G; White, RD. Incidence of EMS-treated out-of-hospital cardiac arrest in the United States. *Resuscitation*, 2004, 63, 17-24

[17] Vaillancourt, C; Stiell, IG. Cardiac arrest care and emergency medical services in Canada. *Can J Cardiol*, 2004, 20, 1081-1090.

[18] Waalewijn, RA; de Vos, R; Koster, RW. Out-of-hospital cardiac arrests in Amsterdam and its surrounding areas: results from the Amsterdam resuscitation study (ARREST) in 'Utstein' style. *Resuscitation*, 1998, 38, 157-167.

[19] Cummins, R; Thies, W. Automated external defibrillators and the Advanced Cardiac Life Support Program: a new initiative from the American Heart Association. *Am J Emerg Med*, 1991, 9, 91-93.

[20] Waalewijn, RA; Nijpels, MA; Tijssen, JG; Koster, RW. Prevention of deterioration of ventricular fibrillation by basic life support during out-of-hospital cardiac arrest. *Resuscitation*, 2002, 54, 31-36.

[21] Paradis, NA; Martin, GB; Rivers, EP; Goetting, MG; Appleton, TJ; Feingold, M; Nowak, RM. Coronary perfusion pressure and the return of spontaneous circulation in human cardiopulmonary resuscitation. *JAMA.*, 1990, 263, 1106-1113.

[22] Meybohm, P; Cavus, E; Dörges, V; Steinfath, M; Sibbert, L; Wenzel, V; Scholz, J; Bein, B. Revised resuscitation guidelines: adrenaline versus adrenaline/vasopressin in a pig model of cardiopulmonary resuscitation-a randomised, controlled trial. *Resuscitation*, 2007, 75, 380-388.

[23] Gazmuri, RJ; von Planta, M; Weil, MH; Rackow, EC. Arterial PCO2 as an indicator of systemic perfusion during cardiopulmonary resuscitation. *Crit Care Med.*, 1989, 17, 237-240.

[24] Duggal, C; Weil, MH; Gazmuri, RJ; Tang, W; Sun, S; O'Connell, F; Ali, M. Regional blood flow during closed-chest cardiac resuscitation in rats. *J Appl Physiol.*, 1993, 74, 147-152.

[25] Huang, L; Tang, W. Vasopressor agents: old and new components. *Curr Opin Crit Care.*, 2004, 10, 183-187.

[26] Betz, AE; Menegazzi, JJ; Logue, ES; Callaway, CW; Wang, HE. A randomized comparison of manual, mechanical and high-impulse chest compression in a porcine model of prolonged ventricular fibrillation. *Resuscitation.*, 2006, 69, 495-501.

[27] Nolan, JP; Dc Latorre, FJ; Steen, PA; Chamberlain, DA; Bossaert, LL. Advanced life support drugs: do they really work? *Curr Opin Crit Care*. 2002, 8, 212-818.

[28] Penson, PE; Ford, WR; Broadley, KJ. Vasopressors for cardiopulmonary resuscitation. Does pharmacological evidence support clinical practice? *Pharmacol Ther.*, 2007, 115, 37-55.

[29] Anonymous. Part 7.2: Management of Cardiac Arrest. *Circulation*, 2005, 112, IV58-IV66.

[30] Herlitz, J; Ekström, L; Wennerblom, B; Axelsson, A; Bång, A; Holmberg, S. Adrenaline in out-of-hospital ventricular fibrillation. Does it make any difference? *Resuscitation.*, 1995, 29, 195-201.

[31] Holmberg, M; Holmberg, S; Herlitz, J. Low chance of survival among patients requiring adrenaline (epinephrine) or intubation after out-of-hospital cardiac arrest in Sweden. *Resuscitation.*, 2002, 54, 37-45.

[32] Woodhouse, SP; Cox, S; Boyd, P; Case, C; Weber, M. High dose and standard dose adrenaline do not alter survival, compared with placebo, in cardiac arrest. *Resuscitation.*, 1995, 30, 243-249.

[33] Olson, DW; Thakur, R; Stueven, HA; Thompson, B; Gruchow, H; Hendley, GE; Hargarten, KM; Aprahamian, C. Randomized study of epinephrine versus methoxamine in prehospital ventricular fibrillation. *Ann Emerg Med.*, 1989, 8, 250-253

[34] Gottlieb, R. Ueber die Wirkung der Nebennieren Extracte auf Herz und Blutdruck. Archiv fur experimentelle Pathologie und Pharmakologie, 1896/97, 38, 99-112

[35] Anonymous. Standards for cardiopulmonary resuscitation (CPR) and emergency cardiac care (ECC). 3. Advanced life support. *JAMA.*, 1974, 227(suppl), 852-860.

[36] Pellis, T; Weil, MH; Tang, W; Sun, S; Xie, J; Song, L; Checchia, P. Evidence favoring the use of an alpha2-selective vasopressor agent for cardiopulmonary resuscitation. *Circulation.*, 2003, 108, 2716-2721.

[37] Cairns, CB; Niemann, JT. Hemodynamic effects of repeated doses of epinephrine after prolonged cardiac arrest and CPR: preliminary observations in an animal model. *Resuscitation*, 1998, 36, 181-185

[38] Michael, JR; Guerci, AD; Koehler, RC; Shi, AY; Tsitlik, J; Chandra, N; Niedermeyer, E; Rogers, MC; Traystman, RJ; Weisfeldt, ML. Mechanisms by which epinephrine augments cerebral and myocardial perfusion during cardiopulmonary resuscitation in dogs. *Circulation*, 1984, 69, 822-835.

[39] Pytte, M; Kramer-Johansen, J; Eilevstjønn, J; Eriksen, M; Strømme, TA; Godang, K; Wik, L; Steen, PA; Sunde, K. Haemodynamic effects of adrenaline (epinephrine) depend on chest compression quality during cardiopulmonary resuscitation in pigs. *Resuscitation.*, 2006, 71, 369-378.

[40] Brown, CG; Werman, HA; Davis, EA; Hobson, J; Hamlin, RL. The effects of graded doses of epinephrine on regional myocardial blood flow during cardiopulmonary resuscitation in swine. *Circulation.*, 1987, 75, 491-497.
[41] Kolarova, J; Yi, Z; Ayoub, IM; Gazmuri, RJ. Cariporide potentiates the effects of epinephrine and vasopressin by nonvascular mechanisms during closed-chest resuscitation. *Chest.*, 2005, 127, 1327-1334.
[42] Ditchey, RV; Lindenfeld, J. Failure of epinephrine to improve the balance between myocardial oxygen supply and demand during closed-chest resuscitation in dogs. *Circulation.*, 1988, 78, 382-389.
[43] Lands, AM; Arnold, A; McAuliff, JP; Luduena, FP; Brown, TG. Differentiation of receptor systems activated by sympathomimetic amines. *Jr. Nature.*, 1967, 214, 597-598.
[44] Lands, AM; Luduena, FP; Buzzo, HJ. Differentiation of receptors responsive to isoproterenol. *Life Sci.*, 1967, 6, 2241-2249.
[45] Rittenberger, JC; Suffoletto, B; Salcido, D; Logue, E; Menegazzi, JJ. Increasing CPR duration prior to first defibrillation does not improve return of spontaneous circulation or survival in a swine model of prolonged ventricular fibrillation. *Resuscitation.*, 2008, 79, 155-160.
[46] Zhong, JQ; Dorian, P. Epinephrine and vasopressin during cardiopulmonary resuscitation. *Resuscitation.*, 2005, 66, 263-269.
[47] Klouche, K; Weil, MH; Tang, W; Povoas, H; Kamohara, T; Bisera, J. A selective alpha(2)-adrenergic agonist for cardiac resuscitation. *J Lab Clin Med*, 2002, 140, 27-34
[48] Dorian, P; Wang, MJ. Defibrillation current and impedance are determinants of defibrillation energy requirements. *Pacing Clin Electrophysiol*, 1988, 11, 1996-2001.
[49] Lindner, KH; Ahnefeld, FW; Schuermann, W; Bowdler, IM. Epinephrine and norepinephrine in cardiopulmonary resuscitation. Effects on myocardial oxygen delivery and consumption. *Chest.*, 1990, 97, 1458-1462.
[50] Tang, W; Weil, MH; Sun, SJ; Noc, M; Yang, L; Gazmuri, RJ. Epinephrine increases the severity of postresuscitation myocardial dysfunction. *Circulation*, 1995, 92, 3089-3093.
[51] Monroe, RG; French, G. Ventricular pressure-volume relationships and oxygen consumption in fibrillation and arrest. *Circ Res*, 1960, 8, 260-266
[52] Lefkowitz, RJ. *Neurotransmission: the autonomic and somatic motor nervous system.* In: J. G. Hardman, & L. E. Limbird (Eds.), Goodman and Gilman's, *The Pharmacological Basis of Therapeutics*. 9th ed. New York, NY: McGraw-Hill, 1996. p. 125.
[53] Gregorini, L; Fajadet, J; Robert, G; Cassagneau, B; Bernis, M; Marco, J. Coronary vasoconstriction following percutaneous transluminal coronary angioplasty is attenuated by antiadrenergic agents. *Circulation.*, 1994, 90, 895-907
[54] Gregorini, L; Marco, J; Palombo, C; Kozakova, M; Anguissola, GB; Cassagneau, B; Bernies, M; Distante, A; Marco, I; Fajadet, J; Zanchetti, A. Post-ischemic left ventricular dysfunction is abolished by alpha-adrenergic blocking agents. *J Am Coll Cardiol.*, 1998, 31, 992-1001.
[55] Gregorini, L; Marco, J; Kozàkovà, M; Palombo, C; Anguissola, GB; Marco, I; Bernies, M; Cassagneau, B; Distante, A; Bossi, IM; Fajadet, J; Heusch, G. alpha-adrenergic

blockade improves recovery of myocardial perfusion and function after coronary stenting in patients with acute myocardial infarction. *Circulation.*, 1999, 99, 482-490.

[56] Baumgart, D; Haude, M; Gorge, G; Liu, F; Ge, J; Grosse-Eggebrecht, C; Erbel, R; Heusch, G. Augmented alpha-adrenergic constriction of atherosclerotic human coronary arteries. *Circulation.*, 1999, 99, 2090-2097.

[57] Heusch, G; Baumgart, D; Camici, PG; Chilian, W; Gregorini, L; Hess, O; Indolfi, C; Rimoldi, O. alpha-adrenergic coronary vasoconstriction and myocardial ischemia in man. *Circulation.*, 2000, 10, 689-694.

[58] Gregorini, L; Marco, J; Farah, B; Bernies, M; Palombo, C; Kozàkovà, M; Bossi, IM; Cassagneau, B; Fajadet, J; Di Mario, C; Albiero, R; Cugno, M; Grossi, A; Heusch, G. Effects of selective alpha1- and alpha2-adrenergic blockade on coronary flow reserve after coronary stenting. *Circulation.*, 2002, 106, 2901-2907.

[59] Killingsworth, CR; Wei, CC; Dell'Italia, LJ; Ardell, JL; Kingsley, MA; Smith, WM; Ideker, RE; Walcott, GP. Short-acting β-adrenergic antagonist esmolol given at reperfusion improves survival following prolonged VF. *Circulation*, 2004, 109, 2469-2474.

[60] Niemann, JT; Garner, D. Post-resuscitation plasma catecholamines after prolonged arrest in a swine model. *Resuscitation.*, 2005, 65, 97-101.

[61] Cobb, LA; Fahrenbruch, CE; Walsh, TR; Copass, MK; Olsufka, M; Breskin, M; Hallstrom, AP. Influence of cardiopulmonary resuscitation prior to defibrillation in patients with out-of-hospital ventricular fibrillation. *JAMA.*, 1999, 281, 1182-1188.

[62] Wayne, MA; Racht, EM; Aghababian, RV; Kudenchuk, PJ; Ornato, JP; Slovis, CM. Prehospital management of cardiac arrest: how useful are vasopressor and antiarrhythmic drugs? *Prehosp Emerg Care.*, 2002, 6, 72-80

[63] Karmazyn, M. Amiloride enhances postischemic ventricular recovery: Possible role of Na+/H+ exchange. *Am J Physiol*, 1988, 255, H608-H615

[64] Tani, M; Neely, JR. Role of intracellular Na+ in Ca2+ overload and depressed recovery of ventricular function of reperfused ischemic rat hearts: possible involvement of H+-Na+ and Na+-Ca2+ exchange. *Circ Res*, 1989, 65, 1045-1056

[65] Avkiran, M. Rational basis for use of sodium-hydrogen exchange inhibitors in myocardial ischemia. *Am J Cardiol*, 1999, 83, 10G-17G

[66] Eigel, BN; Hadley, RW. Antisense inhibition of Na+/Ca2+ exchange during anoxia/reoxygenation in ventricular myocytes. *Am J Physiol*, 2001, 281, H2184-H2190

[67] Tang, W; Weil, MH; Sun, SJ; Gazmuri, RJ; Bisera, J. Progressive myocardial dysfunction after cardiac resuscitation. *Crit Care Med.*, 1993, 21, 1046-1050.

[68] Liberthson, RR; Negal, EL; Hirschman, JC; Nussenfeld, SR. Prehospital ventricular defibrillation: prognosis and follow-up course. *N Engl J Med.*, 1974, 291, 317-321.

[69] Brown, CG; Martin, DR; Pepe, P; Smeven, H; Cummins, R; Gonzalez, E; Jastremaki, M. and the Multicenter High-Dose Epinephrine Study Group. A comparison of standard-dose and high-dose epinephrine in cardiac arrest outside the hospital. *N Engl J Med.*, 1992, 327, 1051-1055.

[70] Lewis, CM; Weil, MH. Hemodynamic spectrum of vasopressor and vasodilator drugs. *JAMA.*, 1969, 208, 1391-1398.

[71] Deantonio, HJ; Kaul, S; Lerman, BB. Reversible myocardial depression in survivors of cardiac arrest. *Pacing Clin Electrophysiol*, 1990, 13, 982-985

[72] Xie, J; Weil, MH; Sun, SJ; Tang, W; Sato, Y; Jin, X; Bisera, J. High-energy defibrillation increases the severity of postresuscitation myocardial dysfunction. *Circulation.*, 1997, 96, 683-688.

[73] Tang, W; Weil, MH; Sun, SJ; Yamaguchi, H; Povoas, HP; Pernat, AM; Bisera, J. The effects of biphasic and conventional monophasic defibrillation on postresuscitation myocardial function. *J Am Coll Cardiol.*, 1999, 4, 815-822.

[74] Kern, KB; Hilwig, RW; Rhee, KH; Berg, RA. Myocardial dysfunction after resuscitation from cardiac arrest: an example of global myocardial stunning. *J Am Coll Cardiol.*, 1996, 28, 232-240.

[75] Liberthson, RR; Nagel, EL; Hirschman, JC. Prehospital ventricular defibrillation: Prognosis and follow-up course. *N Engl Med*, 1974, 291, 317-321

[76] Laurent, I; Monchi, M; Chiche, JD; Joly, LM; Spaulding, C; Bourgeois, B; Cariou, A; Rozenberg, A; Carli, P; Weber, S; Dhainaut, JF. Reversible myocardial dysfunction in survivors of out-of-hospital cardiac arrest. *J Am Coll Cardiol*, 2002, 40, 2110-2116

[77] Wang, HE; Min, A; Hostler, D; Chang, CC; Callaway, CW. Differential effects of out-of-hospital interventions on short- and long-term survival after cardiopulmonary arrest. *Resuscitation.*, 2005, 67, 69-74.

[78] Plamer, BS; Hadziahmetovic, M; Veci, T; Angelos, MG. Global ischemic duration and reperfusion function in the isolated perfused rat heart. *Resuscitation*, 2004, 62, 97-106

[79] Chang, WT; Ma, MH; Chien, KL; Huang, CH; Tsai, MS; Shih, FY; Yuan, A; Tsai, KC; Lin, FY; Lee, YT; Chen, WJ. Postresuscitation myocardial dysfunction: correlated factors and prognostic implications. *Intensive Care Med.*, 2007, 33, 88-95.

[80] Gross, ER; Gross, GJ. Ligand triggers of classical preconditioning and postconditioning. *Cardiovasc Res*, 2006, 70, 212–221.

[81] Piper, HM; Abdallah, Y; Schafer, C. The firstminutes of reperfusion: a window of opportunity for cardioprotection. *Cardiovasc Res*, 2004, 61, 365–371

[82] Tang, W; Weil, MH; Sun, S; Pernat, A; Mason, E. $K_{ATP}$ channel activation reduces the severity of post-resuscitation myocardial dysfunction. *Am J Physiol Heart Circ Physiol*, 2000, 279, 1609-1615.

[83] Niemann, JT; Garner, D; Khaleeli, E; Lewis, RJ. Milrinone facilitates resuscitation from cardiac arrest and attenuates post-resuscitation myocardial dysfunction. *Circulation*, 2003, 108, 1032-1036.

[84] Kern, KB; Hilwig, RW; Berg, RA; Rhee, KH; Sanders, AB; Otto, CW; Ewy, GA. Postresuscitation left ventricular systolic and diastolic dysfunction: treatment with dobutamine. *Circulation*, 1997, 95, 2610-2613

[85] Zhao, L; Zhang, W; Zhang, W; Zheng, Y. The effects of high-dose epinephrine combined with isoprenaline on isolated rabbit heart and cardiomyocytes after cardioversion of ventricular fibrillation. *Mol Cell Biochem*, 2000, 207, 71-75

[86] Angelos, MG; Murray, HN; Waite, MD; Gorsline, RT. Postischemic inotropic support of the dysfunctional heart. *Crit Care Med*, 2002, 30, 410-416

[87] Zaugg, CE; Ziegler, A; Lee, RJ; Barbosa, V; Buser, PT. Postresuscitation stunning: postfibrillatory myocardial dysfunction caused by reduced myofilament Ca2+ responsiveness after ventricular fibrillation-induced myocyte Ca2+ overload. *J Cardiovasc Electrophysiol*, 2002, 13, 1017-1024

[88] Tennyson, H; Kern, KB; Hilwig, RW; Berg, RA; Ewy, GA. Treatment of postresuscitation myocardial dysfunction: aortic counterpulsation versus dobutamine. *Resuscitation*, 2002, 54, 69-75
[89] Vasquez, A; Kern, KB; Hilwig, RW; Heidenreich, J; Berg, RA; Ewy, GA. Optimal dosing of dobutamine for treating post-resuscitation left ventricular dysfunction. *Resuscitation*, 2004, 61, 199-207
[90] Weisfeldt, ML; Becker, LB. Resuscitation after cardiac arrest: a 3-phase time-sensitive model. *JAMA*., 2002, 288, 3035-3038.
[91] Ewy, GA; Kern, KB. Recent advances in cardiopulmonary resuscitation: cardiocerebral resuscitation. *J Am Coll Cardiol*., 2009, 53, 149-157.
[92] Mosesso, VN; Davis, EA; Auble, TE; Paris, PM; Yealy, DM. Use of automated external defibrillators by police officers for treatment of out-of-hospital cardiac arrest. *Ann Emerg Med*, 1998, 32, 200-207.
[93] Valenzuela, T; Roe, D; Nichol, G; Clark, LL; Spaite, DW; Hardman, RG. Outcomes of rapid defibrillation by security officers after cardiac arrest in casinos. *N Engl J Med*, 2000, 343, 1206-1209.
[94] O'Rourke, MF; Donaldson, E; Geddes, JS. An airline cardiac arrest program. *Circulation*, 1997, 96, 2849-2853.
[95] Groeneveld, PW; Kwong, JL; Liu, Y; Rodriguez, AJ; Jones, MP; Sanders, GD; Garber, AM. Cost-effectiveness of automated external defibrillators on airlines. *JAMA*, 2001, 286, 1482-1489.
[96] Kern, KB; Valenzuela, TD; Clark, LL; Berg, RA; Hilwig, RW; Berg, MD; Otto, CW; Newburn, D; Ewy, GA. An alternative approach to advancing resuscitation science. *Resuscitation*., 2005, 64, 261-268.
[97] Page, RL; Joglar, JA; Kowal, RC; Zagrodzky, JD; Nelson, LL; Ramaswamy, K; Barbera, SJ; Hamdan, MH; McKenas, DK. Use of automatic external defibrillators by a U.S. airline. *N Engl J Med*., 2000, 343, 1210 -1216.
[98] Caffrey, SL; Willoughby, PJ; Pepe, PE; Becker, LB. Public use of automatic external defibrillators. *N Engl J Med*., 2002, 347, 1242-1247
[99] The Public Access Defibrillation Trial Investigators. Public-access defibrillation and survival after out-of-hospital cardiac arrest. *N Engl J Med*., 2004, 351, 637- 646.
[100] Berg, RA; Hilwig, RW; Kern, KB; Sanders, AB; Xavier, LC; Ewy, GA. Automated external defibrillation versus manual defibrillation for prolonged ventricular fibrillation: lethal delays of chest compressions before and after countershocks. *Ann Emerg Med*., 2003, 42, 458-467.
[101] Eftestol, T; Sunde, K; Steen, PA. Effects of interrupting precordial compressions on the calculated probability of defibrillation success during out-of-hospital cardiac arrest. *Circulation*., 2002, 105, 2270-2273.
[102] Wik, L; Hansen, TB; Fylling, F; Steen, T; Vaagenes, P; Auestad, BH; et al. Delaying defibrillation to give basic cardiopulmonary resuscitation to patients with out-of hospital ventricular fibrillation: a randomized trial. *J Am Med Assoc*, 2003, 289, 1389-1395.
[103] Niemann, JT; Cairns, CB; Sharma, J; Lewis, FJ. Treatment of prolonged ventricular fibrillation, immediate countershock versus high-dose epinephrine and CPR preceding countershock. *Circulation*, 1992, 85, 281-287.

[104] Menegazzi, JJ; Davis, EA; Yealy, DM; Molner, RL; Nicklas, KA; Hosack, GM; Honingford, EA; Klain, MM. An experimental algorithm versus standard advanced cardiac life support in a swine model of out-of-hospital cardiac arrest. *Ann Emerg Med*, 1993, 22, 235-239.

[105] Menegazzi, JJ; Seaberg, DC; Yealy, DM; Davis, EA; MacLeod, BA. Combination pharmacotherapy with delayed countershock vs. standard advanced cardiac life support after prolonged ventricular fibrillation. *Prehospit Emerg Care*, 2000, 4, 31-37.

[106] Seaberg, DC; Menegazzi, JJ; Check, MacLeod, BA; Yealy, DM. Use of a cardiocerebral-protective drug cocktail prior to countershock in a porcine model of prolonged ventricular fibrillation. *Resuscitation*, 2001, 51, 301-308.

[107] Rittenberger, JC; Menegazzi, JJ; Callaway, CW. Association of delay to first intervention with return of spontaneous circulation in a swine model of cardiac arrest. *Resuscitation*., 2007, 73, 154-160.

[108] Reynolds, JC; Rittenberger, JC; Menegazzi, JJ. Drug administration in animal studies of cardiac arrest does not reflect human clinical experience. *Resuscitation*., 2007, 74, 13-26.

[109] Menegazzi, JJ; Wang, HE; Lightfoot, CB; Fertig, KC; Chengelis, NL; Sherman, LD; Callaway, CW. Immediate defibrillation versus interventions first in a swine model of prolonged ventricular fibrillation. *Resuscitation*, 2003, 59, 261-270.

[110] Wang, HE; Menegazzi, JJ; Lightfoot, CB; Callaway, CW; Fertig, KC; Sherman, LD; Hsieh, M. Effects of biphasic vs. monophasic defibrillation on the scaling exponent in a swine model of prolonged ventricular fibrillation. *Acad Emerg Med*, 2001, 8, 771-780.

[111] Menegazzi, JJ; Callaway, CW; Sherman, LD; Hostler, DP; Wang, HE; Fertig, KC; Logue, ES. Ventricular fibrillation scaling exponent can guide timing of defibrillation and other therapies. *Circulation*., 2004, 109, 926-931.

[112] Nolan, JP; Morley, PT; Vanden Hoek, TL; Hickey, RW; Kloeck, WG; Billi, J; Bottiger, BW; Morley, PT; Nolan, JP; Okada, K; Reyes, C; Shuster, M; Steen, PA; Weil, MH; Wenzel, V; Hickey, RW; Carli, P; Vanden Hoek, TL; Atkins, D. for the International Liaison Committee on Resuscitation. Therapeutic hypothermia after cardiac arrest: an advisory statement by the Advanced Life Support Task Force of the International Liaison Committee on Resuscitation. *Circulation*., 2003, 108, 118 -121.

[113] Beyersdorf, F; Kirsch, M; Buckberg, GG; Allen, BS. Warm glutamate/aspartate-enriched blood cardioplegic solution for perioperative sudden death. *J Thorac Cardiovasc Surg*, 1992, 104, 1141- 1147.

[114] Simpson, PC. Norepinephrine-stimulated hypertrophy of cultured rat myocardial cells is an alpha-1 adrenergic response. *J Clin Invest*, 1983, 72, 732-738

[115] Meidell, RS; Sen, A; Henderson, SA; Slahetka, MF; Chien, KR. Alpha-1 adrenergic stimulation of rat myocardial cells increases protein synthesis. *Am J Physiol*, 1986, 251, H1076-H1084

[116] Landzberg, JS; Parker, JD; Gauthier, DF; Colucci, WS. Effects of myocardial alpha-1 adrenergic receptor stimulation and blockade on contractility in humans. *Circulation*., 1991, 84, 1608-1614.

[117] Fries, M; Weil, MH; Chang, YT; Castillo, C; Tang, W. Microcirculation during cardiac arrest and resuscitation. *Crit Care Med*., 2006, 34, S454-S457

[118] Hashimoto, K; Hashimoto, K. Cardiac irregularities induced by intracoronary injection of epinephrine and acetylcholine into various portions of the canine ventricle. *Am Heart J*, 1972, 83, 197-205
[119] Morady, F; Nelson, SD; Kou, WH; Pratley, R; Schmaltz, S; De Buitleir, M; Halter, JB. Electrophysiologic effects of epinephrine in humans. *J Am Coll Cardiol*, 1988, 11, 1235-1244
[120] Niemann, JT; Haynes, KS; Gardner, D; Rennie, CJ 3rd; Jagels, G; Stormo, O. Post-countershock pulseless rhythms: response to CPR, artificial cardiac pacing, and adrenergic agonists. *Ann Emerg Med.*, 1986, 15, 112-120
[121] Tang, W; Weil, MH; Gazmuri, RJ; Sun, S; Duggal, C; Bisera, J. Pulmonary ventilation/perfusion defects induced by epinephrine during cardiopulmonary resuscitation. *Circulation*, 2001, 84, 2101–2107.
[122] Mally, S; Jelatancev, A; Grmec, S. Effects of epinephrine and vasopressin on end-tidal carbon dioxide tension and mean arterial blood pressure in out-of-hospital cardiopulmonary resuscitation: an observational study. *Crit Care.*, 2007, 11, R39
[123] Lewis, LM; Stothert, J; Standeven, J; Chandel, B; Kurtz, M; Fortney, J. Correlation of end-tidal CO2 to cerebral perfusion during CPR. *Ann Emerg Med*, 1992, 21, 1131-1134.
[124] Idris, AH; Staples, ED; O'Brien, DJ; Melker, RJ; Rush, WJ; Del Duca, KD; Falk, JL. End-tidal carbon dioxide during extremely low cardiac output. *Ann Emerg Med*, 1994, 23, 568-572.
[125] Shibutani, K; Muraoka, M; Shirasaki, S; Kubal, K; Sanchala, VT; Gupte, P. Do changes in end-tidal PCO2 quantitatively reflect changes in cardiac output? *Anesth Analg*, 1994, 79, 829-833.
[126] Grmec, S; Lah, K; Tusek-Bunc, K. Difference in end-tidal CO2 between asphyxia cardiac arrest and ventricular fibrillation/ pulseless ventricular tachycardia cardiac arrest in the prehospital setting. *Crit Care*, 2003, 7, R139-144.
[127] Thrush, DN; Downs, JB; Smith, RA. Is epinephrine contraindicated during cardiopulmonary resuscitation? *Circulation.*, 1997, 96, 2709-2714.
[128] Cameron, HA; Ardlie, NG. The facilitating effects of adrenaline on platelet aggregation. Prostaglandins *Leukot Med*, 1982, 9, 117-128.
[129] Shah, BH; Lashari, I; Rana, S; Saeed, O; Rasheed, H; Arshad Saeed, S. Synergistic interaction of adrenaline and histamine in human platelet aggregation is mediated through activation of phospholipase, map kinase and cyclo-oxygenase pathways. *Pharmacol Res*, 2000, 42, 479–483.
[130] Parikh, V; Singh, M. Possible role of adrenergic component and cardiac mast cell degranulation in preconditioning-induced cardioprotection. *Pharmacol Res*, 1999, 40, 129–137.
[131] Berg, RA; Otto, CW; Kern, KB; Sanders, AB; Hilwig, RW; Hansen, KK; et al. High-dose epinephrine results in greater early mortality after resuscitation from prolonged cardiac arrest in pigs: a prospective, randomized study. *Crit Care Med*, 1994, 22, 282-290.
[132] Lindner, KH; Strohmenger, HU; Ensinger, H; Hetzel, WD; Ahnefeld, FW; Gerogieff, M. Stress hormone response during and after cardiopulmonary resuscitation. *Anesthesiology*, 1992, 77, 662-668.

[133] Behringer, W; Kittler, H; Sterz, F; Domanovits, H; Schoerkhuber, w; Holzer, M; Mülner, M; Laggner, AN. Cumulative epinephrine dose during cardiopulmonary resuscitation and neurologic outcome. *Ann Intern Med*, 1998, 129, 450-456
[134] Cowlen, MS; Toews, ML. Effects of agonist and phorbol ester on adrenergic receptors of DDT1 MF-2 cells. *J Pharmacol Exp Ther*, 1987, 243, 527-533
[135] Insel, PA. Seminars in medicine of the Beth Israel Hospital, Boston. Adrenergic receptors evolving concepts and clinical implications. *N Engl J Med*, 1996, 334, 580-585.
[136] Wikberg, JE; Akers, M; Caron, MG; Hagen, PO. Norepinephrine-induced down regulation of alpha 1 adrenergic receptors in cultured rabbit aorta smooth muscle cells. *Life Sci.*, 1983, 33, 1409-1417.
[137] Anonymous. 2005 American Heart Association guidelines for cardiopulmonary resuscitation and emergency cardiovascular care. *Circulation*, 2005, 112(Suppl. IV), 19-34.
[138] Bossaert, L; Van Hoeyweghen, R. The Cerebral Resuscitation Study Group. Bystander Cardiopulmonary Resuscitation (CPR) in out-of-hospital cardiac arrest. *Resuscitation*, 1989, 17, S55-S69.
[139] Andreka, P; Frenneaux, MP. Haemodynamics of cardiac arrest and resuscitation. *Curr Opin Crit Care.*, 2006, 12, 198-203.
[140] Abella, BS; Sandbo, N; Vassilatos, P; Alvarado, JP; O'Hearn, N; Wigder, HN; Hoffman, P; Tynus, K; Vanden Hoek, TL; Becker, LB. Chest compression rates during cardiopulmonary resuscitation are suboptimal: a prospective study during in-hospital cardiac arrest. *Circulation*, 2005, 111, 428-434.
[141] Van Hoeyweghen, RJ; Bossaert, LL; Mullie, A; Calle, P; Martens, P; Buylaert, WA; Delooz, H. Quality and efficiency of bystander CPR. Belgian Cerebral Resuscitation Study Group. *Resuscitation*, 1993, 26, 47-52.
[142] Abella, BS; Alvarado, JP; Myklebust, H; Edelson, DP; Barry, A; O'Hearn, N; Vanden Hoek, TL; Becker, LB. Quality of cardiopulmonary resuscitation during in-hospital cardiac arrest. *JAMA*, 2005, 293, 305-310.
[143] Wik, L; Kramer-Johansen, J; Myklebust, H; Sørebø, H; Svensson, L; Fellows, B; Steen, PA. Quality of cardiopulmonary resuscitation during out-of-hospital cardiac arrest. *JAMA*, 2005, 293, 299-304.
[144] Olasveengen, TM; Tomlinson, AE; Wik, L; Sunde, K; Steen, PA; Myklebust, H; Kramer-Johansen, J. A failed attempt to improve quality of out-of-hospital CPR through performance evaluation. *Prehosp Emerg Care*, 2007, 11, 427-433.
[145] Kern, KB; Hilwig, RW; Berg, RA; Sanders, AB; Ewy, GA. Importance of continuous chest compressions during cardiopulmonary resuscitation: improved outcome during a simulated single lay-rescuer scenario. *Circulation.*, 2002, 105, 645-649.
[146] Sunde, K; Eftestol, T; Askenberg, C; Steen, PA. Quality assessment of defribrillation and advanced life support using data from the medical control module of the defibrillator. *Resuscitation*, 1999, 41, 237-247.
[147] Valenzuela, TD; Kern, KB; Clark, LL; Berg, RA; Berg, MD; Berg, DD; Hilwig, RW; Otto, CW; Newburn, D; Ewy, GA. Interruptions of chest compressions during emergency medical systems resuscitation. *Circulation*, 2005, 112, 1259-1265
[148] Becker, L; Berg, RA; Pepe, P; Idris, AH; Aufderheide, TP; Barnes, TA; Stratton, SJ; Chandra, NC. A reappraisal of mouth-to-mouth ventilation during bystander-initiated

cardiopulmonary resuscitation: a statement for healthcare professionals from the ventilation working group of the basic life support and pediatric life support subcommittees, American Heart Association. *Circulation.*, 1997, 96, 2102-2112.

[149] Locke, CJ; Berg, RA; Sanders, AB; Davis, MF; Milander, MM; Kern, KB; Ewy, GA. Bystander cardiopulmonary resuscitation: concerns about mouth-to-mouth contact. *Arch Intern Med.*, 1995, 155, 938-943.

[150] Ewy, GA. Cardiopulmonary resuscitation-strengthening the links in the chain of survival. *N Engl J Med*, 2000, 342, 1599-61

[151] Mashiko, K; Otsuka, T; Shimazaki, S; Kohama, A; Kamishima, G; Katsurada, K; Sawada, Y; Matsubara, I; Yamaguchi, K. An outcome study of out-of-hospital cardiac arrest using the Utstein template-a Japanese experience. *Resuscitation*, 2002, 55, 241-246.

[152] Iwami, T; Hiraide, A; Nakanishi, N; Hayashi, Y; Nishiuchi, T; Yukioka, H; Yoshiya, I; Sugimoto, H. Age and sex analysis of out-of-hospital cardiac arrest, Japan. *Resuscitation*, 2003, 57, 145-152

[153] Anonymous. Cardiopulmonary resuscitation by bystanders with chest compression only (SOS-KANTO): an observational study. SOS-KANTO study group. *Lancet.*, 2007, 369, 920-926.

[154] Rittenberger, JC; Bost, JE; Menegazzi, JJ. Time to give the first medication during resuscitation in out-of-hospital cardiac arrest. *Resuscitation*, 2006, 70, 201-206

[155] Vilke, GM; Chan, TC; Dunford, JV; Metz, M; Ochs, G; Smith, A; Fisher, R; Poste, JC; McCallum-Brown, L; Davis, DP. The three-phase model of cardiac arrest as applied to ventricular fibrillation in a large, urban emergency medical services system. *Resuscitation*, 2005, 64, 341-346.

[156] Vukmir, RB. Survival from prehospital cardiac arrest is critically dependent upon response time. *Resuscitation*, 2006, 69, 229-234.

[157] Wyer, PC; Perera, P; Jin, Z; Zhou, Q; Cook, DJ; Walter, SD; Guyatt, GH. Vasopressin or epinephrine for out-of-hospital cardiac arrest. *Ann Emerg Med.*, 2006, 48, 86-97.

[158] Plaisance, P; Adnet, F; Vicaut, E; Hennequin, B; Hennequin, B, Magne, P, Prudhomme, C; Lambert, Y; Cantineau, JP; Léopold, C; Ferracci, C; Gizzi, M; Payen, D. Benefit of active compression-decompression cardiopulmonary resuscitation as a prehospital advanced cardiac life support. *Circulation*, 1997, 95, 955-961.

[159] Lombardi, G; Galagher, EJ; Gennis, P. Outcome of out-ofhospital cardiac arrest in New York City: the pre-hospital arrest survival evaluation study. *JAMA*, 1994, 271, 678-683.

[160] Bernard, SA; Gray, TW; Buist, MD; Jones, BM; Silvester, W; Gutteridge, G; Smith, K. Treatment of comatose survivors of out-of-hospital cardiac arrest with induced hypothermia. *N Engl J Med*, 2002, 346, 557-63.

[161] Fan, KL; Leung, LP. Prognosis of patients with ventricular fibrillation in out-of-hospital cardiac arrest in Hong Kong: prospective study. *Hong Kong Med J*, 2002, 8, 318-821.

[162] Berg, RA; Otto, CW; Kern, KB; Sanders, AB; Hilwig, RW; Hansen, KK; Ewy, GA. High-dose epinephrine results in greater early mortality after resuscitation from prolonged cardiac arrest in pigs: a prospective, randomized study. *Crit Care Med.*, 1994, 22, 282-290.

[163] Vandycke, C; Martens, P. High dose versus standard dose epinephrine in cardiac arrest - a meta-analysis. *Resuscitation.*, 2000, 45, 161-166.

[164] Hoekstra, JW; Griffith, R; Kelley, R; Cody, RJ; Lewis, D; Scheatzle, M; Brown, CG. Effect of standard-dose versus high-dose epinephrine on myocardial high-energy phosphates during ventricular fibrillation and closed-chest CPR. *Ann Emerg Med.*, 1993, 22, 1385-1391.

[165] Hornchen, U; Lussi, C; Schuttler, J. Potential risks of high-dose epinephrine for resuscitation from ventricular fibrillation in a porcine model. *J Cardiothorac Vasc Anesth.*, 1993, 7, 184 -187.

[166] Rivers, EP; Wortsman, J; Rady, MY; Blake, HC; McGeorge, FT; Buderer, NM. The effect of the total cumulative epinephrine dose administered during human CPR on hemodynamic, oxygen transport, and utilization variables in the postresuscitation period. *Chest.*, 1994, 106, 1499 -1507.

[167] Guyton, AC. *Textbook of Medical Physiology* 8th edition. Philadelphia, PA: Saunders, 1991.

[168] Thiebonnier, M; Bayer, AL; Leng, Z. Cytoplasmic and nuclear signaling pathways of V1-vascular vasopressin receptors. *Regul Pept*, 1993, 45, 79-84.

[169] Cooke, CR; Wall, BM; Huch, KM; Mangold, T. Cardiovascular effects of vasopressin following V1 receptor blockade compared to effects of nitroglycerin. *Am J Physiol Regul Integr Comp Physiol*, 2001, 281, 887-893

[170] Lindner, KH; Prengel, AW; Brinkmann, A; Strohmenger, HU; Lindner, IM; Lurie, KG. Vasopressin administration in refractory cardiac arrest. *Ann Intern Med*, 1996, 124, 1061-1064.

[171] Wenzel, V; Lindner, KH; Krismer, AC; Miller, EA; Voelckel, WG; Lingnau, W. Repeated administration of vasopressin but not epinephrine maintains coronary perfusion pressure after early and late administration during prolonged cardiopulmonary resuscitation in pigs. *Circulation*, 1999, 99, 1379-1384

[172] Lindner, KH; Brinkmann, A; Pfenninger, EG; Lurie, KG; Goertz, A; Lindner, IM. Effect of vasopressin on hemodynamic variables, organ blood flow, and acid-base status in a pig model of cardiopulmonary resuscitation. *Anesth Analg*, 1993, 77, 427-35.

[173] Lindner, KH; Prengel, AW; Pfenninger, EG; Lindner, IM; Strohmenger, HU; Georgieff, M; Lurie, KG. Vasopressin improves vital organ blood flow during closed chest cardiopulmonary resuscitation in pigs. *Circulation*, 1995, 91, 215-221.

[174] Wenzel, V; Lindner, KH; Prengel, AW; Maier, C; Voelckel, W; Lurie, KG; Strohmenger, HU. Vasopressin improves vital organ blood flow after prolonged cardiac arrest with postcountershock pulseless electrical activity in pigs. *Crit Care Med*, 1999, 27, 486-492.

[175] Voelckel, WG; Lurie, KG; McKnite, S; Zielinski, T; Lindstrom, P; Peterson, C; Wenzel, V; Lindner, KH. Comparison of epinephrine and vasopressin in a pediatric porcine model of asphyxial cardiac arrest. *Crit Care Med*, 2000, 28, 3777-3783.

[176] Babar, SI; Berg, RA; Hilwig, RW; Kern, KB; Ewy, GA. Vasopressin versus epinephrine during cardiopulmonary resuscitation: a randomized swine outcome study. *Resuscitation*, 1999, 41, 185-192.

[177] Wenzel, V; Lindner, KH; Krismer, AC; Voelckel, WG; Schocke, MF; Hund, W; Witkiewicz, M; Miller, EA; Klima, G; Wissel, J; Lingnau, W; Aichner, FT. Survival with full neurologic recovery and no cerebral pathology after prolonged cardiopulmonary resuscitation with vasopressin in pigs. *J Am Coll Cardiol*, 2000, 35, 527-533.

[178] Popp, E; Vogel, P; Teschendorf, P; Bottiger, BW. Vasopressors are essential during cardiopulmonary resuscitation in rats: Is vasopressin superior to adrenaline? *Resuscitation*, 2007, 72, 137-144.
[179] Biondi-Zoccai, GG ; Abbate, A ; Parisi, Q ; Agostoni, P ; Burzotta, F ; Sandroni, C ; Zardini, P ; Biasucci, LM. Is vasopressin superior to adrenaline or placebo in the management of cardiac arrest? A meta-analysis. *Resuscitation*, 2003, 59, 221-224.
[180] Prengel, AW; Lindner, KH; Keller, A; Lurie, KG. Cardiovascular function during the post-resuscitation phase after cardiac arrest in pigs: a comparison of epinephrine versus vasopressin. *Crit Care Med*, 1996, 24, 2014-2019.
[181] Lindner, KH; Dirks, B; Strohmenger, HU; Prengel, AW; Lindner, IM; Lurie, KG. Randomised comparison of epinephrine and vasopressin in patients with out-of-hospital ventricular fibrillation. *Lancet*, 1997, 349, 535-537.
[182] Stiell, IG; Hebert, PC; Wells, GA; Vandemheen, KL; Tang, AS; Higginson, LA; Dreyer, JF; Clement, C; Battram, E; Watpool, I; Mason, S; Klassen, T; Weitzman, BN. Vasopressin versus epinephrine for inhospital cardiac arrest: a randomised controlled trial. *Lancet*, 2001, 358, 105-109.
[183] Wenzel, V; Krismer, AC; Arntz, HR; Sitter, H; Stadlbauer, KH; Lindner, KH. For the European Resuscitation Council Vasopressor during Cardiopulmonary Resuscitation Study Group: A comparison of vasopressin and epinephrine for out-of-hospital cardiopulmonary resuscitation. *N Engl J Med*, 2004, 350, 105-113.
[184] Aung, K; Htay, T. Vasopressin for cardiac arrest: a systematic review and meta analysis. *Arch Intern Med*, 2005, 165, 17-24.
[185] Krismer, AC; Wenzel, V; Mayr, VD; Voelckel, WG; Strohmenger, HU; Lurie, K; Lindner, KH. Arginine vasopressin during cardiopulmonary resuscitation and vasodilatory shock: current experience and future perspectives. *Curr Opin Crit Care*, 2001, 7, 157-169.
[186] Little, CM; Marietta, MH; Peng, K; Heard, K; Fragoso, M; Severyn, FA; Bebarta, VS; Paradis, NA. Vasopressin alone or with epinephrine may be superior to epinephrine in a clinically relevant porcine model of pulseless electrical activity cardiac arrest. *Am J Emerg Med*, 2006, 24, 810-814.
[187] Stadlebauer, KH; Wagner-Berger, HG; Wenzel, V; Voelckel, WG; Krismer, AC; Klima, G; Rheinberger, K; Pechlaner, S; Mayr, VD; Lindner, KH. Survival with full neurologic recovery after prolonged cardiopulmonary resuscitation with a combination of vasopressin and epinephrine in pigs. *Anesth Analg*, 2003, 96, 1743-1749.
[188] Mayr, VD; Wenzel, V; Voelckel, WG; Krismer, AC; Mueller, T; Lurie, KG; Lindner, KH. Developing a vasopressor combination in a pig model of adult asphyxial cardiac arrest. *Circulation*, 2001, 104, 1651-1656
[189] Stroumpoulis, K; Xanthos, T; Rokas, G; Kitsou, V; Papadimitriou, D; Serpetinis, I; Perrea, D; Papadimitriou, L; Kouskouni, E. Vasopressin and epinephrine in the treatment of cardiac arrest: an experimental study. *Crit Care*, 2008, 12, R40.
[190] Mulligan, KA; McKnite, SH; Lindner, KH; Lindstrom, PJ; Detloff, B; Lurie, KG. Synergistic effects of vasopressin plus epinephrine during cardiopulmonary resuscitation. *Resuscitation*, 1997, 35, 265-271.
[191] Lurie, KG; Voelckel, WG; Iskos, DN; McKnite, SH; Zielinski, TM; Sugiyama, A; Wenzel, V; Benditt, D; Lindner, KH. Combination drug therapy with vasopressin,

adrenaline (epinephrine) and nitroglycerin improves vital organ blood flow in a porcine model of ventricular fibrillation. *Resuscitation*, 2002, 54, 187-194.
[192] Grmec, S; Mally, S. Vasopressin improves outcome in out-of-hospital cardiopulmonary resuscitation of ventricular fibrillation and pulseless ventricular tachycardia: a observational cohort study. *Crit Care*, 2006, 10, R13.
[193] Ruffolo, RR Jr.; Nichols, AJ; Stadel, JM; Hieble, JP. Pharmacological and therapeutic applications of alpha2-adrenoceptor subtypes. *Ann Rev Pharmacol Toxicol*, 1993, 32, 243-279.
[194] Schäfers, RF; Nürnberger, J; Herrmann, B; Wenzel, RR; Philipp, T; Michel, MC. Adrenoceptors mediating the cardiovascular and metabolic effects of α-methylnoradrenaline in humans. *J Pharmacol Exp Ther*, 1999, 289, 918-925.
[195] Klouche, K; Weil, MH; Sun, S; Tang, W; Zhao, DH. A comparison of alpha-methylnorepinephrine, vasopressin and epinephrine for cardiac resuscitation. *Resuscitation.*, 2003, 57, 93-100
[196] Schäfers, RF; Nürnberger, J; Herrmann, B; Wenzel, RR; Philipp, T; Michel, MC. Adrenoceptors mediating the cardiovascular and metabolic effects of alpha-methylnoradrenaline in humans. *J Pharmacol Exp Ther.*, 1999, 289, 918-25.
[197] Callaham, M; Madsen, CD; Barton, CW; Saunders, CE; Pointer, J. A randomized clinical trial of high-dose epinephrine and norepinephrine vs standard-dose epinephrine in prehospital cardiac arrest. *JAMA.*, 1992, 268, 2667-72.
[198] Cammarata, G; Weil, MH; Sun, S; Tang, W; Wang, J; Huang, L. Beta1-adrenergic blockade during cardiopulmonary resuscitation improves survival. *Crit Care Med.*, 2004, 32, S440-S443.
[199] Huang, L; Weil, MH; Cammarata, G; Sun, S; Tang, W. Nonselective beta-blocking agent improves the outcome of cardiopulmonary resuscitation in a rat model. *Crit Care Med.*, 2004, 32, S378-S380.
[200] Bassiakou, E; Xanthos, T; Koudouna, E; Goulas, S; Prapa, V; Papadimitriou, D; Rokas, G; Papadimitriou, L. Atenolol in combination with epinephrine improves the initial outcome of cardiopulmonary resuscitation in a swine model of ventricular fibrillation. *Am J Emerg Med.*, 2008, 26, 578-584
[201] Hollenberg, SM. Vasodilators in acute heart failure. *Heart Fail Rev*, 2007, 12, 143-147.
[202] Murrel, W. Nitroglycerine as a remedy for angina pectoris. *Lancet.*, 1879, 276, 80-81.
[203] Kleschyov, AL; Oelze, M; Daiber, A. Does nitric oxide mediate the Vasodilator activity of nitroglycerin? *Circ Res*, 2003, 93, e104-12.
[204] Kitsou, V; Xanthos, T; Stroumpoulis, K; Rokas, G; Papadimitriou, D; Serpetinis, I; Dontas, I; Perrea, D; Kouskouni, E. Nitroglycerin and Epinephrine Improve Coronary Perfusion Pressure in a Porcine Model of Ventricular Fibrillation Arrest: A Pilot Study. *J Emerg Med.*, 2008 (Epub ahead of print).
[205] Gazmuri, RJ; Ayoub, IM; Hoffner, E; Kolarova, JD. Successful ventricular defibrillation by the selective sodium-hydrogen exchanger isoform-1 inhibitor cariporide. *Circulation*, 2001, 104, 234-239
[206] Ayoub, IM; Kolarova, JD; Yi, Z; Trevedi, A; Deshmukh, H; Lubell, DL; Franz, MR; Maldonado, FA; Gazmuri, RJ. Sodium-hydrogen exchange inhibition during ventricular fibrillation: beneficial effects on ischemic contracture, action potential duration, reperfusion arrhythmias, myocardial function, and resuscitability. *Circulation*, 2003, 107, 1804-1809

[207] Ayoub, IM; Kolarova, J; Kantola, RL; Sanders, R; Gazmuri, RJ. Cariporide minimizes adverse myocardial effects of epinephrine during resuscitation from ventricular fibrillation. *Crit Care Med.*, 2005, 33, 2599-605.

[208] Kolarova, JD; Ayoub, IM; Gazmuri, RJ. Cariporide enables hemodynamically more effective chest compression by leftward shift of its flow-depth relationship. *Am J Physiol Heart Circ Physiol.*, 2005, 288, H2904-11.

[209] Brendt, P; Behrends, M; Peters, J. Myocardial stunning following no flow ischaemia is diminished by levosimendan or cariporide, without benefits of combined administration. *Resuscitation.*, 2008, 76, 95-102.

[210] Cammarata, GA; Weil, MH; Sun, S; Huang, L; Fang, X; Tang, W. Levosimendan improves cardiopulmonary resuscitation and survival by K(ATP) channel activation. *J Am Coll Cardiol.*, 2006, 47, 1083-1085.

[211] Lehmann, A; Kiessling, AH; Isgro, F; Zeitler, C; Thaler, E; Boldt, J. Levosimendan in patients with acute myocardial ischaemia undergoing emergency surgical revascularization. *Eur J Anaesthesiol.*, 2008, 25, 224-229.

[212] Koudouna, E; Xanthos, T; Bassiakou, E; Goulas, S; Lelovas, P; Papadimitriou, D; Tsirikos, N; Papadimitriou, L. Levosimendan improves the initial outcome of cardiopulmonary resuscitation in a swine model of cardiac arrest. *Acta Anaesthesiol Scand.*, 2007, 51, 1123-1129.

[213] Huang, L; Weil, MH; Sun, S; Cammarata, G; Cao, L; Tang, W. Levosimendan improves postresuscitation outcomes in a rat model of CPR. *J Lab Clin Med.*, 2005, 146, 256-261.

In: Advances in Cardiovascular Research, Volume 1
Editors: L. Schmitt, T. Konig, pp. 153-169
ISBN: 978-1-60741-720-0


*Chapter V*

# Defibrillation: Mechanisms, Waveforms, Energy Levels, Transthoracic Impedance and Automated External Defibrillators

***Theodoros Xanthos, Eleni Bassiakou and Lila Papadimitriou***
University of Athens, Greece

## Abstract

Cardiac arrest still remains a daunting medical emergency in Western societies and is the cause of approximately 250,000-600,000 deaths annually in the United States, with ventricular fibrillation being the initial rhythm in 20-38% of cases. Defibrillation is the only treatment available to terminate this life-threatening arrhythmia. This chapter deals initially with the mechanisms of defibrillation, the waveforms and the recommended energy levels of defibrillation. Furthermore, factors influencing transthoracic impedance, which is a major determinant of successful defibrillation, are analysed. Finally, this chapter discusses the use of automated external defibrillators and the early access to defibrillation by lay personnel in out-of-hospital cardiac arrest

## Definition and Mechanisms

Defibrillation is defined as the termination of fibrillation or, the absence of ventricular fibrillation (VF) 5 sec after shock delivery [1]. VF involves a state of unorganized electrical activity within the myocardium. This unorganized activity results in a multitude of electrical impulses that are ineffective for generating a coordinated myocardial contraction that can sustain life. The goal of defibrillation is to stun the myocardium, stopping all electrical activity within the myocardium to allow one of the organized pacemakers to initiate an organized rhythm. Defibrillation is the only treatment available to terminate VF [2-4] but to this day, understanding the mechanisms by which electric shocks halt this life-threatening arrhythmia, remains incomplete.

Mapping studies have demonstrated that defibrillation shocks can halt all wave fronts on the heart, but fibrillation will begin again with an initial activation pattern that is different from the activation pattern on the heart just after the shock is delivered [5, 6]. Fabiato *et al* [7] were the first to suggest that the mechanisms of induction and termination of VF may be similar and a large body of research has demonstrated that an electric shock can induce ventricular arrhythmias if it is given during the 'vulnerable window' within the normal cardiac cycle. Thus, the mechanisms of defibrillation have been strongly linked to cardiac vulnerability to electric shocks. As shocks that result in induction of arrhythmia are bound by a minimum and a maximum strength, termed the lower and upper limits of vulnerability, the upper limit of vulnerability hypothesis for defibrillation has been formed [8]. According to this hypothesis a successful defibrillation attempt must do two things: First, the shock must stop the fibrillation wave fronts in the heart and second, the defibrillation shock must not restart fibrillation.

The mechanism of defibrillation is complex and can be considered at many different levels, starting at the level of the whole patient and extending to the level of cellular membranes and ion channels [9]. At the patient level, shock strength delivered through the defibrillation electrodes is used to describe defibrillation efficacy. However, there are several factors that affect the magnitude of shock necessary to defibrillate the heart. One such factor is the shape of the defibrillation waveform (see below). A second factor is the location of the defibrillation electrodes. In transthoracic defibrillation, 200-360 J are necessary for successful defibrillation, whereas when paddles are placed directly to the heart 20-34 J are usually required. This difference occurs because only about 4%-20% of the current delivered from transthoracic defibrillation electrodes ever reaches the heart [10]. Furthermore, how that current is distributed throughout the heart is an important factor for defibrillation, due to the fact that different amount of current flow through different parts of the heart during a shock.

Just as there is a minimum shock strength needed to defibrillate the fibrillating myocardium, there appears to be a minimum of potential gradient that must be created throughout the ventricles by the shock. The potential gradient generated throughout the heart by the shock is thus another important factor in the mechanisms of defibrillation [9]. It is well known that the minimum potential gradient necessary for defibrillation is not the same for different waveforms. For example, it is approximately 6 V/cm for a typical monophasic waveform, but is approximately 4 V/cm for a typical biphasic waveform [11]. Therefore, one of the reasons that some biphasic waveforms require a smaller shock to achieve defibrillation than some monophasic waveforms is that they must create a lower minimum potential gradient throughout the heart.

The mechanism of defibrillation extends further in the level of cellular membranes. During the shock, changes in the transmembrane potential either initiate new or prolong the action potential. It has been estimated that only one quarter of the total current traversing the heart crosses the membrane to enter the cells [12]. Since the defibrillation electrodes are located extracellularly, current from the shock that enters myocardial cells in some regions must exit the cells in other regions. These currents, which flow through the cell membrane, will introduce changes in the transmemhrane potential that include depolarization or hyperpolarization during the shock pulse [13]. Several mathematical formulations have been proposed to describe which regions of the heart are depolarized and which are hyperpolarized during shocks, but all of them are theoretical and with several limitations.

In the subcellular level, defibrillation involves the response of ion channels to shock delivery. It is known that both fast and slow $Na^+$ and $Ca^{2+}$ channels are active during early fibrillation and that most probably activation of $Na^+$ channels are responsible in initiating a new action potential [14]. Results from computer models have suggested that the role of the first phase of a biphasic defibrillation waveform is to hyperpolarize the cardiac cell membrane from -65 mV that is typically its most negative transmembrane voltage during fibrillation to its resting transmembrane voltage (-90mV). This decrease in transmembrane potential is hypothesized to allow $Na^+$ channels to recover, allowing thus easier tissue stimulation at the second phase of the biphasic waveform [15].

## Waveforms and Energy Levels

Written history of fibrillation and defibrillation goes back to the pioneering work in Carl Ludwig's laboratory [16]. In 1849, Ludwig's student M. Hoffa was the first to witness and, most importantly, document the onset of VF, which he induced by electrical stimulus. Defibrillation was pioneered for internal use by Claude Beck in 1947, when he successfully applied defibrillation therapy and saved the first human life by this method. Originally, defibrillators delivered monophasic energy, defined as energy that flow from one paddle to the other in a single direction. Currently, there are 2 main types of monophasic waveform, the monophasic damped sinusoidal (MDS) (Fig 1), which gradually returns to zero current flow, and the monophasic truncated exponential (MTE) (Fig 2) which is electronically terminated before the current flow reaches zero.

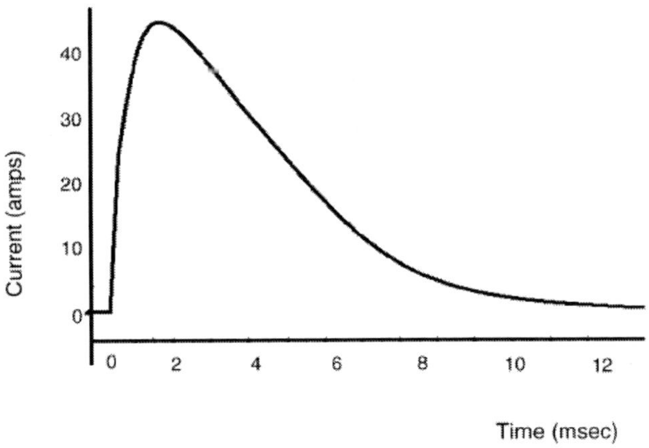


Figure 1. The monophasic damped sinusoidal waveform (modified from Deakin, CD; Nolan, JP. European Resuscitation Council Guidelines for Resuscitation 2005. Section 3. Electrical therapies: Automated external defibrillators, defibrillation, cardioversion and pacing. *Resuscitation* 2005; 67:S25-S37)

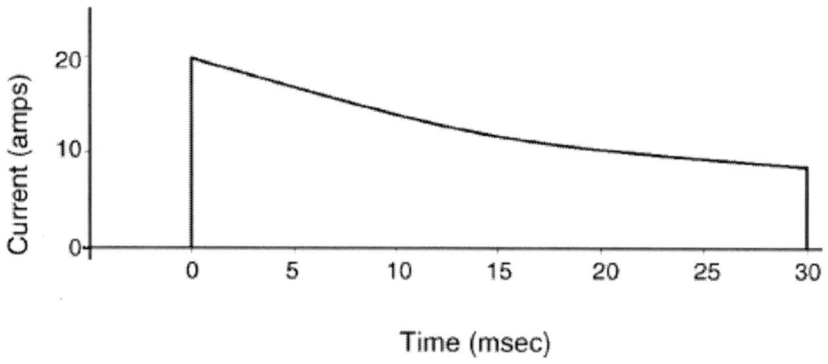


Figure 2. The monophasic truncated exponential waveform (modified from Deakin, CD; Nolan, JP. European Resuscitation Council Guidelines for Resuscitation 2005. Section 3. Electrical therapies: Automated external defibrillators, defibrillation, cardioversion and pacing. *Resuscitation* 2005; 67:S25-S37)

However, in the last decade, biphasic defibrillators have been developed that deliver current that flows in a positive direction for a specified duration before reversing and flowing in a negative direction. There are 2 types of biphasic waveforms currently approved for use in external defibrillation: biphasic truncated exponential (BTE) (Fig 3), which may be used with a ‘‘low-energy protocol’’ or ‘‘high-energy protocol,’’ and rectilinear biphasic (RLB) (Fig 4) currently used with a low-energy protocol. The clinical difference between the low and high-energy protocols relates to the amount of energy available to the provider. Low-energy defibrillators have a maximum setting of 200 J. In contrast, high-energy defibrillators have a maximum setting of 360 J [17]. It is still under debate among the scientific society whether one of this two ‘types’ of energy is superior to the other and research shows equivalent performance between BTE and RLB, across similar energy levels [18, 19]. A third biphasic waveform is also available in Europe that is pulsed at a high frequency is awaiting US Food and Drug Administration approval. This waveform is designed to achieve high shock efficacy at reduced energy by chopping the waveform. Finally, triphasic and quadraphasic types of waveform have entered experimental evaluation [20-22].

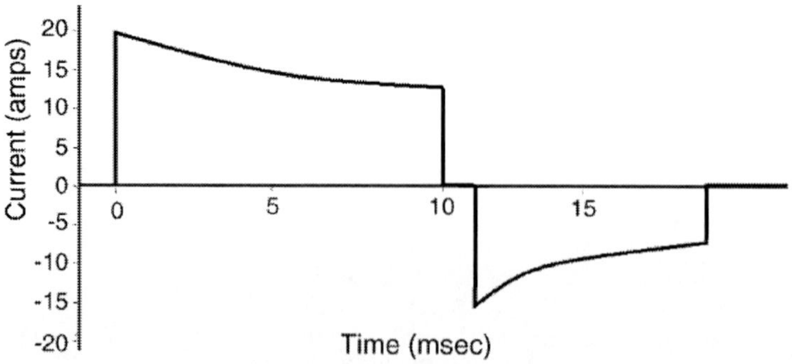


Figure 3. The biphasic truncated exponential waveform (modified from Deakin, CD; Nolan, JP. European Resuscitation Council Guidelines for Resuscitation 2005. Section 3. Electrical therapies: Automated external defibrillators, defibrillation, cardioversion and pacing. *Resuscitation* 2005; 67:S25-S37)

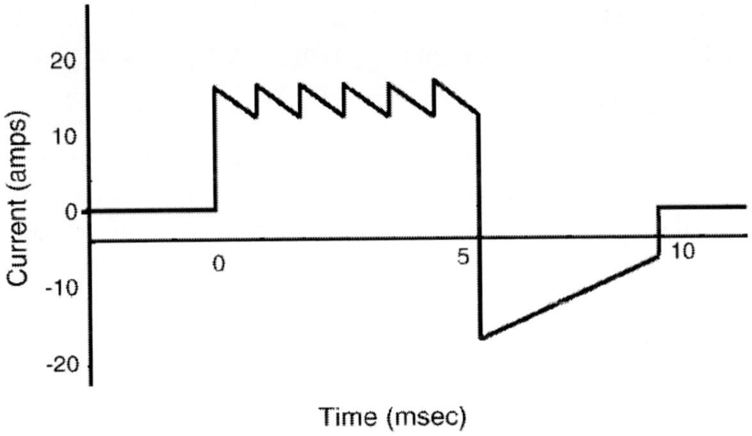


Figure 4. The rectilinear biphasic waveform (modified from Deakin, CD; Nolan, JP. European Resuscitation Council Guidelines for Resuscitation 2005. Section 3. Electrical therapies: Automated external defibrillators, defibrillation, cardioversion and pacing. *Resuscitation* 2005; 67:S25-S37)

Successful external defibrillation depends upon delivering an appropriate amount of electrical current to the heart. Levels of current that are too low are likely to fail, while those that are too high may result in myocardial damage [23]. The optimal energy for defibrillation is that which achieves defibrillation, while causing the minimum myocardial damage. Selection of an appropriate energy level also reduces the number of repetitive shocks, which in turn limits myocardial damage [24]. Optimal energy levels for teminating VF for both monophasic and biphasic waveforms are unknown and practitioners need to be aware that a single, standardized approach to defibrillation does not exist [25].

The recommendations for the energy levels by the European resuscitation council (ERC) and American Heart Association (AHA) are based on a consensus following review of the current literature. Currently, the recommended initial energy level for the first and subsequent shocks using a monophasic defibrillator is 360 J. As far as biphasic waveforms are concerned, the provider choosing the appropriate energy selection for the termination of VF requires information about (a) the waveform utilized within the device and (b) whether the manufacturers subscribe a fixed-joules protocol (eg, 200, 200, 200 J) or an escalating-joules protocol (eg, 200, 300, 360 J) [26].Therefore, manufacturers should display the effective waveform dose range on the face of the biphasic device. If the provider is unaware of the effective dose range of the device, the use of 200 J is recommended. This amount of energy (200J) was selected as it falls within the reported range of doses effective for initial and subsequent biphasic shocks and can be provided by every biphasic manual machine available in 2005, regardless of manufacturer [17]. As far as subsequent shocks are concerned there is no evidence to support either a fixed or escalating energy protocol. Both energy protocols can be used safely and effectively to terminate short-duration and long-duration VF. Nevertheless, none of the available evidence has shown superiority of either non-escalating or escalating energy biphasic waveform defibrillation for termination of VF. Both strategies are acceptable; however, if the first shock is not successful and the defibrillator is capable of delivering shocks of higher energy, it may be appropriate to increase the energy for subsequent shocks [1]. The safety and efficacy data related to specific biphasic waveforms, the most effective initial shock, and whether to use non-escalating or escalating sequences require additional studies in both in-hospital and out-of-hospital settings. Ongoing research is necessary to firmly establish the most appropriate initial settings for both monophasic and biphasic defibrillators. Unfortunately, although the manufacturers offer defibrillator-specific recommendations for the energy use, they always defer to the medical providers for the final decision, therefore leaving a clinician with little concrete direction. Therefore, in clinical practice, users are commonly perplexed about the energy selection for biphasic defibrillators. There is clearly a knowledge deficit in clinical practice with regard to this topic, and energy selection for biphasic defibrillators remains a topic of heated debate [26].

Currently, there is virtually universal agreement that biphasic waveforms, regardless of design, have greater efficacy in defibrillation of ventricular fibrillation when compared with monophasic waveforms [3, 27-32]. Research has demonstrated that biphasic waveforms improve defibrillation efficacy via 2 distinct mechanisms: the reduction of shock-induced myocardial dysfunction and the reduction of the defibrillation threshold [33, 34]. Furthermore, biphasic delivery requires less energy than monophasic delivery to achieve conversion of VF [28, 35] making its use theoretically safer. Moreover, they have the ability to self-adjust, after measuring impedance, to ensure that the patient is receiving the desired current. Due to the aforementioned reasons, biphasic waveforms have supplanted monophasic waveforms and monophasic defibrillators are no longer manufactured, although many remain in use. It remains unresolved, however, whether any specific biphasic waveform has greater clinical superiority than others [3, 36]. Likewise, it remains to be demonstrated whether any biphasic waveform is less injurious to myocardial function than another and whether injury is secondary to peak delivered current or to delivered energy [37]. Nevertheless, no specific waveform (either monophasic or biphasic) is consistently associated with a higher rate of return of spontaneous circulation or rates of survival to hospital discharge after cardiac arrest.

## One Versus 3 Shock Protocol

Analyses of VF waveform characteristics predictive of shock success have documented that the shorter the time between a chest compression and delivery of a shock, the more likely the shock will be successful due to the fact that a brief period of chest compressions can deliver oxygen and energy substrates to the fibrillating myocardium [38] and can increase coronary perfusion pressure, the only proven prognostic factor to predict successful defibrillation [39]. Furthermore, animal studies have shown that frequent or long interruptions in precordial chest compressions for rhythm analysis or rescue breathing are associated with postresuscitation myocardial dysfunction and reduced survival rates [40, 41]. In the context of a 3-shock protocol being recommended in the 2000 guidelines, interruptions in cardiopulmonary resuscitation (CPR) to enable rhythm analysis by AEDs resulted in delays of up to 37 seconds between delivery of the first shock and delivery of the first post-shock compression [42]. With first shock efficacy of biphasic waveforms documented to exceed 90%, failure to terminate VF successfully is more likely to suggest the need for a period of CPR rather than a further shock [3].

Due to the aforementioned reasons the single shock strategy has been recommended by the 2005 Consensus Conference. The single shock strategy is applicable to both monophasic and biphasic defibrillators.

# Transthoracic Impedance and Optimal Defibrillation

Transthoracic impedance (TTI) is a major determinant of successful defibrillation. It has been shown that patients with high TTI will require more voltage to ensure the delivery of the charge and more shocks to achieve a perfusing rhythm in defibrillation, due to the fact that TTI decreases transmyocardial current [23]. TTI can be determined by commercially available defibrillators [43]. Moreover, methods for predicting TTI by applying high-frequency current to the chest in advance prior to any defibrillation attempt have been described in experimental models of VF [44, 45]. TTI varies considerably with body mass, being approximately 70—80 Ω in adults [23, 46], and is comprised of three components: A) extra-corporeal sources including the defibrillator and paddles, B) tissue sources, including intracardiac and extra-cardiac tissue and C) the electrode-skin interface. Tissue sources are the greatest source of overall impedance. Optimal defibrillation technique aims in delivering current across the fibrillating myocardium in the presence of minimal TTI [1].

Concerning the extra-corporeal sources, two types of electrode are commonly used; paddles in which a metal plate is applied to the skin with a conductive pad interposed, and self-adhesive pads in which a thin electrode coated with gel is stuck onto the skin. Several different types of defibrillation paddles and self-adhesive defibrillation pads are currently available for clinical use but the TTI achieved with each type has not been established [47, 48]. The Association for the Advancement of Medical Instrumentation recommends a minimum electrode size, the sum of the areas being of 150 $cm^2$ [49]. Larger electrodes have lower impedance but may result in less transmyocardial current flow. Small electrodes (4.3 cm) may be harmful and may cause myocardial necrosis [50].

The major difference between paddles and self-adhesive defibrillation pads is that the use of defibrillator paddles requires the operator to apply pressure to paddles for the duration of the procedure, while the use of self-adhesive defibrillation pads do not require so. It is suggested that optimal paddle force is approximately 8.0 kg in adults and 5.0 kg in children > 10 kg weight [51, 52]. Appling pressure decreases TTI and one of the mechanisms by which this occurs has been assumed to be due to improved electrical contact at the paddle-skin interface [53]. Conversely, self-adhesive defibrillation pads may reduce TTI by providing better contact with the convex chest wall.

A second mechanism, by which applying pressure to the pads reduces TTI, is that air is expelled from the lungs as the chest is compressed reducing thus thoracic volume that also affects TTI [54]. TTI is minimal at end-expiration. It is suggested therefore to attempt defibrillation at the end expiration phase of the respiratory cycle. TTI has been further shown to increase in a linear fashion with increasing positive end-expiratory pressure (PEEP) [55]. In severe asthma for example that auto-PEEP is a common finding, particularly during acute exacerbations (levels of auto-PEEP as high as 20 cm H2O have been documented), successful defibrillation of those patients may require energy levels above those currently recommended [56]. Defibrillators that first measure TTI and adjust the delivered energy accordingly may have significant advantages over defibrillators with manually selected energy levels in situations where PEEP has caused an increase in TTI.

Finally, concerning the electrode/skin surface effect in TTI, it has been shown that chest hair contributes significantly. It is generally accepted that chest hair increases TTI and reduces defibrillation efficacy, due to the fact that air is trapped beneath the electrode and only poor electrode-to-skin contact is possible. A marked variation in impedance has been also shown in different gels used [57].

## Electrode Position

Although no human studies have evaluated the electrode position as a determinant of survival from VF cardiac arrest, transmyocardial current during defibrillation is likely to be maximal when the electrodes are placed so that the area of the heart that is fibrillating lies directly between them. The European Resuscitation Council (ERC) recommends 4 paddle/pad positions for defibrillation: A) the anterior-apex (right sternum- left midaxillary line) (Fig 5, Fig 6), B) the biaxillary (right and left lateral chest wall), C) anterior-posterior (left precordium-inferior to left scapula) and D) apex-posterior (left midaxillary line- right or left upper back) [1].

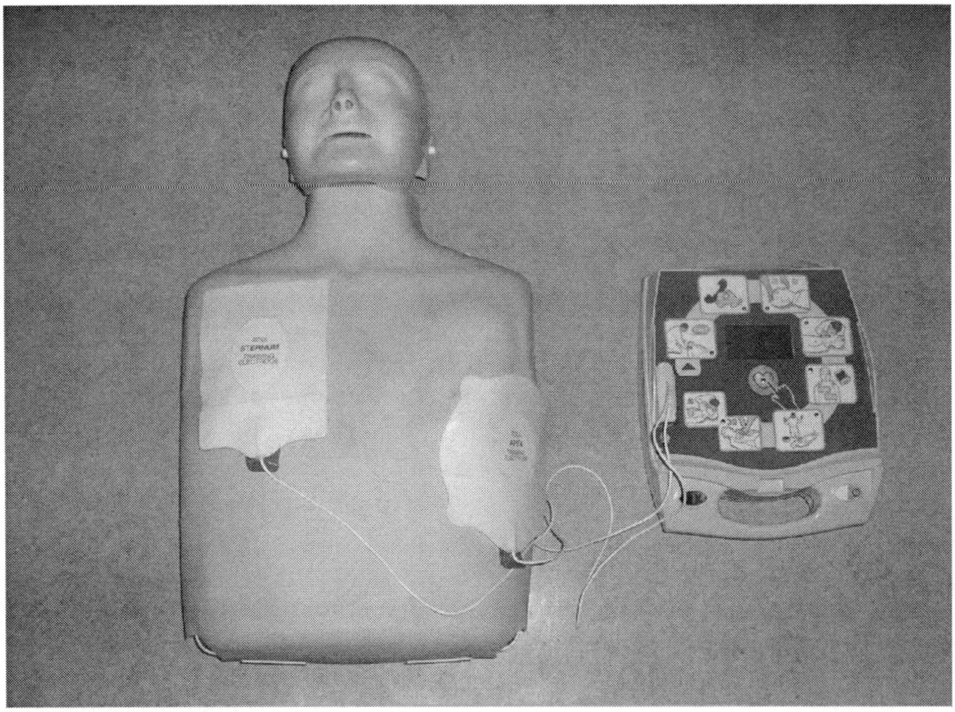

Figure 5. Pad positions for the automated external defibrillator

However, there is only limited data available comparing TTI associated with these various pad/paddle positions [58, 59]. A study that sought to determine any differences among TTI of the various electrode positions using self adhesive defibrillator pads, concluded that there was no difference in TTI between those recommended paddle/pad positions [59]. It is further suggested that pad/paddles should be clear of any breast tissue because TTI has been shown to be minimised when the apical paddle/pad is not placed over the female breast [60]. Asymmetrically shaped apical paddle/pad has been shown to have lower impedance when placed longitudinally rather than transversely [61]. The long axis of the apical paddle/pad should therefore be orientated in a craniocaudal direction.

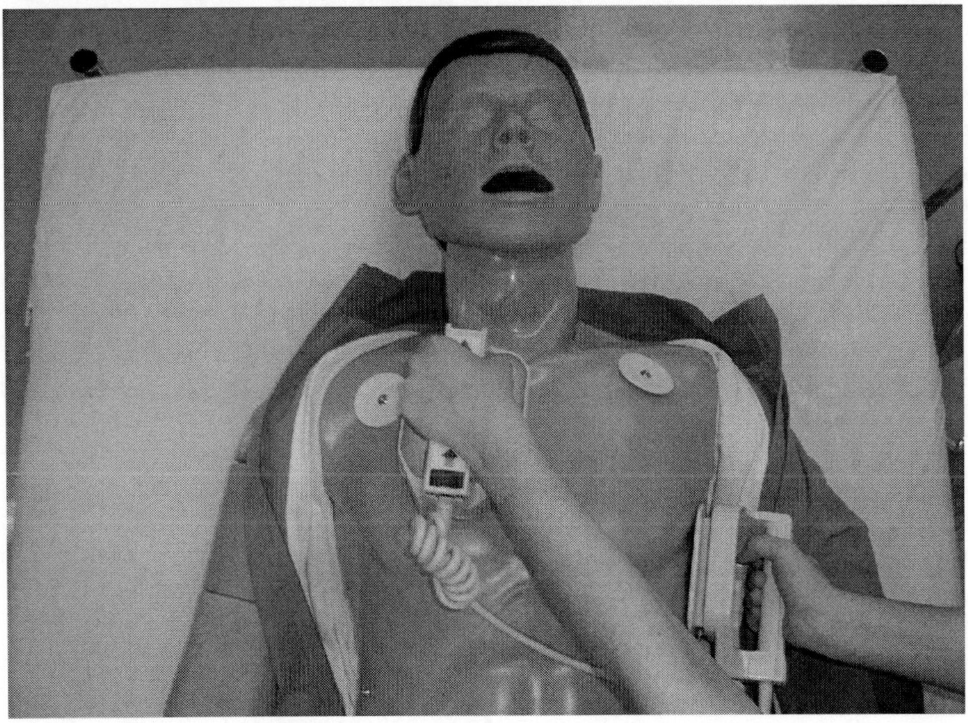

Figure 6. Paddle positions for the manual defibrillator

## Automated External Defibrillators

Cardiac arrest (CA) still remains a daunting medical emergency in Western societies and is the cause of approximately 250,000 deaths annually in the United States, with VF being the initial rhythm in 20-38% of cases [62]. ERC, American Heart Association (AHA) and International Liaison Committee on Resuscitation (ILCOR) have identified early access to defibrillation as a key component to the ''Chain of Survival'' for CA. Studies have shown that the probability of successful defibrillation and subsequent survival to hospital discharge declines rapidly with time and the ability to deliver early defibrillation is one of the most important factors in determining survival from CA [63, 64]. For every minute that passes following collapse and defibrillation, mortality increases 7-10% in the absence of bystander cardiopulmonary resuscitation (CPR) [65]. The practical reality remains that the vast majority of CA events are unanticipated, and that for the victims of these events the best hope of survival is represented by early access to external defibrillators.

Historically, access to external defibrillators for out-of-hospital CA has been provided by specially equipped ambulances and rapid response vehicles, organized as dedicated emergency medical systems (EMS) and staffed by physicians or highly trained paramedics prepared to analyze electrocardiograms and decide whether defibrillation was appropriate. In

1995, in response to the abysmal survival of out-of-hospital cardiac arrest, the AHA challenged the medical industry to develop a defibrillator that could be placed in public settings, used by lay responders, and provide earlier defibrillation to cardiac arrest victims. Requirements for such a device were to include durability, safety, long and reliable battery life, and the ability to perform self-maintenance. These requirements have been met by the modern automated external defibrillator (AED) [66].

AEDs have microprocessors that analyse several features of the electrocardiogram, including frequency and amplitude. These devices defibrillate the heart with a high degree of sensitivity and specificity. Developing technology should soon enable AEDs to provide information about frequency and depth of chest compressions during CPR that may improve basic life support (BLS) performance by all rescuers.

Despite having a well developed EMS system, the survival from out-of-hospital cardiac arrest in many cities is much less than 5% [67]. Several published studies have reported the results of defibrillation by targeted responders, for example persons with a duty to respond to medical emergencies such as police and fire fighters. These studies demonstrated that a 39-71% survival to hospital discharge was associated with a short time to defibrillation [68-70]. In a report from 200 uses on a commercial airline, both the sensitivity and specificity for detection of VF were 100% [68]. In casinos, where security officers operated the AED, 53% of VF victims survived to hospital discharge, and 74% survived when shock occurred within 3 minutes [69]. In Minnesota, addition of a police defibrillation program to conventional EMS services resulted in a 49% survival to discharge rate for patients in VF [70].

Rapid-response programs with AEDs used as part of the "chain of survival" have achieved marked improvements in survival rates in selected localities. AED use requires much less training than use of a manual defibrillator and it has been demonstrated to be remarkably effective in the hands of trained lay responders. In communities that lay personnel were trained in the use of AED the results were promising. For example, 27% of patients with witnessed out-of-hospital arrest due to VF in Seattle, Washington, survived to leave the hospital when bystanders performed CPR. Only 13% of similar cases survived without bystander CPR [71]. In Piacenza, Italy, lay defibrillation was associated with a threefold increase in survival following a witnessed arrest, as compared with EMS resuscitation [72]. Such communities to this day represent the exception rather than the rule [73].

ERC, AHA and ILCOR have advocated the widespread dissemination of AEDs. Since 1995, AHA has recommended the development of lay rescuer AED programs to improve survival rates from out-of-hospital CA. These programs are also known as public access defibrillation (PAD) programs [74]. The survival strategy of AHA is early recognition, early CPR, early defibrillation, and early advanced life support care in order to optimize a patient's chance for surviving out-of-hospital arrest. It has been shown that in New York City the median time to first shock was 12.4 min in 1991 [75]. In rural areas where emergency services are nonexistent or remote and travel time is long, time to defibrillation access is even more. In order to decrease time to defibrillation community-based response program composed of non-medical volunteer responders, who typically are not expected to respond to medical emergencies, would be trained to use, and have access to AEDs. The goal of these programs is to shorten the time from onset of VF until CPR and shock delivery by ensuring that AEDs and trained lay rescuers are available in public areas where CA is likely to occur.

Unfortunately, the PAD program is not universally acknowledged. A critical factor in the success of a PAD program is public awareness and widespread training in basic life support.

To increase the likelihood that a bystander will be trained in CPR, communities should have a strong public awareness program with frequent and convenient courses on BLS/AED. AHA suggests that AEDs should be placed at location where at least one CA is likely to occur every two years. An obstacle to an effective PAD program is the fear of civil lawsuits that might arise from organizations providing an AED and from laypersons becoming involved in the care of a cardiac arrest victim. To protect layperson responders involved in the resuscitation attempts of a cardiac arrest victim, the Cardiac Arrest Survival Act (CASA) was passed into federal law (Public Law 106-505) in 2000. In the USA CASA has played a pivotal role in setting the standards for immunity protection for rescuers using AEDs and for those who acquire an AED. Since then, several other countries incorporated similar acts.

Although AEDs have been shown to reduce time to first shock [70, 76] and improve survival in out-of-hospital VF arrest [73, 77], outcomes in in-hospital cardiac arrest have been relatively unchanged for the past 40 years [78]. Delayed defibrillation may occur when patients sustain cardiac arrest in unmonitored hospital beds. Use of AEDs has been proposed as a strategy to improve in-hospital cardiac arrest survival via prompt defibrillation by floor personnel who witness a VF arrest. Despite limited evidence AHA guidelines recommend consideration of AED use in the in-hospital setting as a means to shorten time to first shock to within 3 minutes of collapse [79]. Nevertheless, a relative study showed that AEDs failed to improve survival to discharge for in-hospital VF arrest when compared with standard monophasic defibrillators [80]. Further studies are necessary in order to incorporate or not AEDs in hospital setting.

The automated external defibrillator is a safe and effective tool that can significantly improve survival for CA victims, but the effectiveness of this device depends on it being present or immediately delivered to the site of arrest. A well established PAD program is worthwhile and it should be universally acknowledged.

# Conclusion

Cardiac arrest still remains a daunting medical emergency in Western societies and is the cause of approximately 250,000-600,000 deaths annually in the United States, with ventricular fibrillation being the initial rhythm in 20-38% of cases. Defibrillation is the only treatment available to terminate this life-threatening arrhythmia.

The mechanism of defibrillation is complex and can be considered at many different levels of explanation, starting at the level of the whole patient and extending to the level of cellular membranes and ion channels. Optimal energy levels for teminating VF for both monophasic and biphasic waveforms are unknown and practitioners need to be aware that a single, standardized approach to defibrillation does not exist. Furthermore, TTI is a major determinant of successful defibrillation and optimal defibrillation technique aims in delivering current across the fibrillating myocardium in the presence of minimal TTI. Early access to defibrillation is a key component to the ''Chain of Survival''. Rapid-response programs have achieved marked improvements in survival rates in selected localities. A well established PAD program is worthwhile and it should be universally acknowledged.

# References

[1] Deakin, CD; Nolan, JP. European Resuscitation Council Guidelines for Resuscitation 2005. Section 3. Electrical therapies: Automated external defibrillators, defibrillation, cardioversion and pacing. *Resuscitation* 2005; 67:S25-S37.

[2] Gliner, BE; Jorgenson, DB; Poole, JE; White, RD; Kanz, KG; Lyster, TD; Leyde, KW; Powers, DJ; Morgan, CB; Kronmal, RA; Bardy, GH. Treatment of out-of-hospital *Biomed Instrum Technol.* 1998; 32:631-644.

[3] Schneider, T; Martens, PR; Paschen, H; Kuisma, M; Wolcke, B; Gliner, BE; Russell, JK; Weaver, WD; Bossaert, L; Chamberlain, D. Multicenter, randomized, controlled trial of 150-J biphasic shocks compared with 200- to 360-J monophasic shocks in the resuscitation of out-of-hospital cardiac arrest victims. Optimized response to cardiac arrest (ORCA) investigators. *Circulation* 2000; 102:1780—7.

[4] Zepf, B. Long-term follow-up after rapid defibrillation. *Am Fam Physician.* 2004; 69:1-2.

[5] Trayanova, N. Defibrillation of the heart: insights into mechanisms from modelling studies. *Exp Physiol* 2006; 91:323–337

[6] Wiggers, CJ. Studies of ventricular fibrillation caused by electric shock: cinematographic and Electrocardiographic observations of the natural process in the dog's heart: its inhibition by potassium and the revival of coordinated beats by calcium. *Am J Physiol* 1930; 5: 351–365.

[7] Fabiato, A ; Coumel, P; Gourgon, R ; Saumont, R. Le seuil de response synchrone des fibres myocardiques: application a la comparaison experimentale de l'efficacite des differentes formes de chocs electriques de defibrillation. *Arch des Mal du Coeur* 1967; 60:527-544.

[8] Walcott, GP; Walcott, KT; Ideker, RE. Mechanisms of Defibrillation. Critical Points and the Upper Limit of Vulnerability. *J Electrocardiol.* 1995; 28 Suppl:1-6.

[9] Walgott, GP; Knisley, SB; Zhou, X; Newton, JG; Ideker, RE. On the mechanism of ventricular defibrillation. *PACE* 1997; 20:422-431.

[10] Karlon, WJ; Eisenherg, SR; Lehr, JL. Effects of paddle placement and size on defibrillation current distribution: A three-dimensional finite element model. *IEEE Trans Biomed Eng* 1993; 40:246-255.

[11] Zhou, X; Daubert, JP; Wolf, PD; Smith, WM; Ideker, RE. Epicardial mapping of ventricular defibrillation with monophasic and biphasic shocks in dogs. *Circ Res* 1993; 72:145-160.

[12] Wharton, JM; Wolf, PD; Smith, WM; Chen, PS; Frazier, DW; Yabe, S; Danieley, N; Ideker, RE. Cardiac potential and potential gradient fields generated by single, combined, and sequential shocks during ventricular defibrillation. *Circulation* 1992; 85:1510-1523

[13] Lerman, BB; Deale, OC. Relation between transcardiac and transthoracic current during defibrillation in humans. *Circ Res* 1990; 67:1420-1426.

[14] Zhou, X; Smith, W; Rollins, D; Ideker, RE. Transmombrane potential changes caused by shocks in guinea pig papillary muscle, *Am J Physiol* 1996; 40:2536-2546.

[15] Jones, JL; Jones, RF. Threshold reduction with biphasic defibrillator waveforms: Role of excitation channel recovery in computer model of the ventricular action potential. *J Eloctrocardiol* 1991; 23:30-35

[16] Furman, S. Early history of cardiac pacing and defibrillation. *Indian Pacing Electrophysiol J.* 2002; 2:2-3.

[17] Finamore, S; Turris, SA. Biphasic External Defibrillation for Adults in Ventricular Fibrillation or Pulseless Ventricular Tachycardia *J Cardiovasc Nurs* 2008; 23:326-329

[18] Kim, ML; Kim, SG; Park, DS; Gross, JN; Ferrick, KJ; Palma, EC; Fisher, JD. Comparison of rectilinear biphasic waveform energy versus truncated exponential biphasic waveform energy for transthoracic cardioversion of atrial fibrillation. *Am J Cardiol.* 2004; 94:1438-1440.

[19] Neal, S; Ngarmukos, T; Lessard, D; Rosenthal, L. Comparison of the efficacy and safety of two biphasic defibrillator waveforms for the conversions of atrial fibrillation to sinus rhythm. *Am J Cardiol.* 2003; 92:810-814.

[20] Kidwai, BJ; McIntyre, A; Anderson, J; Adgey, AA. Optimization of transthoracic ventricular defibrillation-biphasic and triphasic shocks, waveform rounding, and synchronized shock delivery. *J Electrocardiol* 2002; 35:235–244.

[21] Zhang, Y; Ramabadran, RS; Boddicker, KA; Bawaney, I; Davies, LR; Zimmerman, MB; Wuthrich, S; Jones, JL; Kerber, RE. Triphasic waveforms are superior to biphasic waveforms for transthoracic defibrillation. *J Am Coll Cardiol* 2003; 42:568–575.

[22] McDaniel, WC; Magin, T; Madsen, RW; Bonagura, JD; Schuder, JC; Curtis, JJ. Transthoracic defibrillation of dogs with Edmark, biphasic, and quadriphasic waveforms. *J Electrocardiol* 2002; 35:45–52

[23] Kerber, RE; Kouba, C; Martins, J; Kelly, K; Low, R; Hoyt, R; Ferguson, D; Bailey, L; Bennett, P; Charbonnier, F. Advance prediction of transthoracic impedance in human defibrillation and cardioversion: importance of impedance in determining the success of low-energy shocks. *Circulation* 1984; 70:303-8.

[24] Joglar, JA; Kessler, DJ; Welch, PJ; Keffer, JH; Jessen, ME; Hamdan, MH; Page, RL. Effects of repeated electrical defibrillations on cardiac troponin I levels. *Am J Cardiol* 1999; 83:270-2.

[25] Jacobs, IG; Tibballs, J; Morley, PT; Dennett, J; Wassertheil, J; Callanan, V; Hall, J. Australian Resuscitation Council. Energy levels for biphasic defibrillation. *EMJA.* 2003; 179:451.

[26] Adgey, AAJ; Spence, MS; Walsh, SJ. Theory and practice of defibrillation: (2) defibrillation for ventricular fibrillation. *Heart.* 2005; 91:118-125.

[27] Higgins, SL; O'Grady, SG; Banville, I; Chapman, FW; Schmitt, PW; Lank, P; Walker, RG; Ilina, M. Efficacy of lower-energy biphasic shocks for transthoracic defibrillation: a follow-up clinical study. *Prehosp Emerg Care* 2004; 8:262-7.

[28] Faddy, SC; Powell, J; Craig, JC. Biphasic and monophasic shocks for transthoracic defibrillation: a meta analysis of randomised controlled trials. *Resuscitation* 2003; 58:9-16.

[29] Clark, CB; Zhang, Y; Davies, LR; Karlsson, G; Kerber, RE. Transthoracic biphasic waveform defibrillation at very high and very low energies: a comparison with monophasic waveforms in an animal model of ventricular fibrillation. *Resuscitation* 2002; 54:183-6.

[30] White, RD; Hankins, DG; Atkinson, EJ. Patient outcomes following defibrillation with a low energy biphasic truncated exponential waveform in out-of-hospital cardiac arrest. *Resuscitation* 2001; 49:9-14.

[31] Martens, PR; Russell, JK; Wolcke, B; Paschen, H; Kuisma, M; Gliner, BE; Weaver, WD; Bossaert, L; Chamberlain, D; Schneider, T. Optimal Response to Cardiac Arrest study: defibrillation waveform effects. *Resuscitation* 2001; 49:233-43.

[32] Higgins, SL; Herre, JM; Epstein, AE; Greer, GS; Friedman, PL; Gleva, ML; Porterfield, JG; Chapman, FW; Finkel, ES; Schmitt, PW; Nova, RC; Greene, HL. A comparison of biphasic and monophasic shocks for external defibrillation. Physio-Control Biphasic Investigators. *Prehosp Emerg Care* 2000; 4:305-13.

[33] Vikas, CJ; Wheelan ,K. Successful cardioversion of atrial fibrillation using 360-joules biphasic shock. *Am J Cardiol*. 2002; 90:331-332.

[34] Walcott, GP; Killingsworth, CR; Ideker, RE. Do clinically relevant transthoracic defibrillation energies cause myocardial damage and dysfunction? *Resuscitation*. 2003; 59:59-70.

[35] Mittal, S; Ayati, S; Stein, KM; Knight, BP; Morady, F; Schwartzman, D; Cavlovich, D; Platia, EV; Calkins, H; Tchou, PJ; Miller, JM; Wharton, JM; Sung, RJ; Slotwiner, DJ; Markowitz, SM; Lerman, BB. Comparison of a novel rectilinear biphasic waveform with a damped sine wave monophasic waveform for transthoracic ventricular defibrillation. ZOLL investigators. *J Am Coll Cardiol*. 1999; 34:1595-1601.

[36] Stiell, IG; Walker, RG; Nesbitt, LP; Chapman, FW; Cousineau, D; Christenson, J; Bradford, P; Sookram, S; Berringer, R; Lank, P; Wells, GA. BIPHASIC trial: a randomized comparison of fixed lower versus escalating higher energy levels for defibrillation in out-of-hospital cardiac arrest. *Circulation*. 2007; 115:1511-1517.

[37] White, RD. Waveforms for defibrillation and cardioversion: recent experimental and clinical studies. *Curr Opin Crit Care* 2004; 10:202–207.

[38] Weaver, WD; Copass, MK; Bufi, D; Ray, R; Hallstrom, AP; Cobb, LA. Improved neurologic recovery and survival after early defibrillation. *Circulation*. 1984; 69:943–948.

[39] Paradis, NA; Martin, GP; Rivers, EP; Goetting, MG; Appleton, TJ; Feingold, M; Nowak, RM. Coronary perfusion pressure and the return of spontaneous circulation in human cardiopulmonary resuscitation. *JAMA* 1990; 263:1106 –1113.

[40] Berg, RA; Sanders, AB; Kern, KB; Hilwig, RW; Heidenreich, JW; Porter, ME; Ewy, GA.Adverse hemodynamic effects of interrupting chest compressions for rescue breathing during cardiopulmonary resuscitation for ventricular fibrillation cardiac arrest. *Circulation* 2001;104:2465—70.

[41] Kern, KB; Hilwig, RW; Berg, RA; Sanders, AB; Ewy, GA. Importance of continuous chest compressions during cardiopulmonary resuscitation: improved outcome during a simulated single lay-rescuer scenario. *Circulation* 2002; 105:645-9.

[42] van Alem, AP; Sanou, BT; Koster, RW. Interruption of cardiopulmonary resuscitation with the use of the automated external defibrillator in out-of-hospital cardiac arrest. *Ann Emerg Med* 2003; 42:449-57.

[43] Jones, VC; Charbonnier, FM; Long, P. Determining transthoracic impedance, delivered energy, and peak current during defibrillation episodes. *Med Instr* 1981;15: 380-2.

[44] Geddes, LA; Tacker, WA; Schoenlein, W; Minton, M; Grubbs, S; Wilcox, P. The prediction of the impedance of the thorax to defibrillating current. *Med Instr* 1976;10: 159-62.

[45] Armayor, MR; Savino, G; Valentinuzzi, ME; Clavin, DE; Monzon, JE; Arrendondo, MT. Ventricular defibrillation thresholds with capacitor discharge. *Med Biol Eng Comput* 1979;17: 435-42

[46] Kerber, RE; Grayzel, J; Hoyt, R; Marcus, M; Kennedy, J. Transthoracic resistance in human defibrillation: influence of body weight, chest size, serial shocks, paddle size and paddle contact pressure. *Circulation*. 1981; 63:676–682.

[47] KenKnight, BH; Eyuboglu, BM; Ideker, RE. Impedance to defibrillation countershock: does an optimal impedance exist? *Pacing Clin Electrophysiol* 1995; 18:2068-87.

[48] Stults, KR; Brown, DD; Cooley, F; Kerber, RE. Self-adhesive monitor/ defibrillation pads improve prehospital defibrillation success. *Ann Emerg Med*. 1987; 16:872– 877.

[49] American National Standard: Automatic External Defibrillators and Remote Controlled Defibrillators (DF39). Arlington, Virgina: Association for the Advancement of Medical Instrumentation; 1993.

[50] Dahl, CF; Ewy, GA; Warner, ED; Thomas, ED. Myocardial necrosis from direct current countershock: effect of paddle electrode size and time interval between discharges. *Circulation*. 1974; 50:956 –961.

[51] Deakin, CD; Sado, DM; Petley, GW; Clewlow, F. Determining the optimal paddle force for external defibrillation. *Am J Cardiol* 2002; 90:812–3.

[52] Deakin, CD; Bennetts, S; Petley, GW; Clewlow, F. What is the optimal paddle force during paediatric external defibrillation? *Resuscitation* 2003;5 9:83–8.

[53] Zipes, D; Fisher, J; King, R; Nicoll, A; Jolly, W. Termination of ventricular fibrillation in dogs by depolarising a critical amount of myocardium. *Am J Cardiol* 1975; 36:37-44

[54] Sirna, S; Ferguson, D; Charbonnier, F; Kerber, R. Factors affecting trans-thoracic impedance during electrical cardioversion. *Am J Cardiol* 1988; 62:1048–52.

[55] Deakin, CD; McLaren, RM; Petley, GW; Dalrymple-Hay, MJR; Clewlow, F. Effects of positive end-expiratory pressure on transthoracic impedance—implications for defibrillation. *Resuscitation* 1998; 37:9–12.

[56] Leatherman, J; Ravenscraft, S. Low measured auto-positive end-expiratory pressure during mechanical ventilation of patients with severe asthma: Hidden auto-positive end-expiratory pressure. *Crit Care Med* 1996; 24:541–6.

[57] Ewy, G; Taren, D. Impedance to transthoracic direct current discharge: a model for testing interface material. *Med Instrum* 1978; 12:47–8..

[58] Kerber, RE; Jensen, SR; Grayzel, J; Kennedy, J; Hoyt, R. Elective cardioversion: Influence of paddle-electrode location and size on success rates and energy requirements. *New Engl J Med* 1981; 305:658–62.

[59] Garcia, LA; Kerber, RE. Transthoracic defibrillation: does electrode adhesive pad position alter transthoracic impedance? *Resuscitation* 1998; 37:139–143

[60] Pagan-Carlo, LA; Spencer, KT; Robertson, CE; Dengler, A; Birkett, C; Kerber, RE. Transthoracic defibrillation: importance of avoiding electrode placement directly on the female breast. *J Am Coll Cardiol* 1996; 27:449-52.

[61] Deakin, CD; Sado, DM; Petley, GW; Clewlow, F. Is the orientation of the apical defibrillation paddle of importance during manual external defibrillation? *Resuscitation* 2003;56:15-18

[62] American Heart Association Statistics Committee. Heart disease and stroke statistics, 2007 Update. *Circulation.*2007; 115:1-105.

[63] Larsen, MP; Eisenberg, MS; Cummins, RO; Hallstrom, AP. Predicting survival from out-of-hospital cardiac arrest: a graphic model. *Ann Emerg Med* 1993; 22:1652-8.

[64] Valenzuela, TD; Roe, DJ; Cretin, S; Spaite, DW, Larsen MP. Estimating effectivness of cardiac arrest interventions: a logistic regression survival model. *Circulation* 1997; 96:3308-13

[65] Waalewijn, RA; de Vos, R; Tijssen, JGP; Koster, RW. Survival models for out-of-hospital cardiopulmonary resuscitation from the perspectives of the bystander, the first responder, and the paramedic. *Resuscitation* 2001; 51:113-22.

[66] Rho, RW; Page, RL. The Automated External Defibrillator. *J Cardiovasc Electrophysiol* 2007; 18:896-899.

[67] Nichol, G; Detsky, AS; Stiell, IG; Or, K; Wells, G; Laupacis, A. Effectiveness of emergency medical services for victims of out-ofhospital cardiac arrest: a metaanalysis. *Ann Emerg Med* 1996; 27:700-10.

[68] Page, RL; Joglar, JA; Kowal, RC; Zagrodzky, JD; Nelson, LL; Ramaswamy, K; Barbera, SJ; Hamdan, MH; McKenas, DK. Use of automated external defibrillators by a U.S. airline. *N Engl J Med* 2000; 343:1210-1216.

[69] Valenzuela, TD; Roe, DJ; Nichol, G; Clark, LL; Spaite, DW; Hardman, RG. Outcomes of rapid defibrillation by security officers after cardiac arrest in casinos. *N Engl J Med* 2000; 343:1206-1209.

[70] Mosesso, VN Jr; Davis, EA; Auble, TE; Paris; Yealy, DM. Use of automated external defibrillators by police officers for treatment of out-of-hospital cardiac arrest. *Ann Emerg Med* 1998; 32:200–207

[71] Cummins, RO; Eisenberg, MS; Hallstrom, AP; Litwin, PE. Survival of out-of-hospital cardiac arrest with early initiation of cardiopulmonary resuscitation. *Am J Emerg Med* 1985; 3:114-9.

[72] Capucci, A; Aschieri, D; Piepoli, MF. Out-of-hospital *Ital Heart J.* 2002; 3:721-5.

[73] The Public Access Defibrillation Trial Investigators. Public-access defibrillation and survival after out-of-hospital cardiac arrest. *N Engl J Med* 2004; 351:637–646

[74] The PAD Trial Investigators. The Public Access Defibrillation (PAD) Trial Study design and rationale. *Resuscitation* 2003; 56:135-147

[75] Lombardi, G; Gallagher, J; Gennis, P. Outcome of out of hospital cardiac arrest in New York City. The Pre Hospital Arrest Survival Evaluation (PHASE) study. *J Am Med Assoc* 1994; 271:678-83.

[76] White, RD; Asplin, BR; Bugliosi, TF; Hankins, DG. High discharge survival rate after out-of-hospital ventricular fibrillation with rapid defibrillation by police and paramedics. *Ann Emerg Med* 1996; 28:480–485.

[77] Capucci, A; Aschieri, D; Piepoli, MF; Bardy, GH; Iconomu, E; Arvedi, M. Tripling survival from sudden cardiac arrest via early defibrillation without traditional education in cardiopulmonary resuscitation. *Circulation* 2002; 106:1065–1070

[78] Weil, MH; Fries, M. In hospital cardiac arrest. *Crit Care Med* 2005; 33:2825-2830

[79] 2005 American Heart Association Guidelines for Cardiopulmonary Resuscitation and Emergency Cardiovascular Care, Part 5: Electrical Therapies. *Circulation* 2005; 112:IV-35–IV-46

[80] Forcina, MS; Farhat, AY; O'Neill, WW; Haines, DE. Cardiac arrest survival after implementation of automated external defibrillator technology in the in-hospital setting. *Crit Care Med* 2009; 37:1229-1236.

In: Advances in Cardiovascular Research, Volume 1
Editors: L. Schmitt, T. Konig, pp. 171-198
ISBN: 978-1-60741-720-0


*Chapter VI*

# Acute Kidney Injury after Coronary Artery Bypass

***M. Guillouet, B.V. Nguyen, F. Lion, R. Deredec, C.C. Arvieux and G. Gueret*** *

Pôle Anesthésie Réanimation, Centre Hospitalier Universitaire, 29609 Brest, France

## Abstract

Acute kidney injury (AKI) is common after cardiac surgery with cardiopulmonary bypass (CPB). Previous studies have reported an incidence from 3 to 30% according to the authors and the different criteria considered [1-4]. The percentage of patients with AKI requiring dialysis may vary from 0.5 to 3% according to certain studies [5-12]. Post-operative AKI after cardiac surgery with CPB correlates with an increased length of stay in the intensive care unit (ICU) [5]. It is also associated with a high mortality rate (up to 60%) when dialysis is required [3,5,13]. Risk factors like female gender, diabetes, chronic obstructive pulmonary disease, congestive heart failure, length of surgery and age have been identified [14], and one of the most important factors seems to be chronic renal failure before surgery, even if this last association although requiring further research, has been universally accepted [15].

Recently, studies have demonstrated the association of genetic polymorphisms with a risk of renal injury. The genetic variants identified are associated with increases in renal inflammatory response through exagerated synthesis in the IL6 protein [16]. There is also genetic predisposition.

AKI in CPB is the consequence of a mixture of several physiopathological phenomena, among which we find systemic inflammatory response syndrome (SIRS).

Cardiac bypass surgery activates the inflammatory cascade and leads to systemic inflammatory response syndrome through the phenomenon of ischemia-reperfusion. Indeed, initially, we can observe an imbalance between pro- and anti-inflammatory factors as well as between factors of vasoconstriction. Secondly, neutrophils, vascular

* Corresponding author: Gildas Gueret, Pôle Anesthésie Réanimation, Centre Hospitalier Universitaire, 29609 Brest, France. Phone: 33 2 98 34 72 88; Fax: 33 2 98 34 78 10; Email: gildas.gueret@chu-brest.fr

endothelium and platelets are activated. These events lead to capillary microthrombosis and the elaboration of inflammatory mediators such as IL-6, IL-8 and TNF α. These cytokines are both synthetised systemically and locally in the kidney. They are responsible for tubular necrosis, apoptosis, and glomerular injury. Serum creatinine and perioperative urinary output which are routinely used to evaluate the underlying renal status of the patient are not sensitive and specific enough in the detection of the early phases of this condition. New biomarkers, including neutrophil gelatinase, associated lipocalin, interleukin 18 and kidney injury molecule 1 seem promising.

Thus, we can hope that a better knowledge of all of the mechanisms leading to acute renal dysfunction after coronary artery bypass and the use of new renal injury biomarkers may reduce the negative consequences of AKI.

## Introduction

Acute kidney injury (AKI) after coronary artery bypass has an incidence varying between 3 to 30% [1-4] and is associated with substantial morbidity and mortality [5].

Risk factors including those of a genetic nature have been identified in recent studies.

The mechanisms involved are both inflammatory, haemodynamic and nephrotoxic leading to tubular and glomerular injury.

Practice modifications and earlier diagnoses of acute renal injury may provide with some guidelines in its prevention and successful management

## Incidence and Prognosis of Acute Kidney Injuries after Bypass Surgery

Cardiac surgery has a high AKI risk due to perioperative hemodynamic disorders [7]. It is a common yet serious complication: depending on the definition of AKI, the incidence varies across studies from 3 to 30% [1-4]. A need for dialysis occurs in approximately 1 to 2% of patients [5-12]. Even a small postoperative increase of creatinine has been associated with the worst outcome [17-19]. However, the incidence of AKI after cardiac surgery has increased over time [20]. The adjusted risk of mortality decreased in patients with AKI without other postoperative complications but not in those with multiorgan system failure (MOF) [20].

There is an independent association between AKI and mortality following cardiac surgery [13,21]. The associated mortality rate is up to 60%, when dialysis is required, and it is also associated with worse hospital outcomes and a higher risk of infection complications. AKI is often the organ failure which occurs the earliest in the MOF post-operative sequence.

It appears to be increasing in frequency regardless of the clinical severity of the patients undergoing surgery, possibly related to more sensitive and accurate diagnosis [3]. In addition, this also represents an additional financial burden even after allowances for age, gender and co-morbidity factors. Reducing the incidence and the severity of this complication would hopefully lead to a reduction in hospital and health-care costs [31].

# Risk Factors Associated with Acute Kidney Injury

Acute kidney injury is a multifactorial event that involves pre-, peri- and post-operative factors. They are linked to the patient, to the surgical procedure, to the CPB and to the postoperative period.

## A. The Patient

Advanced age, black ethnicity, increased body weight, arterial hypertension, atherosclerotic vascular disease, diabetes and elevated preoperative serum glucose, reduced left ventricular function and chronic obstructive pulmonary disease have been identified as predisposing risk factors [7,13,22-25].

Chronic renal failure has been identified as one of the most important risk factors of post-operative AKI [1,6,8,25,26]. This association has recently been challenged in several studies; some authors have attempted to demonstrate no greater risk for patients with preexisting renal impairement [8,27], but most authors have found that preexisting renal impairment is an important risk factor of AKI [23]. With regards to patients who require dialysis after cardiac surgery, the hemodynamic peri-operative disorders are a more important prognostic factor than pre-existing chronic renal insufficiency [28].

Pre-operative lower-left ventricular ejection fraction or congestive heart failure is a major risk factor of post-operative AKI [1,6,22,23]. Left-ventricle dysfunction is responsible for a reduction in the urinary ejection fraction of sodium due to decrease in renal blood flow [29].

The effect of diabetes mellitus on post-operative renal failure may be the result of renal parenchymal disease, such as glomerulonephritis and glomerulosclerosis. Furthermore, diabetic patients often suffer from renal artery stenosis [30] and microangiopathy. Elevated preoperative hemoglobin A1c levels are associated with increased AKI incidence and mortality [31].

Emergency surgery [23], hemodynamic instability and the recourse to intra aortic conterpulsion are also independant risk factors of AKI [7,32].

The female gender is known to have a lower baseline hematocrit and lower blood volume, which increase the risk of hemodilution and transfusion during surgery. Preoperative anemia is associated with an increase in renal complications depending on the haemoglobin level [33].

Recently, the association between genetic polymorphisms and risks of renal injury have been demonstrated. This may help to explain a two- to three-fold higher variation than clinical risk. Identified genetic variants have been associated with an increase in renal inflammatory response by exaggerated synthesis in the IL-6 protein. There are also vasoconstriction polymorphim factors. In Caucasians, the composition of the IL6 572C and angiotensinogen 842C polymorphisms have been identified to be a predictor of four-fold greater creatinine rises after coronary artery bypass. In Afro-Caribbean ethnicities, findings concern eNOS 894T and angiotensin-converting enzyme deletion polymorphisms [16].

## B. Surgical Procedure

*Emergency surgery* [23] is described as an independent risk factor of post-operative AKI [7,32].

*Combined surgery [11]:* Coronary artery bypass grafting has the lowest incidence of ARF after cardiac surgery [34], combined coronary and valvulary surgery are of a higher risk of AKI. Valvular heart operations are an independant risk for AKI [34].

*Off-pump versus on-pump CABG:* However, the effect of off-pump coronary bypasses on renal dysfunction is still being discussed [35] as it depends on the preoperative renal function [36]. It has been suggested that myocardial revascularization by off-pump coronary artery bypass grafting surgery could reduce the morbidity compared with the on-pump technique [37,38]. Concerning the effects on the renal function, the studies are contradictory; a study on patients at a high risk for renal failure after coronary artery bypass surgery concluded that off-pump techniques did not reduce the risk of postoperative renal AKI [39]. Similar results have been found with patients who had normal renal preoperative functions. Conversely, Ascione et al. [40], in his 1999 study, suggested that off pump coronary revascularization would offer superior renal protection when compared with conventional coronary revascularization with CPB. Furthermore, systemic inflammation is also observed in patients undergoing cardiac surgery off- pump coronary artery bypass with a pattern different to CPB [41].

*Aortic cross-clamping time, duration of surgery:* As with aortic cross clamping duration, longer CPB time [42] seems to be an independant risk factor of AKI; the critical time delays vary according to the studies, superior to 90 minutes [12], 140 minutes [43], or three hours [5].

Operative bleeding (> 1000 ml) and massive blood replacement [44] are risk factors that are classically identified with post-operative AKI [11,32]. Furthermore, transfusion itself is also a risk factor of AKI [44].

## C. CPB

Risk factors related to the bypass procedure itself have been linked to the development of AKI, such as mean arterial pressure during CPB [32,42], perfusion flow [32,42], hypothermia, hemolysis, hemodilution, a high transfusion requirement, use of antifibrinolytic agents, off-pump versus on-pump cardiopulmonary bypass. They have been the subject of debates.

AKI can be influenced by peroperative haemodynamic parameters such as arterial pressure and pump flow during CPB as well as the use of amines during the procedure. However, previous studies have not yet established a relationship between CPB and clinical AKI (increase in creatinine and persistant oliguria) [45] and do not often give prominence to the clear correlation between the hemodynamic factors of CPB and post-operative clinical [11,32].

In fact, experimental studies have established a correlation between the constitution of renal infraclinical lesions and hemodynamic microcirculatory intrarenal modifications [46,47]: CPB leads to modifications in renal blood flow and microcirculatory vascular renal resistance without a clear correlation with the macrocirculatory parameters of CPB: the maintenance of mean arterial pressure by the vasoconstrictors does not improve renal perfusion at a microcirculatory level and only improves the biological criteria of the renal function (clearance and creatininaemia) in per-operation although not in post-operation [48]. Renal blood flow is closely related to blood pressure and pump flow, and urinary flow is primary determined by systemic blood pressure [25]. During CPB, there is a reduction in renal blood flow associated with an increase in renal vascular resistance which contributes to the constitution of a constant tubular necrosis, mostly infraclinical [47].

Hypothermia is not often mentioned as a major risk factor [49]. In CPB surgical patients with or without hypothermia, the evolution of the clearance of creatinine was similar regarding the groups [50,51], as long as the level of hypothermia in CPB was mild (32-34°C).

Non pulsatile flow would not affect clinical renal functioning after CPB [52].

Hemodilution reduces blood viscosity and improves regional blood flow to compensate reduced oxygen carrying capacity compared with prebypass levels. In addition, a moderate hemodilution seems to reduce the risk of kidney injury, although hematocrit below 22, 23 or 24 % is associated with post-operative AKI [24,53,54]. The current practice is to avoid extreme hemodilution which it has been linked to adverse outcomes. Indeed, hematocrit is directly related to tissue oxygen delivery, so severe hemodilution may contribute to severe ischemic tubular necrosis, particularly in the renal medulla which is a hypoxic environment [55].

Administration of an antifibrinolytic agent like aprotinine has been standard practice until recently. Because of the kidney's metabolization rate of the aprotinine, damage to the renal system has been discussed. Temporary renal dysfunction is caused by an overload of tubular reabsorption mechanisms. Patients with normal renal function preoperatively are able to compensate [56]. The dosage of aprotinin for patients with reduced renal function should certainly be adapted. Furthermore aprotinin reduces the need for blood transfusion [57] which increases risk of death, perioperative infection and renal failure. A recent revaluation of aprotinine shows that its administration did not negatively impact renal outcome [57-60]. However, aprotinine has been associated with an increased mortality after cardiac surgery [61,62]. Compared to aprotinine, the use of tranaxemic acid does not modify the incidence rate of AKI after cardiac surgery but is associated with an increased use of blood transfusion [63].

The use of loop diuretics (furosemide) during procedure allows the maintenance of urinary flow which satisfies the treating physician, but will have adverse effects on renal function after cardiac surgery [64].

Mini-CBP attenuates inflammatory response and hemodilution [65,66]. It has also been associated with a decrease in renal injuries [67-69].

### D. Post-Operative Period

Bleeding after cardiac surgery is also a major perioperative complication.

If the hemodynamic parameters during CPB are not clearly correlated with clinical AKI, post-operative hemodynamic instability with prolonged arterial hypotension, left heart failure and low post-operative heart rate, required use of intra aortic conterpulsation causing ischemic lesions are established risk factors [5,10,11,25,43,70].

Extracorporal circulation can be associated with post-operative multi-factorial cardiac dysfunction (insufficient myocardic protection, coronary embolus...) which affects renal functioning. The occurrence of a post-operative myocardic ischemia is an independant risk factor of AKI [32].

## Mechanisms Leading to Acute Kidney Injury

Four mechanisms coexist: hemodynamic and microcirculatory effects, systemic inflammation and ischemia-reperfusion, embolism and toxicity.

### A. Specificity of Renal Vascularisation

On account of the kidney's physiopathology, it is an organ at particular risk of ischemic and endothelial injury.

Because of the kidney's terminal vascularisation, the obstruction of a vessel causes ischemia of any area that is devascularised without any replacement network. The renal perfusion represents 20% of the total cardiac blood flow with marked regional differences in oxygen delivery, 99% of the blood flow is for the cortical and outer medullary areas and only 1 % for the inner medullary zone which is much more sensitive to a low perfusion rate.

In addition, the adaptation of renal capillary vasomotricity to its metabolic needs, to pressure, to renal flow and to the introduction of $O_2$ is mostly humoral and therefore is influenced by the mediators created by the syndrome of ischemia reperfusion and inflammatory reactions.

Finally two serial capillary networks an arterio-arterial glomerular and an arterio-veinous peritubular one, characterize kidney microcirculation. Thus large endothelial contact surface expands the filtration and absorption area. Ischemia-reperfusion provokes an endothelial lesion which greatly affects renal functioning.

Inefficient oxygen delivery to the kidney and a high metabolic rate renders the kidney vulnerable to ischemia-reperfusion injury.

### B. Hemodynamic Effects and Microcirculatory Disruption

CPB is associated with hemodynamic changes. Its role is to maintain regional perfusions at a level that supports optimal cellular and organ functions. Perfusion pressure during cardiopulmonary bypass has two functions: oxygen delivery and nutrient delivery.

The maintenance of cardiovascular stability needs a balance between the settings of the pump and the vascular characteristics of the patient such as venous compliance, systemic vascular resistance and various vascular beds.

Renal perfusion and autoregulation are maintained as long as these hemodynamic goals are reached, and any perturbation may lead to ischemia and cell damage.

Indeed micro-circulatory disruptions during CPB in experimental models are correlated with infra-clinical glomerular and tubular lesions [46,47].

At the micro-circulatory level, hypothermia causes a reduction in vascular renal resistance due to inadequate vasodilation of the afferent and efferent arterioles in some nephrons, and in others, the opening of aglomerular capillary shunts by preglomerular vasoconstriction. There is a loss of autoregulation. The microcirculatory vasomotor tonicity can not adapt to the pressure of the glomerular perfusions and to the metabolic needs of the nephrons [46]. The glomerular filtration rate can be lowered while renal blood flow remains the same and the vascular renal resistances are reduced. During the re-warming process, the vasomotor response on the nephron level is heterogenous and the microcirculatory disturbances lead to tubular and glomerular lesions.

The non pulsatile nature of the procedure decreases the elastance, inertial and reflective components of arterial resistance.

On the capillary level, the suppression of the pulsatility of the blood flow provokes a disturbance in microcirculatory tonicity through dyshomeostasis of the endothelial basal secretion of NO.

The incomplete recovery of the perfusion at the end of procedure, mainly at the superficial cortex layer and the internal medullar leads to acute necrotic tubular ischemic lesions. These lesions will have unfavorable clinical consequences if they are associated with hypotension or a prolonged low-blood flow in immediate post-operative situations.

In post-operative situations, the absolute or relative hypovolemia can also increase the functional part of AKI constituted during the CPB.

### C. Systemic Inflammation and Ischemia-Reperfusion

Both innate and adaptative immune reponses are activated by CPB.

Cardiac bypass surgery activates the inflammatory cascade and leads to systemic inflammatory response through the phenomenon of ischemia-reperfusion [71]. During cardiac bypass surgery we can observe an imbalance between pro- and anti-inflammatory factors with a difference of the glomerular filtration of these mediators [71-73]. Indeed, pro-inflammatory factors moleculars weights are less than 20 kDa, allowing for their rapid glomerular filtration. The pro-inflammatory cytokines are excreted on the tubular level where they exert their cytotoxic effects, participating in the pathogenesis of acute ischemic tubular necrosis (AITN) lesions.

Stimuli during the surgical procedure such as surgical trauma, blood contact with cardiopulmonary surfaces (biocompatibility), endotoxemia, ischemia and reperfusion activate a host of inflammatory mediators, adhesion molecules and proinflammatory transcription factors (such as NFkB) [74].

All manifestations of the acute phases of inflammation are activated; the cellular phase, the humoral phase and the vascular phase. These inflammatory phenomena are directly linked to the activation of coagulation systems, of fibrinolysis and of the complement system. The central phenomenon of physiopathology of the inflammation in CPB is endothelial dysfunction [25,75,76] and the abnormal homeostasis of the NO metabolism plays a key role in the constitution of tubular ischemic lesions [77,78].

Inflammatory mediators such as cytokines (IL-6, IL-8, TNF$\alpha$), chemokines, proteases and cytotoxic oxygen-derived free radicals are released by endothelial cells, circulating monocytes, and tissue-fixed macrophages [74]. TNF–$\alpha$ is responsible for glomerular lesions and it also induces IL-6 and IL-1$\beta$ synthesis. IL-6 stimulates the hepatocytes which synthesize proteins of the acute phase of the inflammation (CRP, MBP (mannose binding protein), orosomucoid, haptoglobin), it also leads to lymphocytic activation. The inflammatory cytokins have a major role in inflammatory glomerular injury [79]. A recent study found an IL-6 increase in patients suffering from severe renal dysfunction after coronary artery bypass [80].

A polymorphism at the gene level of the inflammation, in particular the IL6, has been associated with an increase in myocardial infarction and strokes after cardiac surgery [44,81] and sets up a predisposition to MOF [82].

Adhesion molecules such as selectines, integrines (CD11b, CD41), Ig superfamily are unregulated and activate neutrophils and vascular endothelium. Platelets also undergo activation, degranulation and adhesion to vascular endothelium [83,84]. Intrinsic coagulation systems, kallikrein systems and fibrinolytic systems are initiated by factor XIIa. Complement proteins are also activated. This humoral response leads to capillary microthrombosis and amplifies cellular responses leading to neutrophil, endothelial and monocyte activation and then to further elaboration of proinflammatory cytokines. The phenomenon of ischemia-reperfusion is the main initial trigger of the inflammatory cascade [85,86].

Hypoxemia also leads to a decrease in ATP with first provokes the production of adenosine, arteriolar constriction and tubular cell toxicity. Secondly it increases intracellular calcium and thus production of proinflammatory cytokines, proapoptotic factors and NO. At least, it inhibits active transport leading to edema and cellular death.

All of the above lead to acute necrotic tubular ischemic lesions. In the early phase of reperfusion, leucocytes stick to endothelial cells leading to vascular congestion. Then, they initiate the reflow phenomena, triggering the activation of endothelial and polynuclear cells which release proteolytic factors, cytotoxic oxygen-derived free radicals and proinflammatory cytokines.

The expression of adhesion membrane molecules to the endothelium CD11b by the neutrophilic polynuclears is associated to a renal lesion of AITN in post-operative cardiac surgery with CPB [86].

Finally, a cardio-renal connection is created: the heart develops TNFα and IL-6 which induce their own renal autosecretion [87] and exert their local tubular and glomular cytotoxicity.

Blood contact with the pericardial cavity induces strong hemolysis, inflammatory mediator release, and coagulation activation, driven by tissue factor pathway activation [88]. Elevated proinflammatory cytokines in cardiotomy blood suction are eliminated by cell salvage [89]. However, in off pump coronary artery bypass, retransfusion of washed shed blood decreases the systemic inflammatory response but does not have an impact on subclinical renal injury or dysfunction in low risk patients [89].

The end result of the Systemic Inflammatory Response Syndrome is tubular necrosis with apoptotic cell death, and glomerular injury. Renal ischemia is due to an obstruction of the tubules by the cellular debris and to microcirculatory vasomotor disturbances with inappropriate arteriolar vasoconstriction.

We can also examine back leak of the glomerular filtrate that results from impaired functional integrity of tight junctions caused by disruption of the actin cytoskeleton and loss of cell polarity [90].

Tubular lesions are not specific to coronary artery bypass surgery, they are associated with acute tubular necrosis with death cell agglutination leading to tubular obstruction [91,92].

Thus, coronary artery bypass leads to AKI through Systemic Inflammatory Response Syndrome for which the immune system of certain patients has an inappropriate response.

## D. Embolism

Macroscopic and microscopic embolism, both fat droplets and particles (thrombus, platelet fibrin debris, normal vessel wall, bulla), are often generated during cardiac surgery [93]. Gas emboli form scaffolds for the platelet activation which leads to coagulation and fibrinoformation.

In 2004, Sreeram, Stafford-Smith et al. highlighted a correlation between the numbers of Doppler-detected emboli during coronary artery bypass graft surgery and post-operative renal failure (rise in creatinine) [94].

Aortic plaque disruption because of intra-aortic balloon pump counterpulsion is likely to be a contributor to AKI.

Furthermore, lipid droplet contamination of reinfused blood may affect renal cortical blood flow, in particular during pericardic aspiration, however the importance of this phenomenon is unknown. The double capillary network (glomeruli and tubuli) found in the kidneys may be especially susceptible to lipid microemboli [95] and a correlation between the total number of emboli and postoperative changes in glomerular filtration rate was reported [96].

## E. Toxicity

In pre-operative situations, the renal function of patients can already be altered by antibiotics and non-steroidal anti-inflammatory drugs (NSAIDs). Diuretics, which are commonly prescribed for patients with cardiac failure, modify the autoregulation of renal blood flow and can lead to pre-operative hypovolemia. The use of peri- and post-operative diuretics to increase diuresis can contribute to an aggravation of functional acute renal failure.

Peri-operative use of contrast products (for coronarography) contributes to AKI.

Hemoglobin and myoglobin, which are released during CPB [97], avidly bind nitric oxide, causing AKI through direct cytotoxicity, vasoconstrictor effects and tubular obstruction [98]. Cardiotomy suction is a major cause of hemolysis and contributes significantly to the systemic inflammatory response [99].

During surgery, the use of drugs may be toxic. Catecholamine influences renal perfusion through $\alpha 1$- mediated vasoconstriction, dopaminergic and $\alpha 2$-mediated vasodilatation.

Furthermore, an association can be made between the necessity of transfusion, the use of drugs and an intra-operative instability.

Finally, the peri- and post-operative volemic expansion by hydroxyethylstarch (HES) can increase post-operative renal dysfunction even if its role remains debated [100-104]. The uses of a light-weight molecular 130/0.4 HES does not alter renal function compared to human albumin [105] or gelatin [102,104]. In elderly patients with pre-operative hypoalbuminemia, albumin had no benefit with regard to inflammatory response and renal function compared to 6% HES 130/0.4 [106].

## Diagnosis of Acute Kidney Injury after Coronary Artery Bypass

Early diagnosis of postoperative AKI is difficult, particularly after cardiac surgery. Although the role of early diagnosis of AKI remains to be determined, clinical trials may however be useful to establish effective protocols for possible therapeutic strategies.

The first obstacle in the diagnosis AKI is caused by the numerous existing conflicting definitions and parameters currently in use. Definition of acute renal injury differs between studies. The Thoracic Surgeons Society defines it as a two-fold (minimum required value) creatinine level rise to a value exceeding 2 mg/dL and/or new dialysis. An excessive rise of creatinine is another definition commonly used with different values quoted. A range of 20% [17], 25% [107-109], 30% [11], 35% [5], 50% [110-113] to 100% increase in creatinine was used to define the pathology. Post-operative serum creatinine levels above 177 μmol/L with a pre- to post-operative increase of above 62 μmol/L) [5] or increase in serum creatinine level greater than 0.5 mg/dL or a 25% increase from baseline [109] were also mentioned. Most of the studies included two groups (with or without AKI), but some studies included different groups according to the amount of creatinine increase [114-116]. The Length of clinical observation was also different among the first two [107], five [117] or seven [118] post-operative days.

Peri-operative urinary output of more than 1 ml/kg/h is not an outstanding reflection of renal function after cardiopulmonary bypass whereas a low urinary output during CPB has been associated with postoperative AKI [80].

The plasma creatinine dosage provides insufficient clinical data, particularly in older patients. Furthermore, serum creatinine concentration is greatly influenced by changes in muscle mass, race, age, sex, drugs, muscle metabolism, protein intake and tubular secretion. In AKI, serum creatinine is an even poorer index of kidney function because the patients are not stable, and serum creatinine changes occurs later than the onset of renal injury. Creatinaemia can remain normal, even in cases of serious damage to the renal function [119]. In spite of these limitations the changes of plasma creatinine are still widely used [6,17,25,107,109,115,116].

Many methods exist to evaluate the glomerular flow rate: the inulin clearance and the isotopic methods (125 Iode p aminohippurate, 51Cr-EDTA) [47] remain the methods of reference. They are not routinely used because of their cost, the difficulty of implementation and the availability of equipment.

Creatinine clearance measurement aims to evaluate glomerular filtration and it remains widely used even in cardiac surgery. It needs a stable state during 24 hours, particularly on a metabolic level and depends on the quality of urine collection. The renal excretion of creatinine can vary throughout the day [120]. Its clinical performance is reduced for values below 20 ml/min. The measurement of creatinine clearance has been proposed for shorter periods [121-127], but a minimum collection during four to eight hours is recommended [121,128]. Goldberg et al observed large daily variations of secondary urinary creatinine excretion for unreliability of urine collections [129] and O'Riordan et al have shown that more than 50% of the variations of creatinine clearance could not be explained by glomerular filtration rate (GFR) modifications [119].

Oliguria, increase in creatinine levels and the measured clearance of creatinine are different parameters used depending on the studies. Measured creatinine clearance is not reliable in the early post-operative period after cardiac surgery with CPB [128].

Estimated glomerular filtration rate was first developed by Cockcroft et al [130]. In this work, it was more sensitive than creatinine for renal diagnosis. Studies have demonstrated that a post-operative estimated glomerular filtration rate of less than 60 ml/min/1,73m$^2$ is associated with the worse 5-years survival [131]. After CPB, the MDRD formula [132] is more reliable than the Cockcroft Gault formula [128].

New biomarkers which can diagnose acute renal injury earlier are promising. They include the use of Plasma and urinary markers (α1 microglobulin, Gro-alpha, meprin, β2 microglobulin).

Urinary excretion of brush border tubular proximal cell glycoproteins during ischemia have often been used as markers of infra-clinical kidney injuries [47,73,133,134].

The NAG (N Acetyl β D glucosaminidas) is a lysosomial enzyme specific to proximal tubular cells which are neither secreted nor reabsorbed on a tubular level; the NAG urinary/creatinine report is a sensitive and specific marker of tubular injury [133].

The ADBP (brush border antigen adenosin desaminase binding protein) glycoprotein of the surface of tubular proximal cells, plasma and urinary β2 microglobulin and α1 microglobulin, are low molecular weight molecules which are filtered by the glomerulus and reabsorbed at 95% by tubular in normal conditions (excepting tubular injury). These are sensitive markers for tubular failure and have long been used in experimental studies [135] and in cardiac surgery [136].

The RBP (retinol binding protein) is also a low molecular weight glycoprotein that is reabsorbed by tubular and used as a urinary marker of tubular injury [137], and could be a more practical and reliable index of proximal tubular function than β2 microglobulin [138].

The neutrophil gelatinase-associated lipocalcin (NGAL) is generated by ischemic renal tubular cells and appears in the urine and in the plasma of cardiac surgery patients in less than six hours [45,76,79,110,111]. The two-hours NGAL urine collection levels correlated with severity and duration of AKI, length of stay, dialysis requirement and death [110]. Mishra et al have also shown an early increase of urinary NGAL concentration in children with AKI after pediatric cardiac surgery [79].

The Cystatine C is a low molecular weight protein (13.343 kDa) produced by all nucleus cells of the organism at a constant rate [139]. Cystatine C is freely filtered through the glomerular membrane and then metabolised by tubular cells (>99%). Its plasma concentration seems to be independent from physiological conditions, particularly size, weight and age of the patient, but it varies with thyroid pathology, high-dose corticotherapy, inflammatory syndrome (it increases with fibrinogen and CRP) or tobacco use [140,141]. Its concentration is higher in hospitalized patients for acute coronary syndrome. A genetic polymorphism is accompanied by variations of the Cystatine C/creatinine relationship [142]. Its short half-life time (estimated at 20 minutes for men) is really an interesting marker for the detection of acute renal failure, even though a large intra-individual variability [143]. It is primilarly a sensitive marker of reduction of glomerular filtration. But it cannot distinguish the different types of AKI. After CPB, Cystatine C increases later than creatinine [128]. The interest of plasma cystatine C is still debated until today [108,128,144]. Moreover urinary cystatine C could be interesting for early diagnosis of AKI [108].

The kidney injury molecule-1 (KIM-1) is a transmembrane protein that is overexpressed in proximal tubules of patients with established acute renal injury [145-147]. This marker seems to be more specific to nephrotoxic or ischemic kidney injury and it is not affected by chronic kidney disease or urinary tract infections. Thus it could represent an important tool for differentiating various types of AKI. However it is limited by its delayed urine increase by 12-24h after renal failure onset. Used in conjunction with other sensitive biomarkers it may add specificity to early diagnosis for AKI. Urinary KIM-1 has not yet been evaluated in cardiac surgery.

IL-18 also represents a promising candidate, it is able to predict AKI within six hours of cardiac surgery and it can discriminate between other types of renal injury [112]. Its role in cardiac surgery remains debatable however [148].

Some enzymes can identify the segmental involvement and ultrastructural origin of renal injury. Alpha and pi isomers of glutathione S-transferase are cytosolic enzymes from respectively proximal and distal tubular cells.

Other enzymuria such as Gama-glutamyl transpeptidase, alkaline phosphatase and ala-aminopeptidase identify general brush border.

Other urinary markers have recently been proposed but have not been studied during cardiac surgery: Fetuin-A [149], NHE3 (Na+/H+ exchanger isoform 3) [150], cysteine rich protein 61 (CYR61, CCN1) [151], netrin-1 [152-154] and lipocalin [155].

In conclusion, these new biomarkers seem to be promising in the AKI diagnosis, but studies are necessary to confirm their role in the cardiac surgery setting.

## How Can We Prevent Acute Kidney Injury after Coronary Artery Bypass?

A recent study has shown that a continuous quality improvement program can decrease sepsis and cardiac tamponnade after cardiac surgery but only marginally decrease AKI [156]. More research concerning AKI should be strongly encouraged.

### A. General Measures

The first important point is the identification of high-risk patients.

Secondly, it is important to avoid nephrotoxins and maintain optimal renal perfusion pressure. In sepsis, there is no evidence to suggest that norepinephrine is associated with an increased risk of AKI when used to treat arterial hypotension [157].

Before surgery, volume depletion and congestive heart failure must be treated.

In the peri-operative period, optimization of bypass flow, perfusion pressure, and oxygen delivery must be obtained through appropriate hydratation and the use of inotropic agents. The role of HES in occurrence of AKI is still being discussed [100-104].

Anesthesia techniques such as perioperative thoracic epidural local anesthetic blockade have been shown to attenuate the catecholamine response to cardiopulmonary bypass and surgery and have been associated with improved cardiac output [158,159], reduced apoptosis [158,159] and a decreased incidence of AKI [160]. However, epidural catheters in patients receiving high dose heparin and aspirin may be hazardous (the incidence of epidural hematoma was estimated to be between 1/150 000 and 1/1500 [161], or between 1/68 000 and 1/2100 [162]).

## B. Pharmacological Interventions

Unfortunately, pharmacological interventions have been attempted with inconsistent clinical results. The failure of these treatments may be related to the complex physiopathology of acute renal injury after coronary artery bypass, late pharmacological intervention and the limited number of studies regarding their benefits.

Thus, we can hope that the new biomarkers for earlier diagnosis along with further research on the subject will help us to progress in this direction.

The choice of the anesthetic agent does not affect the post-operative renal function [163].

Dopamine agonist agents have been used in the preventative and curative treatment of AKI because they increase renal blood flow and inhibit proximal tubule reabsorption. Sumeray et al., in 2001, demonstrated a protective effect of low doses of dopamine on tubular lesions (excretion of NAG and RBP), while maintaining glomerular filtration [137]. However, recent studies have failed to demonstrate benefit of dopamine on renoprotection, but have also shown a number of undesirable side effects [164-166]. Renal-dose dopamine such as routine prophylaxis is not recommended.

Fenoldopam, a selective dopamine receptor-1, has also been used in cardiac surgery [167-169]. Results are inconclusive: Bove et al. [167] have not found any modifications of the post-operative renal function whereas other studies [169-171] have shown an improvement of the creatinine clearance in the fenoldopam group. The difference between these studies may be related to an insufficient dose in the Bove et al. study (0.05 µg/kg/min [167] vs 0.1 [169,170] or 0.1 to 0.3 [171] µg/kg/min). In the Caimmi et al. study [171], fenoldopam was associated with shorter mechanical ventilation time and shorter ICU length of stay, but not in the Baar et al study [169]. No hypotension relative to fenoldopam was reported by Caimmi et al. [171], but fenoldopam contributed to peri-operative hypotension in the Barr et al. study [169]. In a recent meta-analysis, Landoni et al. concluded that fenoldopam may confer significant benefits in preventing renal replacement therapy and reducing mortality in patients undergoing cardiovascular surgery [172].

The effects of dopexamine on the renal function after cardiac surgery are still being discussed: increased creatinine clearance [173] or no effect [174,175]. Only Dehne et al. included patients with abnormal pre-operative renal function, and showed no effect on post-operative renal function [174]. However, dopexamine may induce significant systemic hypotension [173]. Dopexamine cannot be recommended to prevent AKI after cardiac surgery.

As previously mentioned, the use of diuretic agents is widely spread. Furosemide increases the diuresis without decreasing AKI [176]. Furosemide may also worsen kidney outcomes [164].

Mannitol produces an osmotic diuresis with a reduction of tubular obstruction and can scavenge free radicals. It is often added to the priming solution during cardio-pulmonary bypass. Mannitol was associated with an increase of β2 microglobuline excretion [177]. It has no effect on the renal function in patients with [178] or without [179] preexisting renal dysfunction.

Natriuretic peptide hormones have been evaluated in cardiac surgery [180-183]. Continuous low dose hANP perfusion increases urine volume [180] and decreases AKI [181]. In patients with left ventricular dysfunction, nesiritide decreases AKI and mortality [182,183].

Dexamethasone administration before CPB has no protective effect on peri-operative renal dysfunction in low-risk cardiac surgery patients, but was associated with greater glycosuria [184]. On the other hand, methylprednisolone administration significantly reduces inflammatory factors and subclinical renal injury although it has no effect on renal dysfunction [185].

The return of filtered glucose to the circulation by the kidney is an energy-consuming process. Thus, postoperative insulin therapy has been suggested. In an ICU population, mostly after cardiac surgery, decreases in AKI and dialysis were reported after strict control of glycemia [186]. Even if poor intra-operative blood glucose in diabetic patients is associated with a worse outcome [187] and strict glycemic control is safe [188], intra-operative insulin therapy does not decrease AKI after cardiac surgery [189].

An attractive therapeutic target is drugs that block inflammation, as far as it is an important mechanism leading to AKI. Pentoxifylline blocks the activation of neutrophils by TNF-alpha and IL-1. It reduces cardiac dysfunction and TNF-α release in ischemia-reperfusion models but not in elderly patients.

The use of antibodies anti Intercellular Adhesion Molecule-1 (ICAM-1) has also been proposed [190,191] and demonstrated its efficiency on animals to protect the kidney against ischemic injury [192] and ICAM-1 deficient mice have been protected against renal injury [193].

N-acetylcysteine blocks inflammation and oxydant stress (through its glutathione-giving function) in cardiac surgery patients but no evidence of renoprotection has been found in patients with or without chronic renal failure [117,118,169,194-197].

The effect of recently used anti-oxidants (vitamine C [198], Vitamine E [199], tocopherol [198], green tea [200]), which are widely studied in cardiac surgery should be highlighted in the framework of peri-operative renal protection.

A study on piglets demonstrated that the platelet-activating factor receptor antagonism with ginkgolide B before the circulatory arrest period could improve recovery of renal blood flow. The platelet-activating factor causes constriction of arterioles, thus ginkgolide B is reported to protect the kidney against ischemic injury [201].

## C. Management of CPB

Priming with gelatin vs. Ringer's Lactate solution has no significant differences in the inflammatory response in patients undergoing coronary artery bypass grafting with cardiopulmonary bypass [202,203]. Compared to HES, priming with human albumin offers no advantage on renal function after CPB in elderly patients with hypoalbuminemia [106].

The objective is to obtain a hemodynamic state that is as stable as possible. The systemic blood pressure recommended is between 50 and 70 mmHg [204,205], dependent on the pump, which is responsible for regulating the flow and the peripheric resistance determined by the arterial vasomotricity, the degree of hemodilution and temperature.

Hemofiltration during CPB removes some major mediators of the inflammatory response, and improves early post-operative oxygenation and hemodynamics, as during septic shock and pediatric cardiac surgery [203,206,207]. Even if its efficiency on reno-protection in cardiac surgery patients remains to be determined, hemofiltration should be applied to treat fluid overload during procedure and immediate post-operative oliguric renal failure.

During weaning from CPB, the patient's temperature should remain close to 37°C and hematocrit maintained over has to be over an optimal threshold that remains to be challenged: 22% [53], 23% [24] or 24% [54].

Hemodynamic stability in CPB and immediate post-operative situations is the best guarantee of the preservation of the renal function.

The improvement of the means of biocompatibility and the development of mini-CPB, which limits the inflammatory reaction, will most likely have an unspecified beneficial effect on renal function.

## Conclusion

AKI after CPB remains a serious complication which often cannot be treated. This condition is associated with substantial mortality and morbidity.

The pathogenesis is complex and dominated by a systemic inflammatory response syndrome for which the human immune system does not have an appropriate response.

The role of genetic predisposition is an interesting area to expand our knowledge and require further exploration.

The attempts to move towards a common definition of AKI and the continuation of the initiative to develop biomarkers for earlier diagnosis are other important goals to be reached.

Finally, further studies on kidney protection intervention and therapy, which must be initiated as soon as possible, will help us to lower the incidence of this common complication.

## References

[1] Novis, BK; Roizen, MF; Aronson, S; Thisted, RA. Association of preoperative risk factors with postoperative acute renal failure. *Anesth. Analg.*, 1994, 78, 143-149

[2] Stafford-Smith, M; Patel, UD; Phillips-Bute, BG; Shaw, AD; Swaminathan, M. Acute kidney injury and chronic kidney disease after cardiac surgery. *Adv. Chronic Kidney Dis.*, 2008, 15, 257-277

[3] Swaminathan, M; Shaw, AD; Phillips-Bute, BG; et al. Trends in acute renal failure associated with coronary artery bypass graft surgery in the United States. *Crit. Care Med.*, 2007, 35, 2286-2291

[4] Stallwood, MI; Grayson, AD; Mills, K; Scawn, ND. Acute renal failure in coronary artery bypass surgery: independent effect of cardiopulmonary bypass. *Ann. Thorac. Surg.*, 2004, 77, 968-972

[5] Mangano, CM; Diamondstone, LS; Ramsay, JG; et al. Renal dysfunction after myocardial revascularization: risk factors, adverse outcomes, and hospital resource utilization. The Multicenter Study of Perioperative Ischemia Research Group. *Ann. Intern. Med.*, 1998, 128, 194-203

[6] Bove, T; Calabro, MG; Landoni, G; et al. The incidence and risk of acute renal failure after cardiac surgery. *J. Cardiothorac. Vasc. Anest.*, 2004, 18, 442-445

[7] Zanardo, G; Michielon, P; Paccagnella, A; et al. Acute renal failure in the patient undergoing cardiac operation. Prevalence, mortality rate, and main risk factors. *J. Thorac Cardiovasc. Surg.*, 1994, 107, 1489-1495

[8] Mangos, GJ; Brown, MA; Chan, WY; et al. Acute renal failure following cardiac surgery: incidence, outcomes and risk factors. *Aust.N. Z. J. Med.*, 1995, 25, 284-289

[9] Conlon, PJ; Stafford-Smith, M; White, WD; et al. Acute renal failure following cardiac surgery. *Nephrol. Dial. Transplant.*, 1999, 14, 1158-1162

[10] Ostermann, ME; Taube, D; Morgan, CJ; Evans, TW. Acute renal failure following cardiopulmonary bypass: a changing picture. *Intensive Care Med.*, 2000, 26, 565-571

[11] Provenchere, S; Plantefeve, G; Hufnagel, G; et al. Renal dysfunction after cardiac surgery with normothermic cardiopulmonary bypass: incidence, risk factors, and effect on clinical outcome. *Anesth. Analg.*, 2003, 96, 1258-1264

[12] Boldt, J; Brenner, T; Lehmann, A; et al. Is kidney function altered by the duration of cardiopulmonary bypass? *Ann. Thorac. Surg.*, 2003, 75, 906-912

[13] Chertow, GM; Levy, EM; Hammermeister, KE; Grover, F; Daley, J. Independent association between acute renal failure and mortality following cardiac surgery. *Am. J. Med.*, 1998, 104, 343-348

[14] Rosner, MH; Okusa, MD. Acute kidney injury associated with cardiac surgery. *Clin. J. Am. Soc. Nephrol.*, 2006, 1, 19-32

[15] Loef, BG; Henning, RH; Navis, G; et al. Changes in glomerular filtration rate after cardiac surgery with cardiopulmonary bypass in patients with mild preoperative renal dysfunction. *Br. J. Anaesth.*, 2008, 100, 759-764

[16] Stafford-Smith, M; Podgoreanu, M; Swaminathan, M; et al. Association of genetic polymorphisms with risk of renal injury after coronary bypass graft surgery. *Am. J. Kidney Dis.*, 2005, 45, 519-530

[17] Ryckwaert, F; Boccara, G; Frappier, JM; Colson, PH. Incidence, risk factors, and prognosis of a moderate increase in plasma creatinine early after cardiac surgery. *Crit. Care Med.*, 2002, 30, 1495-1498

[18] Provenchere, S; Plantefeve, G; Hufnagel, G; et al. Renal dysfunction after cardiac surgery with normothermic cardiopulmonary bypass: incidence, risk factors, and effect on clinical outcome. *Anesth. Analg.*, 2003, 96, 1258-1264, table of contents

[19] Loef, BG; Epema, AH; Smilde, TD; et al. Immediate postoperative renal function deterioration in cardiac surgical patients predicts in-hospital mortality and long-term survival. *J. Am. Soc. Nephrol.*, 2005, 16, 195-200

[20] Thakar, CV; Worley, S; Arrigain, S; Yared, JP; Paganini, EP. Improved survival in acute kidney injury after cardiac surgery. *Am. J. Kidney Dis.*, 2007, 50, 703-711

[21] Simmons, PI; Anderson, RJ. Increased serum creatinine: a marker for adverse outcome before and after cardiac surgery. *Crit. Care Med.*, 2002, 30, 1664-1665

[22] Chertow, GM; Lazarus, JM; Christiansen, CL; et al. Preoperative renal risk stratification. *Circulation.*, 1997, 95, 878-884

[23] Landoni, G; Bove, T; Crivellari, M; et al. Acute renal failure after isolated CABG surgery: six years of experience. *Minerva Anestesiol.*, 2007, 73, 559-565

[24] Ranucci, M; Biagioli, B; Scolletta, S; et al. Lowest hematocrit on cardiopulmonary bypass impairs the outcome in coronary surgery: An Italian Multicenter Study from the National Cardioanesthesia Database. *Tex. Heart Inst. J.*, 2006, 33, 300-305

[25] Andersson, LG; Ekroth, R; Bratteby, LE; Hallhagen, S; Wesslen, O. Acute renal failure after coronary surgery--a study of incidence and risk factors in 2009 consecutive patients. *Thorac. Cardiovasc. Surg.*, 1993, 41, 237-241

[26] Anderson, RJ; O'Brien, M; MaWhinney, S; et al. Mild renal failure is associated with adverse outcome after cardiac valve surgery. *Am. J. Kidney Dis.*, 2000, 35, 1127-1134

[27] Doddakula, K; Al-Sarraf, N; Gately, K; et al. Predictors of acute renal failure requiring renal replacement therapy post cardiac surgery in patients with preoperatively normal renal function. *Interact. Cardiovasc. Thorac. Surg.*, 2007, 6, 314-318

[28] Gaudino, M; Luciani, N; Giungi, S; et al. Different profiles of patients who require dialysis after cardiac surgery. *Ann. Thorac. Surg.*, 2005, 79, 825-829

[29] de Moraes Lobo, EM; Burdmann, EA; Abdulkader, RC. Renal function changes after elective cardiac surgery with cardiopulmonary bypass. *Ren. Fail.*, 2000, 22, 487-497

[30] Bucerius, J; Gummert, JF; Walther, T; et al. On-pump versus off-pump coronary artery bypass grafting: impact on postoperative renal failure requiring renal replacement therapy. *Ann. Thorac. Surg.*, 2004, 77, 1250-1256

[31] Halkos, ME; Puskas, JD; Lattouf, OM; et al. Impact of preoperative neurologic events on outcomes after coronary artery bypass grafting. *Ann. Thorac. Surg.*, 2008, 86, 504-510, discussion 510

[32] Slogoff, S; Reul, GJ; Keats, AS; et al. Role of perfusion pressure and flow in major organ dysfunction after cardiopulmonary bypass. *Ann. Thorac. Surg.*, 1990, 50, 911-918

[33] Kulier, A; Levin, J; Moser, R; et al. Impact of preoperative anemia on outcome in patients undergoing coronary artery bypass graft surgery. *Circulation.*, 2007, 116, 471-479

[34] Grayson, AD; Khater, M; Jackson, M; Fox, MA. Valvular heart operation is an independent risk factor for acute renal failure. *Ann. Thorac. Surg.*, 2003, 75, 1829-1835

[35] Bainbridge, D; Cheng, D; Martin, J; Novick, R. Does off-pump or minimally invasive coronary artery bypass reduce mortality, morbidity, and resource utilization when compared with percutaneous coronary intervention? A meta-analysis of randomized trials. *J. Thorac. Cardiovasc. Surg.*, 2007, 133, 623-631

[36] Di Mauro, M; Gagliardi, M; Iaco, AL; et al. Does off-pump coronary surgery reduce postoperative acute renal failure? The importance of preoperative renal function. *Ann. Thorac. Surg.*, 2007, 84, 1496-1502

[37] Nathoe, HM; van Dijk, D; Jansen, EW; et al. A comparison of on-pump and off-pump coronary bypass surgery in low-risk patients. *N. Engl. J. Med.*, 2003, 348, 394-402

[38] Loef, BG; Epema, AH; Navis, G; et al. Off-pump coronary revascularization attenuates transient renal damage compared with on-pump coronary revascularization. *Chest.*, 2002, 121, 1190-1194

[39] Chukwuemeka, A; Weisel, A; Maganti, M; et al. Renal dysfunction in high-risk patients after on-pump and off-pump coronary artery bypass surgery: a propensity score analysis. *Ann. Thorac. Surg.*, 2005, 80, 2148-2153

[40] Ascione, R; Lloyd, CT; Underwood, MJ; Gomes, WJ; Angelini, GD. On-pump versus off-pump coronary revascularization: evaluation of renal function. *Ann. Thorac. Surg.*, 1999, 68, 493-498

[41] Tomic, V; Russwurm, S; Moller, E; et al. Transcriptomic and proteomic patterns of systemic inflammation in on-pump and off-pump coronary artery bypass grafting. *Circulation.*, 2005, 112, 2912-2920

[42] Fischer, UM; Weissenberger, WK; Warters, RD; et al. Impact of cardiopulmonary bypass management on postcardiac surgery renal function. *Perfusion.*, 2002, 17, 401-406

[43] Suen, WS; Mok, CK; Chiu, SW; et al. Risk factors for development of acute renal failure (ARF) requiring dialysis in patients undergoing cardiac surgery. *Angiology.*, 1998, 49, 789-800

[44] Podgoreanu, MV; White, WD; Morris, RW; et al. Inflammatory gene polymorphisms and risk of postoperative myocardial infarction after cardiac surgery. *Circulation.*, 2006, 114, I275-281

[45] Weinstein, GS; Rao, PS; Vretakis, G; Tyras, DH. Serial changes in renal function in cardiac surgical patients. *Ann. Thorac. Surg.*, 1989, 48, 72-76

[46] Pathi, VL MJ; Mc Phaden, A; Martin, W; McQuiston, AM; Wheastley, DL. Alterations in renal microcirculation during cardiopulmonary bypass. *Ann. Thorac. Surg.*, 1998, 65, 993-998

[47] Lema, G; Meneses, G; Urzua, J; et al. Effects of extracorporeal circulation on renal function in coronary surgical patients. *Anesth. Analg.*, 1995, 81, 446-451

[48] Urzua, J; Troncoso, S; Bugedo, G; et al. Renal function and cardiopulmonary bypass: effect of perfusion pressure. *J. Cardiothorac. Vasc. Anesth.*, 1992, 6, 299-303

[49] Regragui, IA; Izzat, MB; Birdi, I; et al. Cardiopulmonary bypass perfusion temperature does not influence perioperative renal function. *Ann. Thorac. Surg.*, 1995, 60, 160-164

[50] Swaminathan, M; East, C; Phillips-Bute, B; Newman, MF; Reves, MF; Smith, PK; Stafford-Smith, M. Report of a substudy on warm versus cold cardiopulmonary bypass: changes in creatinine clearance. *Ann. Thoac. Surg.*, 2001, 72, 1603-1609

[51] Regragui, IA; Izzat, MB; Birdi, I; Lapsey, M; Bryan, AJ; Angelini, GD. Cardiopulmonary bypass perfusion temperature does not influence perioperative renal function. *Ann. Thoac. Surg.*, 1995, 60, 160-164

[52] Abramov, D; Tamariz, M; Serrick, CI; et al. The influence of cardiopulmonary bypass flow characteristics on the clinical outcome of 1820 coronary bypass patients. *Can. J. Cardiol.*, 2003, 19, 237-243

[53] Habib, RH; Zacharias, A; Schwann, TA; et al. Adverse effects of low hematocrit during cardiopulmonary bypass in the adult: should current practice be changed? *J. Thorac. Cardiovasc. Surg.*, 2003, 125, 1438-1450

[54] Habib, RH; Zacharias, A; Schwann, TA; et al. Postoperative renal dysfunction after on-pump versus off-pump coronary revascularization: role of on-pump hemodilution and transfusions. *Ann. Thorac. Surg.*, 2006, 81, 1548-1549, author reply 1549-1550

[55] Swaminathan, M; Phillips-Bute, BG; Conlon, PJ; et al. The association of lowest hematocrit during cardiopulmonary bypass with acute renal injury after coronary artery bypass surgery. *Ann. Thorac. Surg.*, 2003, 76, 784-791, discussion 792

[56] Feindt, PR; Walcher, S; Volkmer, I; et al. Effects of high-dose aprotinin on renal function in aortocoronary bypass grafting. *Ann. Thorac. Surg.*, 1995, 60, 1076-1080

[57] Lindvall, G; Sartipy, U; Ivert, T; van der Linden, J. Aprotinin is not associated with postoperative renal impairment after primary coronary surgery. *Ann. Thorac. Surg.*, 2008, 86, 13-19

[58] Maslow, AD; Chaudrey, A; Bert, A; Schwartz, C; Singh, A. Perioperative renal outcome in cardiac surgical patients with preoperative renal dysfunction: aprotinin versus epsilon aminocaproic acid. *J. Cardiothorac. Vasc. Anesth.*, 2008, 22, 6-15

[59] Furnary, AP; Wu, Y; Hiratzka, LF; Grunkemeier, GL; Page, US, 3rd. Aprotinin does not increase the risk of renal failure in cardiac surgery patients. *Circulation.*, 2007, 116, I127-133

[60] Dietrich, W; Busley, R; Boulesteix, AL. Effects of aprotinin dosage on renal function: an analysis of 8,548 cardiac surgical patients treated with different dosages of aprotinin. *Anesthesiology.*, 2008, 108, 189-198

[61] Shaw, AD; Stafford-Smith, M; White, WD; et al. The effect of aprotinin on outcome after coronary-artery bypass grafting. *N. Engl. J. Med.*, 2008, 358, 784-793

[62] Mangano, DT; Miao, Y; Vuylsteke, A; et al. Mortality associated with aprotinin during 5 years following coronary artery bypass graft surgery. *Jama.*, 2007, 297, 471-479

[63] Dietrich, W; Spannagl, M; Boehm, J; et al. Tranexamic Acid and Aprotinin in Primary Cardiac Operations: An Analysis of 220 Cardiac Surgical Patients Treated with Tranexamic Acid or Aprotinin. *Anesth. Analg.*, 2008, 107, 1469-1478

[64] Lombardi, R; Ferreiro, A; Servetto, C. Renal function after cardiac surgery: adverse effect of furosemide. *Ren Fail.*, 2003, 25, 775-786

[65] Ohata, T; Mitsuno, M; Yamamura, M; et al. Minimal cardiopulmonary bypass attenuates neutrophil activation and cytokine release in coronary artery bypass grafting. *J. Artif. Organs.*, 2007, 10, 92-95

[66] Ohata, T; Mitsuno, M; Yamamura, M; et al. Beneficial effects of mini-cardiopulmonary bypass on hemostasis in coronary artery bypass grafting: analysis of inflammatory response and hemodilution. *Asaio J.*, 2008, 54, 207-209

[67] Huybregts, RA; Morariu, AM; Rakhorst, G; et al. Attenuated renal and intestinal injury after use of a mini-cardiopulmonary bypass system. *Ann. Thorac. Surg.*, 2007, 83, 1760-1766

[68] Remadi, JP; Rakotoarivelo, Z; Marticho, P; Benamar, A. Prospective randomized study comparing coronary artery bypass grafting with the new mini-extracorporeal circulation Jostra System or with a standard cardiopulmonary bypass. *Am. Heart J.*, 2006, 151, 198

[69] Remadi, JP; Rakotoarivello, Z; Marticho, P; et al. Aortic valve replacement with the minimal extracorporeal circulation (Jostra MECC System) versus standard cardiopulmonary bypass: a randomized prospective trial. *J. Thorac. Cardiovasc. Surg.*, 2004, 128, 436-441

[70] Llopart, T; Lombardi, R; Forselledo, M; Andrade, R. Acute renal failure in open heart surgery. *Ren Fail.*, 1997, 19, 319-323

[71] Gormley, SM; McBride, WT; Armstrong, MA; et al. Plasma and urinary cytokine homeostasis and renal function during cardiac surgery without cardiopulmonary bypass. *Cytokine.*, 2002, 17, 61-65

[72] Tashiro, H; Shimokawa, H; Yamamoto, K; et al. Altered plasma levels of cytokines in patients with ischemic heart disease. *Coron Artery Dis.*, 1997, 8, 143-147

[73] Gormley, SM; McBride, WT; Armstrong, MA; et al. Plasma and urinary cytokine homeostasis and renal dysfunction during cardiac surgery. *Anesthesiology.*, 2000, 93, 1210-1216, discussion 1215A

[74] Laffey, JG; Boylan, JF; Cheng, DC. The systemic inflammatory response to cardiac surgery: implications for the anesthesiologist. *Anesthesiology.*, 2002, 97, 215-252

[75] Herskowitz, A; Mangano, DT. Inflammatory cascade. A final common pathway for perioperative injury? *Anesthesiology.*, 1996, 85, 957-960

[76] Molitoris, BA ; Sutton, TA. Endothelial injury and dysfunction in ischemic acute renal failure. *Crit. Care Med.*, 2002, 30

[77] Lieberthal. Biology of ischemic and toxic renal tubular cell injury: role of nitric oxide and the inflammatory response. *Curr. Opin. Nephrol. Hypertens.*, 1998, 7, 289-295

[78] Chatterjee, PK; Hawksworth, GM; McLay, JS. Cytokine-stimulated nitric oxide production in the human renal proximal tubule and its modulation by natriuretic peptides: A novel immunomodulatory mechanism? *Exp. Nephrol.*, 1999, 7, 438-448

[79] Lakkis, FG; Coelho, SN. The role of cytokines in inflammatory glomerular injury. *Miner Electrolyte Metab.*, 1995, 21, 250-261

[80] Gueret, G ; Lion, F ; Guriec, N ; et al. Acute renal failure after cardiac surgery with cardiopulmonary bypass is associated with plasmatic IL6 increase. *Cytokine.*, 2008, 45, 92-98

[81] Grocott, HP; White, WD; Morris, RW; et al. Genetic polymorphisms and the risk of stroke after cardiac surgery. *Stroke.*, 2005, 36, 1854-1858

[82] Reid, CL PC; Pravica, V; Hutchinson, IV; Campbell, IT. Genetic variation in proinflammatory and anti-inflammatory cytokine production in muliple organ dysfunction syndrome. *Crit. Care Med.*, 2002, 30, 2216-2221

[83] Grunenfelder, J; Zund, G; Schoeberlein, A; et al. Modified ultrafiltration lowers adhesion molecule and cytokine levels after cardiopulmonary bypass without clinical relevance in adults. *Eur. J. Cardiothorac. Surg.*, 2000, 17, 77-83

[84] Klausner, JM PI; Goldman, G; Kobzik, L; Rodzen, C; Lawrence, R; Valeri, R; Shepro, D; Hehtman, HB. Postischemic renal injury is mediated by neutrophols and leukotrienes. *Am. J. Physiol.*, 1989, 256, F794-802

[85] Wan, S; LeClerc, JL; Vincent, JL. Inflammatory response to cardiopulmonary bypass: mechanisms involved and possible therapeutic strategies. *Chest.*, 1997, 112, 676-692

[86] Rinder, CS; Fontes, M; Mathew, JP; Rinder, HM; Smith, BR. Neutrophil CD11b upregulation during cardiopulmonary bypass is associated with postoperative renal injury. *Ann. Thorac. Surg.*, 2003, 75, 899-905

[87] Meldrum, DR; Donnahoo, KK. Role of TNF in mediating renal insufficiency following cardiac surgery: evidence of a postbypass cardiorenal syndrome. *J. Surg. Res.*, 1999, 85, 185-199

[88] Fabre, O; Vincentelli, A; Corseaux, D; et al. Comparison of blood activation in the wound, active vent, and cardiopulmonary bypass circuit. *Ann. Thorac. Surg.*, 2008, 86, 537-541

[89] Allen, SJ; McBride, WT; McMurray, TJ; et al. Cell salvage alters the systemic inflammatory response after off-pump coronary artery bypass grafting surgery. *Ann. Thorac. Surg.*, 2007, 83, 578-585

[90] Lieberthal, W; Nigam, SK. Acute renal failure. II. Experimental models of acute renal failure: imperfect but indispensable. *Am. J. Physiol. Renal. Physiol.*, 2000, 278, F1-F12

[91] McBride, WT. Mechanisms of renal dysfunction at cardiac surgery. *Ann. Fr. Anesth. Réan.*, 2001, 22, 40-42

[92] Thadhani, R; Pascual, M; Bonventre, JV. Acute renal failure. *N. Engl. J. Med.*, 1996, 334, 1448-1460

[93] van der Linden, J; Casimir-Ahn, H. When do cerebral emboli appear during open heart operations? A transcranial Doppler study. *Ann. Thorac. Surg.*, 1991, 51, 237-241

[94] Sreeram, GM; Grocott, HP; White, WD; Newman, MF; Stafford-Smith, M. Transcranial Doppler emboli count predicts rise in creatinine after coronary artery bypass graft surgery. *J. Cardiothorac.Vasc. Anesth*, 2004, 18, 548-551

[95] Bronden, B; Dencker, M; Allers, M; Plaza, I; Jonsson, H. Differential distribution of lipid microemboli after cardiac surgery. *Ann. Thorac. Surg.*, 2006, 81, 643-648

[96] Edmonds, HL Jr. Emboli and renal dysfunction in CABG patients. *J. Cardiothorac. Vasc. Anesth.*, 2004, 18, 545-547

[97] Wright, G. Haemolysis during cardiopulmonary bypass: update. *Perfusion.*, 2001, 16, 345-351

[98] Haase, M; Haase-Fielitz, A; Bagshaw, SM; Ronco, C; Bellomo, R. Cardiopulmonary bypass-associated acute kidney injury: a pigment nephropathy? *Contrib. Nephrol.*, 2007, 156, 340-353

[99] Skrabal, CA; Khosravi, A; Choi, YH; et al. Pericardial suction blood separation attenuates inflammatory response and hemolysis after cardiopulmonary bypass. *Scand. Cardiovasc. J.*, 2006, 40, 219-223

[100] Sakr, Y; Payen, D; Reinhart, K; et al. Effects of hydroxyethyl starch administration on renal function in critically ill patients. *Br. J. Anaesth.*, 2007, 98, 216-224

[101] Davidson, IJ. Deleterious renal effects of hydroxyethyl starch 130/0.4 and 200/0.5 solutions. *Eur. J. Anaesthesiol.*, 2007, 24, 892-893

[102] Boldt, J; Brenner, T; Lehmann, A; et al. Influence of two different volume replacement regimens on renal function in elderly patients undergoing cardiac surgery: comparison of a new starch preparation with gelatin. *Intensive Care Med.*, 2003, 29, 763-769

[103] Mahmood, A; Gosling, P; Vohra, RK. Randomized clinical trial comparing the effects on renal function of hydroxyethyl starch or gelatine during aortic aneurysm surgery. *Br. J. Surg.*, 2007, 94, 427-433

[104] Boldt, J; Brosch, C; Rohm, K; Papsdorf, M; Mengistu, A. Comparison of the effects of gelatin and a modern hydroxyethyl starch solution on renal function and inflammatory response in elderly cardiac surgery patients. *Br. J. Anaesth.*, 2008, 100, 457-464

[105] Boldt, J; Brosch, C; Ducke, M; Papsdorf, M; Lehmann, A. Influence of volume therapy with a modern hydroxyethylstarch preparation on kidney function in cardiac surgery patients with compromised renal function: a comparison with human albumin. *Crit. Care Med.*, 2007, 35, 2740-2746

[106] Boldt, J; Brosch, C; Röhm, K; et al. Is Albumin Administration in Hypoalbuminemic Elderly Cardiac Surgery Patients of Benefit with Regard to Inflammation, Endothelial Activation, and Long-Term Kidney Function? *Anesth. Analg.*, 2008, 107, 1496-1503

[107] Tuttle, KR; Worrall, NK, Dahlstrom LR, et al. Predictors of ARF after cardiac surgical procedures. *Am. J. Kidney Dis.*, 2003, 41, 76-83

[108] Koyner, JL; Bennett, MR; Worcester, EM; et al. Urinary cystatin C as an early biomarker of acute kidney injury following adult cardiothoracic surgery. *Kidney Int.*, 2008.

[109] Barrett, BJ; Parfrey, PS. Prevention of nephrotoxicity induced by radiocontrast agents. *N. Engl. J. Med.*, 1994, 331, 1449-1450

[110] Bennett, M; Dent, CL; Ma, Q; et al. Urine NGAL predicts severity of acute kidney injury after cardiac surgery: a prospective study. *Clin. J. Am. Soc. Nephrol.*, 2008, 3, 665-673

[111] Dent, CL ; Ma, Q ; Dastrala, S ; et al. Plasma neutrophil gelatinase-associated lipocalin predicts acute kidney injury, morbidity and mortality after pediatric cardiac surgery: a prospective uncontrolled cohort study. *Crit. Care.*, 2007, 11, R127

[112] Parikh, CR; Mishra, J; Thiessen-Philbrook, H; et al. Urinary IL-18 is an early predictive biomarker of acute kidney injury after cardiac surgery. *Kidney Int.*, 2006, 70, 199-203

[113] Mishra, J ; Dent, C ; Tarabishi, R ; et al. Neutrophil gelatinase-associated lipocalin (NGAL) as a biomarker for acute renal injury after cardiac surgery. *Lancet.*, 2005, 365, 1231-1238

[114] Brown, JR; Cochran, RP; Dacey, LJ; et al. Perioperative increases in serum creatinine are predictive of increased 90-day mortality after coronary artery bypass graft surgery. *Circulation.*, 2006, 114, I409-413

[115] Kuitunen, A; Vento, A; Suojaranta-Ylinen, R; Pettila, V. Acute renal failure after cardiac surgery: evaluation of the RIFLE classification. *Ann. Thorac. Surg.*, 2006, 81, 542-546

[116] Lassnigg, A; Schmid, ER; Hiesmayr, M; et al. Impact of minimal increases in serum creatinine on outcome in patients after cardiothoracic surgery: do we have to revise current definitions of acute renal failure? *Crit. Care Med.*, 2008, 36, 1129-1137

[117] Burns, KE; Chu, MW; Novick, RJ; et al. Perioperative N-acetylcysteine to prevent renal dysfunction in high-risk patients undergoing cabg surgery: a randomized controlled trial. *Jama.*, 2005, 294, 342-350

[118] Adabag, AS; Ishani, A; Koneswaran, S; et al. Utility of N-acetylcysteine to prevent acute kidney injury after cardiac surgery: a randomized controlled trial. *Am. Heart J.*, 2008, 155, 1143-1149

[119] O'Riordan, SE; Webb, MC; Stowe, HJ; et al. Cystatin C improves the detection of mild renal dysfunction in older patients. *Ann. Clin. Biochem.*, 2003, 40, 648-655

[120] Cho, MM; Yi, MM. Variability of daily creatinine excretion in healthy adults. *Hum. Nutr. Clin. Nutr.*, 1986, 40, 469-472

[121] Cherry, RA; Eachempati, SR; Hydo, L; Barie, PS. Accuracy of short-duration creatinine clearance determinations in predicting 24-hour creatinine clearance in critically ill and injured patients. *J. Trauma.*, 2002, 53, 267-271

[122] Herget-Rosenthal, S; Kribben, A; Pietruck, F; Ross, B; Philipp, T. Two by two hour creatinine clearance--repeatable and valid. *Clin. Nephrol.*, 1999, 51, 348-354

[123] Markantonis, SL; Agathokleous-Kioupaki, E. Can two-, four- or eight-hour urine collections after voluntary voiding be used instead of twenty-four-hour collections for the estimation of creatinine clearance in healthy subjects? *Pharm. World Sci.*, 1998, 20, 258-263

[124] Nichols, L. Can 12-hour creatinine clearances be substituted for 24-hour creatinine clearances in monitoring for nephrotoxicity from cancer chemotherapy? A pilot study and preliminary data. *Am. J. Clin. Pathol.*, 1988, 90, 373-374

[125] O'Connell, MB; Wong, MO; Bannick-Mohrland, SD; Dwinell, AM. Accuracy of 2- and 8-hour urine collections for measuring creatinine clearance in the hospitalized elderly. *Pharmacotherapy.*, 1993, 13, 135-142

[126] Sladen, RN; Endo, E; Harrison, T. Two-hour versus 22-hour creatinine clearance in critically ill patients. *Anesthesiology.*, 1987, 67, 1013-1016

[127] Wilson, RF; Soullier, G. The validity of two-hour creatinine clearance studies in critically ill patients. *Crit. Care Med.*, 1980, 8, 281-284

[128] Gueret, G; Kiss, G; Bezon, E; et al. [Evaluation of the renal function in cardiac surgery with CPB: role of the cystatin C and the calculated creatinine clearance]. *Ann. Fr. Anesth. Reanim.*, 2007, 26, 412-417

[129] Goldberg, TH; Finkelstein, MS. Difficulties in estimating glomerular filtration rate in the elderly. *Arch. Intern. Med.*, 1987, 147, 1430-1433

[130] Cockcroft, DW; Gault, MH. Prediction of creatinine clearance from serum creatinine. *Nephron.*, 1976, 16, 31-41

[131] Brown, JR; Cochran, RP; MacKenzie, TA; et al. Long-term survival after cardiac surgery is predicted by estimated glomerular filtration rate. *Ann. Thorac. Surg.*, 2008, 86, 4-11

[132] Levey, AS; Bosch, JP; Lewis, JB; et al. A more accurate method to estimate glomerular filtration rate from serum creatinine: a new prediction equation. Modification of Diet in Renal Disease Study Group. *Ann. Intern. Med.*, 1999, 130, 461-470

[133] Jorres, A KO; Hess, S; Farke, S; Gahl, GM; Muller, C; Djurup, R. Urinary excretion of thromboxane and markers for renal injury in patients undergoing cardiopulmonary bypass. *Artif. Organs.*, 1994, 18, 565-569

[134] Westhuyzen, J; McGiffin, DC; McCarthy, J; Fleming, SJ. Tubular nephrotoxicity after cardiac surgery utilising cardiopulmonary bypass. *Clin. Chim. Acta.*, 1994, 228, 123-132

[135] Hall, PW 3rd; Ricanati, ES. Renal handling of beta-2-microglobulin in renal disorders: with special reference to hepatorenal syndrome. *Nephron.*, 1981, 27, 62-66

[136] Fernandez, F; de Miguel, MD; Barrio, V; Mallol, J. Beta-2-microglobulin as an index of renal function after cardiopulmonary bypass surgery in children. *Child Nephrol. Urol.*, 1988, 9, 326-330

[137] Sumeray, M; Robertson, C; Lapsley, M; et al. Low dose dopamine infusion reduces renal tubular injury following cardiopulmonary bypass surgery. *J. Nephrol.*, 2001, 14, 397-402

[138] Bernard, AM; Moreau, D; Lauwerys, R. Comparison of retinol-binding protein and beta 2-microglobulin determination in urine for the early detection of tubular proteinuria. *Clin. Chim. Acta.*, 1982, 126, 1-7

[139] Lamb, EJ ; Webb, MC ; Simpson, DE ; et al. Estimation of glomerular filtration rate in older patients with chronic renal insufficiency: is the modification of diet in renal disease formula an improvement? *J. Am. Geriatr. Soc.*, 2003, 51, 1012-1017

[140] Shlipak, MG; Katz, R; Cushman, M; et al. Cystatin-C and inflammatory markers in the ambulatory elderly. *Am. J. Med.*, 2005, 118, 1416

[141] Knight, EL; Verhave, JC; Spiegelman, D; et al. Factors influencing serum cystatin C levels other than renal function and the impact on renal function measurement. *Kidney Int.*, 2004, 65, 1416-1421

[142] Noto, D; Cefalu, AB; Barbagallo, CM; et al. Cystatin C levels are decreased in acute myocardial infarction: effect of cystatin C G73A gene polymorphism on plasma levels. *Int. J. Cardiol.*, 2005, 101, 213-217

[143] Filler, G; Bokenkamp, A; Hofmann, W; et al. Cystatin C as a marker of GFR--history, indications, and future research. *Clin. Biochem.*, 2005, 38, 1-8

[144] Zhu, J; Yin, R; Wu, H; et al. Cystatin C as a reliable marker of renal function following heart valve replacement surgery with cardiopulmonary bypass. *Clin. Chim. Acta.*, 2006, 374, 116-121

[145] van Timmeren, MM; van den Heuvel, MC; Bailly, V; et al. Tubular kidney injury molecule-1 (KIM-1) in human renal disease. *J. Pathol.*, 2007, 212, 209-217

[146] Han, WK; Bailly, V; Abichandani, R; Thadhani, R; Bonventre, JV. Kidney Injury Molecule-1 (KIM-1): a novel biomarker for human renal proximal tubule injury. *Kidney Int.*, 2002, 62, 237-244

[147] Bonventre, JV. Kidney Injury Molecule-1 (KIM-1): a specific and sensitive biomarker of kidney injury. *Scand. J. Clin. Lab. Invest. Suppl.*, 2008, 241, 78-83

[148] Haase, M; Bellomo, R; Story, D; Davenport, P; Haase-Fielitz, A. Urinary interleukin-18 does not predict acute kidney injury after adult cardiac surgery: a prospective observational cohort study. *Crit. Care.*, 2008, 12, R96

[149] Zhou H, Pisitkun T, Aponte A, et al. Exosomal Fetuin-A identified by proteomics: a novel urinary biomarker for detecting acute kidney injury. *Kidney Int.*, 2006, 70, 1847-1857

[150] du Cheyron, D; Daubin, C; Poggioli, J; et al. Urinary measurement of Na+/H+ exchanger isoform 3 (NHE3) protein as new marker of tubule injury in critically ill patients with ARF. *Am. J. Kidney Dis.*, 2003, 42, 497-506

[151] Muramatsu, Y; Tsujie, M; Kohda, Y; et al. Early detection of cysteine rich protein 61 (CYR61, CCN1) in urine following renal ischemic reperfusion injury. *Kidney Int.*, 2002, 62, 1601-1610

[152] Brian Reeves, W; Kwon, O; Ramesh, G. Netrin-1 and kidney injury. II. Netrin-1 is an early biomarker of acute kidney injury. *Am. J. Physiol. Renal. Physiol.*, 2008, 294, F731-738

[153] Wang, W; Brian Reeves, W; Ramesh, G. Netrin-1 and kidney injury. I. Netrin-1 protects against ischemia-reperfusion injury of the kidney. *Am. J. Physiol. Renal. Physiol.*, 2008, 294, F739-747

[154] Basnakian, AG. Netrin-1: a potential universal biomarker for acute kidney injury. *Am. J. Physiol. Renal. Physiol.*, 2008, 294, F729-730

[155] Mishra, J; Ma, Q; Prada, A; et al. Identification of neutrophil gelatinase-associated lipocalin as a novel early urinary biomarker for ischemic renal injury. *J. Am. Soc. Nephrol.*, 2003, 14, 2534-2543

[156] Stamou, SC; Camp, SL; Reames, MK; et al. Continuous quality improvement program and major morbidity after cardiac surgery. *Am. J. Cardiol.*, 2008, 102, 772-777

[157] Martin, C; Papazian, L; Perrin, G; Saux, P; Gouin, F. Norepinephrine or dopamine for the treatment of hyperdynamic septic shock? *Chest.*, 1993, 103, 1826-1831

[158] Kilickan, L; Gonca, S; Dalcik, C; et al. General anesthesia with thoracic epidural anesthesia in the cardiopulmonary bypass surgery reduces apoptosis by upregulating antiapoptotic protein Bcl-2. *J. Cardiovasc. Surg.* (Torino), 2006, 47, 315-322

[159] Kilickan, L; Solak, M; Bayindir, O. Thoracic epidural anesthesia preserves myocardial function during intraoperative and postoperative period in coronary artery bypass grafting operation. *J. Cardiovasc. Surg.* (Torino), 2005, 46, 559-567

[160] Scott, NB; Turfrey, DJ; Ray, DA; et al. A prospective randomized study of the potential benefits of thoracic epidural anesthesia and analgesia in patients undergoing coronary artery bypass grafting. *Anesth. Analg.*, 2001, 93, 528-535

[161] Ho, AM; Chung, DC; Joynt, GM. Neuraxial blockade and hematoma in cardiac surgery: estimating the risk of a rare adverse event that has not (yet) occurred. *Chest.*, 2000, 117, 551-555

[162] Bracco, D; Hemmerling, T. Epidural analgesia in cardiac surgery: an updated risk assessment. *Heart Surg. Forum.*, 2007, 10, E334-337

[163] Saricaoglu, F; Akinci, SB; Oc, B; et al. The effect of halothane, isoflurane, sevoflurane and propofol infusion on renal function after coronary artery bypass surgery. *Middle East J. Anesthesiol.*, 2006, 18, 955-964

[164] Lassnigg, A; Donner, E; Grubhofer, G; et al. Lack of renoprotective effects of dopamine and furosemide during cardiac surgery. *J. Am. Soc. Nephrol.*, 2000, 11, 97-104

[165] Holmes, CL; Walley, KR. Bad medicine: low-dose dopamine in the ICU. *Chest.*, 2003, 123, 1266-1275

[166] Woo, EB; Tang, AT; el-Gamel, A; et al. Dopamine therapy for patients at risk of renal dysfunction following cardiac surgery: science or fiction? *Eur. J. Cardiothorac. Surg.*, 2002, 22, 106-111

[167] Bove, T; Landoni, G; Calabro, MG; et al. Renoprotective action of fenoldopam in high-risk patients undergoing cardiac surgery: a prospective, double-blind, randomized clinical trial. *Circulation.*, 2005, 111, 3230-3235

[168] Halpenny, M; Lakshmi, S; O'Donnell, A; O'Callaghan-Enright, S; Shorten, GD. Fenoldopam: renal and splanchnic effects in patients undergoing coronary artery bypass grafting. *Anaesthesia.*, 2001, 56, 953-960

[169] Barr, LF; Kolodner, K. N-acetylcysteine and fenoldopam protect the renal function of patients with chronic renal insufficiency undergoing cardiac surgery. *Crit. Care Med.*, 2008, 36, 1427-1435

[170] Cogliati, AA; Vellutini, R; Nardini, A; et al. Fenoldopam infusion for renal protection in high-risk cardiac surgery patients: a randomized clinical study. *J. Cardiothorac. Vasc. Anesth*, 2007, 21, 847-850

[171] Caimmi, PP; Pagani, L; Micalizzi, E; et al. Fenoldopam for renal protection in patients undergoing cardiopulmonary bypass. *J. Cardiothorac. Vasc. Anesth.*, 2003, 17, 491-494

[172] Landoni, G; Biondi-Zoccai, GG; Marino, G; et al. Fenoldopam reduces the need for renal replacement therapy and in-hospital death in cardiovascular surgery: a meta-analysis. *J. Cardiothorac. Vasc. Anesth.*, 2008, 22, 27-33

[173] Berendes, E; Mollhoff, T; Van Aken, H; et al. Effects of dopexamine on creatinine clearance, systemic inflammation, and splanchnic oxygenation in patients undergoing coronary artery bypass grafting. *Anesth. Analg.*, 1997, 84, 950-957

[174] Dehne, MG; Klein, TF; Muhling, J; et al. Impairment of renal function after cardiopulmonary bypass is not influenced by dopexamine. *Ren. Fail.*, 2001, 23, 217-230

[175] Sherry, E; Tooley, MA; Bolsin, SN; Monk, CR; Willcox, J. Effect of dopexamine hydrochloride on renal vascular resistance index and haemodynamic responses following coronary artery bypass graft surgery. *Eur. J. Anaesthesiol.*, 1997, 14, 184-189

[176] Mahesh, B; Yim, B; Robson, D; et al. Does furosemide prevent renal dysfunction in high-risk cardiac surgical patients? Results of a double-blinded prospective randomised trial. *Eur. J. Cardiothorac. Surg.*, 2008, 33, 370-376

[177] Carcoana, OV; Mathew, JP; Davis, E; et al. Mannitol and dopamine in patients undergoing cardiopulmonary bypass: a randomized clinical trial. *Anesth. Analg.*, 2003, 97, 1222-1229

[178] Smith, MN; Best, D; Sheppard, SV; Smith, DC. The effect of mannitol on renal function after cardiopulmonary bypass in patients with established renal dysfunction. *Anaesthesia.*, 2008, 63, 701-704

[179] Yallop, KG; Sheppard, SV; Smith, DC. The effect of mannitol on renal function following cardio-pulmonary bypass in patients with normal pre-operative creatinine. *Anaesthesia.*, 2008, 63, 576-582

[180] Sezai, A; Shiono, M; Orime, Y; et al. Low-dose continuous infusion of human atrial natriuretic peptide during and after cardiac surgery. *Ann. Thorac. Surg.*, 2000, 69, 732-738

[181] Sezai, A; Hata, M; Wakui, S; et al. Efficacy of continuous low-dose hANP administration in patients undergoing emergent coronary artery bypass grafting for acute coronary syndrome. *Circ. J.*, 2007, 71, 1401-1407

[182] Mentzer, RM Jr.; Oz, MC; Sladen, RN; et al. Effects of perioperative nesiritide in patients with left ventricular dysfunction undergoing cardiac surgery:the NAPA Trial. *J. Am. Coll. Cardiol.*, 2007, 49, 716-726

[183] Chen, HH; Sundt, TM; Cook, DJ; Heublein, DM; Burnett, JC Jr. Low dose nesiritide and the preservation of renal function in patients with renal dysfunction undergoing cardiopulmonary-bypass surgery: a double-blind placebo-controlled pilot study. *Circulation.*, 2007, 116, I134-138

[184] Loef, BG; Henning, RH; Epema, AH; et al. Effect of dexamethasone on perioperative renal function impairment during cardiac surgery with cardiopulmonary bypass. *Br. J. Anaesth.*, 2004, 93, 793-798

[185] McBride, WT; Allen, S; Gormley, SM; et al. Methylprednisolone favourably alters plasma and urinary cytokine homeostasis and subclinical renal injury at cardiac surgery. *Cytokine.*, 2004, 27, 81-89

[186] van den Berghe, G; Wouters, P; Weekers, F; et al. Intensive insulin therapy in the critically ill patients. *N. Engl. J. Med.*, 2001, 345, 1359-1367

[187] Ouattara, A; Lecomte, P; Le Manach, Y; et al. Poor intraoperative blood glucose control is associated with a worsened hospital outcome after cardiac surgery in diabetic patients. *Anesthesiology.*, 2005, 103, 687-694

[188] Hovorka, R; Kremen, J; Blaha, J, et al. Blood glucose control by a model predictive control algorithm with variable sampling rate versus a routine glucose management protocol in cardiac surgery patients: a randomized controlled trial. *J. Clin. Endocrinol. Metab.*, 2007, 92, 2960-2964

[189] Gandhi, GY; Nuttall, GA; Abel, MD; et al. Intensive intraoperative insulin therapy versus conventional glucose management during cardiac surgery: a randomized trial. *Ann. Intern. Med.*, 2007, 146, 233-243

[190] Liu, J; Wang, L; Wang, XN. [Experimental study of monoclonal antibody to intercellular adhesion molecule-1 for incipient acute tubular necrosis]. *Di Yi Jun Yi Da Xue Xue Bao.*, 2002, 22, 748-750

[191] Souza-Moraes, MR; David-Filho, R; Baptista-Silva, JC; et al. Effect of antibodies to intercellular adhesion molecule type 1 on the protection of distant organs during reperfusion syndrome in rats. *Braz. J. Med. Biol. Res.*, 2003, 36, 605-612

[192] Kelly, KJ; Williams, WW Jr.; Colvin, RB; Bonventre, JV. Antibody to intercellular adhesion molecule 1 protects the kidney against ischemic injury. *Proc. Natl. Acad. Sci.*, U.S.A., 1994, 91, 812-816

[193] Kelly, KJ WW; Colvin, JB; Meehan, SM; Springer, TA; Guttierrez-Ramos, JC; Bonventre, JV. Intercellular Adhesion Molecule-1-deficient Mice Are Protected against Renal Injury. *J. Clin. Invest.*, 1996, 97, 1056-1063

[194] Sisillo, E; Ceriani, R; Bortone, F; et al. N-acetylcysteine for prevention of acute renal failure in patients with chronic renal insufficiency undergoing cardiac surgery: a prospective, randomized, clinical trial. *Crit. Care Med.*, 2008, 36, 81-86

[195] Haase, M; Haase-Fielitz, A; Bagshaw, SM; et al. Phase II, randomized, controlled trial of high-dose N-acetylcysteine in high-risk cardiac surgery patients. *Crit. Care Med.*, 2007, 35, 1324-1331

[196] Bouman, CC; Schultz, MJ. N-acetylcysteine: multiple organ saver during cardiac surgery? *Crit. Care Med.*, 2008, 36, 338-340

[197] Ristikankare, A; Kuitunen, T; Kuitunen, A; et al. Lack of renoprotective effect of i.v. N-acetylcysteine in patients with chronic renal failure undergoing cardiac surgery. *Br. J. Anaesth.*, 2006, 97, 611-616

[198] Barta, E; Pechan, I; Cornak, V; et al. Protective effect of alpha-tocopherol and L-ascorbic acid against the ischemic-reperfusion injury in patients during open-heart surgery. *Bratisl. Lek. Listy.*, 1991, 92, 174-183

[199] Canbaz, S; Duran, E; Ege, T; et al. The effects of intracoronary administration of vitamin E on myocardial ischemia-reperfusion injury during coronary artery surgery. *Thorac. Cardiovasc. Surg.*, 2003, 51, 57-61

[200] Pajonk, F; Riedisser, A; Henke, M; McBride, WH; Fiebich, B. The effects of tea extracts on proinflammatory signaling. *BMC Med.*, 2006, 4, 28

[201] Langley, SM; Chai, PJ; Jaggers, JJ; Ungerleider, RM. Platelet-activating factor receptor antagonism improves cerebral recovery after circulatory arrest. *Ann. Thorac. Surg.*, 1999, 68, 1578-1584, discussion 1585

[202] Tamayo, E; Álvarez, F; Alonso, O; et al. The inflammatory response to colloids and crystalloids used for pump priming during cardiopulmonary bypass. *Acta Anaesth. Scand.*, 2008, 52, 1204-1212

[203] Journois, D ; Pouard, P ; Greeley, WJ ; et al. Hemofiltration during cardiopulmonary bypass in pediatric cardiac surgery. Effects on hemostasis, cytokines, and complement components. *Anesthesiology.*, 1994, 81, 1181-1189

[204] Ohri, SK; Bowles, CW; Mathie, RT; et al. Effect of cardiopulmonary bypass perfusion protocols on gut tissue oxygenation and blood flow. *Ann. Thorac. Surg.*, 1997, 64, 163-170

[205] Ohri, SK; Bjarnason, I; Pathi, V; et al. Cardiopulmonary bypass impairs small intestinal transport and increases gut permeability. *Ann. Thorac. Surg.*, 1993, 55, 1080-1086

[206] Journois, D; Israel-Biet, D; Pouard, P; et al. High-volume, zero-balanced hemofiltration to reduce delayed inflammatory response to cardiopulmonary bypass in children. *Anesthesiology.*, 1996, 85, 965-976
[207] Journois, D. Hemofiltration during cardiopulmonary bypass. *Minerva Anestesiol.*, 1999, 65, 427-432

In: Advances in Cardiovascular Research, Volume 1
Editors: L. Schmitt, T. Konig, pp. 199-218
ISBN: 978-1-60741-720-0


*Chapter VII*

# Rheumatic Valvulopathy: Current Understanding of Pathogenesis and Perspective of Immunobiological Treatments

***Marcelo Derbli Schafranski[1], Luiza Guilherme[2] and Iara de Messias-Reason[1]***

[1]Departamento de Patologia Médica, Hospital de Clínicas, Federal University of Paraná, Curitiba, Brazil.

[2]Heart Institute (InCor), School of Medicine, University of São Paulo, São Paulo, Brazil.

## Abstract

Chronic rheumatic heart disease (CRHD), the most severe sequelae of rheumatic fever (RF), continues to be the most important cause of acquired valvulopathy among children and young adults worldwide, being responsible for approximately 233000 deaths annually. RF is autoimmune sequelae of a group A streptococcal (*Streptococcus pyogenes*) oropharyngeal infection which develops several weeks after sore throat has gone away. Carditis occurs in approximately 50–60% of acute RF cases, and CRHD develops in 30-50% of these patients. Cross-reactive antibodies and autoreactive T-lymphocytes lead to inflammation, cellular infiltration and valvular scarring. All heart valves may be damaged, but the mitral valve is most frequently affected, followed by the aortic valve. The fact that approximately 0.3-3% of the streptococcal oropharyngeal infections cause RF, provides evidence of genetic predisposition to disease development. A number of studies have linked HLA genes to the susceptibility of both RF and CRHD, especially those related to HLA-DR and –DQ loci, but non-HLA genes seem also to be involved in the disease. Molecular mimicry between *S. pyogenes* and human proteins has been proposed as the main factor leading to autoimmunity in RF/CRHD and studies demonstrate that CD4+ T lymphocytes play an important role in the development and maintenance of valve lesions. The cytokines profile observed in rheumatic heart valve specimens suggests a Th1 driven response and an imbalance between proinflammatory

(IL-1, IL-6, TNF-alpha) and antiinflammatory (IL-4, IL-10) cytokines in these lesions may also contribute to the development of chronic valvulopathy. In addition, a growing body of evidence supports the hypothesis of ongoing inflammation in CRHD. Elevated serum levels of adhesion molecules, high-sensitive C-reactive protein, advanced oxidation protein products (AOPP) and complement components including mannan-binding lectin (MBL) have been observed in RF/CRHD patients. The deposition of complement in heart tissue of RF/CRHD patients has also been reported. Currently, there is no therapy that shows any benefit in reducing the risk of developing heart lesions in patients with acute RF. Although monoclonal antibodies that block IL-1, IL-6, TNF-alpha and B-lymphocytes are already available and successfully used in the treatment of different autoimmune and inflammatory disorders, there is no report recomending the use of those immunomodulators in RF/CRHD. Here we present a review of the current understanding of the underlying mechanisms involved in the pathogenesis of RF and CRHD. We also discuss the possibility of immunobiological treatments, based on data available on other autoimmune diseases, such as rheumatoid arthritis, ankylosing spondylitis and systemic lupus erythematosus.

## Introduction

The sore throat is amongst the most prevalent symptoms that health care professionals need to deal with. There are than 225 pathogens, including nearly 200 viruses that cause upper respiratory tract infections. *Streptococcus pyogenes* (beta-hemolytic streptococci group A) is amongst the most common bacteria that induce oropharyngeal infection in school-aged children living under lower socioeconomic conditions. Rheumatic fever (RF) and its most severe sequela, chronic rheumatic heart disease (CRHD), are autoimmune disorders resulting from throat infections with *S. pyogenes*. The immune damage is considered to be due to molecular mimicry between streptococcal antigens and humans proteins, which ultimately leads to autoimmunity in genetically susceptible individuals. The onset of the disease follows the initial oropharyngeal infection typically after a latency period of 2 to 3 weeks, and consists of a febrile illness that can affect the joints, heart (leading to pericarditis, myocarditis and valvulitis), skin (subcutaneous nodules and erythema marginatum) and the central nervous system (chorea) (William and Alto, 1992; Guilherme, Ramasawmy and Kalil, 2007). The clinical picture is self-limiting, but in susceptible individuals (approximately 2%) there is a continuous and progressive injury to the heart valves, resulting in heart failure and need for valve replacement procedures. CRHD continues to be the most significant cause of acquired valvulopathy among children and young adults worldwide, being responsible for approximately 492.000 deaths annually (Beggs, Peterson and Tompson, WHO, 2008).

It has been estimated that in 2005 more than 2.4 million children aged 5-14 years were affected with CRHD with 79% of them coming from less developed nations. In addition, 336.000 new cases of RF are expected to occur yearly, with 95% of them also coming from less developed countries (Carapetis et al., 2005; Beggs, Peterson and Tompson, WHO, 2008).

# Epidemiology and Etiologic Agent

Epidemiological as well as clinical and laboratorial data support the hypothesis that *S. pyogenes* is the causative agent of RF/CRHD. There is evidence that outbreaks of RF follow epidemics of streptococcal sore throat and scarlet fever and that adequate antibiotic treatment reduces the incidence of subsequent RF. Moreover, antimicrobial prophylaxis clearly prevents the recurrence in patients with history of RF and at least one antistreptococcal antibody (streptolysin O, hyaluronidase, streptokinase) can be found in the sera of RF patients (Gibofsky, Kerwar and Zabriskie, 1998).

The classification of streptococci has long been based in the type of hemolytic reaction displayed on blood agar, with complete lysis of red cells being associated with beta–hemolysis. Based on the composition of polysaccharides cell wall, beta-hemolytic streptococci can be divided into several different groups (A to V), with group A being related with the presence of a polymer of N-acetyl glucosamine and rhamnose. Group A (*Streptococcus pyogenes*) can be further subdivided by molecular biology approach into 150 M types, some of them considered to be more "rheumatogenic" (types 5, 14, 18 and 24). In developing countries, impetigo and oropharyngitis are the most common infections caused by *S. pyogenes*, but only throat infection has been linked to the development of RF/CRHD (Gibofsky, Kerwar and Zabriskie, 1998; Martins, Veasy and Hill, 2006).

Rebecca Lancefield in 1928, was the pioneer in developing a method to serotype *S. pyogenes* based on the reactivity of M protein and in 1946 Lancefield reported the serological classification of *S. pyogenes* according to its T surface antigen of which approximately 20 T serotypes have been described. Nowadays the strains are identified by the N- terminal nucleotide sequences of the emm gene.

In general, most children develop at least one episode of oropharyngitis per year, of which 15–20% are caused by group A streptococci and approximately 80% of these infections are due to viral pathogens, such as enterovirus, Epstein-Barr virus, cytomegalovirus, adenovirus, and herpes simplex virus. The peak age of incidence of RF is 4 to 15 years, but cases can also occur in adults. A child with a non-treated streptococcal throat infection has a 0.3 to 3% chance of developing RF. However, there is no predilection for gender or ethnical background for the occurrence of RF (Gibofsky, Kerwar and Zabriskie, 1998).

In developed countries, the annual incidence of RF started to decrease in the 20th century, with a noticeable fall after the introduction of antibiotics into clinical practice in the 1950s. Currently, the annual incidence of RF it is below 1 per 100.000 in these countries. However, in underdeveloped and developing nations the incidence rates are still high, as it is observed in Sudan (100 per 100.000) and China (150 per 100.000). In Brazil, the incidence of acute RF was 5.000 new cases in 2002 (approximately 290 per 100.000) (data from the Brazilian Health Ministry). The prevalence rates of CRHD also show wide variation among different countries, ranging from 0.2 per 1000 in Cuba (1987) to 77.8 per 1000 in Samoa (1999). The mortality rate for CRHD can vary from 0.5 per 100 000 inhabitants in Denmark to 8.2 per 100 000 in China. It has been estimated that there may be approximately 30 million children with CRHD in developing countries and near 1.5 million in developed countries (Carapetis et al., 2005). In some developing countries, CRHD accounts for up to 12-65% of hospital admissions related to cardiovascular disease (WHO, 2001). In Brazil, RF represents 90% of the surgery indications for heart valve replacement in children (DATASUS, 2007).

Socioeconomic and environmental factors (eg. poverty, malnutrition, overcrowding, poor housing) as well as host genetic factors are known to contribute to the development of RF and CHRD (Kaplan, 1996; Guilherme, Ramasawmy and Kalil, 2007).

## Genetic Susceptibility and Pathogenesis

The pathogenesis of RF/CRHD is complex and both environmental and genetic factors contribute to its etiology. Several HLA-DR and DQ alleles have been reported to be associated with RF and CRHD. Among the class II alleles of susceptibility, the HLA-DR7 was found in association with the disease in patients from four ethnically diverse countries (Brazil, Egypt, Latvia and Turkey) and the association of this allele with some DQ alleles seems to be associated with the development of valvular lesions in CRHD (reviewed by Guilherme, Ramasawmy and Kalil, 2007).

Other associations with different genes such as TNF-alpha and *MBL2* have also been described. Association of the TNF-alpha alleles (-308A and -238A) (Hernandez-Pacheco and cols, 2003; Sallackci et al., 2005; Ramasawmy et al., 2007), as well as different variants of promoter and exon 1 regions of the *MBL2* gene have been reported in patients with RF/CRHD (Messias-Reason et al., 2006; Ramasawmy et al., 2008; Schafranski et al. 2008). Other genes related with immune regulation are now being investigated and certainly will contribute towards the definition of new genetic markers and how these genes act in the complex network of autoimmune reactions that occurs in RF/CRHD.

The molecular mechanism by which MHC class II molecules confer susceptibility to autoimmune diseases is not clear, however the role of HLA molecules is to present antigens to the T cell receptor thus triggering the activation of the adaptive immune response. HLA class II molecules are expressed on the surface of antigen-presenting cells such as macrophages, dendritic cells and B lymphocytes and the presentation of pathogen epitopes, *S. pyogenes* in the case of RF/CRHD, with structural or sequential similarity to self epitopes might activate autoreactive T lymphocytes that have escaped immune tolerance by the molecular mimicry mechanism. These auto reactive T cells can also activate B cells that will produce pathogen and self antigen-specific antibodies.

The TNF-alpha -308A allele is responsible for high production of the TNF-alpha proinflammatory cytokine leading to high concentrations of this cytokine in the plasma (Sallakci et al., 2005, Settin et al., 2007) and a great number of TNF-alpha secreting cells have been found in the heart tissue of both acute and CRHD patients (Guilherme et al., 2004).

Mannan-binding lectin (MBL) is an acute phase inflammatory protein and functions as a soluble pathogen recognition receptor. MBL binds to a wide variety of sugars on the surface of pathogens and plays a major role in innate immunity due to its ability to opsonize pathogens enhancing their phagocytosis and to activate the complement cascade via the lectin pathway (Jack and Klein and Turn, 2001). High concentration of MBL levels as well as the presence of high expressing MBL genotypes were recently found associated with the development of acute and chronic carditis in patients with history of RF from Brazil (Schafranski and cols, 2008). As such the pathogenesis of CRHD seems to result from an overt immune response involving either humoral or cellular reaction or both, triggered by GAS infection.

The presence of human and animal antibodies against streptococcal antigens and human heart-tissue proteins was described more than 50 years ago. However, the role of human cross reactive antibodies in the development of heart lesions was postulated only recently by the *in vitro* demonstration that they bind to the endothelial surface, leading to inflammation (Galvin et al., 2000) and upregulation of the adhesion molecule VCAM-1 that facilitates the cellular infiltration and valve scarring (Roberts et al., 2001). These data established the role of the heart–tissue cross reactive antibodies in the early stages of inflammation and T cell infiltration in both acute and CRHD lesions.

The first evidence of $CD4^+$ T cells involvement in CRHD lesions was described by Raizada et al., 1980. By generating T cell clones from heart lesions-infiltrating T cells of acute and CRHD patients it was demonstrated for the first time the ability of 7.5% of these cells to simultaneously recognize M protein peptides and heart tissue-derived proteins by molecular mimicry (Guilherme et al. 1995). Three M5 regions (residues 1-25, 81-103 and 163-177) cross-reactive with several heart protein fractions, mainly those derived from valvular tissue with molecular masses of 95-150, 43- and 30-43 kDa, have been described (Guilherme et al. 1995). The frequencies of autoreactive T cells were higher in patients in acute phase of the disease (67%) when compared with CRHD (around 25%) (Guilherme et al. 2001). Peptides included in the three immunodominant M5 regions described above and heart tissue proteins fractions were also recognized by peripheral T cells from RF/CRHD patients (Guilherme et al. 2001a). The M5(81-96) epitope was preferentially recognized in patients with severe CRHD that expressed HLA-$DR7^+DR53^+$ (Guilherme et al. 2001a). These data suggest a role for the HLA class II molecules DR7 and DR53 in presenting the streptococcal immunodominant peptide to the T cell receptor (TCR), and show the significance of the propensity of DR7 and/or DR53 to cause severe CRHD in Brazilian patients, and probably in other populations as well in which this class II allele is also associated with RHD, and with the development of valvular lesions.

Yoshinaga et al., 1995 compared the reactivity of PHA-stimulated T cell lines derived from heart-valve specimens and peripheral blood lymphocytes of RF patients and showed that, even though these cells recognized cell wall and membrane streptococcal antigens, they failed to react to the M protein, myosin, or other mammalian cytoskeletal proteins. The absence of reactivity against M protein and self-antigens probably was a result of low frequencies of specific T cells.

Cardiac myosin is one of the major autoantigens involved with rheumatic heart lesions involved with rheumatic heart lesions (Krisher and Cunningham, 1985). Cross reactive peripheral T cell clones from a CRHD patient were responsive to group A recombinant M6 protein, cardiac myosin, tropomyosin and laminin, a valve protein (Ellis et al., 2005). The authors showed that the cross reactive response was MHC class I and II restricted for T cell clones $CD4^+$ and $CD8^+$, respectively. These cells recognized streptococcal M6 epitopes on the B region and S2 and LMM regions of human cardiac myosin (Ellis et al., 2005).

Heart-tissue infiltrating T cell clones were able to recognize cardiac myosin ß chain (LMM peptides) and streptococcal M5 peptides and valve-derived proteins by cross reactivity (Faé et al., 2006). The reactivity against LMM peptides of heart-tissue infiltrating T cells may be attributable to the stimulation of these cells initially by the alpha-helical coiled-coil streptococcal M protein. The myosin cross reactivity with several other valvular proteins may occur first through mimicry (Guilherme et al.; 1995; Ellis et al., 2005) and eventually by an epitope spreading mechanism (Lehmann et al., 1992) in which the evolution of an autoimmune pathology may easily obliterate any evidence of the initial target antigens such as streptococcal M protein and cross reactive self antigens. Both peripheral and rheumatic heart lesions-derived T cell clones studies, demonstrate mimicry at T-cell level between streptococcal M protein and human cardiac myosin epitopes and confirm previous work reported for T cell mimicry in the valve.

It has been observed that IFNγ, TNF-alpha (inflammatory cytokines) and IL-10 (regulatory cytokine) positive cells were consistently predominant in both myocardium and valvular tissue whereas IL-4 (regulatory cytokine) was scarce in the valves from acute and CRHD. The predominance of inflammatory cytokines in the heart lesions confirm that the disease is mediated by inflammatory immune response. In addition, the significant lower IL-4 expression in the valvular tissue may contribute to the progression of CRHD leading to permanent damage in the valves (Guilherme et al., 2004).

Heart-tissue infiltrating T cell repertoire is probably composed by migrating peripheral primed T cells. It was assessed the clonality of T-cells by analyzing the Vß and Jß genes of the T-cell receptor (TCR) in both peripheral blood and intralesional T cell lines obtained from heart tissue from several CRHD patients. The analysis of TCR (Vß and Jß rearrangement) showed clonally the presence of expanded families in the heart-tissue and polyclonal distribution in the peripheral blood (Guilherme et al., 2000).

Taken together, these data demonstrate that T-cell populations are expanded in the CRHD-heart lesions, driven by self antigen recognition, and probably contribute to the maintenance and progression of tissue damage. **Figure 1** summarizes all the major events involved with rheumatic autoimmune reactions.

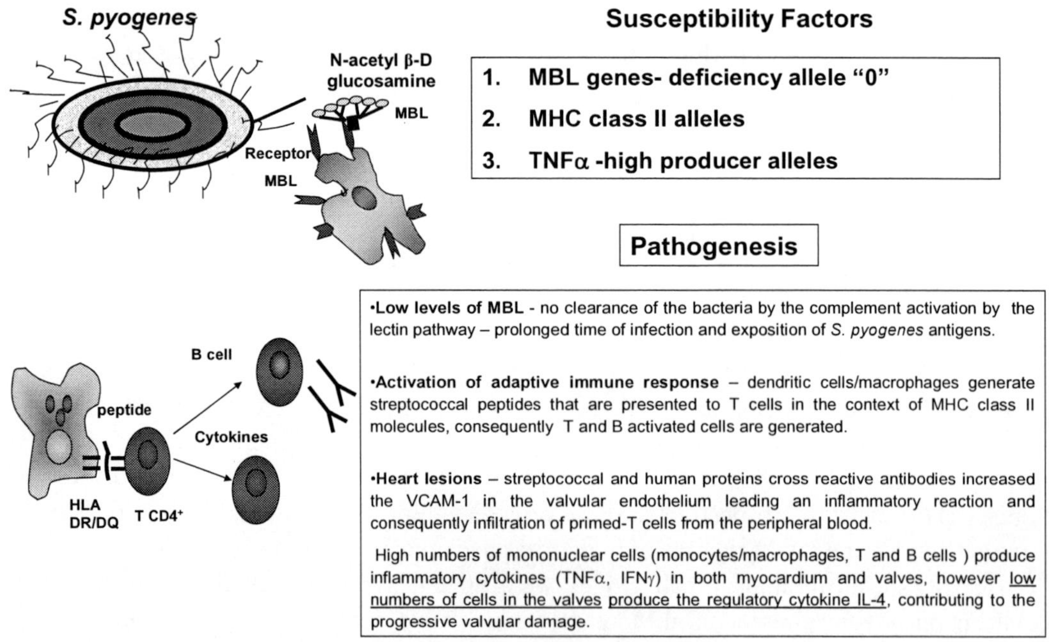


Figure 1. Events leading autoimmune reactions in CRHD.

**Table 1. MODIFIED JONES CRITERIA FOR THE DIAGNOSIS OF ACUTE RHEUMATIC FEVER. For the establishment of the diagnosis, 2 major criteria or 1 major and 2 minors *plus* evidence of a previous streptococcal infection are required (adapted from Gaasch, 1992).**

| Major Criteria | Minor Criteria |
|---|---|
| Arthritis | Arthralgia |
| Carditis | Fever |
| Chorea | Prolonged P-R interval (ECG) |
| Subcutaneous nodules | History or CRHD or previous RF |
| Erythema marginatum | Elevated ESR ou CRP |
| **Evidence of Previous Streptococcal Infection** | |
| Elevated or rising ASO or rapid streptococcal antigen test | |
| Positive streptococcal throat culture | |
| Recent scarlet fever | |

## Diagnosis and Clinical Manifestations

RF is considered a multisystemic disease with involvement of multiple organs: heart, joints, central nervous system and skin. To date, there is no specific clinical or laboratory test that is able to establish the diagnosis of RF. In 1944, Jones developed a set of criteria for the diagnosis of the disease, which was modified and updated in 1992 (Gaasch, 1992). The major criteria include carditis, arthritis, subcutaneous nodules, erythema marginatum and chorea; the minor criteria include arthralgia, fever (ranging from 38.4°C to 40.0°C), elevated acute-phase reactants (erythrocyte sedimentation rate and C-reactive protein), a prolonged electrocardiographic P-R interval and history of previous RF or CHRD. The presence of 2 major criteria or one major and two minor criteria, plus a laboratorial evidence of a previous streptococcal infection (positive throat culture or rapid streptococcal antigen test; or elevated or rising streptococcal antibody titer; or history of recent scarlet fever) are necessary for the diagnosis (**Table 1**). Other minor manifestations such as abdominal pain, epistaxis (Gibofsky, Kerwar and Zabriskie, 1998) and rheumatic pneunomia (Burgert et al., 1995) can also be found although they are not part of the criteria.

### Carditis

Carditis is considered the most specific manifestation of the disease, affecting 30-45% of RF children. Rheumatic carditis affects the pericardium, myocardium and endocardium (valvulitis). All heart valves may be damaged, but the mitral valve is the most frequently affected, followed by the aortic valve (Carapetis, McDonalds and Wilson, 2004). Mitral regurgitation is by far the most common acute valvular lesion. Clinically, it is associated with tachycardia and a murmur of valvulitis. It varies in severity, ranging from mild and transient to very severe, which can lead to cardiac failure and death (Dajani, 1997; Bitar et al., 2000). In some patients there is a silent carditis, a term used to define subclinic carditis, where valve regurgitation can de detected by Doppler echocardiography in the absence of murmur.

However, the use of this test on its own can not be considered as evidence of carditis, according to the latest revised Jones' criteria (Gaasch, 1992). Therefore, the use of echocardiography to evidence acute carditis in the absence of auscultatory findings still remains controversial.

However, the use of echocardiography can increase by 10-fold the sensibility in the detection of CRHD (Marijon et al. 2007). Rheumatic carditis invariably occurs in an RF recurrence, if the initial episode involved the heart (Feinstein and Stern, 1967; Kalim-ud-Din Aziz, Cheema and. Memon, 1992). Repeated episodes of RF and the ongoing inflammatory process in the affected valves lead to progressive valvular scarring, subvalvar thickening and fusion of the valve leaflets **(figure 2)**. As a consequence, after a period of 10-20 years, approximately 30-50% of the patients that presented carditis in the initial episode of RF will develop clinical features of mitral stenosis, the hallmark of CRHD. Other far less common causes of mitral stenosis include rheumatoid arthritis (RA), systemic lupus erythematosus (SLE), mucopolyssacaridosis, congenital abnormalities and carcinoid syndrome.

## Arthritis

In general, approximately 75% of RF children will display arthritis, which is usually incapacitating and affects the major joints. It follows a migratory course: in a matter of days, the inflammation travels from one joint to another. Large joints (knees, ankles, elbows and wrists) are the most common affected sites. Polyarthritis is the most frequent form of presentation, but oligoartrhitis and monoarthritis can also occur (Amigo, Martinez-Lavin and Reyes, 1993). RF arthritis is non-erosive and in most cases non-deforming, except when capsular and periarticular fibrosis develop in the small joints of hands and feet due to repeated episodes of the disease, which is denominated *Jaccoud*'s arthropathy (Bittl and Perloff, 1983).

## Erythema Marginatum

Erythema marginatum, although highly specific, is not a frequent manifestation of RF, affecting less than 5% of the patients (Ravisha, Tullu and Kamat 2003). It is most frequently observed in the trunk and proximal extremities, sparing the face and usually occurs in association with carditis (Amigo, Martinez-Lavin and Reyes, 1993). The clinical picture of erythema marginatum consists on an evanescent, pink, non-pruritic eruption with pale centers and rounded or serpiginous margins.

## Subcutaneous Nodules

Subcutaneous nodules are observed in nearly 20% of RF patients, primarily located on bony prominences of extensor surfaces (elbows, knees, wrists, spinal column). They are firm, painless and movable nodules, with sizes ranging from 0.5 to 2 cm. As it is seen in erythema marginatum, subcutaneous nodules usually appear in association with carditis (Benedek, 1984).

### Chorea

Sydenham´s chorea affects approximately 20% of RF patients and is characterized by involuntary movements, especially of the face and limbs, disturbances of gait, speech and voluntary movements. Patients usually exhibit emotional lability and the abnormal movements are more apparent during periods of anxiety and disappear with sleep. Sydenham´s chorea can be the only manifestation of the disease (Berrios et al., 1985), which is benign, may be and resolved without sequelae. Chorea´s differential diagnosis include atypical seizures, cerebrovascular accidents, collagen vascular diseases (vasculitis, SLE), drug intoxications (amitriptyline, metoclopramide), familiar chorea (e.g. Huntington´s disease), hormonally induced chorea, thyroid disease and Wilson´s Disease (Wild and Tabrizi, 2007).

### Other Manifestations

Fever related to acute RF is defined as an oral or tympanic temperature of 38°C or higher. History of fever in patients taking oral anti-inflammatory drugs also qualifies as minor criteria (Carapetis, McDonalds and Wilson, 2004). Abdominal pain, due to microvascular mesenteric inflammation is nonspecific and can mimic other diseases such as acute appendicitis. Epistaxis is associated with severe rheumatic carditis and can worsen by the usage of salicylates and other anti-inflammatory drugs. Rheumatic pneumonia is a rare manifestation and resembles pulmonary edema or alveolitis caused by other lung diseases (Gibofsky, Kerwar and Zabriskie, 1998).

## Laboratory Investigation

Despite the significant progress in microbiology and molecular biology, to date there is no specific laboratory test for the diagnostic of RF. The laboratory tests used include demonstration of a recent streptococcal infection, the presence of inflammatory process and occurrence and severity of valvular disease.

### Evidence of a Recent Streptococcal Infection

*Throat cultures*: Due to the latent period between the infection and symptoms onset and previous use of antibiotics, it is estimated that only 20% of throat cultures show positivity for *S. pyogenes* in patients with RF.

*Rapid antigen detection test (RADT)*: RADT´s diagnostic value is high (sensitivity of 89.7% and specificity of 97.2%) and can be used safely in populations with suspected streptococcal infections (Camurdan et al., 2008).

*Streptococcal antibody tests*: The presence of streptococcal antibodies must be investigated when there is a suspicion of RF. Streptolysin O (SLO) and S are extracellular hemolysins produced by *S. pyogenes*. Although both are cytolytic toxins, only SLO is antigenic and leads to the production of naturally occurring antibodies. The titers of the antibody produced against SLO, antistreptolysin O (ASO), elevates in more than 80% of individuals affected by a streptococcal infection. About 1 week to 10 days after the initial infection, the ASO antibody response starts to rise. It reaches a peak 3 to 6 weeks later and begins to decline after 6 to 8 weeks. In some individuals, the ASO titers remains elevated for indefinite periods of time. *S. pyogenes* also produces another group of extracellular enzymes, named Dnases (A, B, C and D). Dnase-B antibody concentrations start to rise within 1 to 2 weeks of the initial infection and peak later than ASO titers (usually 6 to 8 weeks after the infection). As it persists in the sera longer than ASO (up to 3 months), Dnase-B antibody is a more consistent test for establishing a previous streptococcal infection (Martins, Veasy and Hill, 2006).

### Inflammatory Markers

Acute-phase reactants, such as erythrocyte sedimentation rate (ESR) and C-reactive protein (CRP) are nearly always abnormal (generally markedly elevated and representing minor criteria for the diagnosis) in acute RF and are useful parameters to monitor disease activity. In CRHD, recent studies demonstrated elevated serum levels of adhesion molecules (Yetkin et al., 2001), pro-inflammatory cytokines (Sallakci et al., 2005, Settin et al., 2007), mannan-binding-lectin (MBL) (Schafranski et al., 2004), CRP and advanced oxygenation protein products (AOPP) (Chiu et al., 2006), suggesting an ongoing inflammatory process, even in the absence of acute RF manifestations.

### Synovial Fluid Analysis

Synovial fluid analysis, which usually shows a profile of acute inflammation (white blood cells count from 20.000 to 40.000 cells/mm$^3$, with a predominance of polymorphonuclear leukocytes) is of importance. Gram stain and culture are indicated in order to rule out septic arthritis.

## Differential Diagnosis

Differential diagnosis of acute RF using laboratorial tests, such as blood and synovial fluid cultures, antinuclear antibody, rheumatoid factor and bone marrow aspiration (when indicated), are essential to exclude other diseases including infections (septic arthritis, bacterial endocarditis, Lyme disease, mycobacterial and fungal arthritis and viral arthritis), reactive arthritis (enteric or urogenital, secondary to inflammatory bowel diseasse), systemic rheumatic disorders (Still´s disease, rheumatoid arthritis, systemic lupus erythematosus, systemic vasculitis, sarcoidosis) and others (especially malignancy) (Pinals, 1994). Some authors support the existence of a distinct entity that shares some features with RF, denominated post-streptococcal reactive arthritis. However this disorder differs from acute RF for several reasons: by presenting a shorter latency period between the oropharyngeal infection and the clinical picture (usually 1 to 2 weeks), poor response to nonsteroidal antiinflammatory agents, absence of carditis and the presence of frequent extra-articular manifestations (as tenosynovitis and renal abnormalities) (Goldsmith and Long, 1982, Barash et al., 2008).

## Treatment

The treatment of acute RF needs to be directed to the suppression of the ongoing inflammatory process at the different clinical presentations of the disease. The therapy also includes the eradication of *S. pyogenes* still present in the throat and the prevention of new infection recurrences that could be harmful in the future **(Table 2)**.

## Treatment of the Clinical Manifestations

The cornerstone in the treatment of RF is the use of antiinflammatory drugs, which commonly lead to dramatic improvement in the clinical symptoms after the initiation of therapy. The most common anti-inflammatory drugs used in the treatment of RF include aspirin, naproxen and steroids.

Arthritis can be managed with aspirin (80-100 mg/kg/day in children and up to 4-8 g/day in adults) or naproxen (15-20 mg/kg/day, bid) (Hashkes et al., 2003). The therapy must be maintained until improvement of clinical symptoms and normalization of laboratorial data.

If severe carditis is present, manifested by cardiac failure or third degree heart block, steroid therapy can be started (prednisone 1 – 2 mg/kg/day), with tapering proportional to the clinical picture (Saxena, 2002). Digitalis, diuretics, angiotensin-converter enzyme (ACE) inhibitors, beta-blockers and invasive procedures (as a pacemaker implant) can also be used, when indicated (James and Smith, 2005).

Sydenham´s chorea generally does not respond well to anti-inflammatory drugs. Benzodiazepines, neuroleptics, and antiepileptics are useful in these cases, in combination with supportive measures such as resting in a silent room. Haloperidol, diazepam, carbamazepine have all been reported to be useful in the management of chorea. Steroids have little or no effect in the treatment of the RF-associated chorea (Rochenzel et al., 1998, Hael et al., 2000).

To date, there is no specific therapy, including non-steroidal antiinflammatory drugs, corticosteroids and intravenous immunoglobulin (IgIV), showing any significant benefit in reducing the risk of developing heart lesions in patients with acute RF (Cilliers, Manyemba and Saloonjee, 2003). In spite of important advances regarding the molecular mechanisms of the disease and the successful results obtained with biologic therapies in many other inflammatory and autoimmune disorders (Furst et al., 2007), only a few randomized controlled trials (RCTs) concerning treatment of acute RF have been published in the recent years (Câmara et al., 2002, Narin et al., 2003). Moreover, no anecdotal cases of immunobiological therapy either in RF or CRHD have been published to date (Furst et al., 2007). Here we suggest different reasonable therapeutic approaches that could be subject for future studies concerning RF and CRHD, based on the known disease mechanisms.

**Table 2. ANTIBIOTICS USED IN THE TREATMENT AND SECONDARY PROPHYLAXIS OR RF. Oral sulfonamides (sulfadiazine, sulfasoxazole) and erythromycin are alternatively used for penicillin allergic patients (adapted from WHO, 2001 and Beggs, Peterson and Tompson, WHO, 2008) IM: intramuscularly.**

| Treatment | | |
|---|---|---|
| **Antibiotic** | **Mode of Administration** | **Dose** |
| Benzathine Penicillin | IM, single dose | <20 kg: 600.000 U |
| | | >20 kg: 1.2 million U |
| Phenoxymethylpenicillin | IM or oral | 250 mg, bid, 10 days |
| Erythromycin | Oral | 10 mg/kg up 500 mg, bid, 10 days |
| Erythromycin ethyl succinate | Oral | 40 mg/kg/day, divided doses, |
| | | (maximum 1 g/day in children |
| Clindamycin | Oral | 10-30 mg/kg/day, in 4 divides do |
| | | Doses |
| Secondary Prophylaxis | | |
| Benzathine Penicillin | IM, single injection every | <30 kg: 600.000 U |
| | 2-3 weeks | >30 kg: 1.2 million U |
| Penicillin V | Oral | 250 mg bid |
| Sulfonamide (sulfadiazine, | Oral | >30 kg: 1 g daily |
| sulfasoxazole) | | <30 kg: 500 mg daily |
| Erythromycin | Oral | 250 mg bid |

# Surgical Treatment

Patients with symptomatic mitral stenosis should be further evaluated by transthoracic and transesophageal echocardiography. According to the *Wilkins-Block Score*, which includes four parameters (leaflet thickening, leaflet mobility, leaflet calcification and involvement of subvalvular apparatus), invasive interventions may be indicated. Those patients with preserved valve morphology are candidates for percutaneous transvenous mitral commissurotomy (balloon valvuloplasty) or surgical commissurotomy. Mitral valve replacement (biologic or metal prosthesis) is recommended for those patients with severe valve deformities (Feldmam, 2000).

In addition, patients with CRHD submitted to invasive procedures that involve manipulation of the periapical region of the teeth or the gingival tissue or perforation of the oral mucosa, procedures on airways, infected skin or musculoskeletal tissues need antibiotic prophylaxis in order to prevent infective endocarditis. As it is well absorbed by the gastrointestinal tract, oral amoxicillin (2g) is the first choice in these circumstances. Patients that cannot take oral antibiotics may receive intravenous or intramuscular ampicillin (2g), ceftriaxone (1g) or cefazolin (1g). Oral clindamycin (600mg), azithromycin (500mg), clarithromycin (600mg), cephalexin (2g) or any other first- or second-generation oral cephalosporin in equivalent dosage may be given to patients that are allergic to penicillin. Moreover, patients who are allergic to penicillin and cannot take oral antibiotics may be given intravenous or intramuscular clindamycin (600 mg), ceftriaxone (1g) or cefazolin (1g) (Khan and Ijaz, 2008). The antibiotics for infective endocarditis prophylaxis mentioned above must be administered 30–60 minutes before the beginning of the intervention.

# Vaccine

Group A beta hemolytic *Streptococcus* causes several diseases, such as: **1**.severe invasive infections, **2**. poststreptococcal nonsuppurative sequel of acute RF and its major clinical manifestation CRHD, **3**.acute glomerulonephritis and also uncomplicated pharyngites and pyoderma. These diseases represent an important cause of morbidity and mortality worldwide.

**Table 3. POSSIBLE MOLECULAR TARGETS IN THE TREATMENT OF RF/CRHD. Interleukin-1 (IL-1), TNF-alpha, interleukin-6 (IL-6), and mannan-binding lectin (MBL) seem to play a role in the pathogenesis of the diseases and can be successfully blocked by molecular agents. B-lymphocytes CD20+ and costimulatory molecules are also potential molecular targets (based on Isaac et al., 1997, Furst et al., 2007 and Schon, 2008).**

| Molecular Targets | Biological Agents | Mechanism of Action |
|---|---|---|
| Interleukin-1 (IL-1) | Anakinra | Interleukin-1 (IL-1) receptor antagonist |
| TNF- alpha | Etanercept | Soluble tumor necrosis factor receptor |
| | Infliximab | Chimeric monoclonal anti-TNF-α antibody |
| | Adalimumab | Humanized monoclonal anti-TNF-alpha antibody |
| B-lymphocytes CD20+ | Rituximab | Human anti-CD20+ monoclonal antibody |
| Interleukin-6 (IL-6) | Tocilizumab | Humanized anti-IL-6 receptor monoclonal antibody |
| Mannan-binding-lectin (MBL) | Anti-MBL mAb | Monoclonal antibody that binds to MBL (experimental) |
| Costimulatory molecules | Abatacept | Fusion protein composed of an immunoglobulin fused to the extracellular domain of CTLA-4 |
| | Efalizumab | Humanized monoclonal antibody (anti-CD11a) that interferes with LFA-1/ICAM-1 binding |
| Lymphocytes T CD4+ | Humanized anti-CD4+ mAb | Lymphocytes T CD4+ depletion |

In order to prevent *S. pyogenes* infections different approaches to develop a vaccine against the bacteria are being undertaken and they differ in their constructions. There are 12 models of vaccine in development. Four models are based on the M protein, the major antigen of *S. pyogenes* and eight on other antigens such as group A CHO, C5a peptidase (SCPA), Cysteine protease (Spe B), binding proteins like fibronectin, opacity factor, lipoproteins, Spe's (superantigens) and streptococcal pili (Jordan Report 2007, NIAID, NIH, USA). Streptococcal N- and C-terminal M protein based vaccines use different approaches. The vaccine model conceived by Prof. Dale combines sequences of the N- terminal portion of 26 strains of GAS, the most frequent in the USA as a recombinant protein and are currently in phase II clinical trial (Hu MC et al., 2001; McNeil et al., 2005; Dale JB et al., 2005). The model of Prof Fischetti, uses the entire C-terminal portion of the M6 strain as recombinant protein (Medaglini et al., 1995). Prof Good defined a minimum B cell epitope (J14) from the

C-terminal portion and the vaccine is constructed as synthetic peptide (Good MF, 2002; Batzloff et al., 2003; Olive C, 2007) and are in the experimental phase. The other model also bound on the C-terminal portion selected both T and B cell protective epitopes by using a large panel of human blood samples, tested against C-terminal M protein overlapping peptides differing by only one amino acid residue (Guilherme et al., 2006) and are currently in the experimental phase.

Since the C- terminal portion of the M protein is conserved among the 150 emm-types the vaccines based on this region are being expected to provide a broader coverage and most probably will change the picture of the diseases caused by *S. pyogenes* in the future.

## Future Perspectives

Considering the important progress made in the knowledge of the mechanisms underlying the pathogenic process of RF and CRHD, and in the recent development of drugs for treatment of inflammatory diseases **(Table 3)**, we would like to stir up interest in the scientific community for the design of future therapeutic studies with these drugs in RF and CRHD.

Elevated serum levels of tumor necrosis factor α (TNF- alpha), a pro-inflammatory cytokine, have been observed in patients with RF/CRHD (Miller et al., 1989, Narin et al., 1995, Yegin, Coskum and Ertug, 1997). Significantly elevated levels of TNF- alpha were also found by analyzing the cytokine secretion profile from lymphocytes of heart valves of CRHD subjects upon streptococcal stimulus and also by the high numbers of positive TNF-alpha heart-tissue infiltrating T cells (GUILHERME et al. (2004). Recently, serum levels of TNF-alpha showed a positive correlation with the severity of mitral valve disease and valvar calcifications (Davotoglu, Celik and Aksoy, 2005) and its plasma and right/left atrial concentrations in patients with rheumatic mitral stenosis were significantly higher than those of healthy volunteers (Chen et al. 2005). As mentioned in the pathogenesis and genetic factors section, polymorphism located within the promoter region of the TNF-alpha gene (-308 *A/A*), which is related to higher levels of the protein represented a significant risk for the development of CRHD in two different populations with OR 3.3 and 56.7 (Sallakci et al., 2005, Settin et al., 2007, Ramasawmy and cols, 2007). As observed in other reactive arthritis, when signs and symptoms of RF develop, the presence of the etiologic agent is no longer observed in the tissue lesions. Infliximab, a chimeric monoclonal anti-TNF-alpha antibody has already been successfully used in the treatment of reactive arthritis secondary to *Yersinia enterocolitica* (Kaipiainen-Seppannen et al., 2003). Considering that anti-TNF drugs (adalimumab, infliximab and etanercept) are widely available, the blockade of this cytokine becomes an interesting subject for future studies in RF/CRHD.

In addition, elevated levels of other pro-inflammatory cytokines, including interleukin-1 (IL-1) and interleukin-6 (IL-6), have also been observed in patients with RF or CRHD (Morris et al., 1993, Narin et al., 1995) (Yegin, Coskum and Ertug, 1997). Similarly to TNF-alpha, IL-6 showed also a positive relationship with the severity of mitral valve disease and valvar calcifications (Davotoglu, Celik and Aksoy, 2005). A soluble blocker of IL-1 (named anakinra) is already commercially available (Furst et al., 2007) and has shown promising results in the treatment of systemic juvenile idiopathic arthritis (Reiff, 2005). Besides that, tocilizumab, a novel IL-6 receptor antagonist (IL-6R inhibitor), has been effectively used in the treatment of RA (Plushner, 2008). The pathogenesis of RF and CRHD involve an abnormal activation of both, humoral and cellular immune response. An exacerbation of humoral response is illustrated by the vast number of cross-reactive antibodies that have been demonstrated in the serum of patients and are believed to have a role in the disease processes (Martins, Veasy and Hill, 2006). Rituximab is a chimeric anti-CD20+ antibody which was approved by the Food and Drugs Administration (FDA) for the treatment of non-Hodgkin lymphoma and RA (Furst et al., 2007). Other studies have shown its efficacy also in the treatment of SLE (Furst et al., 2007), another disease where auto-reactive antibodies play an important role (Anolyk, 2007). The B-cell depletion in patients with acute RF represents an interesting topic for future trials.

In recent studies, high levels of MBL, a pattern-recognition protein capable of complement activation in an antibody independent manner, was observed in patients with CRHD (Schafranski et al., 2004). The polymorphisms of MBL gene (*MBL2*) associated with expression of high levels of this protein represented a risk factor of OR 2.48 and 2.42 for acute and chronic rheumatic carditis, respectively (Messias-Reason et al., 2006; Schafranski et al., 2008). Nayar, Nayar and Cherian (2006) observed myxomatous degeneration in a significant number of valves of patients with CRHD. Myxomatous tissue is rich in hyaluronic acid, a high molecular weight polysaccharide consisting of repeated sequences of glucuronic acid and N-acetylglucosamine. The fact that MBL binds to N-acetylglucosamine supports the hypothesis that activation of the complement system in acute and chronic rheumatic carditis occurs in part through interaction with this molecule. Under normal conditions, MBL does not bind to self-tissues; however, in stressful situations such as process mediated by oxidative stress, glycosylation of cell surfaces may occur which leads to the deposition of MBL and complement activation. Kumar et al. (1991) studied the activity of NADPH oxidase, an enzyme directly involved in the production of oxygen free radicals, and observed elevated enzymatic activity in patients with acute RF and CRHD. The increased levels of IL-6 observed in RF and CRHD patients can also contribute to higher levels of MBL seen in these patients, as it is know that IL-6 modulates *MBL2* gene expression (Arai, Tabona and Summerfield, 1993). Anti-MBL therapy based on the use of monoclonal anti-MBL antibodies has been experimentally used in rats submitted to coronary artery occlusion and showed markedly reduction in the myocardial infarction area and in the expression of pro-inflammatory genes (intercellular adhesion molecule-1, vascular cell adhesion molecule-1 and IL-6) (Jordan, Montalto and Stahl, 2003). Thus, anti-MBL therapy could also be another interesting investigative therapeutic option in RF/CRHD experimental models.

Unlike other autoimmune diseases, the etiologic agent of RF/CRHD is fairly well known, as well as the period of time required for the development of the clinical manifestations following the initial infection. The usage of blocking molecules, such as abatacept and efalizumab, which interfere in the process of antigen presentation, would be another thinkable strategie in this pre-clinical stage, aiming to avoid the recognition of self-antigens and also the antigen spreading phenomenon. The costimulatory blocking molecules abatacept and efalizumab are already widely used in the treatment of rheumatoid arthritis (Vital and Emery, 2006) and psoriasis (Schon, 2008), respectively.

Finally, considering that CD4+ T cells seem to be the major mediators involved in the pathogenesis of CRHD, experimental depletion of those cells may be of interest. Although this approach has already been tried with only transient satisfactory effects in other autoimmune diseases such as rheumatoid arthritis, systemic lupus erythematosus, psoriasis and multiple sclerosis (Isaac et al., 1997).

Based on the recent advances in the field of molecular-based therapies, a new era of research in the management of RF/CHRD can begin, in order to evaluate and establish the value of available immunobiological therapies in diseases that, although very prevalent in some parts of the world, still lack effective treatments.

RF and CRHD are a major health problem in several developing countries and still occur in developed countries. As a systemic disorder whose effects, especially cardiac, can be devastating, we look forward to prevention strategies that may benefit millions of people world wide.

# References

Amigo, M; Martinez-Lavin, M; Reyes, P. Acute Rheumatic Fever. *Rheum Dis Clin N Am,* 1993, 19, 333-351.

Anolyk, JH. B-cell biology and dysfunction in SLE. *Bull NYU Hosp Jt Dis,* 2007, 65(3), 182-6.

Arai, T; Tabona, P; Summerfield, JA. Human mannose-binding protein gene is regulated by interleukins, dexamethasone and heat shock. *QJM,* 1993, 86, 575-82.

Barash, J; Mashiach, E; Navon-Elkan, P; Berkun, Y; Harel, L; Tauber, T; et al. Differentiation of post-streptococcal reactive arthritis from acute rheumatic fever. *Pediatr,* 2008, 153(5), 696-9.

Batzloff, MR; Hayman, WA; Davies, MR; Zeng, M; Pruksakorn, S; Brandt, et al. protection against goup A streptococcus by immunization with J8-diphetheria toxoid: contribution of J8-diphtheria toxoid-specific antibodies to protection. *J Infect Dis,* 2003, 187(10), 1598-608.

Beggs, S; Peterson, G; Tompson, A. WHO 2008. Report of the 2nd Meeting of World Health Organization´s Subcommittee of the Expert Committee of the Selection and Use of Essential Medicine. Geneva.

Benedek, TG. Subcutaneous nodules and the differentiation of rheumatoid artritis from rheumatic fever. *Semin Arthritis Rheum,* 1984, 13, 305-21.

Berrios, X; Quesnay, F; Morales, A; Blazquez, J; Bisno, AL. Are all recurrences of "pure" Sydenham's chorea true recurrences of acute rheumatic fever? *J Pediatr,* 1985, 107, 867-872.

Bisno, AL. Acute pharyngitis: etiology and diagnosis. *Pediatrics*, 1996, 97(6), S949-S954

Bitar, FF; Hayek, P; Obeyd, M; Gharzedinne, W; Mikati, M; Dbaibo, GS. Rheumatic Fever in Children: A 15-Year Experience in a Developing Country. *Pediatr Cardiol,* 2000, 21(2), 119-22.

Bittl, JA; Perloff, JK. Chronic Post-Rheumatic Fever Arthropathy of *Jaccoud. Am Heart J,* 1983, 105(3), 515-7.

Burgert, SJ; Classen, DC; Burke, JP; Veasy LG. Rheumatic pneumonia: reappearance of a previously recognized complication of acute rheumatic fever. *Clin Infect Dis,* 1995 21(4), 1020-2.

Câmara, EJ; Braga, JC; Alves-Silva, LS; Câmara, GF; da Silva-Lopes, AA. Comparison of an intravenous pulse of methylprednisolone versus oral corticosteroid in severe acute rheumatic carditis: a randomized clinical trial. *Cardiol Young,* 2002, 12(2), 119-24.

Camurdan, AD; Camurdan, OM; Ok, I; Sahin, F, Ilhnan, MN; Beyazova, U. Diagnostic value of rapid antigen detection test for streptococcal pharyngitis in a pediatric population. *Int J Pediatr Otorhinolaryngol,* 2008, 72(8), 1203-6.

Carapetis, JR; McDonald, M; Wilson, NJ. Acute Rheumatic Fever. *Lancet,* 2005, 366, 155-68

Carapetis, JR; Steer, AC; Mulholland, EK; Weber, M. The global burden of group A streptococcal diseases. *Lancet Infect Dis,* 2005, 5, 685-94.

Chen, MC; Chang, HW; Wu, CJ; Yang, CH; Yu, TH; Chen, C; Hung, WC. Balance between Plasma Levels of Tumor Necrosis Factor- α and Interleukin-10 in Rheumatic Mitral Stenosis. *Cardiology,* 2005, 104, 171-5.

Chiu, YY; Hayashi, M; Schafranski, M; Mesias-Reason, IJT. Further evidence of inflammation in chronic rheumatic valve disease (CRVD): High levels of advanced oxidation protein products (AOPP) and high sensitive C-reactive protein (hs-CRP). *Int J Cardiol,* 2006, 109, 275-6.

Cilliers, AM; Manyemba, J; Saloonjee, H. Anti-inflammatory treatment for carditis in acute rheumatic fever. *Cochrane Database Sys Rev,* 2003.

Dajani, A. Rheumatic Fever. In: Braunwald, E. *Heart Disease: a Textbook of Medicine*. Philadelphia: Saunders WB; 1997, 1769-1775.

Dale, JB; Penfound, T; Chiang, EY; Long, V; Shulman, ST; Beall, B. Multivalent group A streptococcal vaccine elicits bactericidal antibodies against variant M subtypes. *Clin DiagLab Immunol,* 2005, 12(7), 833-6.

DATASUS. Available from: <http://www.tabnet.datasus.gov.br>

Davutoglu, V; Celik, A; Aksoy, M. Contribution of selected serum inflammatory mediators to the progression of chronic rheumatic valve disease, subsequent valve calcification and NYHA functional class. *J Heart Valve Dis,* 2005, 14, 251-6.

Ellis, NM; Li, Y; Hildebrand, W; Fischetti, VA; Cunningham, MW. T cell mimicry and epitope specificity of cross-reactive T cell clones from rheumatic heart disease. *J Immunol,* 2005, 175, 5448-56.

Fae, KC; Silva, DD; Oshiro, SE. Mimicry in Recognition of Cardiac Myosin Peptides by Heart-Intralesional T Cell Clones from Rheumatic Heart Disease. *J Immunol,* 2006, 176, 5662-70.

Feinstein, AR; Stern, EK. Clinical effects of recurrent attacks of acute rheumatic fever: a prospective epidemiologic study of 105 episodes. *J Chron Dis,* 1967, 20, 13-27.

Feldman, T. Rheumatic Mitral Stenosis. *Curr Treat Options Cardiovasc Med,* 2000, 2, 93-103.

Furst, DE; Breedveld, FC; Kalden, JR; Smolen, JS; Burmester, GR; Sieper, J. et al. Updated consensus statement on biological agents for the treatment of rheumatic diseases, *Ann Rheum Dis,* 2007, 66 (suppl 3), iii2-iii22.

Gaasch, WH. Guidelines for the Diagnosis of Rheumatic Fever. *JAMA,* 1992, 268(15), 2069-73.

Galvin, JE; Hemric, ME; Ward, K; Cunningham, M. Cytotoxic mAb from rheumatic carditis recognizes heart valves and laminin. *J Clin Invest,* 2000, 106, 217-24.

Gibofsky, A; Kerwar, A; Zabriskie, J. Rheumatic Fever: The Relationship Between Host, Microbe and Genetics. *Rheum Dis Clin N Am,* 1998, 24, 237-59.

Gibofsky, A; Zabriskie, JB. Rheumatic Fever and poststreptococcal reactive arthritis. *Curr Opin Rheum*, 1995, 7, 299-305.

Goldsmith, DP; Long, SS. Post-streptococcal disease of childhood: A changing syndrome. *Arthritis Rheum,* 1982, 25, S18.

Good, MF. Progress towards developing a vaccine for group A streptococcus based on the M protein. *Intern Med J,* 2002, 32 (4); 132-3.

Guilherme, L; Dulphy, N; Douay, C ; et al. Molecular evidence for antigen-driven immune responses in cardiac lesions of rheumatic heart disease patients. *Int Immunol,* 2000, 12, 1063-74.

Guilherme, L; Cunha-Neto, E; Coelho, V. Human heart-infiltrating T-cell clones from rheumatic heart disease patients recognized both streptococcal and cardiac proteins. *Circulation,* 1995, 92, 415-20.

Guilherme, L; Cunha-Neto, E; Tanaka, AC; Dulphy, N; Toubert, A; Kalil J. Heart-directed autoimmunity: the case of rheumatic fever. *J Autoimmun,* 2001, 16, 363-67.

Guilherme, L; Cury, P; Demarchi, LM; Coelho, V; Abel., L; Loppez, AP; et al. Rheumatic heart disease: proinflammatory cytokines play a role in the progression and maintenance of valvular lesions. *Am J Pathol,* 2004, 165(5), 1583-91.

Guilherme, L; FAE, KC; Higa, F; Chaves, L; Oshiro, SE; Freschi, de Barros, et al. Towards a vaccine against rheumatic fever. *Clin. Dev Immunol*, 2006, 13(2-4), 125-32.

Guilherme, L; Oshiro, SE; Fae, KC; et al. T cell reactivty against streptococcal antigens in the periphery mirrors reactivity of heart-infiltrating T lymphocytes in rheumatic heart disease patients. *Infect Immun,* 2001a, 69, 5345-51.

Guilherme, L; Ramasawmy, R; Kalil, J. Rheumatic Fever and Rheumatic Heart Disease: Genetics and Pathogenesis. *Scand J Immunol,* 2007, 66, 199-207.

Harel, L; Zecharia, HL; Straussber, R; Volovitz, B; Amir, J. Successful treatment of rheumatic chorea with carbamazepine. *Pediatr Neurol,* 2000, 23(2), 147–151.

Hashkes, PJ; Tauber, T; Somekh, E., Brik, R; Barash, J; Mukamel, M; et al. Naproxen as an alternative to aspirin for the treatment of arthritis of rheumatic fever: a randomized trial. *J Pediatr,* 2003, 143(3), 399-401.

Hernandez-Pacheco, G; Aguilar-Garcia, J; Flores-Dominguez, C; et al. MHC class II alleles in Mexican patients with rheumatic heart disease. *Int J Cardiol*, 2003, 92, 49-54.

Hu, MC; Walls, MA; Stroop, SD; Reddish, MA; Beall, B; Dale, JB. Immunogenicity of a 26-valent group A streptococcus vaccine. *Infect Immun,* 2002, 70(4), 2171-7.

Isaacs, JD; Burrows, N; Wing, M; Keogan, MD; Rebello, PRUB; Watts, RA; et al. Humanized anti-CD4 monoclonal antibody therapy in autoimmune and inflammatory diseases. *Clin Exp Immunol,* 1997, 110, 158-66.

Jack, DL; Klein, NJ; Turner, MW. Mannose-binding lectin: targeting the microbial world for complement attack and opsonophagocytosis. *Immunol Rev,* 2001, 180, 86-99.

James, N; Smith, M. Treatment of Heart Failure in Children. *Curr Paediatr,* 2003, 15(7), 539-48.

Jordan, JE; Montalto, MC; Stahl, GL. Inhibition of mannose-binding lectin reduces postischemic myocardial reperfusion injury. *Circulation,* 2003, 104, 1413-18.

Kahn IA; Ijaz, N. Prophylaxis of infective endocarditis: Current perspectives. *Int J Cardiol*, 2008. In press.

Kaipiainen-Seppannen, O; Niinisalo, H; Korpilahde, T; Virolainen, J. Treatment of reactive arthritis with infliximab 2003. *Scandn J Rheumatol*, 32(2), 122-4.

Kalim-ud-Din Aziz, L; Cheema, L; Memon, AD. Long-term observations or rheumatic carditis. *Cardiol Young,* 1992, 2, 254-60.

Kaplan, E. Recent epidemiology of Group A streptococcal infections in North America and abroad: an overview. *Pediatrics,* 1996, 97(6), S945-S948.

Krisher, K; Cunningham, MW. Myosin: a link between streptococci and heart. *Science*, 1985, 227, 413-5.

Kumar, V; Ganguly, NK; Anand, IS; Wahi, PL; NADPH oxidase activity in the monocytes and neutrophils of patients with rheumatic fever. *Cardioscience,* 1991, 2 (2), 93-7.

Lancefield, RC. The antigenic complex of Streptococcus hemolyticus. *J Exp Med,* 1928, 47, 9–10.

Lancefield, RC; Dole, VP. The properties of T antigen extracted from group A hemolytic streptococci. *J Exp Med,* 1946, 84, 449-71.

Lehmann, PV; Forsthuber, T; Miller, A; Sercarz, EE. Spreading of T-cell autoimmunity to cryptic determinants of an autoantigen. *Nature*, 1992, 358, 155-57.

Marijon, E; Oli, E; Celermajer, DS; Ferreira, B; Mocumbi, AO; Jani, D; et al. Prevalence of Rheumatic Heart Disease Detected by Echocardiographic Screening. *NEJM,* 2007, 357, 470-6.

Martins, TB; Veasy, LG; Hill, HR. Antibody Responses to Group A Streptococcal Infections in Acute Rheumatic Fever. *Immunology for the Pediatrician*, 2006, 5(9), 832-7.

McNeil, SA; Halperin, SA; Langley, JM; Smith, B; Warren, A; Sharrat, GP; et al. Safety and immunogenicity of a 26-valent group A vaccine in healthy adult volunteers. *Clin Infect Dis,* 2005, 41 (8), 1114-22.

Medaglini, D; Pozzi, G; King, TP; Fischetti, VA. Mucosal and systemic immune response to a recombinant protein expressed on the surface of the oral commensal bacterium *Streptococcus gordonii* after oral colonization. *Proc Natl Acad Sci.*, USA, 1995, 92, 6868-72.

Messias-Reason, I; Schafranski, M; Jensenius, JC; Steffensen, R. The association between mannose-binding lectin gene polymorphism and rheumatic heart disease. *Hum Immunol,* 2006, 67(12), 991-8.

Miller, LC; Gray, ED; Mansour, M; Abdin, ZH; Kamwel, R; Zaher, S; et al. Cytokines and Immunoglobulins in Rheumatic Heart Disease: Production by Blood and Tonsilar Mononuclear Cells. *J Rheumatol,* 1989, 16, 1436-42.

Morris, K; Mohan, C; Wahi, PL; Anand, IS; Ganguly, NK. Enhancement of Il-1 and IL-2 production and IL-2 receptor generation in patients with acute rheumatic fever and active rheumatic heart disease; a prospective study. *Clin Exp Immunol,* 1993, 91(3), 429-36.

Narin, N; Karakukcu, M; Narin, F; Akcakus, M; Erez, R; Halici, C. Is pentoxifylline therapy effective for the treatment of acute rheumatic carditis? A pilot study. *J Paediatr Child Health,* 2003, 39(3), 214-8.

Narin, N; Kutukculer, N; Ozyerek, R; Bakiler, AR; Parlar, A; Arcasoy, M. Lymphocyte subsets and plasma IL-1 alpha, IL-2 and TNF-alpha concentrations in acut rheumatic fever and chronic rheumatic heart disease. *Clin Immunol Immunopathol,* 1995, 77(2), 172-6.

Nayar, S; Nayar, PG; Cherian, KM. Heart valve structure: a predisposing factor for rheumatic heart disease. *Heart,* 2006, 92, 1151-2.

Olive, C. Progress in M-protein-based subunit vaccines to prevent rheumatic fever and rheumatic heart disease. *Curr Opin Mol Ther,* 2007, 9(11), 25-34.

Pinals, RS. Polyarthritis and fever. *N Eng J Med,* 1994, 330,769-774.

Plushner, SL. Tocilizumab: an interleukin-6 receptor inhibitor for the treatment of rheumatoid arthritis. *Ann Pharmacother,* 2008, 42(11),1660-8.

Raizada, V; Williams, RC Jr.; Chopra, P; et al. Tissue distribution of lymphocytes in rheumatic heart valves as defined by monoclonal anti-T cells antibodies. *Am J Med,* 1983, 74, 90-6.

Ramasawmy, R; Fae, KC; Spina, G; et al. Association of polymorphisms within the promoter region of the tumor necrosis factor-alpha with clinical outcomes of rheumatic fever. *Mol Immunol,* 2007, 44, 1873-8.

Ravisha, MS; Tullu, MS; Kamat, JR. Rheumatic fever and rheumatic heart disease: clinical profile of 550 cases in India. *Arch Med Res,* 2003, 34(5), 382-7.

Reiff, A. The use of anakinra in juvenile arthritis. *Curr Rheumatol Rep,* 2005, 7(6), 434-40.

Roberts, S; Kosanke, S; Dunn, TS; Jankelow, D; Duran, CMG; Cunningham, MW. Pathogenic Mechanism in Rheumatic Carditis: Focus on Valvular Endothelium. *J Infect Diseases,* 2001, 183, 507-11.

Ronchezel, MV; Hilário, MO; Forleo, LHA; Len, CA; Terreri, MT; Vilanova, LCP; et al. The use of haloperidol and valproate in children with Sydenham chorea. *Indian Pediatrics,* 1998, 35(12), 1215-1218.

Sallakci, N; Akcurin, G; Koksoy, S; Kardelen, F; Uguz, A; Coskun, M; et al. TNF-alpha G-308A polymorphism is associated with rheumatic fever and correlates with increased TNF-alpha production. *J Autoimmun,* 2005, 25, 50-4.

Saxena, A. Treatment of Rheumatic Carditis. *Indian J Pediatr,* 2002, 69(6), 513-6.

Schafranski, MD; Stier, A; Nisihara, R; Messias-Reason, IJ. Significantly increased levels of mannose-binding lectin (MBL) in rheumatic heart disease: a beneficial role for MBL deficiency. *Clin Exp Immunol,* 2004, 138(3), 521-5.

Schafranski, MD; Pereira-Ferrari, L; Scherner, D; Messias-Reason, IJ. High-Producing MBL2 Genotypes Increase the Risk of Acute and Chronic Carditis in Patients with History of Rheumatic Fever. *Molecular Immunology,* 2008, 45(14), 3827-31.

Schon, MP. Efalizumab in the treatment of psoriasis: mode of action, clinical indications, efficacy, and safety. *Clin Dermatol,* 2008, 26(5), 509-14.

Settin, A; Abdel-Hardy, H; El-Ba, R; Saber, I. Gene polymorphisms of TNF-alpha (-308), IL-10(-1082), IL-6(-174), and IL-1Ra(VNTR) related to susceptibility and severity of rheumatic heart disease. *Pediatr Cardiol,* 2007, 28(5), 363-71.

Vital, EM; Emery, P. Abatacept in the treatment of rheumatoid arthritis. *Ther Clin Risk Manag,* 2006, 2(4), 365-75.

Wild, EJ; Tabrizi, SJ. The differential diagnosis of chorea. *Pract Neurol,* 2007, 7(6), 360-73.

William, A; Alto, MD. Acute Rheumatic Fever: an Update. *Am Fam Phys,* 1992, 45, 613-620.

World Health Organization (1999). *Drugs used in the treatment of streptococcal pharyngitis and prevention of rheumatic fever*. Geneva.

Yegin, O; Coskum, M; Ertug, H. Cytokines in acute rheumatc fever. *Eur J Pediatr,* 1997, 156, 25-9.

Yetkin, E; Erbay, AR; Ileri, M; Turhan, H; Balci, M; Cehreli, S; et al. Levels of circulating adhesion molecules in rheumatic mitral stenosis. *Am J Cardiol*., 2001 88(10), 1209-11.

Yoshinaga, M; Figueiroa, F; Wahid, MR; Marcus, RH; Suh, E; Zabriskie, JB. Antigenic specificity of lymphocytes isolated from valvular specimens of rheumatic fever patients. *J Autoimmun,* 1995, 8, 601-13. $\overline{X}$

In: Advances in Cardiovascular Research, Volume 1
Editors: L. Schmitt, T. Konig, pp. 219-236
ISBN: 978-1-60741-720-0


*Chapter VIII*

# Microstructure of the Aortic Valve: Implications for Valvular Mechanics and Function

***Hubert Tseng and K. Jane Grande-Allen**** 
Department of Bioengineering, Rice University, Houston, TX 77005, USA

## Abstract

The aortic valve leaflet has long been observed to be a composite tri-layered structure. However, in characterizing native tissue function, the leaflet tissue has frequently been assumed to be simply a single membrane with uniform transmural stress. Considering that extracellular matrix components, mechanical loading, and cellularity differ across leaflet layers, more consideration of the layered microstructure is warranted. Such knowledge would lay the foundation for more accurate mathematical models of tissue mechanics, vascularity, and diffusion, as well as for the design and analyses of successful therapies to treat heart valve pathology. This review will summarize the current knowledge regarding the primary extracellular matrix constituents and individual mechanics of each layer, as well as their synergistic roles in whole leaflet function. The aortic valve leaflet consists of the fibrosa, spongiosa, and ventricularis layers, and is surrounded by an endothelial layer. The collagen structure of the fibrosa dominates its mechanical behavior, giving the leaflet tensile strength, but also extensibility and flexibility. The ventricularis serves to open and close the valve through the extensibility and elastic recoil of its elastin network. Situated between the outer layers, the viscous nature of the spongiosa is believed to allow shearing between layers, resist compression, and confer flexibility. An endothelial cell layer surrounds the leaflet, and while it contributes little to aortic valve mechanics directly, endothelial cell function is regulated by shear stress and can influence valvular interstitial cell function. Possible directions of future research on this topic include clarifying the functional role of the spongiosa. Particular importance must be placed on characterizing the interconnecting fibers spanning the spongiosa that connect the fibrosa and ventricularis. Layer-specific matrix

* Corresponding author: Department of Bioengineering, Rice University, PO Box 1892 - MS 142, Houston, TX USA 77251-1892, Phone: 713-348-3704, Fax: 713-348-5877, Email: grande@rice.edu

organization, interstitial cell phenotype, and proteoglycan and glycosaminoglycan content must also be further investigated.

## Introduction

The ability of the aortic valve to maintain unidirectional blood flow in the systemic circulation is highly dependent on the individual mechanical performances of the three leaflets of the aortic valve. During the opening and closing of the valve, blood flow through the valve exerts a complex array of mechanical forces on the leaflet in one cardiac cycle: tension, compression, and flexure in diastole; and high shear in systole.[1] These forces, repeated over ~$3x10^9$ cardiac cycles in one lifetime, require the aortic valve leaflets and aortic valve replacements to be both durable and strong, making the aortic valve a biomechanically important and unique tissue within the body.

Aortic valve mechanics are also critical to the biological function of the valve leaflet. Mechanical stimulation is transmitted to the valvular interstitial cells (VICs) through the surrounding extracellular matrix (ECM), and is believed to influence valvular cell biology, ECM maintenance and remodeling in a dynamic manner.[2] Consequently, alterations in mechanical loading can affect these cell-mediated processes and contribute to valvular disease. The influence of mechanical loading on valvular disease is most notably demonstrated through the spatial correlation between valvular disease and regions of the valve leaflet that experience distinct mechanical environments. For example, calcific degeneration, the primary condition affecting aortic valves, tends to occur on the aortic side of the valve leaflet in regions of maximum bending and oscillatory shear.[3] Understanding the biological response of the aortic valve to various mechanical loading conditions is thus crucial to understanding valvular function and the etiology of valvular disease.

The aortic valve leaflet has been well characterized as a composite tri-layered structure, consisting of the fibrosa, spongiosa, and ventricularis, which is then surrounded by an endothelial layer (Figure 1). The collagen-rich fibrosa, located on the aortic side, is the thickest layer, dominating the mechanical behavior of the leaflet in biaxial tension as the main load-bearing component. On the ventricular side, the ventricularis is the thinnest layer, and the high elastin content of the layer allows the leaflets to stretch sufficiently to close the valve fully and then retract to open the valve. The gelatinous spongiosa lies between these two outer layers, comprised of aggregates of the water-binding proteoglycan (PG) versican and the glycosaminoglycan (GAG) hyaluronan.[4] Surrounding this composite of three interstitial layers is an endothelial cell layer whose function is regulated by shear stress and whose cells influence VIC function. These layers of the aortic valve leaflet interact to withstand mechanical loads and facilitate normal leaflet function. While observed to be a layered structure, the aortic valve leaflet has frequently been assumed to be a single, uniform membrane in analyses of overall valve function. Considering the differences in ECM, cellularity, and mechanical environment, achieving a better understanding valvular function, disease and therapy requires revising this assumption of a homogeneous valve leaflet with uniform transmural stress. Knowledge of the layered structure would provide a strong basis for more accurate models of valvular function in native and diseased states, as well as for the design of mechanical and bioprosthetic heart valve replacements. This rethinking is currently taking place, as the microstructure of the aortic valve is being investigated for the purposes of improving models of valvular mechanics and diffusion, analyzing failure in bioprosthetic heart valves, and designing tissue engineered heart valve replacements.[5-7]

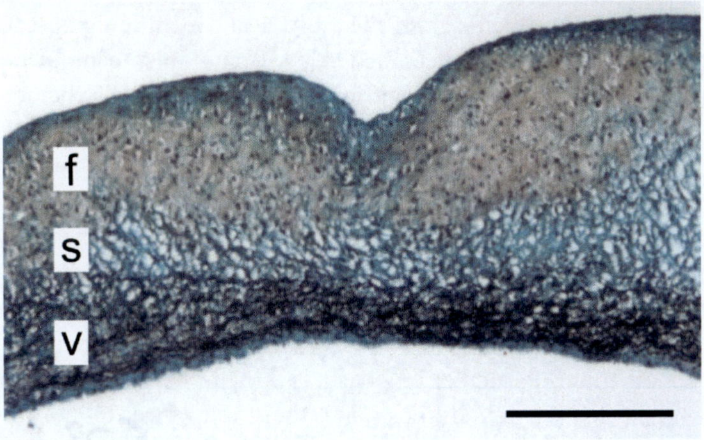


Figure 1. Histology of the aortic valve leaflet, showing the fibrosa (f), spongiosa (s), and ventricularis (v) layers. Leaflet stained with Movat pentachrome (collagen = yellow, PGs/GAGs = blue, elastin = black). Scale bar = 200 μm.

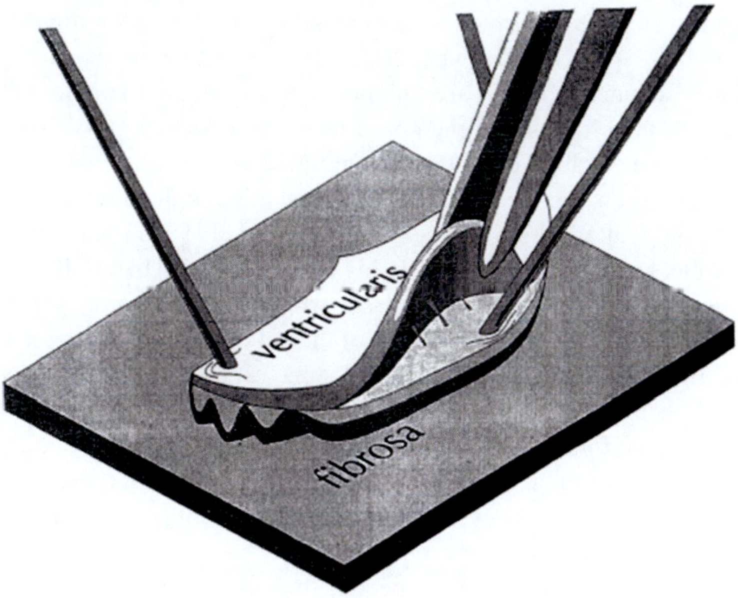


Figure 2. Schematic demonstrating technique for separation of the aortic valve leaflet. The leaflet is pinned down with the fibrosa facing down. The ventricularis is gently lifted and the interconnecting fibers are severed one at a time. Reprinted from Journal of Biomechanics, 25, Vesely, I. and Noseworthy, R., Micromechanics of the fibrosa and the ventricularis in aortic valve leaflets, 757-766 (1992) with permission from Elsevier.[6]

There are few studies that have mechanically tested the individual layers. Research into these properties requires an effective technique to separate the layers of the aortic valve leaflet for subsequent analysis, and only one such technique, which separates the leaflet into the fibrosa and ventricularis, has been reported (Figure 2).[6] In separating the valve, aortic valve leaflets are pinned down with the ventricularis facing upwards. The ventricularis is pulled apart from the fibrosa, and the exposed fibers connecting the outer layers are severed one at a time. This technique yields both the fibrosa and ventricularis, each with minimal damage and some residual spongiosa attached.[5] Using this technique, the mechanical properties of the individual fibrosa and ventricularis have been well characterized. Since no such technique exists to isolate and analyze the spongiosa separate from the intact leaflet, the mechanical behavior of that layer are not clearly understood. Alternatively, histology and microscopy can been used to analyze the microstructure of the valve without separating the leaflet into layers. These techniques can provide information on the extracellular matrix composition, localization, and cellularity of the layers, and can serve as a basis for understanding the mechanical properties of the individual layers.[8-12]

This review will summarize current knowledge on the three interstitial layers as well as the surrounding endothelium. Particular emphasis is placed on the mechanical behavior of the layers under different loading conditions, and their relevance to aortic valve function. Possible directions of future research on this topic will also be discussed.

## Fibrosa

The uppermost interstitial layer, the fibrosa, is comprised primarily of collagen, appearing mostly as Type I and Type III, as is characteristic of most cardiovascular tissues.[13] The collagen fibers are highly organized and predominantly oriented circumferentially, in the prominent direction of tensile stress (Figure 3).[14] In the unloaded state, collagen fibers exist in a crimped and unorganized form. As tensile load is applied through transvalvular pressure, the collagen fibers first align in the direction of stress and then straightens their crimp, after which they start to bear load.[14] Fiber alignment occurs at low tensile loads, while straightening occurs at high tensile loads.[14] Collagen crimp is thus believed to allow small deformations in the tissue while limiting the collagen fibers to bearing actual loads at higher strains only.[6,15] Most of the collagen in the leaflet is crimped; in one report, 60% of the histological cross-sectional area of the entire valve leaflet contained observable crimp when the valve was under no transvalvular pressure.[16] Collagen fibers are further organized into an intermediate, three-dimensional network. These collagen fibers were previously assumed to form a dense collagen network.[17] With the use of elliptically polarized light for contrast, however, the intermediate collagen structure was recently described as a multi-layered network of circumferentially oriented collagen fibers with branching fibers, sub-fibers, and thin connecting membranes in between.[9] This network structure allows collagen fibers to slide past each other while the leaflet is experiencing flexure and biaxial tension, which confers flexibility to the fibrosa while still retaining the circumferential tensile strength provided by the collagen fiber orientation.[9] At the macroscopic scale, the fibrosa is then further folded in the radial direction, giving the fibrosa its corrugated appearance.[6]

Given its collagenous nature, the fibrosa serves as the primary load-bearing layer in tension. The fibrosa mimics the mechanical behavior of the whole leaflet in biaxial tension, although, compared to the whole leaflet, the fibrosa is less compliant and transitions faster between the low and high strain modulus.[5] This layer exhibits anisotropy, as it is stiffer and more elastic in the circumferential direction than in the radial direction, and generally more extensible in the radial direction, though not as extensible as the whole leaflet (Figure 4).[6,18-21] High stiffness, elasticity, and low extensibility in the circumferential direction are results of both the dominant circumferential orientation and the crimp of the collagen fibers.[6] The low extensibility of the fibrosa as compared to the leaflet as a whole seems counterintuitive, considering the need for the leaflet to be able to extend radially and close the valve, but can be explained in multiple ways. As noted previously, the fibrosa is folded in the radial direction. Under tensile load in the radial direction, these folds are straightened, allowing for radial extension.[6] When separated and unfolded from the leaflet, the fibrosa is 28% longer in the radial direction than the attached fibrosa, a detail that can be viewed as a measure of the amount of folding and the additional radial extensibility in the leaflet allowed as a result of folding.[5] In addition, under radial tension, collagen fibers will rotate towards the radial direction. Previously, it was believed that circumferentially oriented collagen fibers would migrate and realign in the radial direction when subjected to radial tension. However, this realignment is not possible *in vivo*, as collagen fiber alignment in the circumferential direction actually increases under increasing transvalvular pressure normal to the leaflet surface.[14] These circumferentially oriented fibers are more likely rotating towards the radial direction, allowing extension and tensile strength in the radial direction (Figure 5).[9,22] The unfolding of collagen crimp also facilitates radial extension within the leaflet.[6] The collagen network of the fibrosa is also influential in deforming VICs, which populate the thickness of the leaflet.[23,24] At peak physiological transvalvular pressure, when collagen fibers are both aligned and straightened in the direction of stress, VICs in the fibrosa are significantly more aligned with collagen fibers than are VICs at zero transvalvular pressure and VICs in the ventricularis.[23]

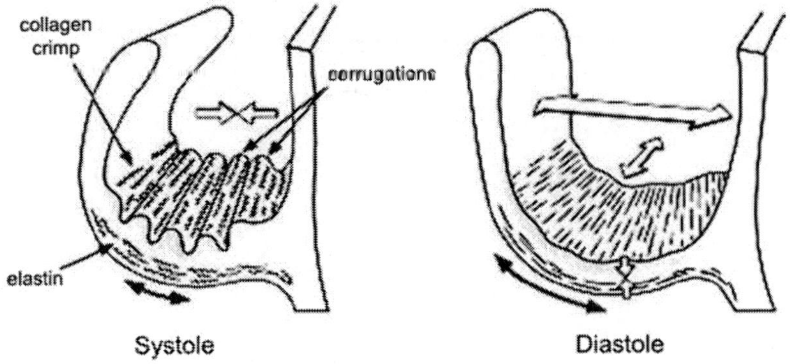


Figure 3. Diagram of the configuration of collagen and elastin during systole and diastole. When tensile load is applied in diastole, collagen fibers uncrimp and the fibrosa unfolds, providing circumferential tensile strength and radial extensibility. Reprinted from Journal of Heart Valve Disease, 6, Schoen, F., Aortic valve structure-function correlations: role of elastic fibers no longer a stretch of the imagination, 1-6 (1997) with permission from ICR Publishers.[27]

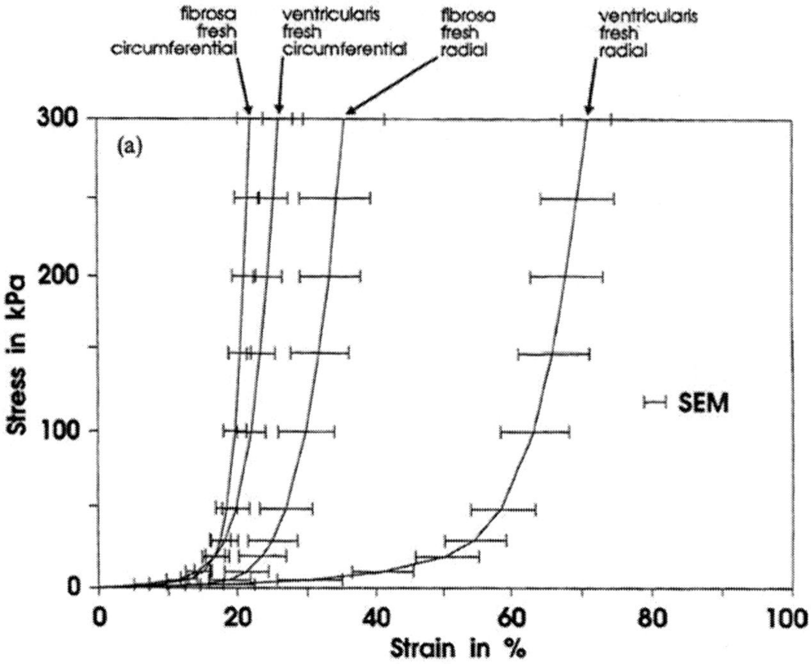


Figure 4. Stress-strain curves of separated fibrosa and ventricularis in circumferential and radial directions. Both the fibrosa and ventricularis exhibit anisotropy, as they are more extensible and less stiff in the radial direction. Reprinted from Journal of Biomechanics, 25, Vesely, I. and Noseworthy, R., Micromechanics of the fibrosa and the ventricularis in aortic valve leaflets, 757-766 (1992) with permission from Elsevier.[6]

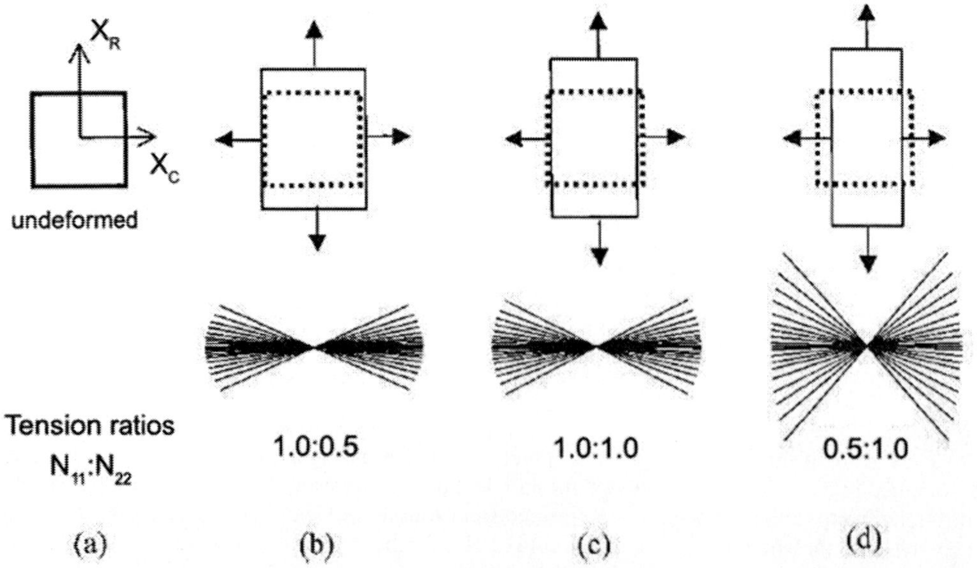


Figure 5. Schematic of collagen fiber orientation. As radial tension increases compared to circumferential tension (b-d), collagen fibers rotate towards the radial direction, allowing for large radial extensibility. Reprinted from Journal of Biomechanical Engineering, 122, Billiar, K. and Sacks, M., Biaxial mechanical properties of natural and glutaraldehyde treated aortic valve cusp - Part I: Experimental Results, 23-30 (2000) with permission from ASME Publications.[22]

Other components of the extracellular matrix also contribute to the mechanical function of the layer. Elastin is present in the fibrosa, but at a very low percentage of mass.[15] Elastic fibers form a mesh surrounding the collagen fiber network, and are oriented circumferentially across the belly region and radially at the annular attachment.[11] The primary role of elastin in the fibrosa is to return the collagen to its original crimped configuration. This action is achieved using energy that is stored by elastin during stretching. When unloaded, the elastin recoils and returns the collagen fiber to its crimped form, as well as folds the fibrosa radially.[11] This mechanism serves to open the aortic valve while unloading in systole. Interactions with the elastin of the ventricularis also contribute to valve function in a similar fashion.[6] Numerous PGs, such as decorin, biglycan, and versican, and GAGs are also present in the layer, but at lower concentrations than found in the other layers.[25]

## Ventricularis

Elastin exists in the ventricularis, the lowermost layer of the valve leaflet, in the form of dense and continuous sheets across the whole of the leaflet, and is the most significant contributor to the mechanical properties of the ventricularis.[11,15] This contribution is shown when all ECM components but elastin are removed when using NaOH digestion; the digested ventricularis matches the mechanical behavior of the undigested ventricularis radially, indicating a strong presence of elastin in the radial direction.[15] The ventricularis, like the fibrosa, is anisotropic, as the digested ventricularis is less stiff and more extensible than the undigested ventricularis in the circumferential direction compared to the radial direction.[15] This difference in stiffness and extensibility between digested and undigested tissue in the circumferential direction suggests that circumferentially oriented collagen within the ventricularis dictates the mechanical behavior in that direction. Further evidence of this collagen presence was shown by the two-fold higher stiffness of separated ventricularis in the circumferential direction than in the radial direction.[6] In addition, elastin content was shown to stay constant in valve leaflets exposed to cyclic circumferential stretch and cultured under flow for 48 hours, suggesting that elastogenesis was not activated during the duration of stretch and that elastin was not important in the mechanical behavior of the leaflet in the circumferential direction.[26] The separated ventricularis was also found to be much more extensible radially than circumferentially.[6,21] Although the morphology of ventricularis elastin as continuous sheets would suggest more isotropic properties, the presence of circumferentially oriented collagen in the ventricularis provides greater stiffness and limits extensibility in that direction. [11] Similar to VICs in the fibrosa, an increase in collagen fiber alignment of the ventricularis results in an increase in VIC deformation. However, VIC alignment in the ventricularis at high transvalvular pressure is significantly lower than in the fibrosa, even with similar collagen fiber alignment. This difference suggests that there are other factors that affect the VIC deformation, such as collagen fiber density and the surrounding matrix.[23] In addition, the connections between elastin and collagen networks may play a role in facilitating radial extensibility of the layer and the leaflet.[6]

Through interactions with the fibrosa, the ventricularis plays a major role in the mechanical behavior of the aortic valve leaflet in the radial direction. At low strains, the elastin of the ventricularis bears the load in the entire leaflet, as the collagen of the fibrosa straightens.[6] Even at high strains, when the collagen is straightened and supposedly dominating mechanical properties, the elastin still plays a significant role. This effect was shown when separated ventricularis was preloaded to mimic its intact configuration; the separated ventricularis was shown to bear load before the separated fibrosa.[5] This response, it has been suggested, acts as a safety mechanism to prevent radial overextension of the aortic valve leaflet. In addition, as previously mentioned, the interactions between the ventricularis and fibrosa serve to use the elastic recoil of the elastin in the ventricularis to return the fibrosa to its original folded and crimped configuration.[27]

Aside from collagen and elastin, the ventricularis shows a significantly greater abundance of decorin and biglycan as compared with the other layers.[25] Both decorin and biglycan are commonly associated with collagen fibrillogenesis, but are also frequently associated with tensile load-bearing regions and the process of elastogenesis.[28-30] Thus, the presence of these PGs reflects the elastin content and cyclic tension experienced in the ventricularis.

## Spongiosa

Because isolation of the spongiosa layer presents a challenge, the true contributions of the spongiosa to aortic valve leaflet mechanics and function have not been fully clarified. There are three main functions that are attributed to the spongiosa: (i) it confers flexibility to the leaflet, (ii) it dampens shock associated with leaflet closing, and (iii) it allows shearing between the outer layers.[27] These perceived functions of the spongiosa are related to the PG and GAG content of the layer. Versican, a large water-binding chondroitin-sulfate PG found in cardiovascular tissue, is localized within the spongiosa.[25] In the spongiosa, versican forms large aggregates with the GAG hyaluronan, which comprises roughly half of total GAG content within the leaflet, and is most abundant within the spongiosa.[25,31] The water-binding nature of these components gives the spongiosa compressive resistance and a gel-like consistency. In contrast, the spongiosa has also been characterized as an agent that resists delamination of the outer layers in biaxial tension conditions.[5] As the innermost and thinnest layer of the aortic valve leaflet, efforts to analyze the layer separately from the whole leaflet have proven difficult without an effective technique of extraction. Techniques for separating fibrosa and ventricularis from the leaflet cannot be used, as those dissection methods cut through the spongiosa.[6]

Studies relevant to spongiosa function have primarily focused on the effects of glutaraldehyde fixation in bioprosthetic heart valves on GAG loss and tissue mechanics.[4,32-35] For example, it has been shown that glutaraldehyde fixation made leaflet tissue stiffer in shear, suggesting a decrease in viscosity of the spongiosa.[33] Glutaraldehyde fixation also causes tissue dehydration, which has been shown to increase shear stiffness in aortic valve leaflets.[34,36] Taken together, it is apparent that the hydrated nature of the spongiosa, by virtue of the high versican and hyaluronan content within the layer, allows some shear between the outer layers. This shearing confers flexibility in the leaflet, allowing the tensing ventricularis to slide past the compressing fibrosa in flexure to accommodate the dynamic motion. Explanted bioprosthetic heart valves exhibit a collapsed spongiosa, a result of the presence of active GAG-degrading enzymes whose activity continues after glutaraldehyde fixation, and significantly depletes GAG content.[4,35] These heart valves also showed a decrease in GAG content when compared to freshly fixed heart valves, with notable losses in chondroitin/dermatan 6-sulfate, the GAG associated with versican, and hyaluronan in particular.[32] GAG loss can accelerate failure in bioprosthetic heart valves, which fatigue tests showed could happen within 10 million cycles with significant GAG loss.[35] Altogether, spongiosa and leaflet function in shear, bending, and compression appears to be highly dependent on the presence of versican and hyaluronan.

Spanning the spongiosa are fibers that connect the collagen and elastin networks of the fibrosa and ventricularis.[5,6] As mentioned previously, the interactions of the outer layers through these fibers fully open the valve during systole by returning collagen in the fibrosa and the leaflet to its original configuration. These fibers are thought to have multiple other roles in aortic valve function as well. They are believed to aid in facilitating flexure of the leaflet by further compressing and folding the fibrosa while at the same time extending the compliant ventricularis, regardless of the presence of vasoconstrictors that force VICs in the ventricularis to contract.[6,24] In compressing the fibrosa and extending the ventricularis, the leaflet accommodates this flexure without significantly increasing tensile stress within the ventricularis.[6] These interconnecting fibers are also believed to exert a preload on the outer layers, specifically a compressive preload on the fibrosa and a tensile preload on the ventricularis. Preload on the outer layers was observed when comparing the extensibilities of layers that were fixed in glutaraldehyde before separation with those fixed afterwards. Samples of fibrosa that were fixed before separation from the leaflet were more extensible than those fixed afterwards. This difference was attributed to collagen fibers being frozen in crimped form when fixed first, indicating the presence of a compressive preload that maintains the crimp in collagen. In contrast, the samples of ventricularis were less extensible when fixed before separation, which indicates a tensile preload that likely limits distention in the leaflet.[21] Preload in the outer layers is also evident by the immediate expansion and contraction of the fibrosa and ventricularis, respectively, in both the circumferential and radial directions after separation.[5] These fibers also exert a compressive preload on both layers through the thickness of the leaflet, as evidenced by the increase in layer thickness after separation. It is unclear as to the purpose of this preload in overall leaflet mechanics.[5]

## Endothelium

In describing the valvular endothelial layer, it is important to distinguish between the vascular and valvular endothelium, as the former is well characterized in the literature. The endothelial layer serves many functions throughout the entire vasculature of the body: as a semipermeable barrier between the circulating blood and underlying tissue; as an inhibitor of inflammation and thrombosis; and as a regulator of valvular tone and remodeling.[37] While continuous with the vascular endothelium, the valvular endothelium shows numerous differences from the vascular endothelium in endothelial cell morphology, focal adhesion pattern, gene expression, and contractility (Figure 6).[38-41] Valvular endothelial cells (VECs) can thus be considered a distinct sub-phenotype of endothelial cells.[42] The valvular endothelial layer appears to have no significant role in the mechanical function of the leaflet aside from the regulation of valvular tone and shape. Like vascular endothelial cells, VECs respond to vasoactive agents such as endothelin-1 and KCl, but valve contraction as a result of endothelin-1 is only 10-25% of the magnitude of arterial contraction.[41,43] This limited contraction in the valve most likely facilitates valve opening in systole, while protecting the valve from large shape changes that could potentially occur during the cardiac cycle.[41,43]

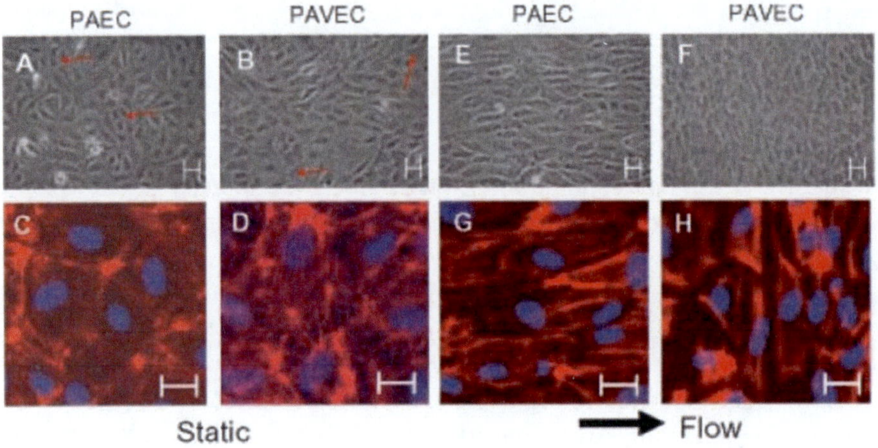


Figure 6. Images of porcine aortic endothelial cells (PAECs – A, E, C, G) and porcine aortic valvular endothelial cells (PAVECs – B, D, F, H) in static and flow environments. A through D, static culture; E through H, after 48 hours of 20 dynes/cm2 steady laminar shear stress. Top panels are phase microscopy images; bottom panels are laser confocal microscopy images. Cells are stained for f-actin (red) and nuclei (blue) Scale = 50 µm. Reprinted from Arteriosclerosis, Thrombosis, and Vascular Biology, 24, Butcher, J. et al., Unique morphology and focal adhesion development of valvular endothelial cells in static and fluid flow environments, 1429-34 (2004) with permission from Lippincott, Williams, & Wilkins.[38]

Blood flow through the aortic valve exerts a shear stress on the leaflets, which is critical for the maintenance and regulation of endothelial phenotype and function. The aortic valve has been reported to experience peak shear stresses between 30-1800 dyne/cm$^2$, though the deleterious effects of shear stress above 400 dyne/cm$^2$ on vascular endothelial cells suggest that the peak shear stress is closer to the lower end of the observed range.[44-49] Regulation of valvular endothelial cell morphology occurs under shear, as VECs align perpendicularly to the direction of flow, rather than in the characteristic cobblestone morphology observed in static culture.[38] Shear stress also affects gene expression in VECs, with the differential expression of 856 genes under flow conditions as compared to static culture, including more than 400 of those genes that were differentially expressed that are unique to valvular endothelial cells.[39] Shear significantly changed expression of groups of genes related to oxioreductase activity, cell migration, cell proliferation, apoptosis, and cell signaling, suggesting a role of shear in inhibiting oxidative and inflammatory responses.[39] When VECs are co-cultured with VICs, the VECs were shown to regulate VIC phenotype and matrix synthesis, and increased regulation of VICs under flow conditions. This result indicates that shear stress on the leaflet plays an active role in regulating the overall leaflet biological response.[50] VECs have also been shown to regulate collagen synthesis and sulfated-GAG content in the leaflet.[16]

The distinct shear and local flow environments that exist on either side of the aortic valve affect local VEC function and phenotype. On the inflow side, blood comes through the valve exerting a high, unidirectional shear on the leaflet, whereas the outflow side experiences a low magnitude, oscillatory flow. It has been shown that a total of 584 genes are differentially expressed between the aortic and ventricular sides of the aortic valve leaflet.[51] These differences in shear environments between the sides have implications in pathology as well. Aortic side VECs show lower expression of inhibitors of vascular and valvular calcification, which is in agreement with the observation that calcification tends to occur on the aortic side in areas of maximum flexure.[3,51] In addition, there is differential expression of mechanoregulated genes between the aortic and ventricular sides.[51] Taken together, local mechanical environments regulate valvular endothelial phenotypes and play a role in the progress of pathology.

## Future Directions

The aortic valve leaflet can no longer be simply assumed to be a homogenous, uniform tissue in analytical studies, but should be considered as a complex, tri-layered tissue. Currently, knowledge of the microstructure is being utilized in a number of applications ranging from developing 3D constitutive models of aortic valve function to acting as a basis for tissue engineered heart valves.[5,7,52,53] There are several directions of interest regarding the layered structure of the leaflet that require further research.

### Determining the Effect of the Hydrated Nature of the Spongiosa on Leaflet Mechanical Behavior in Tension and Compression

As discussed previously, the mechanical role of the spongiosa remains relatively unclear. The importance of the layer to leaflet mechanics is evident; the failure of glutaraldehyde-fixed bioprosthetic heart valves is accelerated by the loss of chondroitin 6-sulfate and hyaluronan, and consequently the loss of viscosity and hydration in the layer.[32,34] Our understanding of the contribution of the spongiosa in flexure and shear is growing because these topics are widely studied, but in other loading conditions experienced in the cardiac cycle, such as tension and compression, the contribution of the spongiosa has not been characterized as well. It has been suggested that the spongiosa can be assumed as resisting delamination within the leaflet under biaxial tension.[5] The role of the viscous, hydrated spongiosa in facilitating the dynamic motion of the outer layers, as well as its role in dampening shock deserves greater attention.

### Characterizing the Composition, Density, and Location of Interconnecting Fibers in the Spongiosa

To date, there has been no study of these interconnecting fibers in terms of their composition, location, or density within the leaflet. Most references to these fibers have been related to simple characterizations during leaflet separation (Figure 7).[5,6] However, there have been curious observations about these fibers that require further investigation. Using scanning electron microscopy to view NaOH-digested, separated ventricularis, branches of elastin were found intertwined in the elastin sheets of the ventricularis like roots along the annular attachment of the leaflet.[11] This finding suggests that the interconnecting fibers between the fibrosa and ventricularis are elastic fibers. Further analysis is required to characterize the fibers fully, and could provide insight into the interactions between the layers and their effect on overall tissue mechanics.

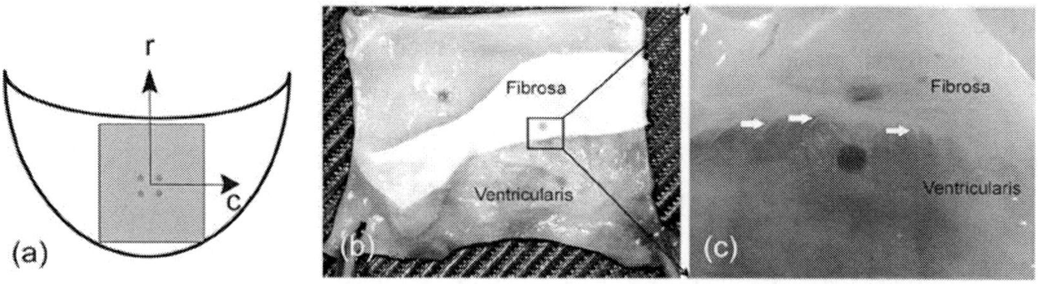


Figure 7. Microdissection of the aortic valve. From the section of the belly region (a) the fibrosa and ventricularis were pulled apart (b). A magnified view (c) of the interface between the fibrosa and ventricularis shows the interconnecting fibers that connects the two outer layers (white arrows). Reprinted from Journal of Biomechanical Engineering, 129, Stella, J. and Sacks, M., On the biaxial mechanical properties of the layers of the aortic valve leaflet, 757-66 (2007) with permission from ASME publications.[5]

## Determining the Effect of the Layered Structure on Diffusion through the Aortic Valve

The adult aortic valve leaflet relies on the diffusion of molecules from its surfaces to meet the metabolic needs of VICs within the leaflet.[54] However, given the thickness of the leaflet, diffusion may not be adequate. [55-57] Understanding and modeling diffusion through the leaflet are crucial for the development of tissue engineered heart valves. Knowledge of the microstructure of the leaflet could play an important role in this research by analyzing the diffusive properties of the viscous layers and transport under dynamic flow conditions. Most models of transport have generally ignored the layered structure, as it was shown that the interstitial layers could be considered as a homogeneous matrix with uniform diffusivity .[58-61] There have nonetheless been interesting discoveries with regards to the microstructure and diffusion. A study of the transport of horseradish peroxidase in aortic valve leaflets indicated the presence of a thin valvular subendothelial intima with larger porosity.[59-61] In addition, another study on modeling oxygen transport in aortic valve leaflets that incorporated the layered structure showed that there must exist some sort of intrinsic circulation that transports nutrients throughout the valve.[55] As most cells reside well within the interstitium of the leaflet in the fibrosa and spongiosa, it is important to consider the diffusive properties of the three layers of the aortic valve.[24] Recent discoveries on the layers' extracellular matrices, such as the discovery of the complex three-dimensional collagen network within the fibrosa, could help to define the diffusive properties of the layers. Further research on the composition and configuration of layer matrices, their effect on molecular transport, and their diffusive properties under dynamic fluid motion will improve future models of diffusion.

## Determining the Effect of the Layered Structure on VIC Phenotype and Function

With differences in substrate composition, rigidity, and mechanical environment across the thickness of the aortic valve, it would be logical for VICs in different layers to have express differential phenotypes. Spatial heterogeneity of VIC phenotype has previously been demonstrated in different regions of the mitral valve that experience distinct mechanical loads.[28,62] Heterogeneity of VEC phenotype, as it pertains to the aortic or ventricular side of the aortic valve leaflet, has also been demonstrated.[51] While VIC phenotype would seem most likely to differ across layers, to date, there has been no comprehensive analysis of such a difference. The limiting factor is the difficulty in isolating the cells of the spongiosa, which is generally the most cellularized of the layers.[16,24] While histology and immunohistochemistry can be used to characterize phenotype without separating the valve into layers, novel techniques to isolate the spongiosa and its constituent cells would greater advance our understanding of layer-specific VIC behavior.[63,64]

## Determining the Influence of GAGs and PGs on Matrix Organization and Mechanical Properties

Finally, the role of GAGs and PGs in the valve needs to be studied in greater detail. There already exists a basic understanding of the locations of these components within the leaflet. (Table 1).[25] There are still questions, however, about the roles of GAGs and PGs, particularly regarding the organization of valvular ECM components such as collagen and elastin. Decorin and biglycan, two small PGs that are associated mostly with collagen fibrillogenesis, are interestingly at their lowest concentrations in the collagen-rich fibrosa.[25] In addition, the complex movement of the layers during normal valve function cannot solely be explained by the presence and morphology of collagen and elastin. Furthermore, the nonuniformity of the layered distribution of PGs and GAGs deserves more attention, with particular emphasis on regions of distinct mechanical environments, such as the coaptation region (flexure) and the commisure region (uniaxial tension). A thorough understanding of the spatial distribution of PGs and GAGs within the aortic valve will be useful for future efforts to characterize aortic valve function and design of aortic valve replacements.

**Table 1. Proteoglycan and hyaluronan distribution within the layers of the aortic valve.**

| | Order of abundance in the aortic valve layers |
|---|---|
| Decorin | v > sp, f‡ |
| Biglycan | v >> sp > f§ |
| Versican | sp > v > f* |
| Hyaluronan | sp > v > f* |

v = ventricularis, sp = spongiosa, f = fibrosa.

*P≤0.001; ‡P≤0.01; §P≤0.05.

Modified from Acta Biomaterialia, 4, Stephens, E., Chu, C., Grande-Allen, K., Valve proteoglycan content and glycosaminoglycan fine structure are unique to microstructure, mechanical load and age: Relevance to an age-specific tissue-engineered heart valve, 1148-1160 (2008) with permission from Elsevier.[25]

# Conclusion

The aortic valve is a composite tri-layered structure, consisting of the fibrosa, ventricularis, spongiosa, and then is surrounded by valvular endothelium. Each layer has a distinct mechanical behavior and function, which synergistically contribute to leaflet mechanics and function as a whole. Further research is needed in clarifying the role of the spongiosa and interconnecting fibers, and determining the effect of layers on diffusion, VIC and VEC phenotype, and the organization of extracellular matrix within the leaflet, especially PGs and GAGs.

# References


[1] Thubrikar, M., Bosher, L. & Nolan, S. (1979). The mechanism of opening of the aortic valve. *Journal of Thoracic and Cardiovascular Surgery*, *77*, 863-870.

[2] Gupta, V. & Grande-Allen, K. (2006). Effects of static and loading in regulating extracellular matrix synthesis by cardiovascular cells. *Cardiovascular Research*, *72*, 375-383.

[3] Thubrikar, M., Aouad, J. & Nolan, S. (1986). Patterns of calcific deposits in operatively excised stenotic or purely regurgitant aortic valves and their relation to mechanical stress. *American Journal of Cardiology*, *58*, 304-308.

[4] Simionescu, D., Lovekamp, J. & Vyavahare, N. (2003). Glycosaminoglycan-degrading enzymes in porcine aortic heart valves: implications for bioprosthetic heart valve degeneration. *Journal of Heart Valve Disease*, *12*, 217-225.

[5] Stella, J. & Sacks, M. (2007). On the biaxial mechanical properties of the layers of the aortic valve leaflet. *Journal of Biomechanical Engineering*, *129*, 757-766.

[6] Vesely, I. & Noseworthy, R. (1992). Micromechanics of the fibrosa and the ventricularis in aortic valve leaflets. *Journal of Biomechanics*, *25*, 101-113.

[7] Shi, Y., Ramamurthi, A. & Vesely, I. (2002). Towards ntissue engineering of a composite aortic valve. *Biomedical Sciences Instrumentation*, *38*, 35-40.

[8] Clark, R. & Finke, E. (1974). Scanning and light microscopy of human aortic leaflets in stressed and relaxed states. *Journal of Thoracic and Cardiovascular Surgery*, *67*, 792-804.

[9] Doehring, T., Kahelin, M. & Vesely, I. (2005). Mesostructures of the aortic valve. *Journal of Heart Valve Disease*, *14*, 679-686.

[10] Schenke-Layland, K., Riemann, I., Opitz, F., König, K., Halbhuber, K. & Stock, U. (2004). Comparative study of cellular and extracellular matrix composition of native and tissue engineered heart valves. *Matrix Biology*, *23*, 113-25.

[11] Scott, M. & Vesely, I. (1996). Morphology of porcine aortic valve cusp elastin. *Journal of Heart Valve Disease*, *5*, 464-471.

[12] Stephens, E. & Grande-Allen, K. (2007). Age-related changes in collagen synthesis and turnover in porcine heart valves. *Journal of Heart Valve Disease*, *16*, 672-82.

[13] Bashey, R., Bashey, H. & Jimenez, S. (1978). Characterization of pepsin-solubilized bovine heart-valve collagen. *The Biochemical Journal*, *173*, 885-894.

[14] Sacks, M., Smith, D. & Hiester, E. (1998). The aortic valve microstructure: effects of transvalvular pressure. *Journal of Biomedical Materials Research*, *41*, 131-141.

[15] Vesely, I. (1998). The role of elastin in aortic valve mechanics. *Journal of Biomechanics*, *31*, 115-123.

[16] Sacks, M. & Yoganathan, A. (2007). Heart valve function: a biomechanical perspective. Philosophical Transactions of the Royal Society of London. Series B, *Biological Sciences*, *362*, 1369-1391.

[17] Gross, L. & Kugel, M. (1931). Topographic anatomy and histology of the valves in the human heart. *The American Journal of Pathology*, *7*, 445-456.

[18] Thubrikar, M., Piepgrass, W., Bosher, L. & Nolan, S. (1980). The elastic modulus of canine aortic valve leaflets in vivo and in vitro. *Circulation Research*, *47*, 792-800.

[19] Billiar, K. & Sacks, M. (2000). Biaxial mechanical properties of the native and glutaraldehyde-treated aortic valve cusp: Part II - A structural constitutive model. *Journal of Biomechanical Engineering*, *122*, 327-335.

[20] Vesely, I., Gonzalez-Lavin, L., Graf, D. & Boughner, D. (1990). Mechanical testing of cryopreserved aortic allografts. Comparison with xenografts and fresh tissue. *Journal of Thoracic and Cardiovascular Surgery*, *99*, 119-123.

[21] Vesely, I. & Lozon, A. (1993). Natural preload of aortic valve leaflet components during glutaraldehyde fixation: effects on tissue mechanics. *Journal of Biomechanics*, *26*, 121-131.

[22] Billiar, K. & Sacks, M. (2000). Biaxial mechanical properties of the natural and glutaraldehyde treated aortic valve cusp - Part I: Experimental Results. *Journal of Biomechanical Engineering*, *122*, 23-30.

[23] Huang, H., Liao, J. & Sacks, M. (2007). In-situ deformation of the aortic valve interstitial cell nucleus under diastolic loading. *Journal of Biomechanical Engineering*, 2007, 6.

[24] Merryman, W., Huang, H., Schoen, F. & Sacks, M. (2006). The effects of cellular contraction on aortic valve leaflet flexural stiffness. *Journal of Biomechanics*, *39*, 88-96.

[25] Stephens, E., Chu, C. & Grande-Allen, K. (2008). Valve proteoglycan content and glycosaminoglycan fine structure are unique to microstructure, mechanical load and age: Relevance to an age-specific tissue-engineered heart valve. *Acta Biomateralia*, *4*, 1148-1160.

[26] Balachandran, K., Konduri, S., Sucosky, P., Jo, H. & Yoganathan, A. (2006). An ex vivo study of the biological properties of porcine aortic valves in response to circumferential cyclic stretch. *Annals of Biomedical Engineering*, *34*, 1655-1665.

[27] Schoen, F. (1997). Aortic valve structure-function correlations: role of elastic fibers no longer a stretch of the imagination. *Journal of Heart Valve Disease*, *6*, 1-6.

[28] Grande-Allen, K., Calabro, A., Gupta, V., Wight, T., Hascall, V. & Vesely, I. (2004). Glycosaminoglycans and proteoglycans in normal mitral valve leaflets and chordae: association with regions of tensile and compressive loading. *Glycobiology*, *14*, 621-33.

[29] Gupta, V., Werdenburg, J., Blevins, T. & Grande-Allen, K. (2007). Synthesis of glycosaminoglycans in differently loaded regions of collagen gels seeded with valvular interstitial cells. *Tissue Engineering*, *13*, 41-9.

[30] Reinboth, B., Hanssen, E., Cleary, E. & Gibson, M. (2001). Molecular interactions of biglycan and decorin with elastic fiber components: biglycan forms a ternary complex

with tropoelastin and microfibril-associated glycoprotein 1. *Journal of Biological Chemistry*, *277*, 3950-7.

[31] Murata, K. & Yokoyama, Y. (1989). Acidic glycosaminoglycans in human atherosclerotic cerebrl arterial tissues. *Atherosclerosis*, *78*, 69-79.

[32] Grande-Allen, K., Mako, W., Calabro, A., Shi, Y., Ratliff, N. & Vesely, I. (2003). Loss of chondroitin 6-sulfate and hyaluronan from failed porcine bioprosthetic valves. *Journal of Biomedical Materials Research: Part A*, *65*, 251-259.

[33] Talman, E. & Boughner, D. (1995). Glutaraldehyde fixation alters the internal shear properties of porcine aortic heart valve tissue. *The Annals of Thoracic Surgery*, *60*, S369-373.

[34] Talman, E. & Boughner, D. (2001). Effect of altered hydration on the internal shear properties of porcine aortic valve cusps. *The Annals of Thoracic Surgery*, *71*, S375-378.

[35] Vyavahare, N., Ogle, M., Schoen, F., Zand, R., Gloeckner, D., Sacks, M. & Levy, R. (1999). Mechanisms of bioprosthetic heart valve failure: fatigue causes collagen denaturation and glycosaminoglcyan loss. *Journal of Biomedical Materials Research*, *46*, 44-50.

[36] Ferrans, V., Spray, T., Billingham, M. & Roberts, W. (1978). Structural changes in glutaraldehyde-treated porcine heterografts used as substitute cardiac valves. Transmission and scanning electron microscopic observations in 12 patients. *The American Journal of Cardiology*, *41*, 1159-1184.

[37] Galley, H. & Webster, N. (2004). Physiology of the endothelium. *British Journal of Anaesthesia*, *93*, 105-113.

[38] Butcher, J., Penrod, A., Garcia, A. & Nerem, R. (2004). Unique morphology and focal adhesion development of valvular endothelial cells in static and fluid flow environments. *Arteriosclerosis, Thrombosis, Vascular Biology*, *24*, 1429-1434.

[39] Butcher, J., Tressel, S., Johnson, T., Turner, D., Sorescu, G., Jo, H. & Nerem, R. (2006). Transcriptional profiles of valvular and vascular endothelial cells reveal phenotypic differences: influence of shear stress. *Arteriosclerosis, Thrombosis, Vascular Biology*, *26*, 69-77.

[40] Deck, J. (1986). Endothelial cell orientation on aortic valve leaflets. *Cardiovascular Research*, *20*, 760-767.

[41] Kershaw, J., Misfeld, M., Sievers, H., Yacoub, M. & Chester, A. (2004). Specific regional and directional contractile responses of aortic cusp tissue. *Journal of Heart Valve Disease*, *13*, 798-803.

[42] Butcher, J., Simmons, C. & Warnock, J. (2008). Mechanobiology of the aortic heart valve. *Journal of Heart Valve Disease*, *17*, 62-73.

[43] Chester, A., Misfeld, M. & Yacoub, M. (2000). Receptor-mediated contraction of aortic valve leaflets. *Journal of Heart Valve Disease*, *9*, 250-254.

[44] Einav, S., Stolero, D., Avidor, J., Elad, D. & Talbot, L. (1990). Wall shear stress distribution along the cusp of a tri-leaflet prosthetic valve. *Journal of Biomedical Engineering*, *12*, 13-18.

[45] Fry, D. (1968). Acute vascular endothelial changes associated with increased blood velocity gradients. *Circulation Research*, *22*, 165-197.

[46] Fry, D. (1969). Certain histological and chemical responses of the vascular interface to acutely induced mechanical stress in the aorta of the dog. *Circulation Research*, *24*, 93-108.

[47] Walburn, F. & Stein, P. (1984). Wall shear stress during pulsatile flow distal to a normal porcine aortic valve. *Journal of Biomechanics*, *17*, 97-102.

[48] Weston, M., LaBorde, D. & Yoganathan, A. (1999). Estimation of the shear stress on the surface of an aortic valve leaflet. *Annals of Biomedical Engineering*, *27*, 572-579.

[49] Woo, Y., Williams, F. & Yoganathan, A. (1983). In-vitro fluid dynamic characteristics of the Abiomed trileaflet heart valve prosthesis. *Journal of Biomechanical Engineering*, *105*, 338-345.

[50] Butcher, J. & Nerem, R. (2006). Valvular endothelial cells regulate the phenotype of interstitial cells in co-culture: effects of steady shear stress. *Tissue Engineering*, *12*, 905-915.

[51] Simmons, C., Grant, G., Manduchi, E. & Davies, P. (2005). Spatial heterogeneity of endothelial phenotypes correlates with side-specific vulnerability to calcification in normal porcine aortic valves. *Circulation Research*, *96*, 792-799.

[52] Ramamurthi, A. & Vesely, I. (2005). Evaluation of the matrix-synthesis potential of crosslinked hyaluronan gels for tissue engineering of aortic heart valves. *Biomaterials*, *26*, 999-1010.

[53] Vesely, I. (2005). Heart valve tissue engineering. *Circulation Research*, *97*, 743-755.

[54] Hammon, J.J., O'Sullivan, M., Oury, J. & Fosburg, R. (1974). Allograft cardiac valves. A view through the scanning electron microscope. *Journal of Thoracic and Cardiovascular Surgery*, *68*, 352-60.

[55] Filion, R. & Ellis, C. (2003). A finite difference model of $O^2$ transport in aortic valve cusps: importance of intrinsic microcirculation. *American Journal of Physiology - Heart and Circulatory Physiology*, *285*, H2099-104.

[56] Weind, K., Ellis, C. & Boughner, D. (2000). The aortic valve blood supply. *Journal of Heart Valve Disease*, *9*, 1-7.

[57] Weind, K., Ellis, C. & Boughner, D. (2002). Aortic valve cusp vessel density: relationship with tissue thickness. *Journal of Thoracic and Cardiovascular Surgery*, *123*, 333-40.

[58] Tompkins, R., Schnitzer, J. & Yarmush, M. (1989). Macromolecular transport within heart valves. *Circulation Research*, *64*, 1213-23.

[59] Zeng, Z., Nievelstein-Post, P., Yin, Y., Jan, K., Frank, J. & Rumschitzki, D. (2007). Macromolecular transport in heart valves. III. Experiment and theory for the size distribution of extracellular liposomes in hyperlipidemic rabbits. *American Journal of Physiology - Heart and Circulatory Physiology*, *292*, H2687-97.

[60] Zeng, Z., Yin, Y., Huang, A., Jan, K. & Rumschitzki, D. (2007). Macromolecular transport in heart valves. I. Studies of rat valves with horseradish peroxidase. *American Journal of Physiology - Heart and Circulatory Physiology*, *292*, H2664-H2670.

[61] Zeng, Z., Yin, Y., Jan, K. & Rumschitzki, D. (2007). Macromolecular transport in heart valves. II. Theoretical models. *American Journal of Physiology - Heart and Circulatory Physiology*, *292*, H2671-86.

[62] Blevins, T., Peterson, S., Lee, E., Bailey, A., Frederick, J., Huynh, T., Gupta, V. & Grande-Allen, K. (2008). Mitral valvular interstitial cells demonstrate regional, adhesional, and synthetic heterogeneity. *Cells Tissue Organs*, *187*, 113-22.

[63] Aikawa, E., Whittaker, P., Farber, M., Mendelson, K., Padera, R., Aikawa, M. & Schoen, F. (2006). Human semilunar cardiac valve remodeling by activated cells from

fetus to adult: implications for postnatal adaptation, pathology, and tissue engineering. *Circulation*, *113*, 1344-52.

[64] Rabkin-Aikawa, E., Farber, M., Aikawa, M. & Schoen, F. (2004). Dynamic and reversible changes of interstitial cell phenotype during remodeling of cardiac valves. *Journal of Heart Valve Disease*, *13*, 841-7.

In: Advances in Cardiovascular Research, Volume 1
Editors: L. Schmitt, T. Konig, pp. 237-250
ISBN: 978-1-60741-720-0


*Chapter IX*

# Morphological Aspects in Analysis of Postoperative Remodeling of Left Ventricle in Patients with Icmp

***V. M. Shipulin, V. A. Kazakov, B. N. Kozlov, A. A. Lezhnev, E. V. Krivoshchekov, I. V. Suhodolo, A. A. Miller***
Tomsk Centre of Cardiology, Russia

## Abstract

Functional morphology of LV myocardium and RA appendage in 48 patients with ICMP was studied based on intraoperative biopsies analysis. In the early postoperative period (1 year) all the patients were divided into 2 groups. Group one was comprised of the patients with positive dynamics of EDI and LV EF, group two – with negative ones. Retrospective analysis of echocardiographical values did not let to reveal predictors of postoperative remodeling of heart in both patients groups. On the contrary, drawing clinical-morphological parallels of negative dynamics in the early postoperative period showed that the presence of diffuse lymphocytic- macrophage inflammatory infiltration of myocardial stroma in combination with pronounced fibrosis, low values of trophic index (TI) (<0,015) and specific volume (SV) of atrial natriuretic peptide granules in atrial cardiomyocytes as well as high values of pericappilar diffusion zone (PDZ) (>1000 mcm) and Kernogan index (KI) (>1,6) of LV myocardium are morphological predictors of postoperative heart remodeling.

**Keywords:** ischemic cardiomyopathy, postinfarction left ventricle remodeling, morphological predictors of postoperative remodeling, myocarditis.

# Introduction

Ischemic heart disease (IHD) remains to be one of the most widely spread, progressing and unfavorable diseases cardio-vascular system. According to different authors, ischemic cardiomyopathy (ICMP), conditioned by significantly pronounced diffuse sclerosis of coronary arteries and manifesting as megalocardia and as symptoms of congestive heart failure, develops in 10-35% of the patients with IHD. [2, 4] The process of heart remodeling is an aggregate of changes of form, volume of heart cavities and mass of postinfarction heart myocardium in response to pronounced inadequate hemodinamic conditions of its functioning, which are not connected with lengthening of sarcomeres [8, 10]. Coronary artery bypass grafting (CABG), correction of shape and volume of left ventricle (LV) and mitral regurgitation (MR) – have become widely-spread as complex surgical treatment of the patients with postinfarction heart remodeling. Nevertheless, according to the worlds' publications, 12-25% of the patients experience secondary LV remodeling in the late follow-up period. During this remodeling, sizes of heart chambers and hemodynamic values reach preoperative level and in some cases exceed it [6, 7, 9]. A thorough selection of the patients based on complex clinical-morphological analysis of prognosis for surgical treatment results will let enhance efficacy of this approach of operative intervention. The patients with potentially unfavorable outcome of surgical treatment of LV remodeling should be refused from the operation in favor of primary heart transplantation.

The question of preoperative prognosis for late follow-up results of operative treatment remains unanswered. Character of LV wall's kinesis, high pressure in the right heart, amount of viable myocardium, presence of mitral regurgitation were considered as possible preoperative parameters connected with the risk of postoperative progressing of LV remodeling. Trustworthy scientists (Batista R.J., 1997; Dowling R.D. et al., 1998), who dealt with the search for clinical and instrumental predictors of postoperative heart remodeling, drew attention to the importance of studying of morphofunctional condition of pre- and intraoperative LV myocardium biopsy samples in the patients with ICD to understand fundamentals of heart failure progressing in the late follow-up period.

Myocardium is a unique tissue which consists of high-differentiated cells (cardiomyocytes) normally having a number of features and reacting with a set of nonspecific structural changes to pathomorphosis of cardio-vascular diseases. It has been 7-10 years since foreign scientists began their search for morphological predictors of postoperative heart remodeling during cardiomyopathies for the first time. They analyzed the course of postoperative period and compared morphofunctional conditions of LV myocardium based on intraoperative biopsy samples. Nevertheless, the results of these isolated studies are very controversial. Moreira L.F.P. et al [6] attribute mean value of LV myocardium cardiomyocytes diameter exceeding 22mcm to the factors connected with unfavorable late results of surgical treatment of the patients with DCMP. On the other hand Popovic Z. et al. [9] did not find correlation between preoperative morphology of myocardium and its postoperative function. This fact, according to the authors (Popovic Z. et al.) was connected with narrow coverage of morphological approaches in their study. We have not found any data concerning search for morphological predictors of postoperative LV remodeling in the patients with ICMP dealing with complex evaluation of morphofunctional condition of different areas of myocardium and comparison of morphological and late clinical outcomes of surgical treatment in the available foreign and Russian literature. In home publications there are solitary articles devoted to the study of morphofunctional condition and morphometrical parameters of LV myocardium and RA auricle in patients with IHD of different functional classes. These articles cannot boast wide coverage of morphological parameters [3]; some authors content themselves with mere descriptive morphology without careful consideration of the mechanisms of possible pathogenesis of heart remodeling [5]. Thus, until today, complex fundamental scientific studies directly based on the clinic have not been carried out in the world.

**OBJECTIVE** of the study is to draw tissue and ultrastructural parallels of LV remodeling in patients with an extensive postinfarction cardiosclerosis underwent complex surgical treatment.

## Materials and Methods

At present 48 patients with previous large-focal myocardial infarctions and systolic LV dysfunction are enrolled into the study. Their survival rate after the operations was not less than 1 year. Clinical characteristics of the enrolled patients are shown in Table 1.

**Table 1. Clinical characteristics of the enrolled patients (n = 48)**

| Characteristics | | Total |
|---|---|---|
| Age (years), X ± x | | 54.3±5.2 |
| Females (%) | | 2 (4.2%) |
| Number of previous MIs | 1 | 29 (60.4%) |
| | 2 | 12 (25.0%) |
| | 3 | 7 (14.6%) |
| Angina class (CCS) | I | 4 (8.3%) |
| | II | 27 (56.3%) |
| | III | 11 (22.9%) |
| | IV | 6 (12.5%) |
| Prescription of MI (months) | | 36±18 |
| Heart failure (HF) class (NYHA) | II | 2 (4.2%) |
| | III | 41 (85.4%) |
| | IV | 5 (10.4%) |
| Disturbance of carbohydrate metabolism | | 9 (18.7%) |
| End diastolic index (EDI) LV (ml/m$^2$) | | 131.3±7.8 |
| End systolic index (ESI) LV (ml/m$^2$) | | 79.1±9.1 |
| Ejection fraction (EF) LV (%) | | 39.4±4.2 |
| Pulmonary artery pressure (PAP) (mmHg) | | 38.5±10.6 |
| Mitral regurgitation grade of 3-4 degrees | | 21 (43.7%) |
| Scintigraphy perfusion defect | | 32.7±7.6 |
| Number of affected vessels | | 2.4±0.7 |

Intraoperative biopsy samples of RA auricle myocardium and LV myocardium were taken from all the patients (n=48). The spectrum of the performed surgical procedures is shown in Table 2.

Preparation of histological samples was made according to the standard method including their fixing in 10% solution of neutral formalin, dehydration in ethanol of grade-concentration and saturation of the material with paraffin. Histological samples of intraoperative biopsy material, dyed with hematoxylin-eosin and by Mallory method, were studied with the use of common light and polarized microscopy. Myocardium of similar parts of the heart from 25 patients was studied with the help of electron-microscopy. For this purpose samples of myocardium of not more that 2 $mm^3$ size were fixed in 2.5% solution of glutaraldehyde in 0.2M cacodilate buffer with pH = 7,2 at +4°C temperature and postfixed in 1% solution of $OsO_4$ in the cold during 4 hours. Then biopsy samples were dehydrated in ethanol of grade-concentration and embedded with the mixture of epone and araldite. Ultrathin sections prepared on the ultratome LKB III (Sweden) were contrasted with lead citrate and with uranylacetate and studied in electronic microscope JEM-100 CX (Japan). Such factors as parenchymo-stromal ratio (PSO), trophic index (TI) and pericappilar diffusion zone (PDZ) were evaluated for quantitative characteristic of relationship of myocardial parenchyma, organ's stroma and exchanging area of microcirculatory bed to reveal risk factors for postoperative heart remodeling. Kernogan index (KI) was calculated for quantitative characteristic of microcirculatory vessels' bed condition and their carrying capacity. Calculation of mitochondrial-myofibrillar ratio (MMR) and specific volume (SV) of granules of atrial natriuretic peptide was made with the help of electron-diffraction pattern. PSO is a ratio between myocardial parenchyma SV and stromal SV; TI (giving the most complete picture of myocardial trophy condition) is the ratio between capillary SV and parenchymal SV; PDZ (area of tissue supplied with the blood by one capillary) is the ratio between capillaries diameter and their SV; KI (parameter of carrying capacity of microcirculatory bed) is the ratio between arterioles' vascular wall thickness and the radius of their lumen; MMR is the ratio between mitochondrial SV and SV of myofibrils [1]. "Coronary reserve" (CR) was measured for microcirculatory area of vascular bed. CR is the ratio of number of nonfunctioning capillaries to their general number, area of capillaries' lumen, density of free pinocytic vesicles, and number of pinocytic vesicles attached to the surface of capillary endotheliocytes.

**Table 2. The spectrum of the performed surgical treatment of the patients enrolled into the study.**

| surgical procedure | Total |
|---|---|
| Dor procedure + CABG (%) | 34 (70.8%) |
| CABG with mitral annuloplasty (%) | 8 (16.6%) |
| Tricuspid valve repair (%) | 4 (8.3%) |
| Isolated CABG (%) | 8 (16.6%) |
| No. of distal anastomoses | 2.2±0.4 |

Diameters of cardiomyocytes on longitudinal section on the level of myocardial cells' nuclei were measured.

To compare morphometrical parameters myocardium of similar heart's parts was taken from hearts of 25 corpses (22 male and 3 female) of comparable age died from acute injure with no signs of cardio-vascular pathology. The given study was approved by Local Ethical Committee of Tomsk Institute of Cardiology.

Pre- and postoperative echocardiographical examination was performed in all the patients (100%). Numerous examinations were carried out before the operation and during a year after the operation on «PHILIPS EnVisor C HD».

Tissue and cellular stereological parameters were calculated basing on the data of light and electronic microscopy such as specific volumes of parenchyma, stroma, general myocardial edema, vascular and capillary area of microcirculatory bed, mitochondria, myofibrils, nuclei and granules of atrial cardiomyocytes. PSO, TI, PDZ, KI and MMR were calculated by the aforementioned formulas. Results were given as a mean value (M) and as an error of mean (m). Reliability of the obtained data was checked with the help of Van-der-Varden nonparametric test. Difference of the values in comparing groups was considered significant at $p<0,05$. Reliability of differences of relative occurrence of myocarditis signs was assessed in the groups of the patients with positive and negative dynamics of late follow-up outcomes of surgical treatment for ICMP.

## Results and Discussion

Basing on the results of surgical treatment all the patients were divided into two groups. The 1st group consisted of 36 patients which had LV EDI on postoperative level in a year after surgical intervention. The 2nd group was formed of 12 patients with repeated LV remodeling whose EDI was on preoperative level or exceeded it. In a year after surgical treatment LV EF was significantly higher in the 1st group of the patients and values of LV EDI and ESI were significantly lower than initial ones. In the 2nd group, on the contrary, statistically significant decrease of LV EF due to increase of LV EDI and ESI in comparison with preoperative values was noticed. In the 1st group values of circulation insufficiency FC were significantly lower and in the 2nd group – significantly higher than the initial preoperative values. Spectrum of surgical treatment procedures performed in the patients with positive and negative dynamic of late follow-up period as well as patients' EchoCG data and clinical picture are shown in tables 3 and 4 accordingly.

Retrospective analysis of the initial clinical patients' characteristic enrolled in the given study revealed that the majority of the 1st group patients had had a single previous myocardial infarction, while the majority of the 2nd group patients had previously had multiple myocardial infarctions. In both groups the patients had predominantly III FC NYHA, but the patients of the 1st group had carbohydrate metabolism disturbance more often.

Morphological study of intraoperative biopsy samples of LV and RA auricle showed that in ICMP patients density of vessels distribution is dramatically lowered in comparison with control samples of autopsies from people died from acute injure with no signs of cardio-vascular pathology. Irrespectively of blood vessels' diameters signs of hemodynamic disturbance, such as perivascular and interstitial edemas (Figure 1), venous plethora (Figure 1B), desolation and spasm of arterioles and small vessels were noticed everywhere.

**Table 3. Spectrum of surgical procedures performed in the patients with positive and negative dynamic of late follow-up period**

| Surgical procedure | no postoperative remodeling (n=36) | postoperative remodeling (n=12) |
|---|---|---|
| Dor procedure + CABG | 29 (85.3%) | 5 (14.7%) |
| Dor procedure + CABG + MV repair | 1 (50.0%) | 1 (50.0%) |
| CABG + MV repair | 1 (25.0%) | 3 (75.0%) |
| Isolated CABG | 5 (62.5%) | 3 (37.5%) |
| TOTAL | 36 (75.0%) | 12 (25.0%) |

**Table 4. EchoCG data and circulation insufficiency FC in control terms of follow-up period**

| Value | 1 Preoperatively | Comparison of Value P in columns 1, 2 | Comparison of Value P in columns 1, 3 | One year after surgical treatment | | Comparison of Value P in columns 2, 3 |
|---|---|---|---|---|---|---|
| | | | | 2 Effective surgical treatment (n=36) | 3 Ineffective surgical treatment (n=12) | |
| EDI (ml/m2) | 131.3±7.8 | 0.043 | 0.048 | 112.8±5.4 | 147.0±10.2 | 0.002 |
| ESI (ml/m2) | 79.1±9.1 | 0.037 | 0.046 | 61.4±11.1 | 87.1±7.1 | 0.004 |
| EF, % | 39.4±4.2 | *0.065* | *0.054* | 41.9±2.3 | 38.1±1.7 | 0.047 |
| MI (months) | 1.9±0.4 | *0.051* | *0.063* | 1.7±0.2 | 2.1±0.7 | 0.036 |
| PAP (mmHg) | 38.5±10.6 | 0.020 | *0.059* | 21.5±7.6 | 30.2±5.2 | 0.003 |
| Scintigraphic perfusion defect (%) | 32.7±7.6 | 0.039 | 0.042 | 23.0±1.6 | 25.0±5.1 | *0.053* |
| FC NYHA | 2.4±0.6 | *0.071* | 0.047 | 2.3±0.3 | 3.3±0.4 | 0.047 |

Note: insignificant differences are in italics

Microvasculature was plethoric, occurrence of erythrocytes stasis in capillaries, pericapillaries and arterioles was often observed. In some capillaries bulging of endothelial cells' nuclei to the inside of capillaries lumen was noticed which weakened their carrying capacity and myocardial trophy level.

Mixed lymphocytic-macrophage infiltrate (> 14 for 1mm$^2$ of tissue according to Marburg classification) [11] was found in LV myocardial stroma in all the patients of the 2$^{nd}$ (100%) and in 23 patients (63.9%) of the 1$^{st}$ group. We categorized it as myocarditis (Figure 2).

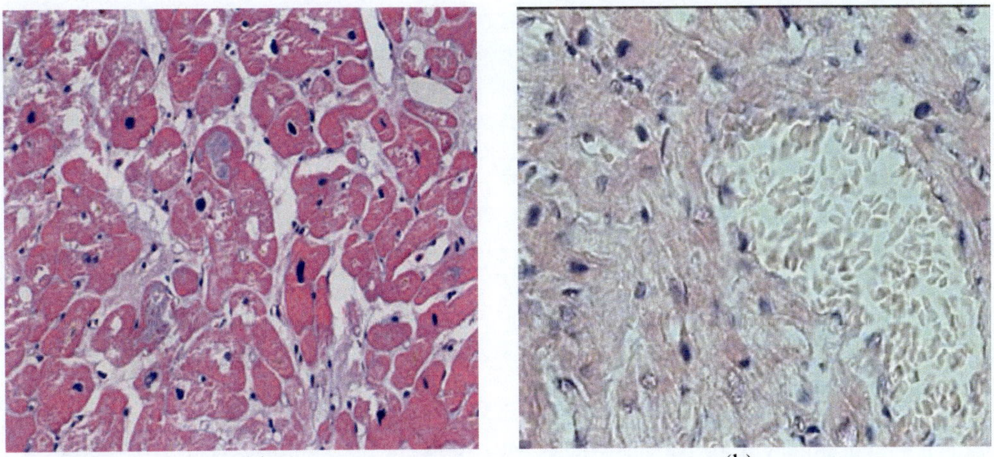

(a) (b)

Figure 1. LV myocardium of the patients with ICMP. Interstitial edema (A), venous plethora (B). Dyed with hematoxyline and eosine. X 700 (A) and 500 (B).

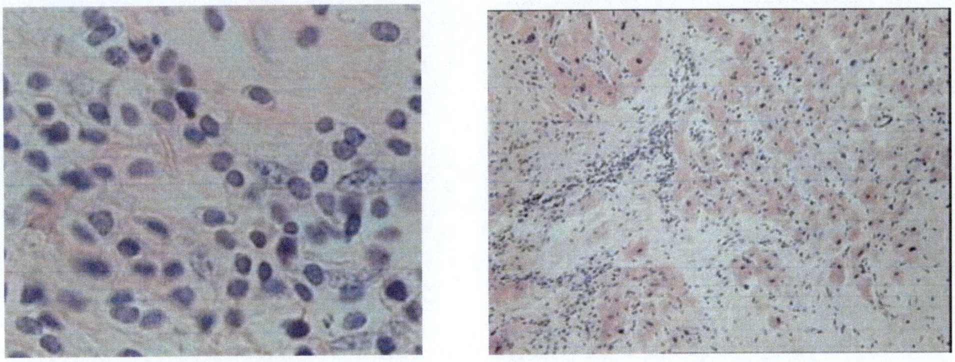

Figure 2. LV myocardium of the patients with ICMP. Mixed (lymphocytic-macrophage) infiltration of stroma. Dyed with hematoxylin and eosin. X 150 (A) and 800 (B).

At the same time fibrosis (according to Marburg classification) [11] in LV myocardium was, as a rule, moderate of insignificant in the 1st group and predominantly pronounced (unfavorable) and in rare cases moderate in the 2nd group patients with ICMP. In half of the cases among the patients of the 1st group and in 100% cases in the 2nd group patients infiltration had diffuse character, less often – focal or confluent. Besides, in 7 patients with repeated LV remodeling (58.3%) and in 10 patients with favorable late outcome of surgical treatment (27.8%) infiltrate of identical character was found in myocardium of RA auricle. In the mean time fibrosis in RA auricle myocardium was I-II degrees lower than in LV myocardium [11]. In the polarized light alongside with unchanged parts of cardiomyocytes' cytoplasm of LV myocardium and myocardium of RA auricle there were noticed affected parts, in which segmental contractions (Figure 3A), contractions of I, II, less often of III degree, isolated areas of intracellular myocytolysis and primary clump disintegration of myofibrils as well as cytolysis of cardiomyocytes were prevalent. These changes had mosaic character.

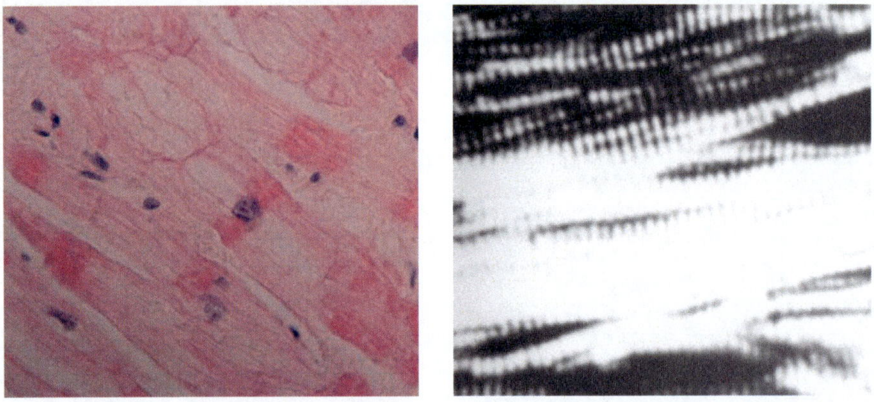

Figure 3. LV myocardium of the patients with ICMP. Subsegmental contractions (A), III degree contractions (B). Dyed with hematoxylin and eosin. Polarized light (B). X. 400.

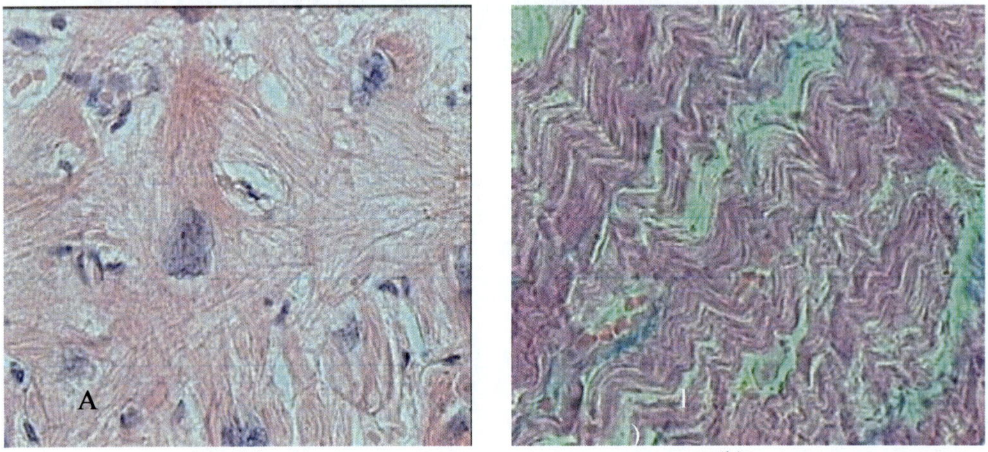


(a) (b)

Figure 4. LV myocardium of the patients with ICMP: A – cellular structure of myocardium, stellar shape CMC; B – wave-like deformation of myocardial cells. Dyed with hematoxylin and eosin (**a**) and by Malory method (b). X. 700 (**a**) and 500 (b)

Very interesting features were observed during studying of morphofunctional condition of LV myocardium in patients with ICMP: disturbance of cardiomyocytes' arrangement in muscle fibers and poor direction of heart fibers in relation to one another, disintegration of myocardial cells along intercalated disk, elimination of cardiomyocytes along muscle fibers. In these cases myocardium had not fiber but cellular structure that resulted in its contractility disturbance. Sometimes heart myocytes had stellar shape (Figure 4A). Moreover, in longitudinal sections of LV myocardium in the patients with ICMP wave-like deformation of CMC along myocardial fibers was observed (Figure 4B).

During electron-microscopic study of CMC of LV and RA auricle, myocardium polymorphism of myocardial cells' ultrastructure drew our attention. Nuclei, often having an awkward scalloped shape with multitude intussusceptums and **выростов** of nuclear membrane, were situated in the center of myocardial cells but were displaced into subsarcolemmic zone in some cases. Genetic material was presented more often as euchromatin and took central position. In some CMC nuclei, vice versa, heterochromatin prevailed and was situated mostly in perimembranous zone. Quite often aggregation of chromatin was noticed (Figure 5). Nuclear membrane was uninterrupted and had pores.

Widening of perinuclear space was noticed which was not filled with mitochondrias, granular reticulumand with the elements of Golgi apparatus but contained to a great extent rarefied matrix with β-glycogen of round or oblong shape (monogranular glycogen). α-glycogen rosettes were present in a very insignificant amount in intermyofibrillar spaces.

We also noticed dispersed nuclei, segregation of fibrillar and granular components of nucleolonema, ring-shaped nuclei that evidenced depression of rRNA biosynthesis.

Variety of different lesion forms of cardiomyocytes' myofibrilla of LV and RA auricle myocardium such as contractile lesions of myofibrilla of I, less often of II and III degrees (Figure 6), isolated areas of their primary clump disintegration drew our attention. In the majority of CMC small-focal and diffuse lysis of myofibrillar bundles and "melting" of myofibrilla were observed (Figure 7). I-stripes, in which thin (actinic) filaments were situated, were lysed to a greater extent. Myofibrilla became less dense, interstice appeared in many sarcomeres and in some cases total lysis of myofilaments within sacromeres was noticed. In the area of intercalated disks and in perinuclear zone sarcomeres were significantly destructed.

In LV and RA auricle myocardial cardiomyocytes we found focuses of intercellular regeneration of ultrastructures extremely seldom. We judged about them by accumulation of free ribosomes on stumps of survived myofibrilla which contributed to synthesis and new growth of contractile proteins. Newly formed myofilaments gathered into bundles of myofibrilla as they grew and synthesized on polyribosomes. But disturbance of their normal direction and extra elongation takes place during the process of a new growth manifesting by extension of distance between adjacent Z-stripes.

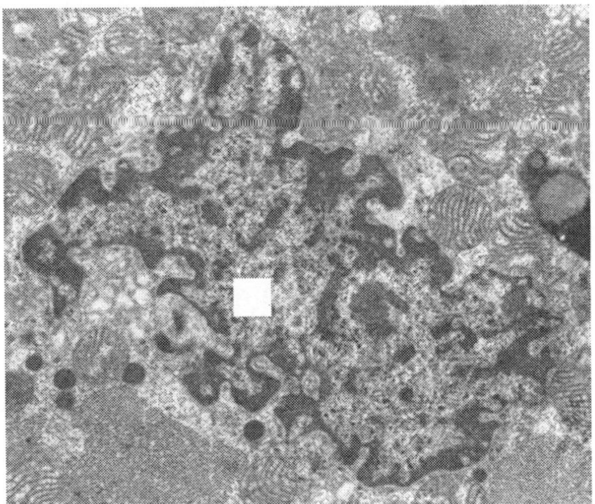

Figure 5. Cardiomyocyte of RA myocardium of a patient with ICMP: chromatin aggregation (ChA) in the nucleolus core (N) and in the perimembranous zone; MF – myofibrilla; MCh – mitochondria. X. 25000.

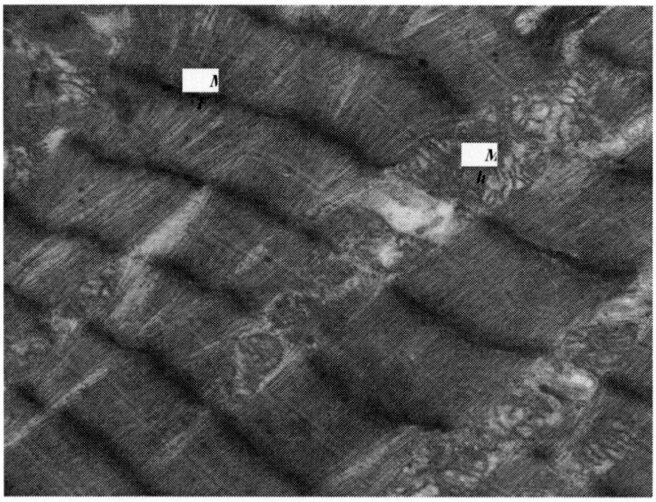

Figure 6. Ultrastructure of cardiomyocyte of LV myocardium of a patient with ICMP: contractile lesions of myofibrilla *(MF) II degree; MCh – mitochondria. X. 20000.*

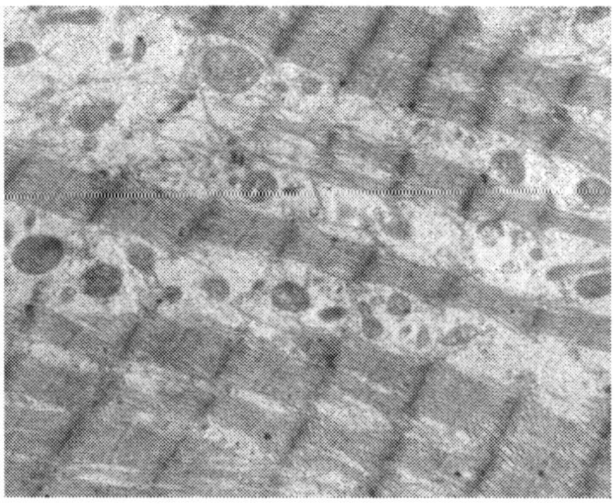

Figure 7. LV cardiomyocyte of a patient with ICMP: diffuse lysis (L) of myofibrilla bundles (MF), «melting» of myofibrilla. X. 20000.

Apart from disturbance of normal direction of newly-formed myofibrilla, chaotic direction of "mature" contractile proteins was noticed (Figure 8). Myofibrilla bundles and even isolated myofilaments were situated under different angles to each other. Besides wave-like deformation of myofibrilla of LV and RA auricle myocardium was registered in the patients with ICMP. All these circumstances, without any doubt, contribute to desynchronization of contractile processes by that determining systolic dysfunction of myocardium.

Cisterns and vacuole of sarcoplasmic reticulum and Golgi apparatus in cardiomyocytes of LV and RA auricle myocardium were reduced and sometimes dilated. Dilatation of cisterns was noticed mostly in perinuclear area and less often in the space between myofibrilla (in Z-stripes area) and mitochondria.

Atrial cardiomyocytes contained electron-dense granules of natriuretic peptide of different sizes.

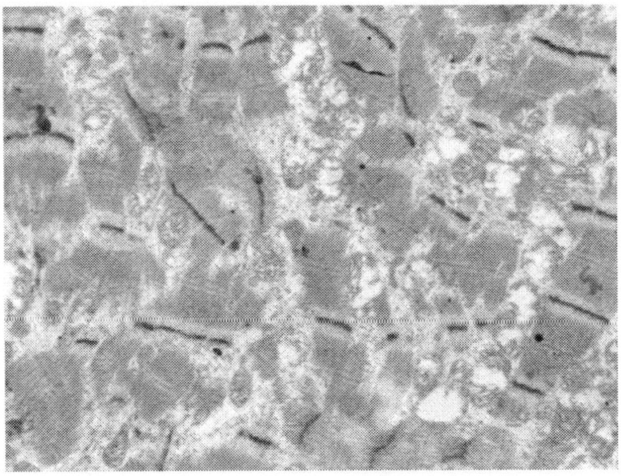

Figure 8. A part of a LV myocardium cardiomyocyte of a patient with ICMP: *MF* – disturbance of normal direction of newly-formed myofibrilla bundles. *X. 18000.*

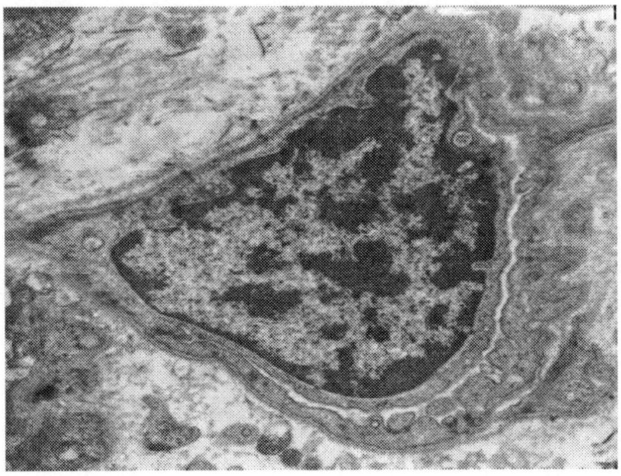

Figure 9. A nonfunctioning capillary of LV myocardium of a patient with ICMP: bulging of endotheliocytes nuclei (N) into capillary lumen. X. 16000.

In microcirculatory area of vascular bed of LV and RA myocardium bulging of endotheliocytes nuclei into capillary lumen (Figure 9), folding of luminal surface of endothelial cell, reduction of vessels' lumen, thickening of basal membrane, reduction of carrying capacity of capillaries and massive fibrosis were noticed. Chromatin in endotheliocytes' nuclei was condensed and had the form of lumps. Pericappilar edemas were seen everywhere.

Thus, morphofunctional condition of LV and RA auricle myocardium in the patients with ICMP fully reflects clinical severity of this nosologic form. Intensity and combination of the main forms of cardiomyocytes' lesions vary in different patients. It is easy to explain, since coronary arteries lesions cause myocardial ischemia which influences contractile function of a heart muscle differently in different patients and depends on a kind of coronary arteries lesion (severity and duration of ischemia), on reperfusion (time and completeness of blood flow recovery) on myocardial response, which, evidently, has significant flexibility in this answer and on morphological features of a heart muscle of an every single patient. Morphofunctional condition of RA auricle myocardium reflects morphofunctional condition of LV myocardium, that is to say is a kind of a "mirror" for the latter. To reveal morphological predictors of postoperative heart remodeling basing only descriptive morphology data is absolutely impossible. To achieve the set objective it is necessary to take into account quantitative values, which allow for complete evaluation of functioning conditions of a cardiomyocyte as a structural unit of heart.

Statistical analysis of the obtained morphometrical data showed that PSO and TI of PA auricle and LV myocardium were significantly lower in the patients with postoperative heart remodeling and their TI was 8-12 times lower than that in the control group. On the contrary, values PDZ and KI of RA auricle and LV myocardium were significantly higher in the 2nd group of the patients and their PDZ value was 14-20 higher than that in the control group. Similar values of the 1st group patients were much more favorable than those of the 2nd group patients, but still they differed very much from the data of control studies. Mean values of diameters of LV and RA auricle myocardium cardiomyocytes did not fifer significantly in the patients with different outcomes of operative treatment, though they exceeded those values of the control group (Table 5).

6 out of 25 patients whose LV and RA auricle myocardium was subjected to electron-microscopic study, had postoperative heart remodeling, while in the rest of them contractile function of LV remained satisfactory. Statistical analysis of morphometrical data of ultrastructure showed that SV of cardiomyocytes myofibrilla was significantly lower and SV of cardiomyocytes mitochondria of both LV myocardium and RA auricle was higher in patients with unfavorable late outcome of surgical treatment.

Increase of mitochondrial- myofibrillar ratio is a consequence of the aforementioned changes. SV of atrial natriuretic peptide granules of RA auricle cardiomyocytes decrease significantly as heart failure progresses which, evidently, reflects depression of all synthetic processes in a cell. SV of cardiomyocytes' nuclei does not change essentially (Table 6).

**Table 5. Parenchymo-stromal ratio (PSO), trophic index (TI), pericappilar diffusion zone (PDZ), Kernogan index (KI) and diameter of cardiomyocytes ($D_{cmc}$) of LV and RA auricle myocardium in patients with ICMP with different late outcomes of surgical treatment. Van-der-Vaden criterion, M±m**

| | Group I (n=36) | | Group II (n=12) | | Control (n=25) | |
|---|---|---|---|---|---|---|
| | *RA* | *LV* | *RA* | *LV* | *RA* | *LV* |
| PSR | 2.40± 0.35* | 2.10± 0.30** | 2.27± 0.43* | 1.32± 0.37** | 6.77± 0.18 | 8.59± 0.24 |
| TI | 0.0485± 0.0184* | 0.0284± 0.0131** | 0.0262± 0.0089* | 0.0087± 0.0039** | 0.0862± 0.0074 | 0.0903± 0.0041 |
| PDZ, mcm | 292.7± 30.4* | 504.2± 58.1** | 600.6± 64.5* | 1295.8± 87.1** | 82.9± 1.8 | 69.5± 2.8 |
| KI | 1.62± 0.42* | 1.56± 0.33** | 1.82± 0.32* | 1.84± 0.22** | 1.15± 0.11 | 1.14± 0.07 |
| $D_{cmc}$, mcm | 14.1± 2.3 | 26.9± 3.1 | 14.1± 2.6 | 26.1± 3.3 | 10.1± 0.9 | 12.3± 0.9 |

*, ** - $p<0.05$ –significance of differences between groups

**Table 6. Morphometrical parameters of ultrastructures of myocardial cardiomyocytes of LV and RA auricle in patients with ICMP with different outcomes of surgical treatment. Van-der-Varden criterion (M±m)**

| Parameters | Group I (n=19) | | Group II (n=6) | |
|---|---|---|---|---|
| | *RA* | *LV* | *RA* | *LV* |
| Myofibrilla SV, $mcm^3/mcm^3$ | 0.416± 0.021* | 0.503± 0.032** | 0.336± 0.025* | 0.419± 0.043** |
| Mitochondria SV, $mcm^3/mcm^3$ | 0.175± 0.023* | 0.208± 0.027** | 0.243± 0.021* | 0.247± 0.022** |
| Mitochondria-myofibrilla ratio | 0.428± 0.071* | 0.414± 0.057** | 0.723± 0.074* | 0.590± 0.087** |
| Cardiomyocytes' nuclei SV, $mcm^3/mcm^3$ | 0.041± 0.004 | 0.041± 0.007 | 0.042± 0.006 | 0.040± 0.006 |
| SV of granules of atrial natriuretic peptide, $mcm^3/mcm^3$ | 0.0032± 0.0004* | - | 0.0024± 0.0007* | - |

*, ** - $p<0.05$ – significance of differences between groups

Ratio of nonfunctioning ("close") capillaries to their general number ("coronary reserve" CR) was statistically significantly higher in the group of the patients with positive dynamics of late postoperative period (Group I). This fact lets consider significant number of nonfunctioning capillaries as favorable forecasting factor for "close" capillaries can turn into "open" condition in critical ischemic moments increasing transcapillary exchange and support myocardial trophy on the necessary level. In the same patients density of free pinocytic vesicles as well as the number of pinocytic vesicles attached to luminal surface of endotheliocytes of functioning capillaries did not differ significantly from similar parameters of the 2nd group patients. We explain these results by insignificant volume of general sampling of patients for by far values of transcapillary exchange have been analyzed in only 14 patients with ICMP.

# Conclusion

In the course of our study in 25% of the cases we obtained unfavorable outcome of complex surgical treatment of LV ischemic remodeling, which corresponds to the data presented by other authors [6, 7, 9]. In a year of postoperative observation in this group irrespective of surgical treatment, LV cavity size exceeded preoperative values. Having divided the groups based on follow-up results of surgical treatment and comparing their initial parameters we did not find significant difference in preoperative examination data and the method of operative treatment. In other words we did not reveal any reliable clinical or echocardiographical predictors of postoperative LV remodeling. At the same time, comparison of these morphometric values, describing quantitative relations of myocardium parenchyma, stroma and microvascular bed, and late follow-up results of surgical treatment let us reveal morphological predictors of postoperative LV remodeling. They were: presence of signs of myocarditis in combination with pronounced fibrosis (parenchymo-stromal ratio<1.6), low trophic index (<0.015) and high values of pericapillarly diffuse zone (>1000 mcm), Kernogan index (>1.5) and mitochondrial-myofibrillar ratio (>0.050).

Presence of myocarditis in the RA auricle myocardium evidences the presence of inflammatory infiltration in LV myocardium in 100%.This fact may also be referred to as a morphological predictor of secondary heart remodeling and heart failure progress in patients with ICMP in the late follow-up period.

Revelation of the mechanisms of heart failure progress after intracardiac correction and revascularisation would allow to narrow indications for complex surgical treatment. In some of the patients standard methods of surgical treatment (total myocardial revascularization, LV volume reduction and mitral regurgitation correction) do not result in involution of this pathological process. The patent № 2310372 of 20.11.2007 for the results of this study was granted to the authors by the Federal Service for Intellectual Property, Patents and Trademarks. The developed approach for prognosis of postoperative heart remodeling based on complex functional morphology of myocardium in preoperative period will let avoid unfavorable late outcomes of surgical treatment in the future. At the same time it remains unclear how to evaluate the degree of intensity of such morphofunctional changes in every case based on clinical and instrumental data.

## References

[1] Avtandilov, G. G. (1990). Medical morphometry / – M.: Medicine, *384*.

[2] Belenkov Ju, N. (2002). Epidemiological studies of heart failure: urgency of the question / Ju.N. Belenkov, V. Ju. Mareev, F. T. Agheev // J Heart Failure. № 2. 57-58.

[3] Kuznetsov, G. E. (2003). Clinical-morphological parallels of left ventricle remodeling at chronic heart failure / Cardiology. №, *12*. 19-22.

[4] Yu, V. (2002). Mareev. Design of the study and characteristics of the patients in the 'FASON' study // J Heart Failure. №, *2*. 97-98.

[5] Salikhova, S. P., Stadnikov, A. A., Semagin, A. P. (2002). Morphlogical aspects of heart remodeling at chronic heart failure // Morphology. T. *122*, №, *5*. 60-62.

[6] Current perspectives of partial left ventriculectomy in the treatment of dilated cardiomyopathy / L.F. Moreira [et al.] // Eur J Cardio-thorac. Surg. 2001, Vol. *19*. 54-60.

[7] Dor, V. (1997). Left ventricular aneurysms: the endoventricular circular patch plasty / V. Dor // Semin Thorac Cardiovasc Surg. Vol., *9*. 123-130.

[8] Extension of borderzone myocardium in postinfarction dilated cardiomyopathy / B.M. Jackson [et al.] // J. Am. Coll. Cardiol. 2002. Vol. *40*. 1160-1167.

[9] Functional capacity late after partial left ventriculectomy: relation to ventricular geometry and performance / Z. Popovic [et al.] // Eur J Cardio-thorac Surg. 2001, Vol., *19*. 61-67.

[10] Maisch, B. (1996). Ventricular remodeling / B. Maisch // Cardiology. Vol. *87*. – Suppl. 1. 2-10.

[11] World Heart Federation Classification and Consensus Conference on the Histo- and Immunohistopathology of Myocarditis, Marburg, April 28-29, 1997 and on Viral Cardiomyopathy, Marburg, October, 3-5, 1997.

In: Advances in Cardiovascular Research, Volume 1
Editors: L. Schmitt, T. Konig, pp. 251-268
ISBN: 978-1-60741-720-0


*Chapter X*

# Functional and Ischemic Mitral Regurgitation

***Marco Pocar, Andrea Moneta, Davide Passolunghi, Alessandra Di Mauro, Alda Bregasi, Roberto Mattioli and Francesco Donatelli***

Unit of Cardiac Surgery & Echo-Lab, Scientific Institute MultiMedica Hospital, University of Milan, Milan, Italy.

## Abstract

Unlike organic mitral regurgitation, so-called "functional" or "secondary" mitral regurgitation (MR) is related to progressive left ventricular dilatation, remodeling, dyssinchrony or distortion involving the mitral apparatus. Thus, there is no primary valve disease and leaflets are basically normal. More in general, valvular function is impaired because of underlying chronic or acute left ventricular dysfunction. As a consequence, functional MR is typically encountered in two clinical scenarios: acute left ventricular failure and chronic cardiomyopathy.

Although the possible causes vary widely, the present chapter will focus on the two most common and best studied etiologies of functional MR: chronic ischemic heart disease with left ventricular dysfunction and non-ischemic, idiopathic dilated cardiomyopathy.

## Introduction

Mitral regurgitation (MR) is commonly observed in patients with heart failure and is associated with a poor prognosis. Mitral valve repair or replacement to restore valve competency is a well-established procedure when there are symptoms of heart failure and the primary disease is of the valve leaflets. Recent interest has focused on so-called "functional" or "secondary" MR in which valve anatomy is basically normal but leaflets do not fully coapt because of annular dilatation and restricted leaflet motion secondary to increased ventricular size and sphericity. More in general, valvular function is impaired because of underlying chronic or acute left ventricular dysfunction, leading to progressive left ventricular dilatation, remodeling, dyssinchrony or distortion of the mitral apparatus. Such a remodeled ventricle is often associated with an ejection fraction of 40% or lower and advanced heart failure symptoms.

Functional MR is typically part of two clinical scenarios: acute left ventricular failure and chronic cardiomyopathy. Although the possible causes vary widely, the present chapter will focus the two most common and best studied etiologies of chronic functional MR, i.e., chronic ischemic heart disease with left ventricular dysfunction, and non-ischemic dilated cardiomyopathy.

# Ischemic Mitral Regurgitation

## Etiology and Epidemiology

Chronic ischemic mitral regurgitation (IMR) represents a possible consequence of evolving ischemic heart disease, and is a common determinant of chronic heart failure and reduced survival after myocardial infarction [1]. IMR is the most commonly observed form of functional MR. Although IMR may be applied to define a broad spectrum of valve dysfunction, the trend in recent years has been to use the term chronic IMR in a more strict sense, referring to functional valve dysfunction preceded by myocardial infarction, at a minimum of 16 days [2]. Thus, the diagnosis of IMR implies the exclusion of organic valve disease, and the presence of left ventricular wall motion abnormalities with corresponding stenotic or occluded coronary tributaries. The prevalence of IMR is very difficult to estimate because published reports refer to heterogeneous definitions, variable time intervals from acute myocardial infarction, and different diagnostic modalities [3,4]. In this respect, IMR is reported in as many as 20% and more than 70% of patients with coronary artery disease, with or without prior myocardial infarction, when diagnosis is based on angiography or echocardiography, respectively. Despite the practical impossibility to exactly define the true prevalence of IMR, it must be stressed that IMR is strongly associated with heart failure and mortality [5-7]. In this scenario, moderate-degree IMR, defined as an effective regurgitant orifice area $\geq 20$ mm$^2$ determines a three-fold incidence of heart failure and a near-double incidence of death after 5 years. Of additional interest is the correlation between a less favourable prognosis and mild mitral insufficiency, which also confirms the detrimental effects of regurgitation on ventricular remodeling [8].

## Pathophysiology and Diagnostic Assessment

### *Experimental IMR*

The first explanatory models of IMR were formulated by Burch in the early Sixties and focused on papillary muscle dysfunction as a determinant of increased annulo-papillary distance during systole and secondary leaflet prolapse [9,10]. However, experimental papillary muscle lesions leaving an intact adjacent free wall were unable to reproduce IMR [11]. Burch also introduced the concept of restricted leaflet motion, which was subsequently developed by others [9,12] showing the importance of ischemic areas including – but not confined to – the papillary muscle(s). Consequently, the latter are displaced outward, do not lie parallel to the longitudinal ventricular axis and perpendicular to the valve leaflets, are unable to balance the intraventricular forces generated by the contracting segments during systole, and ultimately result in restricted leaflet motion and malcoaptation. The distance between the papillary muscle tip and mitral annulus is increased and valve leaflets are tethered in the ventricular cavity (Figure 1). More recent studies performed by Kaul in the Nineties confirmed that papillary muscle ischemia does not cause prolapse or IMR, but that an ischemic or necrotic free wall *and* associated ventricular dilatation *may* generate IMR, despite normally perfused papillary muscles [13]. Furthermore, experimental damage confined to the papillary muscle and the adjacent myocardial segment dose not cause acute IMR, which stresses the importance of left ventricular dysfunction in the understanding of IMR pathophysiology, because reduced contractility implies a reduction of leaflet closure forces, which are outweighed by leaflet tethering, thus generating IMR [14]. Although this approach intrinsically limits the in vitro study of IMR because ventricular dysfunction is associated to dilatation, it served as a base for subsequent more sophisticated measurements (further enhanced by the introduction of three-dimensional echocardiography), including the annulo-papillary distance, which could correlate with the presence of IMR irrespective of ejection fraction or global left ventricular dimensions. In fact, ventricular dilatation per se does not invariably produce IMR, unless ejection fraction falls to less than 20% [15]. Rather, IMR is generated by a more spherical ventricular geometry, which displaces outward the posteromedial papillary muscle.

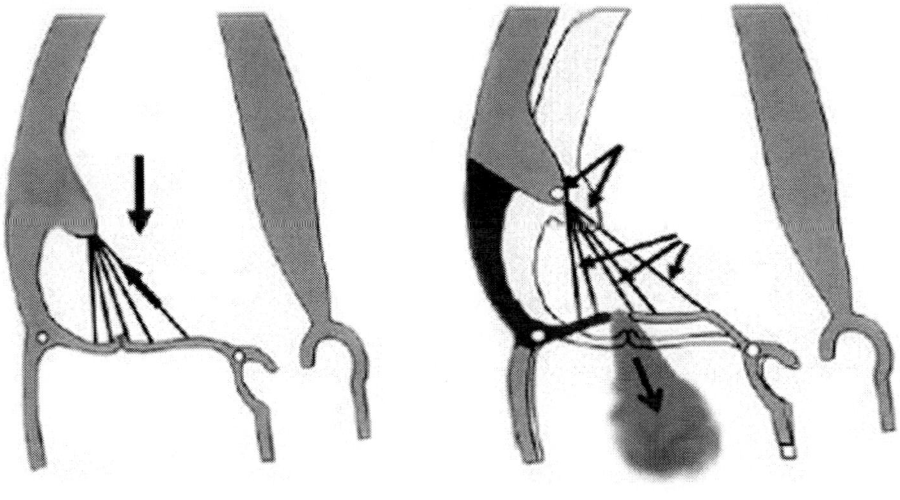

Figure 1. Schematic depiction of functional mitral regurgitation: the subvalvular apparatus is displaced outward and inferiorly causing malcoaptation of anatomically normal leaflets. Arrows indicate tethering forces and the regurgitant jet.

### *Inferior and anterior infarction*

Summarizing, the more recent experimental models distinguish IMR in two main subtypes, related to global or regional left ventricular remodeling [15-19]:

1. a purely dilative model, typical of extensive anterior infarction;
2. a so-called dysfunctional model, characteristic of inferoposterior infarction.

Irrespective of infarct location, the pathophysiological implications of IMR overlap those of mitral regurgitation on a different basis. IMR determines left ventricular volume overload and dilatation, and increased left ventricular wall stress, which further worsen papillary muscle displacement and tethering [20]. In other words, IMR generates IMR in a vicious circle. Echocardiographic analysis of the regurgitant pattern has often outlined how the IMR area and degree typically reach a peak during early and end-systole, and less severe regurgitation during mid-systole, when intraventricular pressure is increased. It may be inferred that tethering forces, rather than closure forces, are the major determinant of IMR. Because apical displacement causes greater tethering forces compared to lateral displacement, this might also explain why inferior infarcts cause IMR more commonly and earlier than anterior lesions, irrespective of global left ventricular dysfunction.

### *Annular dilatation*

Annular dilatation is an additional component of IMR, and causes further malcoaptation in the presence of leaflet tethering [16,21]. IMR alters mitral annular geometry and excursion during the cardiac cycle: the annulus is dilated and deformed caudally, and loses its typical saddle shape [22]. Annular dilatation is generally more severe in patients with IMR following anterior myocardial infarction [23]. Furthermore, although the process is more evident with respect to the posterior annulus, there are observations supporting global involvement of the entire circumference [24], whereas annular area is increased, and sphincter function is greatly reduced because annular contraction is lost [24,25].

### *Left ventricular dyssynchrony*

An additional component of IMR mechanisms is left ventricular dyssynchrony, which determines a conduction delay between the papillary muscle insertions. Prospective studies focused on the analysis of ventricular dyssynchrony in patients with non-organic mitral regurgitation – ischemic and non-ischemic – outlined the severity of leaflet tenting and ventricular remodeling as independent predictors of the severity of regurgitation. This suggests that ventricular remodeling involving the insertion of the papillary muscle is necessary to produce IMR, whereas dyssynchrony is only an aggravating factor [26]. In fact, ventricular dyssynchrony may be present irrespective of a myocardial scar, as commonly observed in patients with non-ischemic dilated cardiomyopathy. Different potential mechanisms may generate IMR in case of dyssynchrony:

- non-coordinated left ventricular contraction in segments supporting the papillary muscles alter mitral leaflet geometry and increase leaflet tethering [27];
- an improper atrio-ventricular relaxation time may generate an atrio-ventricular pressure gradient and IMR during diastole [28];
- most importantly, patients with left ventricular dysfunction closure forces on the mitral leaflets are reduced and are less efficient in case of dyssynchrony.

### *Dynamic IMR*

Despite the considerations listed above, IMR should always be considered *also* a dynamic dysfunction. Thus, variations of IMR severity, depending not only on the interactions between tethering and closure forces, but also on physiologic and pharmacologic factors, are commonly observed in clinical practice, which is of primary importance in the surgical setting. For example, inotropic agents increase left ventricular wall stress ($\partial P/\partial t$) and, consequently, closure forces, reducing IMR [29]. This is even more evident in case of inodilators because afterload and/or preload are also reduced. On the couterpart, general anesthesia, by unloading the left ventricle, reduces tethering forces and IMR [30]. Similar effects are obtained with diuretics.

IMR also varies greatly with physical exertion and the importance of the underestimation of IMR in resting conditions should be emphasized. Increased IMR severity during exercise is caused by an increased deformation of the mitral apparatus, which is directly dependent on the degree of the underlying ventricular remodeling. Conversely, the degree of IMR increase during exercise is inversely correlated with contractile reserve, independently of IMR degree at rest [31]. Stress echocardiography is nowadays an important diagnostic tool to stratify patients with IMR, and stress-induced IMR has been outlined as a prognostic risk factor for death and hospitalization for heart failure [32-34]. This relates to the occurrence of "fluctuating" left ventricular overload as a chronic mechanism of left ventricular remodeling [34]. Finally, acutely increased pulmonary artery pressure has been correlated with mortality [35,36].

### *Echocardiographic measurements*

Doppler echocardiography is the most important diagnostic tool to correctly define IMR clinically, implying a detailed morpho-functional evaluation of the left ventricle, including systolic and diastolic diameters and volumes, left ventricular sphericity, ejection fraction, diastolic function, and regional wall motion analysis.

The quantification of the severity of IMR can be estimated with different measurements, including the effective regurgitant orifice (ERO) area calculated with the proximal isovelocity surface area (PISA) method, which has the advantage of being non dependent of hemodynamic conditions and has been outlined as an independent risk factor for late death after myocardial infarction [37]. Other measurements, such as the vena contracta, although semi-quantitative, are also useful, especially in case of eccentric regurgitant jets. The most important measurements to define the degree of mitral valve apparatus deformation – mitral valve remodeling – are: annular dimensions, coaptation height of the leaflets (normal value in healthy subjets, 0.6 cm), and tenting area (normal, 1 $cm^2$). Recently, tenting volume has also been calculated with three-dimensional echocardiography [38].

The combination of different echocardiographic measurements allows the identification of the 2 main subgroups of patients outlined previously [39]:

1. patients with prior inferoposterior infarction show asymmetric leaflet tethering, so-called anterior leaflet "pseudo-prolapse", and a central and posterior eccentric regurgitant jet directed posteriorly. Left ventricular remodeling is more commonly regional and IMR develops early after infarction;
2. the second type is characterized by symmetric apical tethering of both leaflets, and a central jet, and is the typical presentation of patients with IMR following anterior

myocardial infarction. IMR generally develops late after infarction and ventricular remodeling is extensive.

## Surgical Technique

### *Annuloplasty*

The most commonly performed (and the only standardized) surgical procedure to correct functional MR or IMR is certainly represented by restrictive annuloplasty with implantation of an "undersized" prosthetic ring. Since Bolling first pioneered this therapeutic approach during the Nineties in patients with idiopathic dilated cardiomyopathy and severe functional MR [40], various prosthetic devices have become commercially available to correct different subtypes of valvular tethering [41]. Undersizing refers to the intertrigonal distance and the rationale of the procedure is to force leaflet coaptation by reducing annular diameters. Annuloplasty also directly corrects (posterior) annular dilatation (a common finding in case of IMR), but the most important concept of this strategy is to indirectly address a primarily ventricular problem at the valvular level. Consequently, the more dilated the ventricle, the higher the probability of an incomplete or insufficient (or impossible) correction of mitral malcoaptation [42-45]. The hazard of recurrent MR is also increased in the presence of advanced ventricular remodeling.

The choice of the device for annuloplasty represents a controversial issue and has generated considerable debate, including the opportunity of rigid versus flexible, complete versus incomplete, and symmetric versus asymmetric rings [46-49, Figure 2]. The latter include the ETlogix Carpentier-McCarthy-Adams and GeoForm rings (Edwards Lifesciences, Irvine, CA), and are intended to hyper-correct malcoaptation of the postero-medial and central mitral scallops. Suture posterior annuloplasty has also been performed, especially in conjunction with left ventricular restoration procedures [50].

Annular dynamics are abolished by rigid ring annuloplasty, which may be functionally detrimental, whereas flexible rings allow a more physiologic reconstruction, especially with respect to the posterior annulus [51-53]. Another possible concern of rigid mitral rings is postoperative systolic anterior motion and left ventricular outflow tract obstruction [51,52,54]. However, patients with IMR caused by prior inferior infarction, which represent a vast majority of patients with IMR, have akinetic postero-basal segments and an already compromised annular function. Furthermore, dynamic outflow obstruction is unlikely in patients with ventricular systolic dysfunction, in view of the flattened angle between the mitral and aortic annular planes. On the contrary a (semi-)rigid annular stabilization may better fix the valve, particularly during exercise. Importantly, a recent analysis outlined how prosthetic annular rigidity enhances the probability and earlier timing of left ventricular reverse remodelling after restrictive annuloplasty to correct IMR [55].

Summarizing, although this procedure does not directly address the ventricular causes of functional MR or IMR, restrictive annuloplasty is straighforward, technically reproducible and not time-consuming, and presents low operative mortality [40]. The major drawback is the non-negligible rate of recurrent MR, which may be moderate in over 25% of the patients 6 or 12 months after the operation [45,56-58].

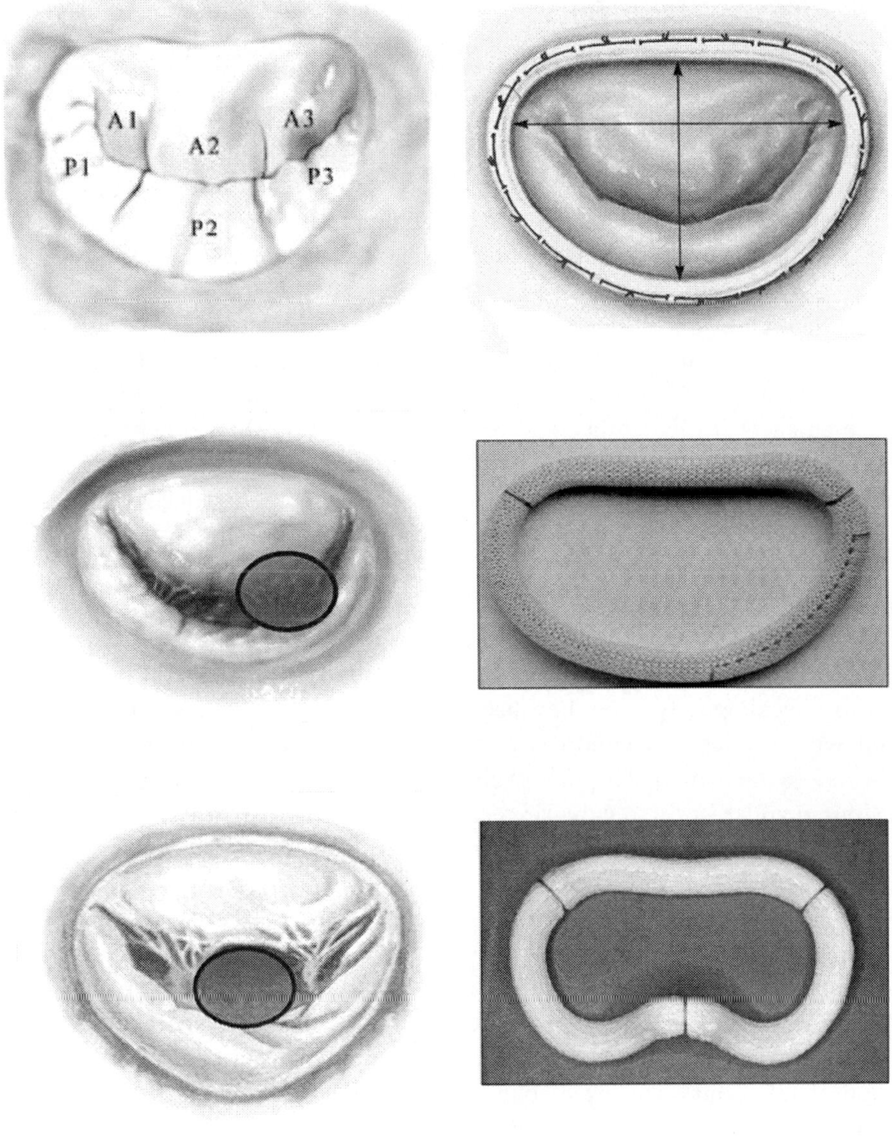


Figure 2. Mitral valve anatomy and annuloplaty prosthetic rings. Anatomy of the mitral scallops as viewed by the operating surgeon and traditional complete symmetric ring (*top*); eccentric regurgitant jet caused by postero-inferior myocardial infarction and asymmetric ring, more restrictive in the P3 region (*middle*); central jet following anterior infarction or dilated cardiomyopathy, and device specifically designed to hyper-correct symmetric leaflet tethering (*bottom*).

## *Procedures on the mitral leaflets*

**Posterior mitral valve restoration**

This technique addresses postero-medial malcoaptation and includes disinsertion of the 2 and P3 scallops at the base, eccentric postero-medial annular plication, and reimplantation of the disinserted leaflet by running suture on the plicated annulus, which is further stabilized with a ring or posterior band [59]. Strut chordae may be cut to enhance anterior leaflet mobilization.

**Anterior leaflet augmentation**

This procedure consists of pericardial patch enlargement of the anterior leaflet, which is incised parallel to the annulus for 3-4 cm [60]. Coaptation is more posterior, in the direction of the tethered papillary muscles. Associated annuloplasty is advisable, but undersizing is avoided. The technique appears most suitable for symmetric tethering patterns.

**Posterior leaflet extension**

This solution exemplifies another possible approach to IMR following posterior infarction. The tethered P2-P3 scallops are detached from the annulus and a pericardial patch is sutured to augment leaflet surface and enhance coaptation. Clinical experience is confined to case reports, always associated with restrictive annuloplasty. An experimental model from the Stanford group has subsequently shown that this approach reduces IMR in the acute phase, but fails to correct posterior leaflet restricted movement [61].

**Edge-to-edge**

Initially described for mitral prolapse in Barlow's disease, this technique creates a double mitral orifice by approximating the mitral leaflets, centrally or eccentrically. The technique is appealing for its simplicity, and has been employed for IMR (and functional MR) in association with restrictive annuloplasty, particularly for symmetric mitral tethering, and includes A2-P2 juxtaposition. This approach has generated considerable debate, and concerns have been raised with respect to valve area reduction.

### *Procedures on the subvalvular apparatus and papillary muscles*

**Chordal cutting**

This technique refers to surgical interruption of the strut chordae of the anterior leaflet to enhance leaflet mobility and thus coaptation. It can easily be combined to annuloplasty. Although concerns have been raised with respect to a possible role of the strut chordae in the preservation of left ventricular architecture and function, particularly between the Stanford and Harvard groups, T. David has shown how this adjunctive maneuver appears to lower the rate of recurrent IMR if compared to annuloplasty alone, with no negative effect on ventricular function [62].

**Papillary muscle sling**

This technique corrects papillary muscle dislocation through the mitral orifice by the implantation of a ring created by suturing the two ends of a 3-mm Gore-Tex prosthesis, which is passed around the papillary muscles' insertions and adjacent trabeculae [63]. It is most suitable for symmetric tethering, and is combined with annuloplasty. Clinical experience is limited to a case series.

**Posterior papillary muscle relocation**

In case of asymmetric tethering after inferior infarction, relocation of the tethered posterior papillary muscle offers another possible technical strategy [64]. Papillary muscle displacement is corrected with a polypropylene traction suture which tractions the papillary muscle tip to the mitral annulus at an established distance. Annuloplasty completes the procedure.

**Ring plus String suture**

Another similar solution has been recently proposed. Relocation is accomplished with a 4-0 polypropylene traction suture passed through the posterior papillary muscle tip and subsequently exteriorized outside the heart, passing through the fibrous body and the aortic root between the non-coronary and left coronary cusps [65]. This support is anatomically equivalent to a third-order neo-chorda. Experience is limited to a case series and the technique has the potential drawback of aortic valve injury. However, this approach offers the unique possibility to determine the length of the neo-chorda under transesophageal echocardiographic guidance on the beating heart.

### *Procedures at the ventricular level*

An exhaustive description of left ventricular reconstructive techniques, and their respective functional effects on the mitral apparatus are beyond the scope of this chapter. Specific procedures aimed at the correction of IMR are listed below.

**Papillary muscle approximation - imbrication**

This technique approximates the dislocated papillary muscle insertions and has originally been proposed with a transventricular approach during left ventricular restoration procedures. It has subsequently been performed transatrially associated with annuloplasty [66].

**Left ventricular infarct transversal plication**

Although experience is limited to a small case series, this technique addresses the primary cause of postero-medial tethering of the mitral apparatus by correcting postinfarction free wall expansion [67]. The infarct is plicated by passing sutures through teflon felt strips. The latter lie parallel to the posterior atrioventricular groove.

**Left ventricular infarct longitudinal plication**

This approach determines papillary muscle approximation and left ventricular volume reduction. Plication is performed parallel to the posterior interventricular groove, and may be performed on the beating (assisted) heart. Experience is confined to experimental models and initial clinical case reports [67,68].

**Coapsys and CorCap devices**

The Coapsys device consists of a midventricular "chorda" which is exteriorized and anchored to two external anterior and posterior pads. The distance between the pads is fixed by the device, the septal-lateral mitral annular diameter is reduced, ultimately enhancing leaflet coaptation [69]. Implantation of the device does not require cardioplegia.

The CorCap is a cardiac support wrapping device designed to prevent further remodeling in patients with dilated cardiomyopathy and has also been implanted in patients with functional MR [70].

### *Minimally invasive and transcatheter procedures*

Minimally invasive approaches, including Port-Access technology and a limited right thoracotomy, have been adopted for functional MR and represent an appealing strategy, particularly for reoperations with patents coronary bypass grafts.

Transcatheter solutions are also under investigation, and include the possibility to restrict the mitral orifice with implantation of a device through the coronary sinus at the subannular level, and by the creation of edge-to-edge repair with percutaneously implanted clips.

## Current Attitudes and Indications for Surgery

> "More than once in history the discovery of paradox has been the occasion for major reconstruction at the foundations of thought".
>
> [W. V. O. Quine, The Ways of Paradox and Other Essays, 1962]

Indications for surgery in case of functional MR are a widely debated issue. In the past, it has been thought that elimination of a low pressure runoff might worsen the overload of the left ventricle and contribute to the high mortality rates observed with mitral valve surgery (replacement) in patients with poor ventricular function. Because functional MR is primarily the consequence and not the cause of left ventricular dysfunction, the prognosis is likely more related to the underlying cardiomyopathic process. Functional MR leads to increased preload, increased wall tension, and increased ventricular workload, all of which contribute in a positive feedback loop to progressive heart failure.

The presence of MR itself is an independent risk factor of poor outcome, both in nonischemic and ischemic etiologies [71-73]. Even uncorrected mild MR, as well as moderate to severe MR associated with ischemic cardiomyopathy, is associated with reduced long-term survival [74]. In addition, it is a progressive disorder in which MR-related ventricular volume overload promotes further ventricular remodeling leading to worsening MR. Although it is clear that the advent of secondary MR is associated with a worse prognosis, it is unclear whether the worse outcomes stem from the MR itself or whether MR is simply a marker of progressive heart failure.

In this scenario, we should ask if there is evidence that correction of functional MR impacts the heart failure syndrome and will improve survival or only palliate symptoms. Operative mortality is also an important issue because a surgery is more likely to be denied in sicker and higher-risk patients. Ultimately, what evidence is there that patient survival is benefited by the elimination of mitral insufficiency in functional MR secondary to idiopathic cardiomyopathy or ischemic cardiomyopathy? Is there evidence that the elimination of MR results in LV reverse remodeling? What is "acceptable early mortality"?

Traditional teaching has been that surgical correction of MR in advanced heart failure with poor left ventricular function was associated with the hypothesis held that the mitral valve functions as a "pop off valve" for the failing ventricle and surgical correction results in prohibitive operative mortality [75] This view was challenged by Bolling during the Nineties [42,43,76-80] The Bolling hypothesis is that there is "*annular solution for ventricular problem…such that reconstruction of the mitral valve annulus geometric abnormality by an undersized ring restores valvular competency, alleviates excessive ventricular workload, improves ventricular geometry, and improves ventricular function.*" Miller and his Stanford colleagues [81] have reported, in an experimental model, that annular undersizing reduces the ventricular radius of curvature at the basal, equatorial and apical levels. This supports the concept that a small ring can restore a more elliptical ventricular shape. Surgical mortality of mitral valve replacement in the past was most likely the result of the loss of the subvalvular apparatus and not secondary to the loss of the pop off valve, as previously thought, underscoring the paramount importance of maintaining the integrity of annular and subvalvular continuity during mitral valve surgery. Bolling was the first to show a reasonable operative mortality (5%) in a series of 140 class III and class IV patients with an ejection fraction of 25% or less. He demonstrated improvement in LV ejection fraction and functional class, and decrease in ventricular volumes at a 3-to-5-year follow-up [76] The Cleveland Clinic group subsequently published similar results [79].

The most comprehensive updated analysis of MR correction in advanced heart failure patients with left ventricular dysfunction comes from Acker [70] and the Acorn trial evaluating the safety and efficacy of mitral surgery with and without implantation of a cardiac wrapping device (CorCap cardiac support device). Although not specifically randomized, this multicenter trial prospectively assessed the safety and efficacy of mitral valve surgery in almost 200 patients with advanced and prolonged heart failure (NYHA III-IV in 75% of the patients; mean duration of heart failure, 5 years; mean ejection fraction <25%; mean LV end-diastolic diameter of 70 mm). The vast majority of the patients had idiopathic or valvular cardiomyopathy, whereas only 10% had IMR. Remarkably, the operative mortality was only 1.6% and 2-year cumulative survival was >85% [43,77,79] Most patients received a complete small annuloplasty ring repair. MR degree was reduced from 2.7 to 0.6 at 18 months and remained stable. Most importantly, there was strong evidence of reverse ventricular remodeling by elimination of MR alone, reflected by decreased ventricular end-diastolic and end-systolic volume, and reduced sphericity, i.e., with the restoration of a more ellipsoid shape, at 2 years.

There is also accumulating evidence that the combination of surgical revascularization and mitral valve repair in patients with IMR will improve quality of life, reflected by an improved NYHA class [74,78,82-87] LV reverse remodeling has also been demonstrated in this context, particularly by Bax et al, as a result of either MV repair alone or in combination with revascularization [55,74,78]. In addition, a randomized study has recently outlined that the addition of mitral valve repair to isolated coronary bypass improves postoperative functional class and ventricular remodeling, decreases pulmonary arterial pressure, and reduces hospitalization rates for heart failure [87]. Updated reports also show that combined surgery for IMR in advanced heart failure patients can be performed with low mortality, generally below 5%.

It is now clear that the obsolete theory that the mitral valve in heart failure patients functions as a pop off valve has been disproven. [70,78,83-87] As Miller states, "*We now recognize that ignoring an important degree of ischemic MR at the time of coronary artery bypass surgery is not prudent because it will only limit the potential functional benefits to be obtained from the operation and compound the patient's poor life's expectancy*" [88]. Multiple studies suggest recurrent MR rates of 30-40% after repair, but generally fail to address ring selection and amount of downsizing as an important consideration for durable results in the ischemic MR population [49,89]. Consequently, current guidelines suggest that "mitral annuloplasty alone with a downsized annuloplasty ring is often effective in relieving IMR," and that "most patients with IMR seem to benefit from valve repair from using an undersized rigid ring annuloplasty". Early failure with recurrent MR reported in ischemic heart failure patients after coronary artery bypass surgery and annuloplasty ring was likely caused by the use of a flexible band or ring [49,89]]. which stands in sharp contrast to no recurrent MR after rigid and undersized ring implantation [55,82,88,90].

Currently, there are no randomized studies comparing mitral valve repair with medical management in patients with advanced heart failure and LV dysfunction. A retrospective analysis of patients with significant MR and ventricular dysfunction compared mitral valve annuloplasty with medical therapy alone [91]. This study did not report changes in ventricular size or function, or quality-of-life improvement, and data regarding recurrent MR or the type of annuloplasty were not included, but valve repair did not predict the clinical outcome with respect to survival, transplantation, or requirement of a ventricular assist device.

## Conclusion

In summary, current evidence suggests that functional MR in patients with advanced heart failure and left ventricular dysfunction can be corrected with low operative mortality in either ischemic or nonischemic cardiomyopathies. There are multiple prospective but nonrandomized series suggesting both a symptomatic benefit, as well as left ventricular reverse remodeling, in patients who undergo mitral valve repair in idiopathic dilated cardiomyopathies and coronary revascularization with mitral valve repair in patients with IMR. Stiffer annular stabilization and aggressive undersizing seem to correlate with a reduced hazard of recurrent MR and a higher probability of reverse remodeling. Despite the current lack of survival benefit conveyed by the elimination of MR, there is accumulating evidence that MV repair is certainly safe and results in symptomatic improvement, improved exercise capacity, and reversed remodeling in NYHA class III patients with nonischemic cardiomyopathy. Whether this is true in patients with ischemic cardiomyopathy is less clear, and robust randomized trials are necessary.

## References

[1] Adams, DH; Filsoufi, F; Aklog, L. Surgical treatment of ischemic mitral valve. *J Heart Valve Disease*, 2002, 11 (Suppl 1), S21-5.

[2] Grigioni, F; Detaint, D; Avierinos, JF; Scott, C; Tajik, J; Enriquez-Sarano, M. Contribution of ischemic mitral regurgitation to congestive heart failure after myocardial infarction. *J Am Coll Cardiol*, 2005, 45, 260-7.

[3] Agricola, E; Oppizzi, M; Pisani, M; Meris, A; Maisano, F; Margonato, A. Ischemic mitral regurgitation: mechanisms and echocardiographic classification. *Eur J Echocardiography*, 2008, 9, 207-21.

[4] Lamas, GA; Mitchell, GF; Flaker, GC; et al. Clinical significance of mitral regurgitation after acute myocardial infarction. Survival and Ventricular Enlargement Investigators. *Circulation*, 1997, 96, 827-33.

[5] Lehmann, KG; Francis, CK; Dodge, HT. Mitral regurgitation in early myocardial infarction. Incidence, clinical detection, and prognostic implications. TIMI Study Group. *Ann Intern Med*, 1992, 117, 10-7.

[6] Neskovic, AN; Marinkovic, J; Bojic, M; Popovic, AD. Early predictors of mitral regurgitation after acute myocardial infarction. *Am J Cardiol*, 1999, 84, 329-32.
[7] Grigioni, F; Enriquez-Sarano, M; Zehr, KJ; Bailey, KR; Tajik, AJ. Ischemic mitral regurgitation: long-term outcome and prognostic implications with quantitative Doppler assessment. *Circulation*, 2001, 103, 1759-64.
[8] Prifti, E; Bonacchi, M; Frati, G; et al. Should mild-to-moderate and moderate ischemic mitral regurgitation be corrected in patients with impaired left ventricular function undergoing simultaneous coronary revascularization? *J Card Surg*, 2001, 16, 473-83.
[9] Silverman, ME; Hurst, JW. The mitral complex: interaction of the anatomy, physiology, and pathology of the mitral annulus, mitral valve leaflets, chordae tendineae, and papillary muscles. *Am Heart J*, 1968, 76, 399-418.
[10] Burch, GE; DePasquale, NP; Phillips, JH. Clinical manifestations of papillary muscle dysfunction. *Arch Intern Med*, 1963, 112, 112-17.
[11] Burch, GE; DePasquale, NP; Phillips, JH. The syndrome of papillary muscle dysfunction. *Am Heart J*, 1968, 75, 399-415.
[12] Mittal, AK; Langston, M Jr.; Cohn, KE; Selzer, A; Kerth, WJ. Combined papillary muscle and left ventricular wall dysfunction as a cause of mitral regurgitation: an experimental study. *Circulation*, 1971, 44, 174-80.
[13] Liel-Cohen, N; Guerrero, JL; Otsuji, Y; et al. Design of a new surgical approach for ventricular remodelling to relieve ischemic mitral regurgitation: insights from 3-dimensional echocardiography. *Circulation*, 2000, 101, 2756-63.
[14] Kaul, S; Spotnitz, WD; Glasheen, WP; Touchstone, DA. Mechanism of ischemic mitral regurgitation: an experimental evaluation. *Circulation*, 1991, 84, 2167-80.
[15] He, S; Fontaine, AA; Schwammenthal, E; Yoganathan, AP; Levine, RA. Integrated mechanism for functional mitral regurgitation: leaflet restriction versus coapting force: in vitro studies. *Circulation*, 1997, 96, 1826-34.
[16] Messas, E; Guerrero, JL; Handschumacher, MD; et al. Paradoxic decrease in ischemic mitral regurgitation with papillary muscle dysfunction: insights from threedimensional and contrast echocardiography with strain rate measurement. *Circulation*, 2001, 104, 1952-7.
[17] Otsuji, Y; Handschumacher, MD; Schwammenthal, E; et al. Insights from three-dimensional echocardiography into the mechanism of functional mitral regurgitation: direct in vivo demonstration of altered leaflet tethering geometry. *Circulation*, 1997, 96, 1999-2008.
[18] Lai, DT; Tibayan, FA; Myrmel, T; et al. Mechanistic insights into posterior mitral leaflet inter-scallop malcoaptation during acute ischemic mitral regurgitation. *Circulation*, 2002, 106(suppl I), I40-5.
[19] Otsuji, Y; Gilon, D; Jiang, L; et al. Restricted diastolic opening of the mitral leaflets in patients with left ventricular dysfunction: evidence for increased valve tethering. *J Am Coll Cardiol*, 1998, 32, 398-404.
[20] Yiu, SF; Enriquez-Sarano, M; Tribouilloy, C; Seward, JB; Tajik, AJ. Determinants of the degree of functional mitral regurgitation in patients with systolic left ventricular dysfunction: a quantitative clinical study. *Circulation*, 2000, 102, 1400-6.
[21] Boltwood, CM; Tei, C; Wong, M; Shah, PM. Quantitative echocardiography of the mitral complex in dilated cardiomyopathy: the mechanism of functional mitral regurgitation. *Circulation*, 1983, 68, 498-508.

[22] Srichai, MB; Grimm, RA; Stillman, AE; et al. Ischemic mitral regurgitation: impact of the left ventricle and mitral valve in patients with left ventricular systolic dysfunction. *Ann Thorac Surg*, 2005, 80, 170-8.

[23] Salgo, IS; Gorman, JH 3rd; Gorman, RC; et al. Effect of annular shape on leaflet curvature in reducing mitral leaflet stress. *Circulation*, 2002, 106, 711-7.

[24] Watanabe, N; Ogasawara, Y; Yamaura, Y; et al. Mitral annulus flattens in ischemic mitral regurgitation: geometric differences between inferior and anterior myocardial infarction: a realtime 3-dimensional echocardiographic study. *Circulation*, 2005, 112, I458-62.

[25] Ahmad, RM; Gillinov, AM; McCarthy, PM; et al. Annular geometry and motion in human ischemic mitral regurgitation: novel assessment with three-dimensional echocardiography and computer reconstruction. *Ann Thorac Surg*, 2004, 78, 2063-8.

[26] De Simone, R; Wolf, I; et al. A clinical study of annular geometry and dynamics in patients with ischemic mitral regurgitation: new insights into asymmetrical ring annuloplasty. *Eur J Cardiothorac Surg*, 2006, 29, 355-61.

[27] Agricola, E; Oppizzi, M; Galderisi, M; et al. Role of regional mechanical dyssynchrony as a determinant of functional mitral regurgitation in patients with left ventricular systolic dysfunction. *Heart*, 2006, 92, 1390-5.

[28] Kanzaki, H 3rd; Bazaz, R; Schwartzman, D; Dohi, K; Sade, LE; Gorcsan, J 3rd. A mechanism for immediate reduction in mitral regurgitation after cardiac resynchronization therapy: insights from mechanical activation strain mapping. *J Am Coll Cardiol*, 2004, 44, 1619-25.

[29] Appleton, CP; Basnight, MA; Gonzalez, MS. Diastolic mitral regurgitation with atrioventricular conduction abnormalities: relation of mitral flow velocity to transmitral pressure gradients in conscious dogs. *J Am Coll Cardiol*, 1991, 18, 843-9.

[30] Keren, G; Katz, S; Strom, J; Sonnenblick, EH; LeJemtel, TH. Dynamic mitral regurgitation. An important determinant of the hemodynamic response to load alterations and inotropic therapy in severe heart failure. *Circulation*, 1989, 80, 306-13.

[31] Bach, DS; Deeb, GM; Bolling, SF. Accuracy of intraoperative transesophageal echocardiography for estimating the severity of functional mitral regurgitation. *Am J Cardiol*, 1995, 76, 508-12.

[32] Lancellotti, P; Lebrun, F; Pierard, LA. Determinants of exercise-induced changes in mitral regurgitation in patients with coronary artery disease and left ventricular dysfunction. *J Am Coll Cardiol*, 2003, 42, 1921-8.

[33] Lancellotti, P; Pierard, LA. Chronic ischemic mitral regurgitation: exercise testing reveals its dynamic component. *Eur Heart J*, 2005, 26, 1816-7.

[34] Lancellotti, P ; Troisfontaines, P ; Toussaint, AC ; Pierard, LA. Prognostic importance of exercise-induced changes in mitral regurgitation in patients with chronic ischemic left ventricular dysfunction. *Circulation*, 2003, 108, 1713-7.

[35] Pierard, LA; Lancellotti, P. The role of ischemic mitral regurgitation in the pathogenesis of acute pulmonary edema. *N Engl J Med*, 2004, 351, 1627-34.

[36] Lebrun, F; Lancellotti, P; Pierard, LA. Quantitation of functional mitral regurgitation during bicycle exercise in patients with heart failure. *J Am Coll Cardiol*, 2001, 38, 1685-92.

[37] Bursi, F; Enriquez-Sarano, M; Jacobsen, SJ; Roger, VL. Mitral regurgitation after nyocardial infarction. A review. *Am J Med*, 2006, 119, 103-12.

[38] Zoghbi, WA; Enriquez-Sarano, M; Foster, E; et al. American Society of Echocardiography. Recommendations for evaluation of the severity of native valvular regurgitation with two-dimensional and Doppler echocardiography. *J Am Soc Echocardiogr*, 2003, 16, 777-802.

[39] Gorman, JH 3rd; Gorman, RC; Plappert, T; et al. Infarct size and location determine development of mitral regurgitation in the sheep model. *J Thorac Cardiovasc Surg*, 1998, 115, 615-22.

[40] Fedak, PWM; McCarthy, PM; Bonow, RO. Evolving concepts and technologies in mitral valve repair. *Circulation*, 2008, 117, 963-74.

[41] Menicanti, L; Di Donato, M; Frigiola, A; et al. Ischemic mitral regurgitation: intraventricular papillary muscle imbrication without mitral ring during left ventricular restoration. *J Thorac Cardiovasc Surg*, 2002, 123, 1041-50.

[42] Bolling, SF; Pagani, FD; Deeb, GM; Bach, DS. Intermediate term outcome of mitral reconstruction in cardiomyopathy. *J Thorac Cardiovasc Surg*, 1998, 115, 381-6.

[43] Gummert, JF; Rahmel, A; Bucerius, J; et al. Mitral valve repair in patients with end stage cardiomyopathy: who benefits? *Eur J Cardiothorac Surg*, 2003, 23, 1017-22.

[44] Gillinov, AM; Wierup, PN; Blackstone, EH; et al. Is repair preferable to replacement for ischemic mitral regurgitation? *J Thorac Cardiovasc Surg*, 2001, 122, 1125-41.

[45] Tahta, SA; Oury, JH; Maxwell, JM; Hiro, SP; Duran, CM. Outcome after mitral valve repair for functional ischemic mitral regurgitation. *J Heart Valve Dis*, 2002, 11, 11-8.

[46] Levine, RA ; Hung, J ; Otsuji, Y ; et al. Mechanistic insights into functional mitral regurgitation. *Curr Cardiol Rep*, 2002, 4, 125-9.

[47] McCarthy, PM. Does the intertrigonal distance dilate? Never say never. *J Thorac Cardiovasc Surg*, 2002, 124, 1078-9.

[48] Daimon, M; Fukuda, S; Adams, DH; et al. Mitral valve repair with Carpentier-McCarthy-Adams IMR ETlogix annuloplasty ring for ischemic mitral regurgitation: early echocardiographic results from a multi-center study. *Circulation*, 2006, 114(Suppl.1), I588-93.

[49] McGee, EC; Gillinov, AM; Blackstone, EH; et al. Recurrent mitral regurgitation after annuloplasty for functional ischemic mitral regurgitation. *J Thorac Cardiovasc Surg*, 2004, 128, 916-24.

[50] Di Donato, M; Castelvecchio, S; Kukulski, T; et al. Surgical ventricular restoration: left ventricular shape influence on cardiac function, clinical status, and survival. *Ann Thorac Surg*, 2009, 87, 455-61.

[51] Kreindel, MS; Schivone, WA; Level, JM; Cosgrove, D. Systolic anterior motion of the mitral valve after Carpentier ring valvuloplasty for mitral valve prolapse. *Am J Cardiol*, 1986, 57, 408-12.

[52] Spence, PA; Peniston, CM; David, TE; et al. Toward a better understanding of the etiology of left ventricular dysfunction after mitral valve replacement: an experimental study with possible clinical implications. *Ann Thorac Surg*, 1986, 41, 363-71.

[53] Van Rijk-Zwikker, GL; Mast, F; Shipperheyn, JJ; et al. Comparison of rigid and flexible rings for annuloplasty of the porcine mitral valve. *Circulation*, 1990, 82(suppl 4), IV58-IV64.

[54] Votta, E; Maisano, F; Bolling, SF; Alfieri, O; Montevecchi, FM; Redaelli, A. The Geoform disease-specific annuloplasty system: a finite element study. *Ann Thorac Surg*, 2007, 84, 92-107.

[55] Pocar, M; Passolunghi, D; Moneta, A; et al. Baseline left ventricular function and surgical annular stiffening to predict outcome and reverse left ventricular remodeling after undersized annuloplasty for intermediate-degree ischemic mitral regurgitation. *J Thorac Cardiovasc Surg*, 2009 Dec 5 [Epub ahead of print] doi:10.1016/j.jtcvs.2009.08.043.
[56] Bolling, SF; Deeb, GM; Bach, DS. Mitral valve reconstruction in elderly, ischemic patients. *Chest*, 1996, 109, 35-40.
[57] Von Oppell, UO; Stemmet, F; Brink, J; Commerford, PJ; Heijke, SA. Ischemic mitral valve repair surgery. *J Heart Valve Dis*, 2000, 9, 64-74.
[58] Hung, J; Papakostas, L; Tahta, SA; et al. Mechanism of recurrent ischemic mitral regurgitation after annuloplasty: continued LV remodeling as a moving target. *Circulation*, 2004, 110(Suppl 2), II85-II90.
[59] Fundarò, P; Pocar, M; Moneta, A; Donatelli, F; Grossi, A. Posterior mitral valve restoration for ischemic mitral regurgitation. *Ann Thorac Surg*, 2004, 77, 729-30.
[60] Kincaid, EH; Riley, RD; Hines, MH; Hammon, WJ; Kon, ND. Anterior leaflet augmentation for ischemic mitral regurgitation. *Ann Thorac Surg*, 2004, 78, 564-8.
[61] Langer, F; Rodriguez, F; Cheng, A; et al. Posterior mitral leaflet extension: an adjunctive repair option for ischemic mitral regurgitation? *J Thorac Cardiovasc Surg*, 2006, 131, 868-77.
[62] Borger, MA; Murphy, PM; Alam, A; et al. Initial results of chordal-cutting operation for ischemic mitral regurgitation. *J Thorac Cardiovasc Surg*, 2007, 133, 1483-92.
[63] Hvass, U; Tapia, M; Baron, F; Pouzet, B; Shafy, A. Papillary muscle sling: a new functional approch to mitral repair in patients with ischemic left ventricular dysfunction and functional mitral regurgitation. *Ann Thorac Surg*, 2003, 75, 809-11.
[64] Kron, IL; Green, GR; Cope, TJ. Surgical relocation of the posterior papillary muscle in chronic ischemic mitral regurgitation. *Ann Thorac Surg*, 2002, 74, 600-1.
[65] RING plus STRING: papillary muscle repositioning as an adjuvant repair technique for ischemic mitral regurgitation. *J Thorac Cardiovasc Surg*, 2007, 133, 247-9.
[66] Rama, A; Praschker, L; Barreda, E; Gandjbakhch, I. Papillary muscle approximation for functional ischemic mitral regurgitation. *Ann Thorac Surg*, 2007, 84, 2130-1.
[67] Ramzi, R; Nawwar, AA; Mohammadi, S; et al. Left ventricular infart plication restores mitral function in chronic ischemic mitral regurgitation. *J Thorac Cardiovasc Surg*, 2005, 129, 440-2.
[68] Garcìa-Fuster, R; Rodrìguez, I; Estornell, J; Martìnez-Leon, J. A combined approach for ischemic mitral valve regurgitation: scar placation and the role of magnetic resonance imaging. *J Thorac Cardiovasc Surg*, 2008, 135, 1169-72.
[69] Grossi, eA; Woo, YJ; Schwartz, CF; et al. Comparison of Coapsys annuloplasty and internal reduction mitral annuloplasty in the randomized treatment of functional ischemic mitral regurgitation: impact on the left ventricle. *J Thorac Cardiovasc Surg*, 2006, 131, 1095-8.
[70] Acker, MA; Bolling, S; Shemin, R; et al. Mitral valve surgery in heart failure: insights from the Acorn clinical trial. *J Thorac Cardiovasc Surg*, 2006, 132, 568-77.
[71] Koelling, TM; Aaronson, KD; Cody, RJ; Bach, DS; Armstrong, WF. Prognostic significance of mitral regurgitation and tricuspid regurgitation in patients with left ventricular systolic dysfunction. *Am Heart J*, 2002, 144, 524-9.

[72] Robbins, JD; Maniar, PB; Cotts, W; Parker, MA; Bonow, RO; Gheorghiade, M. Prevalence and severity of mitral regurgitation in chronic systolic heart failure. *Am J Cardiol*, 2003, 91, 360-2.

[73] Trichon, BH; Felker, GM; Shaw, LK; Cabell, CH; O'Connor, CM. Relation of frequency and severity of mitral regurgitation to survival among patients with left ventricular systolic dysfunction and heart failure. *Am J Cardiol*, 2003, 91, 538-43.

[74] Braun, J; Bax, JJ; Versteegh, MI; et al. Preoperative left ventricular dimensions predict reverse remodeling following restrictive mitral annuloplasty in ischemic mitral regurgitation. *Eur J Cardiothorac Surg*, 2005, 27, 847-53.

[75] Patel, JB; Borgeson, DD; Barnes, ME; Rihal, CS; Daly, RC; Redfield, MM. Mitral regurgitation in patients with advanced systolic heart failure. *J Card Fail*, 2004, 10, 285-91.

[76] Bach, DS; Bolling, SF. Improvement following correction of secondary mitral regurgitation in end-stage cardiomyopathy with mitral annuloplasty. *Am J Cardiol*, 1996, 78, 966-9.

[77] Badhwar, V; Bolling, SF. Mitral valve surgery in the patient with left ventricular dysfunction. *Semin Thorac Cardiovasc Surg*, 2002, 14, 133-6.

[78] Bax, JJ; Braun, J; Somer, ST; et al. Restrictive annuloplasty and coronary revascularization in ischemic mitral regurgitation results in reverse left ventricular remodeling. *Circulation*, 2004, 110(suppl 1), II103-II108.

[79] Bishay, ES; McCarthy, PM; Cosgrove, DM; et al. Mitral valve surgery in patients with severe left ventricular dysfunction. *Eur J Cardiothorac Surg*, 2000, 17, 213-21.

[80] Romano, MA; Bolling, SF. Update on mitral repair in dilated cardiomyopathy. *J Card Surg*, 2004, 19, 396-400.

[81] Tibayan, FA; Rodriguez, F; Langer, F; et al. Undersized mitral annuloplasty alters left ventricular shape during acute ischemic mitral regurgitation. *Circulation*, 2004, 110, II98-II102.

[82] Braun, et al. Long term follow-up confirms left ventricular reverse remodeling following restrictive mitral annuloplasty and CABG in ischemic MR. Presented at the AATS 87th Annual Meeting, San Diego, California, May 2007.

[83] Di Donato, M; Frigiola, A; Menicanti, L; et al. Moderate ischemic MR and CABG: effect of mitral repair on clinical outcome. *J Heart Valve Dis*, 2003, 12, 272-9.

[84] Geidel, S; Schneider, C; Lass, M; et al. Changes of myocardial function after combined coronary revascularization and mitral valve downsizing in patients with ischemic mitral regurgitation and advanced cardiomyopathy. *Thorac Cardiovasc Surg*, 2007, 55, 106.

[85] Westenberg, JJ; van der Geest, RJ; Lamb, HL; et al. MRI to evaluate left atrial and ventricular reverse remodeling after restrictive mitral annuloplasty in dilated cardiomyopathy. *Circulation*, 2005, 112, I437-42.

[86] Ganzoni, LM; Kern, JA; Swenson, BR; et al. A change in perspective: results for ischemic mitral valve repair are similar to mitral valve repair for degenerative disease. *Ann Thorac Surg*, 2007, 84, 750-8.

[87] Fattouch, K; Guccione, F; Sampognaro, R; et al. POINT: Efficacy of adding mitral valve restrictive annuloplasty to coronary artery bypass grafting in patients with moderate ischemic mitral valve regurgitation: a randomized trial. *J Thorac Cardiovasc Surg*, 2009, 138, 278-85.

[88] Miller, DC. Ischemic mitral regurgitation redux—to repair or to replace? *J Thorac Cardiovasc Surg*, 2001, 122, 1059-62.

[89] Mihaljevic, T; Lam, BK; Rajeswaran, J; et al. Impact of mitral valve annuloplasty combined with revascularization in patients with functional ischemic MR. *J Am Coll Cardiol*, 2007, 49, 2191-201.

[90] Spoor, MT; Geltz, A; Bolling, SF. Flexible versus nonflexible mitral valve rings for congestive heart failure: differential durability of repair. *Circulation*, 2006, 114, I67-71.

[91] Wu, AH; Aaronson, KD; Bolling, SF; Pagani, FD; Welch, K; Koelling, TM. Impact of mitral valve annuloplasty on mortality risk in patients with mitral regurgitation and left ventricular systolic dysfunction. *J Am Coll Cardiol*, 2005, 45, 381-7.

In: Advances in Cardiovascular Research, Volume 1
Editors: L. Schmitt, T. Konig, pp. 269-285
ISBN: 978-1-60741-720-0


*Chapter XI*

# Confounding of Genetic and Environmental Factors in Pregnancy-Induced Hypertension

***Gen Kobashi****
Department of Global Health and Epidemiology, Hokkaido University Graduate School of Medicine, Sapporo, Japan

## Abstract

Pregnancy-Induced Hypertension (PIH) is one of the most common causes of maternal and neonatal mortality. It is a multifactorial disease with genetic and environmental factors involved in its etiology. We have carried out molecular epidemiologic research on Japanese subjects in order to identify genetic variants associated with PIH, and to analyze confounding genetic and environmental factors involved in the pathophysiology of PIH. Self-administered questionnaires were returned by the subjects between 1 and 6 months after delivery. The candidate genetic variants were identified by means of a PCR-RFLP method. T235 of *AGT*, C1166 of *AT1* and Asp298 of *NOS3* were respectively associated with PIH, although no significant associations were found between PIH and the common genetic variants of *ACE, FV, MTHFR, B3AR, TNF-A, PAI-1, GSTP1, mEH,* or *LPL*. However, in subgroup analyses, a significant association of the TT genotype of *AGT* was maintained only in women possessing the 4G/4G genotype of *PAI-1*, while that of the GA or AA genotype of *NOS3* was maintained only in women possessing the 5G/5G or 4G/5G genotype, suggesting that there must be at least two kinds of possible pathogenetic pathways for the manifestation of severe PIH.

Furthermore, in analyses using genetic, environmental and lifestyle factors, 9 factors were significantly associated with PIH on univariate analysis, and 5 factors, i.e. "prepregnancy BMI > or = 24 kg/m2", "family history of hypertension", "TT genotype of AGT", "mentally stressful condition during pregnancy," and "salty dishes preferred

* Corresponding author: Research Center for Charged Particle Therapy, National Institute of Radiological Science, 4-9-1 Anagawa, Chiba 263-8555, Japan, E-mail: genkoba@goo.jp, TEL: +81-43-206-3241, FAX: +81-43-206-3245

during pregnancy" were found to be independent and potent risk factors for PIH on multivariate analysis. Dividing the subjects into 2 subgroups according to whether they possessed "TT genotype of AGT" or not, we identified acquired risk factors before and during pregnancy for PIH in each of the groups. A multivariate analysis identified "mentally stressful condition" as a potent significant risk factor during pregnancy in the former subgroup. However, there were no significant risk factors concerning "mental stress" in the latter subgroup. Through further exploration of the risk factors associated with PIH, useful insights should emerge for development of new and effective preventive measures for a range of multifactorial diseases.

## Introduction

Pregnancy-induced hypertension (PIH) is one of the most common causes of maternal and neonatal mortality. It is believed to be a complex syndrome made up of certain pathophysiological pathways, each of which is comprised of a combination of PIH susceptibility genetic variants and environmental risk factors. The analysis of both PIH susceptibility genes and the lifestyle factors associated with PIH has been anticipated to help identify the interaction between these factors, since there is an increasing need for the development of effective preventive measures for PIH that takes into consideration the characteristics of individual patients. Recent developments in genetic epidemiology improved our understanding of the role of genetic and environmental factors in the complex etiology of PIH[1].

We have carried out molecular epidemiologic research in the Japanese subjects in order to identify genetic variants associated with PIH, and to analyze confounding genetic and environmental factors involved in the pathophysiology of PIH. This paper reports the results obtained thus far from this research, and also provides some prospects for future research on PIH.

## Subjects and Methods

Patients with PIH and normal controls were recruited from women aged 20-34 years with primiparous and single-fetus pregnancies delivered at Hokkaido University Hospital and its affiliated hospitals between 1993 and 1998. PIH was diagnosed (following the criteria of the consensus report [2]) when at least one of the following criteria was met: (1) increase of systolic blood pressure of ≥30 mmHg, and/or (2) increase of diastolic blood pressure of ≥15 mmHg, compared to the average value before 20 weeks of gestation, or (3) blood pressure ≥140/90 mmHg after 20 weeks of gestation. Women with blood pressure ≥140/90 mmHg and proteinuria prior to 20 weeks of gestation or at 4 weeks after delivery were excluded from the PIH subjects, because they may have had latent hypertensive or renal diseases. Normal controls were women who did not experience hypertension, proteinuria, or edema during their pregnancies and for 1 month after delivery. Women with HELLP (hemolysis, liver dysfunction, low platelets) syndrome, renal disease, diabetes mellitus, amniotic volume abnormalities, or fetal anomalies were excluded from this study.

Self-administered questionnaires were returned by the subjects between 1 and 6 months after delivery. The semiquantitative questionnaire asked questions about (1) characteristics of mother and baby, (2) symptoms, (3) physical practices and habits during pregnancy, (4) dietary habits, food preferences, and consumption, (5) exercise, sleep, stress, and physical burden, and (6) smoking and drinking (alcohol consumption) before pregnancy and during pregnancy (the 20th to 25th gestational week)[3]. Parity, maternal age, family history (FH) of hypertension and prepregnancy BMI were determined from medical records. Pregnancies with prepregnancyBMI≥24 were defined as prepregnancy high BMI. Written informed consent for the study was obtained from every subject, following the guidelines for informed consent in epidemiologic studies, which was approved by the Institutional Review Board of Hokkaido University.

Genomic DNA was extracted from 1.0 ml of whole blood using DNA Extractor WB Kits (Wako Chemicals, Tokyo, Japan). The variant M235T of the angiotensinogen gene (*AGT*), A1166C of the angiotensin II type 1 receptor gene (*A1R*), Insertion/ Deletion of the angiotensin converting enzyme gene *(ACE*), Leiden mutation of the Factor V gene (*FV*), C677T of the Methylenetetrahydrofolate reductase gene *(MTHFR*), T64A of the beta 3 adrenergic receptor gene (*B3AR*), Glu298Asp of the endothelial nitric oxide synthase gene (*NOS3*), G-308A of the tumor necrosis factor gene (*TNF-A*), 4G/5G of the plasminogen activator inhibitor-1 gene (*PAI-1*), Ile105Val of the glutathione S-transferase P1 gene (*GSTP1*), Tyr113His of the Microsomal epoxide hydrolase gene (*mEH*), and S447X of the Lipoprotein lipase gene (*LPL*) were identified by using the PCR-RFLP methods previously described, respectively, followed by 1.5% agarose electrophoresis or 10% polyacrylamide electrophoresis [4-10].

Statistical analyses were performed after all of variables had been dichotomized. For example, in the analysis using *AGT* genotypes as a genetic factor, the number of T235 homozygous (TT) women was compared with that of M235 homozygous (MM) plus heterozygous (MT) women, and the answers of the questions were first transformed to binary or yes/no type answers by pooling them according to their categories (summarized in the Table footnotes). Univariate analysis was carried out using the chi-squared test (df = 1). Yates' correction for continuity was used when an observed number was ≤5. A stepwise method was applied to identify significant ($p<0.05$) factors in multivariate analysis of the factors which were significantly associated with PIH in univariate analysis. A multiple logistic model was applied to evaluate the odds ratios of the major risk factors. Furthermore, for tree-based analysis, the subjects were divided into 2 subgroups according to whether they possessed “the TT genotype of AGT” (n=175) or not (n=109), and the univariate and the multivariate analyses described above were carried out for these 2 groups. All statistical analyses were conducted using a statistical analysis system package (SAS Institute Inc., Cary, NC).

# Results

## Associations between Pregnancy-Induced Hypertension and the Genetic Variants

The rate of the homozygosity of T235 (TT) with *AGT* was significantly higher in PIH patients than in controls among the subjects aged 20-34 years (Table 1)[4]. The frequency of women with the AC+CC genotypes of *AT1* was significantly higher in PIH cases than controls ($p<0.05$) among primiparous subjects, whereas there were no significant differences found for multiparous subjects (Table 2)[5]. The frequency of GA+AA genotypes of *NOS3* was significantly higher in PIH cases than controls ($p<0.01$) (Table 3)[6]. Multivariate analysis revealed the following 4 potent independent risk factors for PIH: "family history of hypertension (FH of HT) ", " TT genotype of *AGT*", "GA+AA genotype of *NOS3*", and "prepregnancy high body mass (BMI ≥ 24)", after adjusting for maternal age and parity. The odds ratios of the factors were 2.7, 2.3, 2.2 and 2.1, respectively, in a multiple logistic model (Table 4)[6].

Table 1. Distribution of M235T variant of angiotensinogen gene

| Diagnosis | Age | Gravidity | No. | MM | MT | TT | Freq. of TT (%) |
|---|---|---|---|---|---|---|---|
| PIH | 20-34 | G=0 | 51 | 1 | 3 | 47 | 92* |
| | | G>0 | 38 | 0 | 5 | 33 | 87* |
| | | total | 89 | 1 | 8 | 80 | 90* |
| | 35≦ | G=0 | 6 | 0 | 1 | 5 | 83 |
| | | G>0 | 18 | 1 | 6 | 11 | 61 |
| | | total | 24 | 1 | 7 | 16 | 66 |
| Controls | 20-34 | total | 310 | 13 | 123 | 174 | 56 |
| | 35≦ | total | 58 | 5 | 20 | 33 | 57 |

PIH: pregnancy-induced hypertension
* $p<0.001$ vs. 20-34 aged controls by chi-square test

Table 2. Distribution of A1166C variant of angiotensin II type1 receptor gene

| Diagnosis | Parity | No. | AA | AC | CC | Freq. of AA+AC (%) |
|---|---|---|---|---|---|---|
| PIH | P=0 | 82 | 66 | 15 | 1 | 20* |
| | P>0 | 62 | 56 | 6 | 0 | 10 |
| severe PIH | P=0 | 69 | 53 | 15 | 1 | 23** |
| Controls | P=0 | 181 | 165 | 14 | 2 | 9 |
| | P>0 | 134 | 116 | 15 | 3 | 13 |

All subjects are 20-34 years old.
PIH: pregnancy-induced hypertension
* $p<0.05$, ** $p<0.01$ vs. P=0 controls by chi-square test

Table 3. Distribution of Glu298Asp variant of endothelial nitric oxide synthase gene

| Diagnosis | Parity | No. | GG | GA | AA | Freq. of GA+AA (%) |
|---|---|---|---|---|---|---|
| PIH | | 152 | 117 | 35 | 0 | 23** |
| | P=0 | 90 | 71 | 19 | 0 | 21* |
| | P>0 | 62 | 46 | 16 | 0 | 26* |
| Controls | | 335 | 294 | 41 | 0 | 12 |
| | P=0 | 191 | 168 | 23 | 0 | 12 |
| | P>0 | 144 | 126 | 18 | 0 | 13 |

PIH: pregnancy-induced hypertension
* p<0.05, ** p<0.01 vs. controls by chi-square test

Table 4. Odds ratios of selected risk factors existing before pregnancy for pregnancy-induced hypertension calculated by multivariate analysis

| | Odds Ratios (95% Confidence Interval) |
|---|---|
| Family history of hypertension | 2.7 (1.6-4.4)** |
| TT genotype of *AGT* | 2.3 (1.5-3.5)** |
| GA+AA genotype of *NOS3* | 2.2 (1.3-3.7)* |
| Prepregnancy high body mass (BMI≧24) | 2.1 (1.3-3.4)* |
| Maternal Age≧35 | - |
| Primiparity | - |

BMI: Body mass index
* p<0.05, ** p<0.01.

The distribution of candidate genes for hypertension pregnancy is shown in Table 5. There were no significant associations between the common genetic variants and PIH in *ACE*, *FV*, *MTHFR*, *B3AR*, *TNF-A*, *PAI-1*, *GSTP1*, *mEH*, or *LPL*[7-11]. *However,* in the subgroup possessing the 4G/4G genotype of *PAI-1*, the frequency of the TT genotype of *AGT* was significantly higher in severe PIH (77.5%) than controls (56.2%; p=0.008<0.0125), while no significant difference was observed between the two groups (70.8% vs. 61.2%) in the subgroup possessing the 5G/5G or 4G/5G genotypes of *PAI-1* (Table 6). The odds ratios (ORs) and their 95% confidence intervals (95%CIs) in women with the TT genotype of *AGT* without the 4G/4G genotype of *PAI-1*, with the 4G/4G genotype of *PAI-1* but without the TT genotype of *AGT,* and with both of these genotypes compared to those without both of these genotypes were 1.54 (0.89-2.68), 0.73 (0.33-1.61) and 1.84 (1.01-3.34), respectively. On the other hand, in the subgroup possessing the 5G/5G or 4G/5G genotypes of *PAI-1*, the frequency of the GA or AA genotypes of *NOS3* was significantly higher in severe PIH (27.8%) than in controls (13.3%; p=0.008<0.0125), while no significant difference was observed between the two groups (18.3% vs. 11.1%) in the subgroup possessing the 4G/4G genotype of *PAI-1* (Table 7). The ORs and their 95%CIs in women with the GA or AA genotype of *NOS3* without the 5G/5G or 4G/5G genotype of *PAI-1*, with the 5G/5G or 4G/5G genotype of *PAI-1* without the GA or AA genotype of *NOS3,* and with both of these genotypes compared to those without both of these genotypes were 1.80 (0.74-4.39), 0.91 (0.57-1.44) and 2.27 (1.18-4.36), respectively (Kobashi, et al., in preparation).

Table 5 Distributions of variants of candidate genes for pregnancy-induced hypertension

| | PIH | | | Controls | | | |
|---|---|---|---|---|---|---|---|
| Genotypes | AA | Aa | aa | AA | Aa | aa | |
| *AGT* | 40 | 56 *** | 1 | 19 | 80 | | 4 |
| *AT1* | 80 | 19 | 1 | 91 | 8 | 1 * | |
| *NOS3* | 0 ** | | 77 | 23 | 0 | 88 | 12 |
| *ACE* | 42 | 2 | 16 | 1 | 47 | 12 | |
| *FV* | 100 | 0 | 0 | 100 | 0 | 0 | |
| *PAI -* | | 40 | 50 | 10 | 39 | 47 | 14 |
| *TNF-α* | 4 | 0 | 96 | 4 | 0 | | 96 |
| *MTHFR* | 44 | 55 | 11 | 39 | 46 | 15 | |
| *LPL* | 76 | 22 | 2 | 76 | 23 | 1 | |
| *B3AR* | 70 | 24 | 6 | 70 | 28 | 2 | |
| *GSTP1* | 72 | 28 | 0 | 74 | 26 | 0 | |
| *mEH* | 24 | 34 | 42 | 26 | 29 | 45 | |

PIH: pregnancy-induced hypertension

Table 6. Distribution of M235T variant of angiotensinogen gene in women with severe PIH and controls with normal pregnancy according to the genotype of plasminogen activator inhibitor-1 gene

| Diagnosis | No. of cases | Genotype of *AGT* | | | Frequency | |
|---|---|---|---|---|---|---|
| | | MM | MT | TT | TT (%) | |
| 4G/4G genotype of *PAI-1* | | | | | | |
| severe PIH | | 49 | 1 | 10 | 38 | 77.5 |
| controls | 144 | 6 | 53 | 81 | 56.2 | |
| 4G/5G + 5G/5G genotype of *PAI-1* | | | | | | |
| severe PIH | 79 | 3 | 20 | 56 | 70.8 | |
| controls | | 232 | 7 | 83 | 142 | 61.2 |

*p=0.008<0.0125 vs. controls
*PAI-1*: plasminogen activator inhibitor-1 gene
*AGT*: angiotensinogen gene

Table 7. Distribution of Glu298Asp variant of endothelial nitoricoxide synthase gene in women with severe PIH and controls with normal pregnancy according to the genotype of plasminogen activator inhibitor-1 gene

| Diagnosis | No. of cases | Genotype of *NOS3* | | | Frequency of |
|---|---|---|---|---|---|
| | | GG | GA | AA | GA+AA (%) |
| 4G/4G genotype of *PAI-1* | | | | | |
| severe PIH | 49 | 40 | 9 | 0 | 18.3 |
| controls | 144 | 128 | 16 | 0 | 11.1 |
| 4G/5G + 5G/5G genotype of *PAI-1* | | | | | |
| severe PIH | 79 | 57 | 22 | 0 | 27.8* |
| controls | 232 | 201 | 30 | 1 | 13.3 |

*p=0.008<0.0125 vs. controls
*PAI-1*: plasminogen activator inhibitor-1 gene
*NOS3*: endothelial nitoricoxide synthase gene

## Confounding Genetic, Environmental and Lifestyle Factors in Pregnancy-Induced Hypertension

Five factors before pregnancy and 4 factors during pregnancy were significantly ($p<0.05$) associated with PIH on univariate analysis. Further multivariate analysis revealed 3 factors before pregnancy, i.e. "prepregnancy BMI≥24", "family history of hypertension" and "TT genotype of *AGT*", and 2 factors during pregnancy, i.e. "mentally stressful condition" and "salty dishes preferred" were potent independent risk factors for PIH (Table 8 and Table 9)[11].

Table8. Risk factors before pregnancy for pregnancy-induced hypertension

| Factors | Positive answers(%) Cases | Positive answers(%) Controls | Odds ratio (95%CI) Univariate | Odds ratio (95%CI) Multivariate |
|---|---|---|---|---|
| High body mass index (BMI 24) | 29.4 | 9.0 | 4.2 (2.1-8.5)*** | 4.8 (1.5-6.0)*** |
| Family history of hypertension | 39.7 | 20.5 | 2.6 (1.4-4.6)** | 3.0 (1.5-6.0)*** |
| Poor relationship with[1] husband's parents | 29.4 | 15.2 | 2.3 (1.2-4.4)** | - |
| TT genotype of AGT | 75.0 | 59.9 | 2.0 (1.1-3.7)** | 2.6 (1.3-5.0)** |
| Mentally stressful condition[1] | 27.9 | 16.6 | 2.0 (1.0-3.7)* | - |

There were 71 cases and 213 controls. Factors with $p<0.1$ in univariate analysis were subjected to multivariate analysis and are shown. Odds ratios are shown only when a significant difference existed (*p<0.05, **p<0.01, ***p<0.001).
[1]Five possible answers were: a, yes; b, somewhat; c, neutral; d, not much; and e, not at all. In this table, a+b was compared with c+d+e, with a+b considered a risk factor.

Table 9. Risk factors during pregnancy for hypertension in pregnancy

| Factors | Positive answers(%) | | Odds ratio (95%CI) | |
|---|---|---|---|---|
| | Cases | Controls | Univariate | Multivariate |
| Mentally stressful condition[1] | 54.4 | 31.3 | 2.6 (1.5-4.6)*** | 3.5 (2.1-10.6)*** |
| Salty dishes preferred[1] | 36.8 | 19.7 | 2.4 (1.3-4.4)** | 2.5 (1.8-6.7)** |
| Poor relationship with[1] husband's parents | 23.5 | 12.3 | 2.2 (1.1-4.4)* | - |
| Physically demanding work[1] | 47.1 | 33.2 | 1.8 (1.0-3.1)* | - |

There were 71 cases and 213 controls. Factors with p<0.1 in univariate analysis were subjected to multivariate analysis and are shown. Odds ratios are shown only when a significant difference existed (*p<0.05, **p<0.01, ***p<0.001).
[1]Five possible answers were: a, yes; b, somewhat; c, neutral; d, not much; and e, not at all. In this table, a+b was compared with c+d+e, with a+b considered a risk factor.

Dividing the subjects into 2 subgroups according to whether they possessed the "TT genotype of *AGT*" (n=175) or not (n=109), we identified acquired risk factors before and during pregnancy for PIH that were significant (p<0.05) by both univariate and multivariate analyses. The multivariate analysis identified "mentally stressful condition" as a potent significant risk factor during pregnancy in the former subgroup. However, there were no potent significant risk factors concerning and "mental stress" in the latter subgroup (Table 10 and Table 11)[11].

Table 10. Risk factors during pregnancy for pregnancy-induced hy,pertension in the subgroup "TT genotype of *AGT*"

| | Positive answers(%) | | Odds ratio (95%CI) | |
|---|---|---|---|---|
| | Cases | Controls | Univariate | Multivariate |
| ***Factors before pregnancy*** | | | | |
| High body mass index (BMI?24) | 27.4 | 12.1 | 2.7 (1.2-6.2)* | 3.7 (1.4-9.7)** |
| Family history of hypertension | 35.3 | 15.8 | 2.9 (1.4-6.2)** | 2.9 (1.3-6.8)* |
| GA+AA genotypes of *NOS3* | 31.4 | 16.3 | 2.4 (1.1-5.0)* | 3.3 (1.3-8.4)* |
| Poor relationship with husband's parents | 31.4 | 15.3 | 2.5 (1.2-5.4)* | - |
| ***Factors during pregnancy*** | | | | |
| Mentally stressful condition | 54.9 | 30.7 | 2.8 (1.4-5.4)** | 3.8 (1.8-8.3)*** |
| Poor relationship with husband's parents | 25.5 | 12.9 | 2.3 (1.0-5.2)* | - |
| Salty dishes preferred | 35.3 | 20.6 | 2.1 (1.0-4.4)** | - |

There were 51 cases and 124 controls in the subgroup. Factors with p<0.1 in univariate analysis subjected to multivariate analysis and are shown.
Odds ratios are shown only when a significant difference existed (*p<0.05).

Table 11. Risk factors during pregnancy for pregnancy-induced hypertension in the subgroup "MM+MT genotypes of *AGT*"

| | Positive answers(%) | | Odds ratio (95%CI) | |
|---|---|---|---|---|
| | Cases | Controls | Univariate | Multivariate |
| ***Factors before pregnancy*** | | | | |
| High body mass index (BMI?24) | 35.3 | 4.8 | 10.8 (2.6-44.3)* | 10.5 (2.6-43.1)** |
| ***Factors during pregnancy*** | | | | |
| Salty dishes preferred | 41.2 | 15.6 | 3.8 (1.2-11.9)* | - |

There were 20 cases and 89 controls in the subgroup. Factors with $p<0.1$ in univariate analysis subjected to multivariate analysis and are shown.
Odds ratios are shown only when a significant difference existed (*$p<0.05$).

# Discussion

## Candidate Genes and their Possible Pathogeneses in the Development of Pregnancy-Induced Hypertension

The *AGT* variant was the first gene variant associated with the occurrence of PIH. The amino acid located at position 235 in the AGT protein is known to be either methionine (M235) or threonine (T235). Of the two *AGT* variants, T235 has been found to occur at a higher frequency among women with PIH than among women with normal pregnancy outcome[12]. Genetic variants which are candidates in the pathogenesis of PIH, such as the rennin-angiotensin system, the blood coagulation system, and the intravascular system, have been thoroughly studied in terms of their association with PIH[13]. To date, the *AGT* M235T variant, the *AT1* A1166C variant, and the *NOS3* Glu298Asp variant have been found to be associated with PIH in Japanese women[4-6].

Several factors are believed to be associated with PIH, including pressor/depressor mechanisms, the blood coagulation system, lipid metabolism, the intravascular system, placental function, the skeletal system, abdominal wall abnormalities, physical/psychological stress, and the nervous system. Consequently, a number of gene variants have been examined in terms of their contribution to PIH. However, due to genetic differences among races, a gene variant that shows association with PIH in one group, such as Caucasian women, may show no significant association with PIH in Japanese women[8]. Even when a certain gene variant is found to be associated with PIH in a particular group such as Japanese women, the frequency of disease occurrence may vary across patients with different baseline characteristics[9,14]. Despite the genetic differences between the general Japanese population and the general Caucasian population, the contribution of the *AGT* variant to the manifestation of PIH has been demonstrated and proven among Japanese as well as Caucasian populations. A subsequent study reported that *AGT* M235T polymorphism is in tight linkage disequilibrium with a molecular variant in the proximal promoter of the *AGT*, which consists of an adenine instead of a guanine six-nucleotide upstream from the site of transcription initiation (G-6A). In other words, the M235 variant is a marker for -6G and the T235 variant is a marker for -6A[15]. Furthermore, according to an *in-vitro* study, -6A was associated with a lower promoter activity than -6G[15]. T235 (-6A) is reported to be associated with an inadequate trophoblastic invasion of the uterine spiral arteries and a narrowing of the spiral arterioles in early pregnancy, which can trigger the onset of PIH[16].

According to a previous study carried out among Caucasian women to examine the association between the *AGT* T235 variant and preeclampisa (PE) (hypertension with proteinuria), the *AGT* T235 allele frequency was significantly higher among primiparous women with PE with respect to the control group (65% vs. 40%)[12]. On the other hand, in the Japanese population, the T235 variant was found to be strongly associated with the incidence of PIH, regardless of parity. Furthermore, the T235 allele is found at a higher frequency among the Japanese population (94% in patients with PIH and 76% in the control) than among the Caucasian population[4]. The *FV* Leiden mutation is a mutation in the blood coagulation factor *FV*, causing activated protein C resistance. Known as the most common genetic risk factor for thrombosis, it is present in 10% of the Caucasian women with PIH and 4% of the Caucasian women with normal pregnancy[17], but is very rare among the Japanese population[8]. Thus, two main genetic factors may be associated with the onset of PIH among the Caucasian population, namely, the *AGT* variants (PE among primiparous women) and the *FV* Leiden mutation. On the other hand, PIH among the Japanese population is predominantly associated with the *AGT* variants.

Asp298 of *NOS3* has been thought to reduce the stimulation of NO production in the endothelium, since it enhances the vascular reactivity to an $\alpha 1$-adrenergic stimulant, although the Glu298Asp variant is not located in any functional consensus sequence[18]. It was also suggested in our previous association study that the Asp298 of *NOS3*, Val105 of the GSTP1 gene (*GSTP1*) and pregnancy with an advanced maternal age were synergistically associated with the manifestation of PIH via a reduction of NO production[19]. Some experimental studies have reported that NOS inhibition using L-NG nitro arginine-methyl-ester induces vascular PAI-1 expression, which is thought to occur during vascular injury[20,21], although the role of NO in the regulation of PAI-1 expression in humans has not been clarified yet.

PIH has long been known to have various forms and causes. Many researchers currently believe that the symptoms of PIH are the product of the interaction of various genetic as well as environmental factors. In fact, what is clinically termed PIH is actually a multifactorial syndrome comprising a heterogeneous group of diseases. Thus, the results obtained from a study on genetic and environmental risk factors for PIH may provide not only a useful insight into the etiology and pathology of this multifactorial disease, but also provide a basis for more exactly classifying PIH. It is neither practical nor appropriate to use pedigree analysis or sib-pair analysis to identify candidate genes involved in the development of PIH, because the population at risk is limited to pregnant women. The use of a case-control study is more appropriate in this respect. Furthermore, it is important to remember that even when a certain gene is found to have no statistically significant association with the development of PIH among pregnant women in general, a significant association may be found when the association is assessed in patients belonging to specific subgroups.

Caution is needed when interpreting the results obtained from a multivariate analysis because a multivariate approach can only detect potent risk factors for general subjects. For example, no association was initially found between the IV+VV genotypes of *GSTP1* and

PIH among pregnant women in general. However, this genotype turned out to be significantly associated with the development of PIH among primiparous women with severe PIH who belonged to one of the following three groups: 1) women of older age, 2) GA+AA genotypes of *NOS3* (this genotype is known to be associated with PIH), and 3) MM+MT genotypes of *AGT* (this genotype is known to be associated with reduced risk of toxipathy) [10] (data are not shown in the present paper).

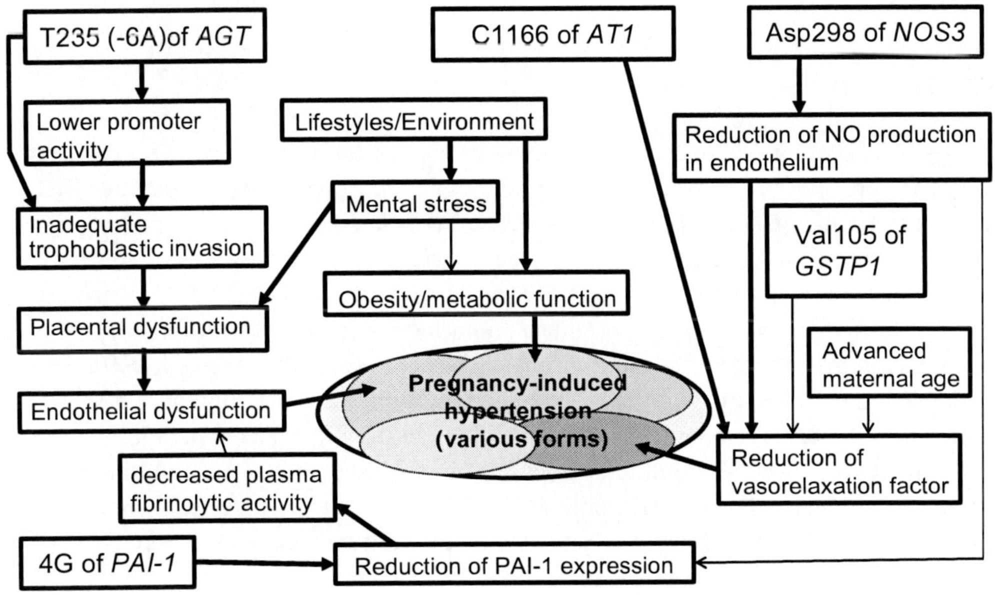


Figure 1. Pregnancy-induced hypertension is a complex syndrome made up of certain pathophysiological pathways, each of which is comprised of a combination of PIH susceptibility genetic variants and environmental risk factors. In this figure, thickness of arrows reflects significance of association.

Furthermore, in the result of the subgroup analysis according to the *PAI-1* genotype, the significant association of the TT genotype of *AGT* was maintained only in the subgroup possessing the 4G/4G genotype, while on the other hand, the significant association of the GA or AA genotypes of *NOS3* was maintained only in the subgroup possessing the 4G/5G or 5G/5G genotypes. One reason may be that the 4G/5G variant of *PAI-1* is a factor which has quite a weak association with severe PIH, while subjects with the 4G/4G of *PAI-1* are reported to have an approximately 20% higher plasma PAI-1 level than those with other genotypes [22,23]. Thus, the detection of a significant difference depends on an interaction with other genetic and environmental factors. This may confound studies of the 4G/5G variants, since factors such as pressor/depressor mechanisms, lipid metabolism, the intravascular system, the placental dysfunction, and the nervous system may be associated with PIH in the form of converging pathways which include the blood coagulation system, and the major characteristics which should be matched between the cases and the controls such as maternal age, gravidity and parity, were not different between the two groups. There were also no differences between them based on the severity of PIH or in terms of obesity.

It is suggested that there are at least two pathogenetic pathways for the manifestation of PIH, in which one consists of synergism of the TT of *AGT*, 4G/4G of *PAI-1* and mental stress during pregnancy, and the other a synergism of the GA or AA of *NOS3*, 4G/5G or 5G/5G of *PAI-1,* Ile/Val or Val/Val of *GSTP1* and pregnancy with advanced maternal age (Figure 1). This hypothesis is concordant with confirmatory reports of an association of the TT genotype of *AGT* in PIH rather than essential hypertension[24-27], and the association of the GA or AA of *NOS3* has been reported not only in PIH, but also atherosclerosis and/or myocardial infarction[28-31].

## A Possibility of Individualized Medicine for Pregnancy-Induced Hypertension

Figure 2 shows a schema for the natural history of PIH in which genetic, environmental, and age factors are involved in the pathogenesis of PIH. Preventive measures for PIH should address environmental as well as lifestyle-related risk factors both during pregnancy and the pre-pregnancy period. In fact, it is widely acknowledged that consulting an obstetrician for advice regarding appropriate lifestyle during pregnancy is effective to some extent in reducing the risk of PIH. However, due to interindividual genetic differences, a lifestyle-related factor that is identified as a strong risk factor for PIH among a certain group of individuals may have no significant association with PIH risk among other groups of individuals. The advancement of molecular biology in the future may potentially improve our understanding of diseases/conditions caused by the interaction of multiple genes or a combination of genetic and environmental risk factors, and it may also contribute to the development of disease prevention and health promotion measures tailored to a specific genotype[3,11].

The present result shows that lifestyle-related factors for PIH, particularly mental stress-related risk factors, vary by the *AGT* genotype, a fact which reflects the multifactorial nature of the disease. The *AGT* TT genotype is reportedly associated with an incomplete trophoblastic invasion of the uterine spiral arteries and a narrowing of the spiral arterioles in early pregnancy. Coupled with the effect of physical and psychological stress during pregnancy, such abnormalities could lead to decreased blood flow in the placenta, potentially triggering PIH (Figure 1). AGT genotyping may be useful for developing individualized measures for relieving physical/psychological stress during pregnancy to prevent PIH among those women whose risk for PIH is seemingly low as measured by conventional criteria[3,11].

The goal of tailor-made/individualized medicine is to utilize genotyping technology to provide effective preventive measures against a range of multifactorial diseases, including cancer, strokes, myocardial infarction, and diabetes. The analytical model constructed in the present study to examine the contribution of genetic and environmental factors to PIH can be applied to other multifactorial diseases as well, which could be useful for understanding the pathogenesis of the disease in question and for developing appropriate preventive measures.

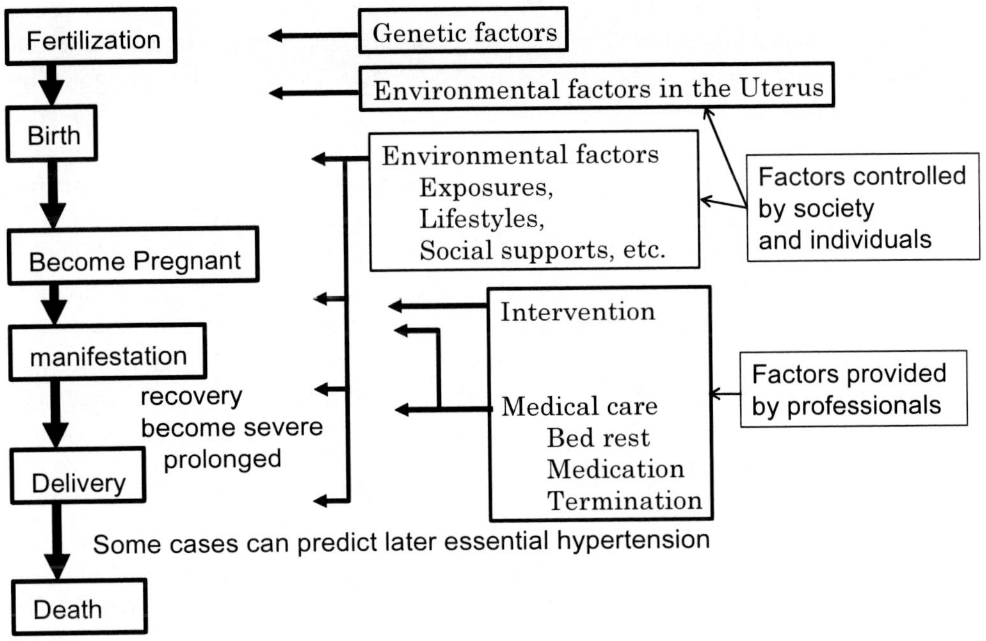


Figure 2. Natural history of pregnancy-induced hypertension in our lifetime influenced by several kinds of factors.

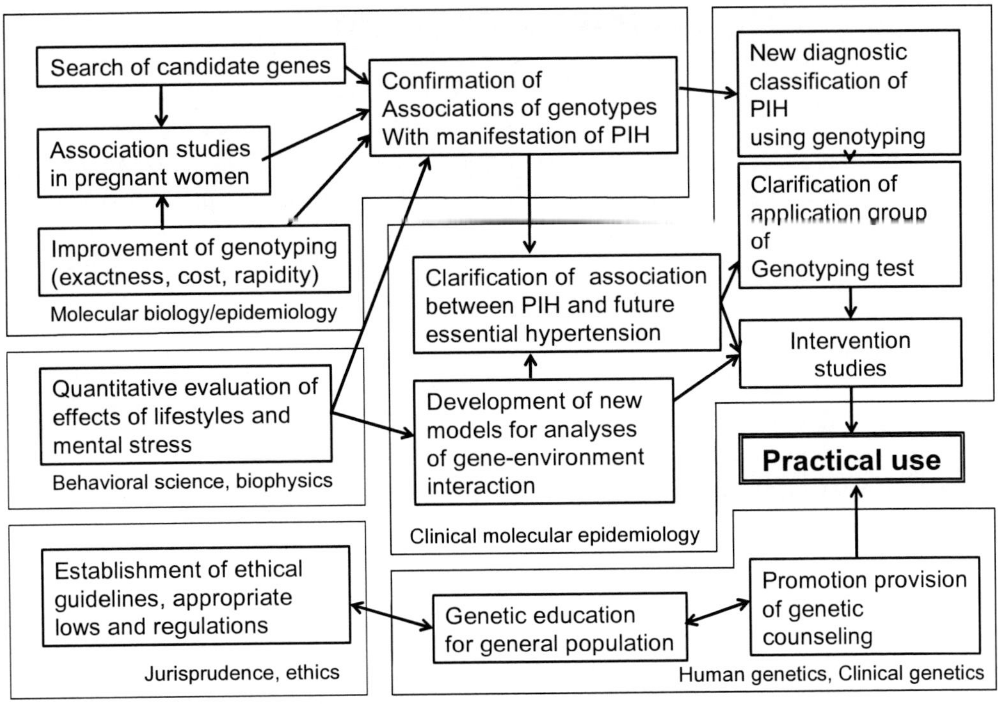


Figure 3. There are several hurdles to overcome with development of each study field before realizing individualized prevention by use of genotyping in early pregnancy.

However, there are several hurdles to overcome before genotyping technology can be applied for PIH prevention and control, which include, i) developing a proper genotyping technology, ii) establishing appropriate epidemiologic methods, iii) developing ethical guidelines iv) establishing appropriate laws and regulations, v) providing education on advantages and disadvantages of genotyping, and vi) promoting the provision of genetic counseling (Figure 3). However, PIH research has the following advantages: (1) Because almost all pregnant women in Japan visit a doctor for regular prenatal care during pregnancy, information regarding pregnant women's lifestyle can be obtained with relative ease and patients have the opportunity to obtain feedback and advice on appropriate lifestyle through prenatal care visits; (2) Because it takes less than 10 months to obtain pregnancy outcomes, the study results can be obtained in a short period of time; (3) In some groups of pregnant women, PIH prediction and prevention during pregnancy may be useful for the early prediction and prevention of development of essential hypertension in the future; and (4) The involvement of obstetricians may facilitate the informed consent process.

Through further exploration of the risk factors associated with PIH, we hope to provide useful suggestions for new and effective preventive measures for a range of multifactorial diseases, carrying out detailed analyses of "gene-environment- mental interaction", i.e. mental power in interaction with genetic and environmental factors in the development of diseases, utilizing experimental data as well as epidemiological data in the near future.

## Acknowledgments

Cordial thanks are due to Drs. Akira Hata, Koichi Shido, Kaori Ohta, Hideto Yamada, Hisanori Minakami, Hiko Tamashiro, Seiichiro Fuimoto, Kiyotaro Kondo, and many collaborators in the Hokkaido University Graduate School of Medicine, Hokkaido University Hospital and its affiliated hospitals. Pacific Edit reviewed the manuscript prior to submission.

## References

[1] Kobashi, G. Genetic and Environmental Factors Associated with the Development of Hypertension in Pregnancy. *J Epidemiol*, 2006, 16, 1-8.

[2] National High Blood Pressure Education Program Working Group. Report on high blood pressure in pregnancy (Consensus Report). *Am J Obstet Gynecol*, 1990, 163, 1689-1712.

[3] Kobashi, G; Hata, A; Shido, K; Ohta, K; Yamada, H; Fujimoto, S; Kondo, K. M235T variant of angiotensinogen gene and body mass index are useful markers for prevention of hypertension in pregnancy; a tree-based analysis of gene-environment interaction. *Seminor Thromb Hemostat*, 2002, 28, 501-505.

[4] Kobashi, G; Hata, A; Shido, K; Kato, EH; Yamada, H; Fujimoto, S; Kishi, R; Kondo, K. Association of a variant of the angiotensinogen gene with pure type of hypertension in pregnancy in the Japanese: implication of a racial difference and significance of an age factor. *Am J Med Genet*, 1999, 86, 232-236.

[5] Kobashi, G; Hata, A; Ohta, K; Yamada, H; Kato, EH; Minakami, H; Fujimoto, S; Kondo, K. A1166C variant of angiotensin II type 1 receptor gene independently associated with severe hypertension in pregnancy from T235 variant of angiotensinogen gene. *J Hum Genet*, 2004, 49, 182-186.

[6] Kobashi, G; Yamada, H; Kato, EH; Ebina, Y; Ohta, K; Fujimoto, S. Glu298Asp variant of the endotherial nitric oxide synthase gene (*NOS3*) and hypertension in pregnancy. *Am J Med Genet*, 2001, 103, 241-244.

[7] Kobashi, G; Hata, A; Shido, K; Ohta, K; Yamada, H; Kato, EH; Minakami, H; Tamashiro, H; Fujimoto, S; Kondo, K; Tamashiro, H. Insertion/deletion polymorphism of angiotensin-converting enzyme gene and preeclampsia in Japanese. *Seminor Thromb Hemostat*, 2005, 31, 346-350.

[8] Kobashi, G; Yamada, H; Asano, T; Nagano, S; Hata, A; Kishi, R; Kondo, K; Fujimoto, S. The factor V Leiden mutation is not a common cause of pregnancy-induced hypertension in Japan. *Semin Thromb Hemost*, 1999, 25, 487-489.

[9] Kobashi, G; Yamada, H; Asano, T; Nagano, S; Hata, A; Kishi, R; Kondo, K; Fujimoto, S. Absence of association between a common mutation in the methylenetetra-hydrofolate reductase gene and preeclampsia in Japanese. *Am J Med Genet*, 2000, 93, 122-125.

[10] Ohta, K; Kobashi, G; Hata, A; Yamada, H; Minakami, H; Fujimoto, S; Kondo, K; Tamashiro, H. Association Between a Variant of the Glutathione S-transferase P1 (GSTP1) gene and Hypertension in Pregnancy in Japanese: Interaction with parity, Age and Genetic Factors. *Seminor Thromb Hemostat*, 2003, 29, 653-659.

[11] Kobashi, G. Gene polymorphisms and preeclampsia in Japanese; analysis for gene-environment interaction. *Acta Obst Gynaec Jpn*, 2003, 55, 817-829.

[12] Ward, K; Hata, A; Jeunemaitre, X; Helin, C; Nelson, L; Namikawa, C; Farrington, PF; Ogasawara, M; Suzumori, K; Tomoda, S; Berrebi, S; Sasaki, M; Corvol, P; Lifton, RP; Lalouel, JM. A molecular variant of angiotensinogen associated witPIHreeclampsia. *Nat Genet*, 1993, 4, 59-61.

[13] Lachmeijer, AM; Dekker, GA; Pals, G; Aarnoudse, JG; ten Kate, LP, Arngrimsson, R. Searching for preeclampsia genes: the current position. *Eur J Obstet Gynecol Reprod Biol*, 2002, 105, 94-113.

[14] Sohda, S; Arinami, T; Hamada, H; Yamada, N; Hamaguchi, H; Kubo, T. Methylenetetrahydrofolate reductase polymorphism and pre-eclampsia. *J Med Genet*, 1997, 34, 525-526.

[15] Inoue, I; Nakajima, T; Williams, CS; Quackenbush, J; Puryear, R; Powers, M; Cheng, T; Ludwig, EH; Sharma, AM; Hata, A; Jeunemaitre, X; Lalouel, JM. A nucleotide substitution in the promoter of human angiotensinogen is associated with essential hypertension and affects basal transcription in vitro. *J Clin Invest*, 1997, 99, 1786-1797.

[16] Morgan, T; Craven, C; Lalouel, JM; Ward, K. Angiotensinogen Thr235 variant is associated with abnormal physiologic change of the uterine spiral arteries in first-trimester decidua. *Am J Obstet Gynecol*, 1999, 180, 95-102.

[17] Grandone, E; Margaglione, M; Colaizzo, D; Cappucci, G; Paladini, D; Martinelli, P; Montanaro, S; Pavone, G; Di Minno, G. Factor V Leiden, C > T MTHFR polymorphism and genetic susceptibility to preeclampsia. *Thromb Haemost*, 1997, 77, 1052-1054.

[18] Philip, I; Plantefeve, G; Vuillaumier-Barrot, S; Vicaut, E; LeMarie, C; Henrion, D; Poirier, O; Levy, BI; Desmonte, JM; Durand, G; Benessiano, J. G894T polymorphism in the endothelial nitric oxide synthase gene is associated with an enhanced vascular responsiveness to phenylephrine. *Circulation*, 1999, 99, 3096-3098.

[19] Ohta, K; Kobashi, G; Hata, A; Yamada, H; Minakami, H; Fujimoto, S; Kondo, K; Tamashiro, H. Association between a variant of the glutathione S-transferase P1 gene (GSTP1) and hypertension in pregnancy in Japanese: interaction with parity, age, and genetic factors. *Semin Thromb Hemost*, 2003, 29, 653-659.

[20] Katoh, M; Egashira, K; Mitsui, T; Chishima, S; Takeshita, A; Narita, H. Angiotensin-converting enzyme inhibitor prevents plasminogen activator inhibitor-1 expression in a rat model with cardiovascular remodeling induced by chronic inhibition of nitric oxide synthesis. *J Mol Cell Cardiol*, 2000, 32, 73-83.

[21] Kaikita, K; Fogo, AB; Ma, L; Schoenhard, JA; Brown, NJ; Vaughan, DE. Plasminogen activator inhibitor-1 deficiency prevents hypertension and vascular fibrosis in response to long-term nitric oxide synthase inhibition. *Circulation*, 2001, 104, 839-844.

[22] Ye, S; Green, FR; Scarabin, PY; Nicaud, V; Bara, L; Dawson, SJ; Humphries, SE; Evans, A; Luc, G; Cambou, JP; Arveiler, D; Henney, AM; Cambien, F. The 4G/5G genetic polymorphism in the promoter of the plasminogen activator inhibitor-1 (PAI-1) gene is associated with differences in plasma PAI-1 activity but not with risk of myocardial infarction in the ECTIM study. *Thromb Haemost*, 1995, 74, 837-841.

[23] Kathiresan, S; Gabriel, SB; Yang, Q; Lochner, AL; Larson, MG; Levy, D; Tofler, GH; Hirschhorn, JN; O'Donnell, CJ. Comprehensive survey of common genetic variation at the plasminogen activator inhibitor-1 locus and relations to circulating plasminogen activator inhibitor-1 levels. *Circulation*, 2005, 112, 1728-1735.

[24] Kato, N; Sugiyama, T; Morita, H; Kurihara, H; Furukawa, T; Isshiki, T; Sato, T; Yamori, Y; Yazaki, Y. Comprehensive analysis of the renin-angiotensin gene polymorphisms with relation to hypertension in the Japanese. *J Hypertens*, 2000, 18, 1025-1032.

[25] Rodriguez-Perez, JC; Rodriguez-Esparragon, FJ; Hernandez-Perera, O; Fiuza-Perez, MD; Anabitarte-Prieto, A; Losada-Cabrera, A. Effects of the angiotensinogen gene M235T and A(-6)G variants on blood pressure and other vascular risk factors in a Spanish population. *J Hum Hypertens*, 2000, 14, 789-793.

[26] Lachmeijer, AM; Dekker, GA; Pals, G; Aarnoudse, JG; ten Kate, LP; Arngrimsson, R. Searching for preeclampsia genes: the current position. *Eur J Obstet Gynecol Reprod Biol*, 2002, 105, 94-113.

[27] Mondry, A; Loh, M; Liu, P; Zhu, AL; Nagel, M. Polymorphisms of the insertion / deletion ACE and M235T AGT genes and hypertension: surprising new findings and meta-analysis of data. *BMC Nephrol*, 2005, 6, 1.

[28] Shimasaki, Y; Yasue, H; Yoshimura, M; Nakayama, M; Kugiyama, K; Ogawa, H; Harada, E; Masuda, T; Koyama, W; Saito, Y; Miyamoto, Y; Ogawa, Y; Nakao, K. Association of the missense Glu298Asp variant of the endothelial nitric oxide synthase gene with myocardial infarction. *J Am Coll Cardiol*, 1999, 100, 1515-1520.

[29] Heltianu, C; Costache, G; Gafencu, A; Diaconu, M; Bodeanu, M; Cristea, C; Azibi, K; Poenaru, L; Simionescu, M. Relationship of eNOS gene variants to diseases that have in common an endothelial cell dysfunction. *J Cell Mol Med*, 2005, 9, 135-142.

[30] Spoto, B; Benedetto, FA; Testa, A; Tripepi, G; Mallamaci, F; Maas, R; Boeger, RH; Zoccali, C; Parlongo, RM; Pisano, A. Atherosclerosis and the Glu298Asp polymorphism of the eNOS gene in white patients with end-stage renal disease. *Am J Hypertens*, 2005, 18, 1549-1555.

[31] Sandrim, VC; Coelho, EB; Nobre, F; Arado, GM; Lanchote, VL; Tanus-Santos, JE. Susceptible and protective eNOS haplotypes in hypertensive black and white subjects. *Atherosclerosis*, 2006, 186, 428-432.

In: Advances in Cardiovascular Research, Volume 1
Editors: L. Schmitt, T. Konig, pp. 287-306
ISBN: 978-1-60741-720-0


*Chapter XII*

# Management of Pregnant Women with Complete Atrioventricular Block

***Nobuhiro Hidaka*[a,c*] *and Yoshihide Chiba*[b,c]**
[a]Department of Obstetrics and Gynecology, Graduate School of Medical Sciences, Kyushu University, Fukuoka, Japan.
[b]Chiba Women's Clinic, Osaka, Japan.
[c]Department of Perinatology, National Cardiovascular Center, Osaka, Japan.

## Abstract

We have summarized the care management of pregnant women with complete atrioventricular block (CAVB) by reviewing the data from previous literature and our experience including 29 births. The management of patients already implanted with a permanent pacemaker does not involve any risks. Some of the patients without permanent pacemaker may develop syncope due to heart failure during pregnancy. Pre-pregnancy prophylactic placement of a permanent pacemaker is not indicated in all asymptomatic patients; however, for symptomatic patients in the first and second trimesters, permanent pacemaker implantation is the therapy of choice. For symptomatic women with CAVB who present at or near term, temporary pacing at the earliest possible time prior to labor induction should be recommended. Most pregnant women with CAVB who do not require a permanent pacemaker before delivery can be managed safely during labor even without temporary pacing. Elective epidural analgesia and forceps delivery are also important components of the care of patients without permanent pacemaker for maintaining stable maternal hemodynamics.

* Corresponding author: Department of Obstetrics and Gynecology, Graduate School of Medical Sciences, Kyushu University, 3-1-1 Maidashi, Higashiku 812-8582, Fukuoka, Japan, Email: n-hidaka@kpa.biglobe.ne.jp, Phone: 81 92 642 5394, FAX: 81 92 642 5414

# Introduction

Complete atrioventricular block (CAVB) is predominantly observed in elderly male than female, and it is rarely observed in pregnant women. However, the incidence of CAVB may increase in younger people with the increase in the number of open heart surgeries for the treatment of congenital heart diseases. Although there have been some reports of CAVB in female patients during pregnancy and labor in the English literature, these have been isolated case reports or small case series [1–21]. There are some other reports of comparatively large series of pregnant women with CAVB [22–24]; however, unfortunately, they have not been reported in English. Therefore, there are no established guidelines for the clinical management of pregnant women with CAVB, especially of those in labor. There are anecdotal case reports that show good outcomes of temporary pacing for CAVB patients in labor [11–14]. Women with CAVB but without a permanent pacemaker surely seemed to receive temporary pacing for the duration of labor and birth; however, the appropriate rationale for the requirement of this temporary pacing has not been provided. In 2006, on the basis of our experience, we presented the largest prospective series to date and discussed the necessity of temporary pacing for women with CAVB who were not implanted with a permanent pacemaker [25]. Our results suggested that women with CAVB who do not require a permanent pacemaker can be managed without temporary pacing during labor.

Here, we have summarized the clinical management techniques for pregnant women with CAVB by using the data of previous case reports and the data from our hospital, including those for 29 births. We hope that the information presented in this report will assist in the establishment of management guidelines for such women in the future.

# Complete Atrioventricular Block

CAVB is the most common cause for the development of permanent bradycardia and is a disorder of the cardiac conduction system in which the atrioventricular conduction is completely absent. In CAVB, the conduction of sinus or atrial impulses is completely interrupted at the level of the atrioventricular node, in the bundle of His, or is associated with an aberrantly located anatomical atrioventricular node that precludes normal anatomical communication with the distal conduction tissue. Atria and ventricles depolarize independently of each other, and the rate of depolarization of the ventricles is typically slower than that of the atria (Figure 1). This disorder may be congenital or acquired secondary to cardiac surgery, coronary spasm, rheumatic heart disease, Lyme disease, syphilis, diphtheria, or other infective disorders. Although CAVB may be associated with some other cardiac anomaly, in many cases, there are no coexisting lesions. Most pediatric patients with postoperative CAVB had undergone intracardiac surgery for atrial septal defect repair, ventricular septal defect repair, valve repair or replacements, or other complex congenital heart surgeries. The incidence of congenital CAVB was determined to be approximately 1 in 22,000 live births [26,27]; however, most of the congenital cases are reported well before childbearing age. Some patients with CAVB experience weakness, dizziness, exercise intolerance, syncope, or congestive heart failure. If the heart rate is inadequate to maintain the blood flow to the brain, patients may experience syncopal episodes, whereas some patients may be asymptomatic. No diagnostic modality has been shown to independently predict mortality in such patients; therefore, the determination of the risk of sudden death and need for pacing is not well defined.

## Maternal Hemodynamic Change during Pregnancy

In normal pregnancies, the cardiac output increases by 5 weeks after the last menstrual period, and continues to increase up to mid-pregnancy, when it is 45% more than the rate in non-pregnant women, to meet the higher hemodynamic requirements [28,29]. After the mid-pregnancy stage, the cardiac output remains stable, and no further significant change is observed. Both heart rate and stroke volume contribute to this increase: the heart rate increases by 5 weeks of gestation and continues to increase up to 32 weeks. The heart rate increases by 25% during pregnancy. The increase in stroke volume occurs slightly later at 8 weeks and reaches its maximum level at about 20 weeks [28]. In addition, further increased hemodynamic requirement is present during delivery, when the cardiac output increases even more, especially during uterine contractions [28,30–32].

Generally, the regulation of cardiac output rate is achieved via changes in both stroke volume and heart rate. However, in CAVB patients, in whom a sufficient increase in heart rate cannot be achieved, the increased cardiac output throughout pregnancy mostly depends on altered stroke volume. Therefore, it is sometimes considered that pregnant women with CAVB can remain asymptomatic during pregnancy but may develop Adams-Stokes attacks during delivery [5]. In addition, it is also unclear whether the hemodynamic status of pregnant women with CAVB who have not been implanted with a permanent pacemaker would remain stable during and immediately after labor and delivery, particularly, considering that there is an increased cardiac workload during labor and since there is acute blood loss post-delivery.

## Review of Literature

The first report of a pregnant woman with CAVB was presented in 1914 by Nanta [33]. In the 1950s, it was considered that pregnancy in women with CAVB who have not been implanted with a pacemaker was associated with high maternal and fetal mortality [17,34]. In fact, Epstein and Altman reported a series of 43 pregnant women with permanent bradycardia, 6 of whom died during pregnancy [17]. The first case of a pregnant woman with a cardiac pacemaker was reported by Shouse and Acker in 1964 [18]. Thus far, there have been several reports of permanent pacemakers implanted before or during pregnancy for the treatment of CAVB. In 1987, Jaffe et al. reviewed 20 such cases with 1 case in their own experience [6], following which, some additional cases have also been reported thus far [4,8,10].

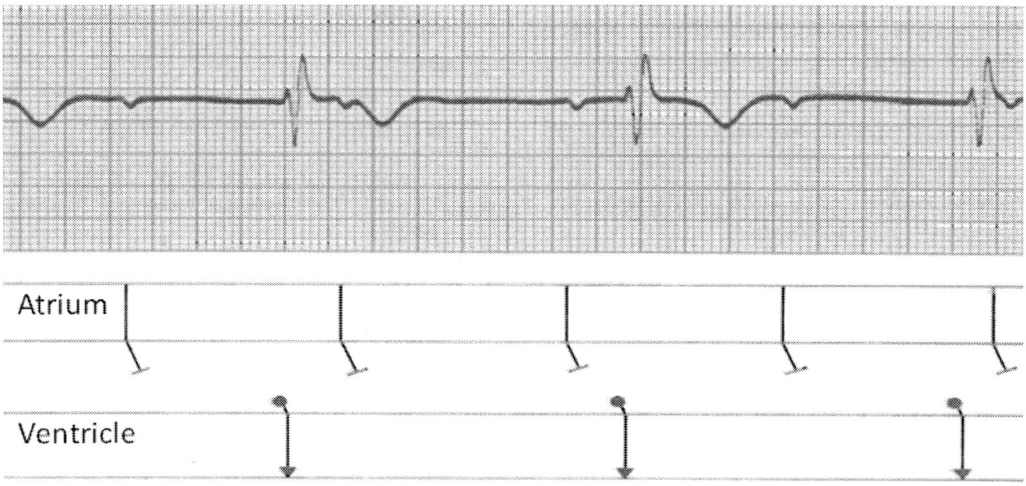


Figure 1. This figure shows an electrocardiogram of a person with complete atrioventricular block. P and QRS waves are present but unrelated.

Today, permanent cardiac pacemakers are increasingly being used in younger women with permanent bradycardia owing to improved implantation techniques, reliable equipment, extensive clinical experience, and better cardiovascular function compared to that achieved by using conventional drugs. Since the use of artificial pacemakers has considerably increased, the prognosis of patients with CAVB has dramatically improved. It is likely that most women of reproductive age with severe bradycardia secondary to CAVB will have a permanent pacemaker implanted before pregnancy. One of the treatment options for patients in whom permanent pacemakers are not implanted, was the use of prophylactic temporary pacing during labor progression. In fact, some case reports have described good outcomes of temporary pacing for CAVB patients in labor [11–14]. However, in these reports, the appropriate time for initiating artificial pacing and the appropriate rate were not discussed. Further, the answer to whether temporary pacing was truly necessary for their patients seemed beyond the scope of these reports.

There have been some reports in the English literature focusing on women with CAVB during pregnancy and labor. Table 1 summarizes such cases reported since 1970. As seen in the table, most recent reports published in the English literature have been anecdotal case reports or small case series [1–16].There are some other studies on comparatively large series of pregnant women with CAVB [22–24]; however, unfortunately, these have not been published in English. Hence, till date, there are no established guidelines for the management of pregnant women with CAVB.

## Cases in Our Experience between 1981 and 1996

From 1981 to 1996, we successfully managed 13 pregnant women with CAVB (21 births) at the National Cardiovascular Center (NCVC), Osaka, Japan. The clinical backgrounds of these patients have been outlined in Table 2. Of these patients, 4 had a previous history of Adams-Stokes attack. No patients showed disease progression to cardiac failure or syncope during pregnancy, and both maternal and neonatal outcomes were favorable.

Of the 13 women, 4 (7 births) had already undergone permanent pacemaker implantation. In the rest 14 deliveries, a permanent pacemaker had not been implanted, and we had no definite guidelines for managing such cases. Maternal heart rates during these 14 deliveries varied from 30 to 56. We inserted a temporary pacing lead immediately before delivery and used an external pacemaker in 11 cases indistinctively. We could manage these patients successfully; however, the necessity of this procedure and the proper timing or rate setting for artificial pacing have not been fully discussed. In most of the cases, forceps delivery was performed, whereas some women delivered without any instrumental intervention. Despite a transvaginal attempt, a cesarean delivery was finally performed in 2 cases because of arrest of labor.

## Clinical Trials in Our Center between 1997 and 2004

Between 1997 and 2004, at NCVC, we managed women who had CAVB but did not have a permanent pacemaker implanted with the regimens briefly described below. This clinical trial has already been reported in 2006 **[25]**. During the abovementioned study period, we intentionally induced labor by injecting oxytocin after achieving sufficient mechanical cervical dilation by using laminarias to allow elective insertion of a temporary pacing lead pre-delivery at a gestational stage of 37–39 weeks in each case. Prior to the induction of labor, a temporary pacing lead was inserted into the right ventricular apex through the right internal jugular vein; however, it was planned that this pacing lead would be used only if the patient became symptomatic. Throughout labor, the maternal blood pressure and central venous blood pressure were recorded via an arterial line and a central venous line, respectively. Epidural anesthesia was used electively to minimize the changes in the hemodynamic conditions caused by labor pain or bearing down. We anesthetized patients by administering lidocaine or bupivacaine after the uterine cervix had dilated more than 5 cm. In the second stage of labor, sufficient vertex descent was allowed to occur spontaneously, following which a forceps-assisted delivery was performed.

We managed 6 women (7 births) in the abovementioned manner during the study period. Table 3 summarizes these patients. None of the patients had a structural cardiac defect or a history of Adams-Stokes attack. A tocolytic agent was administered to 2 patients because of the risk of preterm labor. All the women remained well and symptom free during pregnancy. At admission, the heart rates of the 7 cases ranged from 38 to 55 beats/min. Table 4 summarizes the details of the labor progression for all the women. In 2 cases, we could not prevent preterm labor even after administering ritodrine hydrochloride. In the other 5 women, labor was induced at full term as predicted. In the 5 women, deliveries were performed using forceps, as planned. 1 had a spontaneous vaginal breech delivery, and 1 had a precipitate second-stage delivery that did not require assistance. For all the women, the maternal heart rate did not vary significantly before, during, or after labor and delivery. The average

**Table 1. Summaries of previous cases of pregnant women with CAVB in the English literature.**

| Pt. | Authors | Age | Past history of open heart surgery | History of syncope | Heart rate | Cardiac failure during pregnancy | Obstetrical complication | Pacemaker | Gestational age at delivery | Delivery mode | Indication for CS | Anesthesia | Birth weight | Intrapartum outcome |
|---|---|---|---|---|---|---|---|---|---|---|---|---|---|---|
| 1 | Ginns HM et al. *1)* | 29 | No | Yes | 70 pacing | No | Premature contractions | Permanent pacemaker already implanted before pregnancy | 30 | Forceps | | | 1420 g | uneventful |
| 2 | Middleton EB et al. *2)* | 23 | No | Yes | 75 pacing | No | none | Permanent pacemaker already implanted before pregnancy and generator replaced during pregnancy | full term | CS | marginal placental reserve | | 3473 g | uneventful |
| 3 | Eddy WA et al. *3)* | 21 | No | No | 32 | No | none | No | full term | Forceps | | | 8 pounds and 6 ounces | uneventful |
| 4 | Eddy WA et al. *3)* | 21 | No | Yes | 72 pacing | No | none | Permanent pacemaker already implanted before pregnancy | NA | TVD | | Epidural | NA | widespread passive pulmonary vessel congestion with cardiomegaly immediately following delivery |

**Table 1. (Continued)**

| Pt. | Authors | Age | Past history of open heart surgery | History of syncope | Heart rate | Cardiac failure during pregnancy | Obstetrical complication | Pacemaker | Gestational age at delivery | Delivery mode | Indication for CS | Anesthesia | Birth weight | Intrapartum outcome |
|---|---|---|---|---|---|---|---|---|---|---|---|---|---|---|
| 5 | Amikan S et al. *4)* | 27 | No | Yes | 85 pacing | No | none | Permanent pacemaker already implanted before pregnancy | full term | TVD | | | 2850 g | uneventful |
| 6 | Amikan S et al. *4)* | 32 | Yes (VSD) | Yes | NA pacing | No | none | Permanent pacemaker already implanted before pregnancy | 38 | TVD | | | 2750 g | uneventful |
| 7 | Abramovici H et al. *5)* | 24 | NA | Yes | 80 pacing | No | none | Permanent pacemaker already implanted before pregnancy | NA | Forceps | | | NA | uneventful |
| 8 | Abramovici H et al. *5)* | 32 | Yes | Yes | NA | No | none | Permanent pacemaker already implanted before pregnancy | NA | NA | | | NA | uneventful |
| 9 | Abramovici H et al. *5)* | 38 | NA | No | 46 | No | none | No | NA | NA | | | NA | uneventful |
| 10 | Abramovici H et al. *5)* | 29 | Yes | No | 52 | No | none | No | NA | NA | | | NA | uneventful |

**Table 1. (Continued)**

| Pt. | Authors | Age | Past history of open heart surgery | History of syncope | Heart rate | Cardiac failure during pregnancy | Obstetrical complication | Pacemaker | Gestational age at delivery | Delivery mode | Indication for CS | Anesthesia | Birth weight | Intrapartum outcome |
|---|---|---|---|---|---|---|---|---|---|---|---|---|---|---|
| 11 | Jaffe R et al. *6)* | 39 | Yes (ASD) | Yes | 70 pacing | No | Premature contractions | Permanent pacemaker already implanted before pregnancy | 37 | Forceps | | | 2730 g | uneventful |
| 12 | Guldal M et al. *7)* | 30 | NA | Yes | 40 | NA | NA | Permanent pacemaker implanted at 10 weeks of gestation | NA | NA | | | NA | NA |
| 13 | Andersen C et al. *8)* | 24 | Yes (ASD, VSD) | No | 70 pacing | No | none | Permanent pacemaker already implanted before pregnancy | full term | CS | NA | | 3200 g | NA |
| | | 27 | | | 70-102 pacing | No | none | Pacemaker already implanted before pregnancy and replaced with rate-responsive pacemaker during pregnancy | 39 | CS | NA | | 2945 g | uneventful |
| 14 | Lau CP et al. *9)* | 33 | NA | No | 30 | Yes | none | Permanent pace-maker implanted at 29 weeks of gestation | 39 | CS | previous CS | | 2860 g | favorable |
| 15 | Matorras R et al. *10)* | 21 | NA | NA | 74 pacing | No | none | Permanent pacemaker already implanted before pregnancy | 39 | Vacuum | | | 2870 g | uneventful |

**Table 1. (Continued)**

| Pt. | Authors | Age | Past history of open heart surgery | History of syncope | Heart rate | Cardiac failure during pregnancy | Obstetrical complication | Pacemaker | Gestational age at delivery | Delivery mode | Indication for CS | Anesthesia | Birth weight | Intrapartum outcome |
|---|---|---|---|---|---|---|---|---|---|---|---|---|---|---|
| | | 28 | | | 74 pacing | No | none | Permanent pacemaker already implanted before pregnancy | 38 | Forceps | | Spinal | NA | fetal distress and neonatal acidemia |
| 16 | Dalvi BV et al. *11)* | 22 | No | Yes (GA 38w) | 30 | No | none | Temporary pacemaking during labor progresion in view of symptoms | 38 | Forceps | | | NA | developed blackouts, permanent pacemaker implanted before discharge |
| 17 | Dalvi BV et al. *11)* | 20 | No | Yes (GA 36w) | 38 | No | none | Temporary pacemaking during labor progresion in view of symptoms | 36 | Forceps | | | NA | developed blackouts, permanent pacemaker implanted before discharge |
| 18 | Dalvi BV et al. *11)* | 24 | No | No | 52 | No | none | Prophylactic temporary pacemaking during labor progresion | full term | TVD | | | NA | uneventful |
| 19 | Ramsewak S et al. *12)* | 22 | NA | no | 42 | No | twin pregnancy | Prophylactic temporary pacemaking during labor progresion | 36 | CS | breech presentation | | 2420 g<br>2340 g | uneventful |

**Table 1. (Continued)**

| Pt. | Authors | Age | Past history of open heart surgery | History of syncope | Heart rate | Cardiac failure during pregnancy | Obstetrical complication | Pacemaker | Gestational age at delivery | Delivery mode | Indication for CS | Anesthesia | Birth weight | Intrapartum outcome |
|---|---|---|---|---|---|---|---|---|---|---|---|---|---|---|
| 20 | Sharma JB et al. *13)* | 24 | No | No | 40 | No | IUGR and oligohydramnios | Prophylactic temporary pacemaking during labor progresion | 39 | TVD | | | 1960 g | uneventful |
| 21 | Mehta S et al. *14)* | 30 | No | No | 44 | No | none | Prophylactic temporary pacemaking during labor progresion | 39 | TVD | | | 2630 g | uneventful |
| 22 | Avasthi K et al. *15)* | 26 | No | No | 52 | No | triplet pregnancy, hypertension, proteinuria | No (with arrangements for a temporary pacemaker) | 36 | CS | triplet pegnancy | | 2400 g, 2100 g, 1200 g | uneventful |
| 23 | Adekanye O et al. *16)* | 28 | No | No | 40 | No | hypertension | No (with arrangements for a temporary pacemaker) | 38 | TVD | | Epidural | 3850 g | uneventful |

Pt: patient, CS: cesarean section, ASD: atrial septal defect VSD: ventricular septal defect, GA: gestational age, NA: not available, IUGR: intrauterine growth restriction, TVD: transvaginal delivery.

## Table 2. Summaries of 21 deliveries in women with CAVB between 1981 and November 1997 at the National Cardiovascular Center.

| Pt. | Year | Age | Age at diagnosis of CAVB | History of Adams-Stokes attack or cardiac arrest | Heart rate on admission (/min) | Obstetrical complication | Pacemaker | Gestational age at delivery (week) | Delivery mode | Indication for CS | Birth weight (g) | Apgar score | Cord arterial pH | Total blood loss(g) |
|---|---|---|---|---|---|---|---|---|---|---|---|---|---|---|
| 1 | 1981 | 24 | 22 | (-) | N.A. | (-) | temporary | N.A. | N.A | | N.A. | N.A. | N.A. | N.A. |
| | 1987 | 30 | | | 46 | (-) | temporary | 37 | forceps | | 2820 | 9,9 | 7.325 | 220 |
| 2 | 1982 | 27 | 24 | (+) | 78 | mild toxemia | permanent | 39 | emergent CS | arrest of labor | 2710 | 8,10 | 7.294 | 250 |
| | 1985 | 30 | | | 75 | previous C/S | permanent | 37 | elective CS | previous CS | 2674 | 8,9 | N.A. | 1100 |
| 3 | 1984 | 25 | 15 | (-) | 56 | (-) | temporary | 39 | forceps | | 2748 | 8,9 | 7.247 | 725 |
| | 1987 | 27 | | | 56 | IUGR | no | 36 | spontaneous TVD | | 1974 | 8,8 | 7.388 | 240 |
| 4 | 1984 | 26 | 1 | (-) | 50 | threatened preterm labor | temporary | 37 | forceps | | 2736 | 9,9 | 7.266 | 950 |
| 5 | 1984 | 28 | 15 | (-) | 48 | threatened preterm labor | no | 38 | forceps | | 2773 | 8,9 | 7.265 | 450 |
| | 1986 | 31 | | (-) | 45 | breech presentation | temporary | 38 | spontaneous TVD | | 2460 | 9,9 | 7.333 | 400 |
| | 1991 | 35 | | | 46 | threatened preterm labor | no | 38 | forceps | | 2882 | 8,9 | 7.372 | 420 |
| 6 | 1985 | 26 | 12 | (+) | 53 | (-) | temporary | 37 | spontaneous TVD | | 2478 | 8,9 | 7.345 | 910 |
| 7 | 1987 | 24 | 5 | (+) | 90 | (-) | permanent | 38 | forceps | | 3088 | 9,9 | 7.338 | 800 |
| | 1989 | 26 | | | 90 | threatened preterm labor | permanent | 38 | forceps | | 2828 | 10,10 | 7.280 | 500 |
| 8 | 1991 | 24 | 15 | (+) | 78 | (-) | permanent | 39 | forceps | | 2886 | 9,9 | 7.233 | 1720 |
| | 1993 | 26 | | | 80 | (-) | permanent | 38 | forceps | | 2894 | 8,9 | 7.281 | 660 |
| 9 | 1992 | 29 | 14 | (-) | 48 | threatened preterm labor | temporary | 37 | forceps | | 2616 | 8,9 | 7.334 | 1578 |

**Table 2. (Continued)**

| Pt. | Year | Age | Age at diagnosis of CAVB | History of Adams-Stokes attack or cardiac arrest | Heart rate on admission ( /min) | Obstetrical complication | Pacemaker | Gestational age at delivery (week) | Delivery mode | Indication for CS | Birth weight (g) | Apgar score | Cord arterial pH | Total blood loss(g) |
|---|---|---|---|---|---|---|---|---|---|---|---|---|---|---|
| | 1993 | 30 | | | 54 | (-) | temporary | 37 | forceps | | 3166 | 9,9 | 7.293 | 740 |
| 10 | 1993 | 28 | 3 | (-) | 84 | excessive weight gain | permanent | 37 | emergent CS | arrest of labor | 3050 | 8,9 | 7.220 | 260 |
| 11 | 1995 | 26 | 7 | (-) | 56 | (-) | temporary | 40 | forceps | | 3516 | 8,9 | 7.310 | 1551 |
| 12 | 1997 | 32 | 0 | (-) | 30 | IUGR | temporary | 39 | forceps | | 2308 | 9,9 | 7.285 | 580 |
| 13 | 1997 | 32 | 0 | (-) | 46 | threatened preterm labor | temporary | 37 | forceps | | 2916 | 7,8 | 7.343 | 1638 |

Pt: patient, CAVB: complete atrioventricular block, CS: cesarean section, TVD: transvaginal delivery.

(range) of the estimated total blood loss was 949 (158–2414) mL. One woman (Patient 4) developed hypotension (84/47 mmHg) after significant postpartum hemorrhage (2414 mL) caused by uterine atony. However, her blood pressure was normalized by means of simple resuscitation with intravenous crystalloid, and artificial pacing was not required. In this series, the minimum maternal heart rate observed in a patient after delivery was 32 beats/min. This woman remained well throughout the study period with no syncopal or hypotensive episodes even though she had an estimated blood loss of 678 mL. Hence, none of the cases experienced syncope during labor or puerperium and did not require temporary pacing. These results indicate that women with CAVB who do not require a permanent pacemaker can be managed during labor without temporary pacing.

**Table 3. The outcomes of the 6 patients included in our study.**

| Patient | Age (y.o.) | Age at diagnosis of CAVB (y.o.) | History of Adams-Stokes attacks | Obstetric complication | HR on admission ( /min) | Edema | Cardiomegaly |
|---|---|---|---|---|---|---|---|
| 1 | 26 | 0 | (-) | | 48 | (-) | (-) |
| | 28 | | | | 52 | (-) | (-) |
| 2 | 29 | 7 | (-) | | 55 | (-) | (-) |
| 3 | 33 | 0 | (-) | threatened preterm labor | 45 | (-) | (+) |
| 4 | 28 | 0 | (-) | | 46 | (+) | (+) |
| 5 | 38 | 0 | (-) | | 40 | (-) | (+) |
| 6 | 21 | 1 | (-) | threatened preterm labor | 38 | (-) | (-) |
| mean ± SD | 29.6 ± 4.3 | | | | 49.9 ± 7.4 | | |

CAVB: complete atrioventricular block
HR: heart rate

**Table 4. Summary of labor progression in CAVB women.**

| Patient | Gestational age at delivery | Labor onset | HR before delivery (/min) | Delivery mode | Birth weight (g) | Total blood loss (g) | HR after delivery (/min) | Minimum blood pressure (mmHg) | Pacing |
|---|---|---|---|---|---|---|---|---|---|
| 1 | 37w2d | induced | 50 | forceps | 2656 | 416 | 38 | 118/56 | (-) |
| | 38w4d | induced | 40 | forceps | 3016 | 680 | 40 | 113/54 | (-) |
| 2 | 39w6d | induced | 45 | forceps | 3116 | 798 | 48 | 116/58 | (-) |
| 3 | 26w6d | spontaneous | 45 | sp.TVD | 1027 | 1500 | 53 | 90/40 | (-) |
| 4 | 38w2d | induced | 48 | forceps | 2291 | 2412 | 45 | 84/47 | (-) |
| 5 | 38w4d | induced | 40 | sp.TVD | 2594 | 158 | 36 | 112/42 | (-) |
| 6 | 36w0d | spontaneous | 38 | forceps | 2234 | 678 | 32 | 118/58 | (-) |
| mean ± SD | | | 52.0 ± 14.1 | | 2522.0 ± 566.5 | 935.8 ± 642.5 | 49.6 ± 15.1 | | |

HR: heart rate, TVD: transvaginal delivery

# Management of Pregnant Women with Permanent Pacemaker

Owing to improved implantation techniques, reliable equipment, extensive clinical experience, and better cardiovascular function than that achievable by using conventional drugs, permanent cardiac pacemakers are increasingly being used in younger women with CAVB. As a result, the number of women who become pregnant with heart pacemakers is also growing. Clearly, the development of the permanent cardiac pacemakers has significantly reduced the perinatal risk associated with CAVB. Generally, pacing is indicated in CAVB patients who have exercise intolerance. Moreover, if the escape rhythm is less than 50 beats/min in infants or 45 beats/min in adolescents, permanent pacemaker therapy may be indicated even in asymptomatic patients to prevent the development of syncope or symptoms of congestive heart failure.

As shown in Table 1, there are 10 published reports of cases (12 deliveries) in which permanent pacemakers had already been implanted prior to delivery. In our research center, there have been 4 such cases (7 births). Analysis of all of these cases demonstrates that such patients have favorable perinatal outcomes. The maternal heart rate increases by approximately 25% during pregnancy [28]. Of course, this increased heart rate cannot be obtained in women who are implanted with fixed rate pacemakers. However, increase in cardiac output is achieved in such patients at the expense of an increase in stroke volume. This is the probable reason for the rare incidences of heart failure during pregnancy and delivery in such patients. The heart rate in such patients varies considerably, as shown in Table 1. The maternal hemodynamic condition varies with the progression of gestation. Hence, it is possible to further discuss the most appropriate rate setting depending on each gestational and intrapartum stage.

The most frequent complication of permanent pacemaker implantation in pregnant women is skin irritation and ulceration at the site of implantation, which is caused by stretching of the skin due to enlargement of the breasts and abdomen during pregnancy [2,4,19,35]. Ginns et al. have reported a case of breast skin ulceration at 16 weeks of gestation as a complication of implantation of a permanent pacemaker due to the increase in breast size [4]. They reimplanted the battery unit of the pacemaker in the subpectoral pocket (chest wall under the breasts). Hence, implanting pacemakers in the abdominal or breast areas of young women should be avoided because of the changes theses areas undergo during pregnancy. The subpectoral pocket is a good choice for pacemaker implantation since it does not cause strain to the skin during pregnancy and does not cause hindrance in the abdominal area in the cases wherein cesarean procedure needs to be performed [4]. Other complications of permanent pacemakers in pregnant women, such as pain, battery failure, and extrasystoles have also been reported [6,35,36].

# Management of Pregnant Women without Permanent Pacemakers

The requirement of pacing in symptomatic patient has been clearly discussed. However, the guidelines for determining whom to pace and when to pace if the patient is asymptomatic have not been established. Although the risk of sudden death is unpredictable even in patients who are asymptomatic, some experts recommend that implantation of a permanent pacemaker should be avoided as possible in young asymptomatic patients because of the risk of infection and the requirement of frequent yearly changes of pacemakers. Therefore, some asymptomatic patients are not implanted with a permanent pacemaker before pregnancy.

Some such patients may develop syncope due to heart failure during pregnancy. Needless to say, in pregnant CAVB patients, a sufficient increase in heart rate cannot be achieved although an increased cardiac output is required to cope with the hyper-hemodynamic condition during pregnancy. Indeed, Grand et al. have reported that there is an increase in the number of syncopes during pregnancy (4 out of their 12 series) **[23]**, and Bouvrain et al. evaluated 36 pregnant women with CAVB and reported that 4 of them suffered Adams-Stokes attack **[22]**. For symptomatic patients in the first and second trimesters, permanent pacemaker implantation therapy is generally suggested; it can be performed under echocardiographic control [7,9]. Lau et al. reported a case of a woman with CAVB (pulse rate 30 beats/min) who complained of recurrent dizzy episodes and exertional dyspnea at 29 weeks of gestation and hence required pacemaker implantation [9]. Güldal et al. have reported a case of a woman with CAVB who developed syncope that lasted for about 2 min following dizziness and exertion since the early stages of pregnancy [7]. In this case, a permanent pacemaker was successfully implanted at 10 weeks of gestation, and her subsequent perinatal course was uneventful. Although all of our cases fortunately remained functionally latent during their pregnancies, careful regular follow-up throughout pregnancy is advised. For symptomatic CAVB women who present at or near term, temporary pacing followed by labor induction at the earliest possible time should be recommended.

Ramsewak et al. have reported a CAVB case of twin pregnancy **[12]**. The cardiac work load in a twin pregnancy is greater than that in a singleton pregnancy, and the increased maternal heart rate and contractility in twin pregnancies suggest that the cardiovascular reserve is reduced [37,38]. In general, the cardiac output in a twin pregnancy is reported to be on average 15% higher throughout pregnancy compared to that in a singleton pregnancy [37]. Echocardiographic finding of the abovementioned case reported by Ramsevak et al. demonstrated a borderline cardiac output, suggesting that the stroke volume would be unable to compensate for the increased heart rate. Further, Avasthi et al. have recently described a case of CAVB with triplet pregnancy [15]. Even though a favorable outcome was achieved eventually, their patient experienced chest pain and cardiomegaly was detected on chest X-ray at 32 weeks of gestation. In multiple pregnancies, additional attention should be paid to monitor the maternal hemodynamic changes at the earliest possible stage.

# Intrapartum Management of Women without Permanent Pacemaker

In pregnant women with CAVB, hospital admission a few days before the expected date of delivery is desirable so that any procedure that is electively required can be performed. Some reports have stated good outcomes of temporary pacing for CAVB patients in labor **[11–14]**. Women with CAVB but who have not been implanted with a permanent pacemaker seemed to certainly receive temporary pacing during labor and birth; however, the absolute justification of this temporary pacing has not been provided. Our clinical analysis, which included 7 cases, suggested that women with CAVB who do not require a permanent pacemaker can be managed in labor even without temporary pacing, and thus, the risks associated with such procedures can be avoided **[25]**. Recently, 2 case reports have described similar management **[15–16]**.

We also believe that other aspects of labor management such as elective epidural analgesia and invasive monitoring of arterial blood pressure or central venous blood pressure are important as components of the care of these women and for maintaining stable maternal hemodynamics [16,25,39]. In normal labor without epidural anesthesia, essentially during the first stage of labor, a 12% increase is observed in the basal cardiac output rate between contractions. Further, cardiac output during contraction increases progressively as labor advances; it increases by a mean value of 34% at full dilatation of the cervix **[28]**.Considering these hemodynamic changes during labor progression, epidural anesthesia should be recommended to reduce labor pain and to minimize the hemodynamic changes. If anesthesia is not administered, it is preferable to perform delivery in a lateral decubitus position in order to avoid or minimize bearing down. Elective instrumental delivery is also an important method to shorten the duration of the active phase of the second stage of labor.

After delivery, some hemodynamic changes during pregnancy, including increase in blood volume, hemodilution, and peripheral vascular resistance revert to the levels of pre-pregnant state. These altered hemodynamic variables can contribute to the CAVB symptoms of patients during pregnancy; therefore, the symptomatic status should be reassessed in the postpartum period. If the symptoms are persistent or reappear, the requirement of permanent pacemaker implantation should be carefully discussed.

# Obstetric Complications in Women with CAVB

A previous report has described that intrauterine growth restriction (IUGR) is associated with CAVB [40]. IUGR was defined as a birth weight below the $10^{th}$ percentile for the given gestational age in our study [41]. As shown in Tables, IUGR was observed in only 2 of the overall 28 pregnancies at our hospital. On the basis of the analysis of previous literature and our series, we found that there was no correlation between maternal CAVB and IUGR.

In our series, threatened preterm delivery was defined as frequent uterine contractions with progressive cervical maturation requiring intravenous administration of tocolytic agents. As a result, threatened preterm delivery was diagnosed in 8 (29%) out of the overall 28 pregnancies. This incidence seems higher than that observed in the general population. In 2 cases, we could not prevent preterm labor even after administering tocolytic agents. In contrast, an analysis of previous literature suggests that the incidence of preterm delivery in CAVB patients is not very high. One report has described the case of a pregnant woman with CAVB, in which spontaneous preterm delivery occurred at 30 weeks of gestation without any obvious obstetric cause [1]. However, all the other cases in previous literature show that gestation stage progressed to at least 36 weeks. Therefore, CAVB is possibly not associated with spontaneous preterm delivery.

Furthermore, maternal hypertension or preeclampsia was observed in some cases; however, the incidence was not very high. Fetal distress, low Apgar scores, or acidemia in the neonatal stage were rarely observed; a sole case was described by Matorras et al. [10]. Hence, CAVB appears to be rarely associated with any specific obstetric problem.

## Long Term Follow-up after Delivery

Eddy et al. have reported 2 cases of pregnant women with CAVB who required permanent pacemaker implantation several months after an uneventful transvaginal delivery **[3]**. In their report, 1 woman showed syncope episodes 1 year after delivery, and the other showed decreased ventricular contraction 3 months after delivery. In 2005, we encountered a case of a woman with CAVB who developed syncope and died suddenly 1 month after an uneventful elective cesarean delivery, although this case has not been listed in this study. Generally, postpartum women experience considerable physical stress owing to the responsibility of parenting and breast feeding. Hence, the course of clinical symptoms and cardiac contractility of patients should be carefully followed by echocardiography, even in the cases of uneventful pregnancies and deliveries.

## Conclusion

Obstetric management of women who have permanent pacemakers implanted before conception have been sufficiently reported thus far, and that the management of such patients can be considered to be nearly free of any risks. Since CAVB usually does not cause any specific obstetric problems during pregnancy, pre-pregnancy prophylactic placement of a permanent pacemaker is not indicated in all asymptomatic patients. The current increase in the use of permanent pacemakers in young women with symptomatic CAVB will certainly limit the need for intrapartum temporary pacing in patients who can survive without pace makers before pregnancy. In fact, most women with CAVB who do not require a permanent pacemaker before delivery can be safely managed during labor even without temporary pacing. CAVB is not an indication for therapeutic abortion, and young women with CAVB with or without pacemakers should not be discouraged from attempting pregnancy.

# References


[1] Ginns, HM; Hollinrake, K. Complete heart block in pregnancy treated with an internal cardiac pacemaker. *J Obstet Gynaecology Br Commonw*, 1970, 77, 710-712.

[2] Middleton, EB; Lee, YC. Pregnancy associated with cardiac pacemaker generator implanted in the abdominal wall. *Obstet Gynecol*, 1971, 38, 272-275.

[3] Eddy, WA; Frankenfeld, RH. Congenital complete heart block in pregnancy. *Am J Obstet Gynecol*, 1977, 128, 223-225.

[4] Amikam, S; Abramovici, H; Brandes, JM; Peleg, H; Riss, E. Pregnancy in the presence of an implanted pacemaker. *Int Surg*, 1981, 66, 369-371.

[5] Abramovici, Dimfeld, M; Weisman, Z; Sorokin, Y; Lissak, A; Rofe, A; Sheinfeld, M. Maternal permanent bradycardia: pregnancy and delivery. *Obstet Gynecol*, 1984, 63, 381-383.

[6] Jaffe, R; Gruber, A; Fejgin, M; Altaras, M; Ben-Aderet, N. Pregnancy with an artificial pacemaker. *Obstet Gynecol Surv*, 1987, 42, 137-139.

[7] Gudal, M; Kervancioglu, C; Oral, D; Gurel, T; Erol, C; Sonel, A. Permanent pacemaker implantation in a pregnant woman with the guidance of ECG and two-dimensional echocardiography. *Pacing Clin Electrophysiol*, 1987, 10, 543-545.

[8] Anderson, C; Oxho, H; Arnsbo, P; Lybecker, H. Pregnancy and cesarean section in a patient with a rate-responsive pacemaker. *Pacing Clin Electrophysiol*, 1989, 12, 386-391.

[9] Lau, CP; Lee, CP; Wong, CK; Cheng, CH; Leung, WH. Rate responsive pacing with a minute ventilation sensing pacemaker during pregnancy and delivery. *Pacing Clin Electrophysiol*, 1990, 13, 158-163.

[10] Matorras, R; Diez, J; Saez, M; Montoya, F; Aranguren, G; Rodriguez-Escudero, FJ. Repeat pregnancy associated with cardiac pacemaker. *Int J Obstet Gynecol*, 1991, 36, 323-327.

[11] Dalvi, BV; Chandhuri, A; Kulkarni, HL; Kale, PA. Therapeutic guidelines for congenital complete heart block. *Obstet Gynecol*, 1992, 79, 802-804.

[12] Ramsewak, S; Persad, P; Perkins, S; Narayansingh, G. Twin pregnancy in a patient with complete heart block. *Clin Exp Obstet Gynecol*, 1992, 19, 166-167.

[13] Sharma, JB; Malhotra, M; Purdir, P. Successful pregnancy outcome with cardiacpacemaker after complete heart block. *Int J Gynecol Obstet*, 2000, 68, 145-146.

[14] Mehta, S; Goswami, D; Temple, A. Successful pregnancy outcome in a patient with complete heart block. *J Postgrad Med*, 2003, 49, 98.

[15] Avasthi, K; Gupta, S; Avasthi, G. An unusual case of complete heart block with triplet pregnancy. *Indian Heart J*, 2003, 55, 641-642.

[16] Adekanye, O; Srinivas, K; Collis, RE. Bradyarrhythmias in pregnancy: a case report and review of management. *Int J Obstet Anesth*, 2007, 16, 165-170.

[17] Epstein, JR; Altman, HE. Heart block in pregnancy; report of two cases *Med Ann Dist Columbia*, 1951, 20, 660-663.

[18] Shouse, EE; Acker, JE. Pregnancy and delivery in a patient with external-internal cardiac pacemaker. *Obstet Gynecol*, 1964, 24, 817-818.

[19] Schonbrun, M; Rowland, W; Quiroz, AC. Complete heart block in pregnancy. *Obstet Gynecol*, 1966, 27, 243-246.

[20] Kenmure, AC; Cameron, AJ. Congenital complete heart block in pregnancy. *Br Heart J*, 1967, 29, 911-913.

[21] Berestka, SA; Spellacy, WN. Complete heart block associated with pregnancy and treated with an internal pacemaker. *J Lancet*, 1967, 87, 461-463.

[22] Bouvrain, Y; Kpodonu, J; Butruille, C; Slama, R; Muqica, J. Pregnancy in women with atrioventricular block. 13 cases (in French) *Nouv Presse Med*, 1976, 9, 2141-2143.

[23] Grand, A; Huret, JF; Farge, C; Ferry, M; Perret, SP. Auriculo-ventricular block and pregnancy. (in French) *Arch Mal Coeur Vaiss*, 1981, 74, 909-916.

[24] Huang, H; Lin, Q; Zhang, L. Clinical observation of cardiac pacemaker in pregnant women. (in Chinese) *Zhonghua Fu Chan Ke Za Zhl*, 1997, 32, 345-346.

[25] Hidaka, N; Chiba, Y; Kurita, T; Satoh, S; Nakano, H. Is intrapartum temporary pacing required for women with complete atrioventricular block? An analysis of seven cases. *BJOG*, 2006, 113, 605-607.

[26] Gochberg, SH. Congenital heart block. *Am J Obstet Gynecol*, 1964, 88, 238-241

[27] Camm, AJ; Bexten, RS. Congenital complete heart block. *Eur Heart J*, 1984, 5, 115-117.

[28] Hunter, S; Robson, SC. Adaptation of the maternal heart in pregnancy. *Br Heart J*, 1992, 68, 540-543.

[29] Duvekot, JJ; Peeters, LL. Maternal cardiovascular hemodynamic adaptation to pregnancy. *Obstet Gynecol Surv*, 1994, 49, S1-14.

[30] Robson, SC; Dunlop, W; Boys, RJ; Hunter, S. Cardiac output during labour. *Br Med J*, 1987, 7, 1169-1172.

[31] Ueland, K. Maternal cardiovascular dynamics II Posture and uterine contractions. *Am J Obstet Gynecol*, 1969, 103, 1-7.

[32] Ueland, K. Maternal cardiovascular dynamics III Labor and delivery under local and caudal analgesia. *Am J Obstet Gynecol*, 1969, 103, 8-18.

[33] Nanta, A. *Arch. Mal. Coeur.*, 1914, 7, 305.

[34] Mendelson, CL. Disorders of the heart beat during pregnancy. *Am J Obstet Gynecol*, 1956, 72, 1268-1301.

[35] Büchner, Bilger, R; Overbeck, W; Miklaw, H; Reindel, H. Delivery in a patient with an artificial heart pacemaker (in German). *Dtsch Med Wochenschr*, 1964, 89, 1932-1933.

[36] Smirnova, LM; Glukhova, PA; Paulova, SS; Ivanova, IG. Pregnancy and labor in patients with artificial pacemakers (in Russian). *Akush Ginelol (Mosk)*, 1982, 5, 31-34.

[37] Robson, SC; Hunter, S; Boys, RJ; Dunlop, W. Hemodynamic changes during twin pregnancy. A Doppler and M-mode echocardiographic study. *Am J Obstet Gynecol*, 1989, 161, 1273-1278.

[38] Veille, JC; Morton, MJ; Burry, KJ. Maternal cardiovascular adaptations to twin pregnancy. *Am J Obstet Gynecol*, 1985, 153, 261-263.

[39] Baron, JF; Decaux-Jacolot, A; Edouard, A; Berdeaux, A; Samii, K. Influence of venous return on baroreflex control of heart rate during lumbar epidural anesthesia in humans. *Anesthesiology*, 1986, 64, 188-193.

[40] Plesse, R; During, R. A case of intrauterine fetal retardation with polycythemia in a patient with pacemaker. (in German) *Zentralbl Gynakol*, 1984, 106, 1547-1550.

[41] Ogawa, Y; Iwamura, T; Kuriya, N; Nishida, H; Takeuchi, H; Takada, M; Itabashi, K; Imura, S; Isobe, K. Birth size standards by gestational age for Japanese neonates. (in Japanese) *Acta Neonatologica Japonica*, 1998, 34, 624-63.

In: Advances in Cardiovascular Research, Volume 1
Editors: L. Schmitt, T. Konig, pp. 307-320
ISBN: 978-1-60741-720-0


*Chapter XIII*

# Cardiovascular Risk Following Hypertensive Pregnancy

***Giancarlo Paradisi**, *Terryann Spagnuolo, Francesca Ianniello, Marina Bracaglia, Antonietta Labianca, Lorena Quagliozzi, Augusto Di Vico and Alessandro Caruso***

Department of Obstetrics & Gynecology, Università Cattolica del Sacro Cuore - Policlinico Agostino Gemelli, Largo Vito 8, 00168 – Roma, Italy

## Abstract

More and more are the evidence that identify hypertensive disorders in pregnancy as an important factor of cardiovascular risk. Compared to women who have had a prior physiological pregnancy we can see that those who had pregnancy complicated by hypertensive disorders show an increased predisposition for cardiovascular diseases in the following years, with a higher risk of myocardial infarction and cerebral ictus. The close correlation between hypertensive dysfunction in pregnancy-particularly preeclampsia-and cardiovascular diseases can be in part explained since they have factors of risk in common, such as obesity, diabetes and dyslipidemia, which cause as a whole the so-called "metabolic syndrome".

In addition, the altered endothelial function, *primum movens* of the micro and macro vascular damage, is either present in the metabolic syndrome or in the hypertension in pregnancy. So there are numerous analogies between the two pathologic conditions, and the clinical epidemiological data, almost univocal, shows that hypertension in pregnancy must be considered by the gynaecologist as a factor of risk for women's health, not only during gestation but also to the years to come.

**Keywords:** Pregnancy, preeclampsia, endothelial dysfunction, metabolic syndrome, cardiovascular risk.

* Corresponding author: Mobile: 39 335 5335787, Fax: 39 06 3051160, E-mail: giancarlo.paradisi@tin

# Introduction

Hypertensive disorders represent the most frequent pathology in pregnancy and, nowadays in the World, the main cause of maternal and perinatal morbility and mortality [1]. The incidence oscillate among 1 and 10%, with a variable prevalence mostly due to the different ethnic group, geographical areas, but also according to age and body mass index. In United States it affects an estimated 5-8% of pregnant women annually [2]. The economical impact is enormous: just consider the periodical, and at times long necessary hospitalization, during pregnancy, in order to guarantee an effective monitoring of the maternal conditions and an adequate prenatal surveillance. Moreover, the frequent fetal complications associated to such pregnancies – as fetal growth restriction and the preterm delivery -or maternal-such as eclampsia and the abruptio placentae-on the whole involve a high rate of premature babies, need an adequate care in the Neonatal Intensive Care Unit.

On a hemodynamic point of view, physiological pregnancy is typically characterized by an increase of the cardiac output and of the plasmatic volume, a general vasodilatation, a reduced arterial pressure and a resistance to vasopressor agents, such as noroadrenaline and angiotensin II. It is considered as an atherogenous condition, in the light of metabolic modifications as hyperlipidemia and a mild thrombophylia. These modifications are physiologically present in pregnancy, but turn out to be particularly accentuate in the hypertensive pregnant status and similar to those present in high cardiovascular risk patients.

Until a few years ago hypertensive dysfunctions in pregnancy were considered particularly important for the maternal-fetal negative effects during pregnancy. However, numerous scientific evidence have recently led up to identifying hypertension in pregnancy as an important factor of risk in cardiovascular diseases. Both the conditions show in fact factor of risk in common, such as obesity, diabetes and dyslipidemia; so we could hypothesize that hypertension in pregnancy can be itself the cause of vascular and metabolic alterations responsible of an increased cardiovascular risk in the future years [3]. From a study carried out by our Group [4] it has emerged that healthy women with previous gestation hypertension presented an altered endothelial function, able to justify at least in part, the increased risk of cardiovascular diseases. Similar results came out from a study that correlated hypertension in pregnancy with the risk of death by myocardial ischemia in adulthood [5], as well as by wide-ranging and recent trials, which we will be talking about later [6,7,8].

The epidemiological evidence of the correlation between previous hypertensive diseases in pregnancy and subsequent cardiovascular events as ictus, myocardial infarction, hypertension is therefore well consolidated. But which are the mechanism beneath such association?

During this treatise it will be taken in consideration above all the classification of hypertensive disorders, then their association with the cardiovascular disease which may appear in adulthood, finally the common etiopathogenical mechanism.

# Hypertension in Pregnancy and Implications in the Cardiovascular Diseases

A part from the classify criterion adopted, it is basically important to feature in 2 groups the broad spectrum of hypertension disorders in pregnancy, since their etiopathogenesis is different:

- those pre-existent pregnancy *(30%)* →chronic hypertension;
- those that emerge in pregnancy *(70%)*→gestation hypertension/preeclampsia.

However the diagnosis of hypertension in pregnancy –and even more the differential diagnosis of the various hypertensive disorders in pregnancy – not always appears either evident or clear. Together with the *National High Blood Pressure Educational Program* [9] 4 groups are distinguished:

1. chronic hypertension;
2. preeclampsia-eclampsia;
3. preeclampsia superimposed to chronic hypertension;
4. gestation hypertension that, in turn, may differentiate in :

    - **transitory** → in absence of preeclampsia at the time of delivery and in the case of normalization of the pressure value within the $12^{th}$ week after the delivery;
    - **chronic** → in the presence of pressure value persistently enhanced over the $12^{th}$ week after the delivery ( both retrospective diagnosis ).

      We talk about **chronic hypertension** with values *of* PAS ≥ 140 mmHg or of PAD ≥ 90 mmHg in two consecutive observations, carried out 6 hours gap one from the other, before pregnancy, or before the $20^{th}$ gestation week. We also consider chronic hypertension diagnosed for the first time in pregnancy, which doesn't spontaneously solve over the $12^{th}$ week after the delivery.

**Preeclampsia** is the pathological condition, specific of pregnancy and exclusive of the human species, which appears after the $20^{th}$ gestation week, engendered by:

- **hypertension** ( meaning the increase of the pressure in pregnancy, i.e. → observation of a PAS ≥ 140 mmHg or of a PAD ≥ 90 mmHg in two further measurement, 6 hours gap one from the other, in a normal blood pressure woman till the $20^{th}$ gestation week, marking hypertension "mild" for values of PAD < 110 mmHg and *"serious"* for values of PAD ≥ 110 mmHg), the more constant constituent, associated to
- **proteinuria,** the more sure sign, although sometimes absent or late developer outset;
- **oedemas**, the more aspecific and not necessary sign.

We call **eclampsia** the emerging of convulsive fit, till coma, not related to neurologic causes, in pregnant women suffering from preeclampsia.

5. We call **gestation hypertension** the increase of the pressure which appears for the first time after the $20^{th}$ gestation week, in absence of proteinuria. It is often the

prelude of chronic hypertension which will develop in the next decades, but it can be the first symptom of preeclampsia. Therefore to this category belong either women with isolated hypertension or women with preeclampsia who haven't developed proteinuria yet. If preeclampsia hasn't developed and the pressure has become again standard within the $12^{th}$ week after the delivery, we will talk about gestation hypertension (it's, therefore, a diagnosis of exclusion, that can be only emphasized a posteriori); if hypertension persists after such time, we will talk about chronic hypertension.

## Hypertension in Pregnancy and Subsequent Chronic Hypertension

It goes back to 1936 the first record of an association between preeclampsia and long term risk for developing arterial hypertension [10], however restricted to the fact of being retrospective, to checking on a relatively small pattern and to the inadequate lasting of the follow-up.

Researches carried out among 1960's and the beginning of 1980's have fully confirmed such hypothesis [11, 12]. Afterwards other prospect [13, 14] and retrospective [15, 16] trials have emphasized a close relationship between gestation hypertension, preeclampsia/eclampsia and subsequent arterial hypertension as already shown by Sibai in 1986 [17]. In confirmation to such data a more recent cohort study [18] have shown that women with severe preeclampsia, diagnosed at the beginning of the third trimester of pregnancy, have more than ever double risk to develop hypertension, 30-50 years later, compared with women with past physiological pregnancy.

The present knowledge about factors that affect the pressure normalization immediately after delivery and during postpartum is still scarce. From a past study made on a group of 90 women with hypertension disorders in pregnancy [19] it has emerged that the normalization of pressure levels during post-partum depends from the type of disorder: in fact it results slower in patients with pressure disorders associated to *proteinuria*, such as preeclampsia or the HELLP-syndrome, while faster in patients with hypertension disorders not associated to *proteinuria*, i.e. chronic hypertension or gestation hypertension. Therefore in the light of such data *proteinuria in pregnancy may have a predictive value for the evolvement of a chronic hypertension or of future cardiovascular diseases.*

## Hypertension in Pregnancy and Cardiovascular Diseases

It is interesting to underline that the effects of hypertension in pregnancy on the morbility in the following years are not exclusively limited to the evolvement of hypertension. It goes back to 1976 the first study [20] that showed the increased of mortality caused by cardiovascular diseases in women with previous eclampsia compared with the whole population.

More recently [6] a large epidemiological study confirmed the above association. Women with history of past "placental syndrome" (Figure 1) – such as preeclampsia, gestation hypertension, abruptio placentae, placental infarction (75.380 women, the 7% of the total) – have pointed out a doubled risk of the insurgence of cardiovascular diseases. Such risk was further increased in case of concomitant fetal growth restriction, intrauterine death or pre-existing factors of cardiovascular risks, such as smoke or other characteristic features of the metabolic syndrome: obesity, chronic hypertension, diabetes, dyslipidemia (Figure 2). Other authors [7, 8] have on the other hand underlined how preeclampsia and fetal growth restriction could be most likely considered marker precocious of high cardiovascular risk. Preeclampsia would increase 5 times more the risk, fetal growth restriction, circa 7-11 times.

The already known relationship between preeclampsia, low weight at birth and high risk of death of cardiovascular diseases [21, 22] it has been later confirmed by large studies.

In order to better analyze the relationship between hypertension in pregnancy and the subsequent cardiovascular risk (Table 1), some Authors have examined cohorts of women with history of cardiovascular diseases and compared their obstetric story with those of a control group [24]. A positive history of eclampsia, either for the nullipara or for the multipara, was associated to an increased mortality for cardiovascular diseases [20]. More in detail Sibai *et all* [25] have underlined the importance of a severe preeclampsia arisen at the beginning of the third trimester as a factor of cardiovascular risk. Consistent with these results, other authors [5] studying the incidence of myocardial acute heart attack, have noticed an increase of death in case of previous gestational hypertension, with a further increase in women with past preeclampsia, in particular in the group at early onset [26, 27, 28].

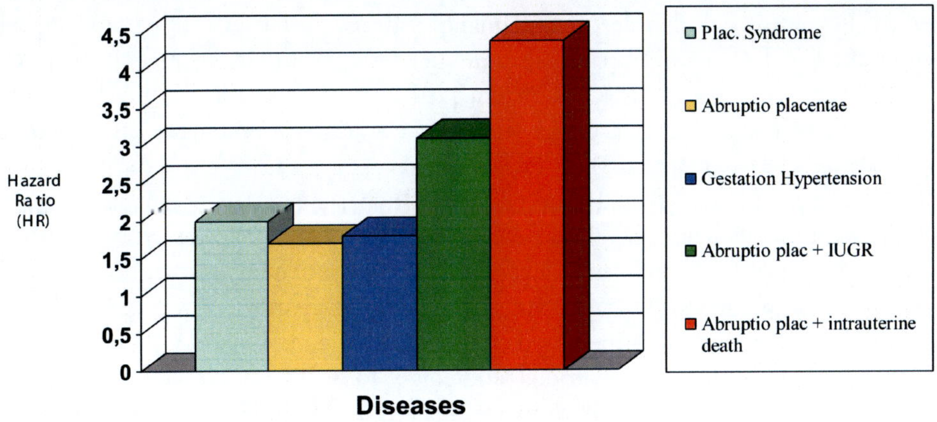


Rielaborated by: Ray JG, Vermeulen MJ, Schull MJ and Redelmeier DA. Cardiovascular health after maternal syndromes (CHAMPS): population-based retrospective cohort study. Lancet 2005; 366: 1797-1803.

Figure 1. Maternal cardiovascular risk according to the type of "placental syndrome" associated to fetal growth restriction (IUGR) or intrauterine death.

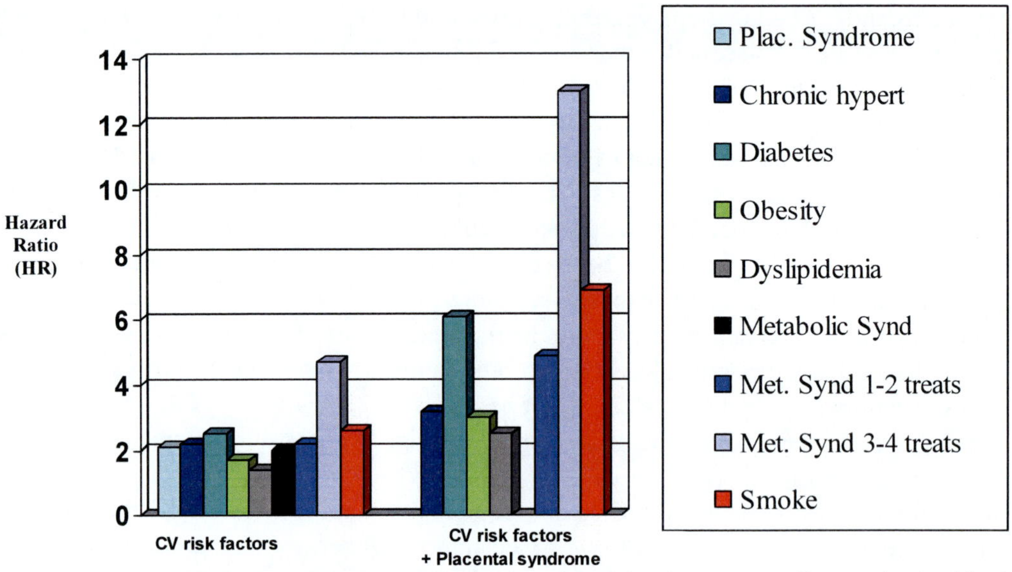


Rielaborated by: Ray JG, Vermeulen MJ, Schull MJ and Redelmeier DA. Cardiovascular health after maternal syndromes (CHAMPS): population-based retrospective cohort study. Lancet 2005; 366: 1797-1803.

Figure 2. Cardiovascular risk and placental syndrome either in presence or not of the traditional cardiovascular risk factors (arterial hypertension, diabetes, obesity dysplidemia).

It seems that the risk of myocardial acute heart attack is increasing, according to the severity of hypertensive disorder in pregnancy, from gestational hypertension without proteinuria (IRR = 1.6), to mild preeclampsia (IRR = 1.9), to severe preeclampsia (IRR = 2.8), as shown by the Groups of Kestenbaum [29] and of Wikstrom [30]. Also the risk of cerebral ictus has resulted increased in women with past preeclampsia, as shown in the studies of Wilson [18] and Brown [31].

It is interesting to note that the only systolic hypertension in pregnancy may have a leading role in the incidence of death of cardiovascular diseases [32]. Recently a study with a follow-up of 44 years made on a sample group of 4090 women has shown how women with systolic hypertension arisen in precocious times of pregnancy – but not associated to proteinuria – have a significantly increased risk of death of cardiovascular diseases.

The conclusions to which the various studies get to are quite overlapping: hypertensive disorders in pregnancy- in particular severe and recurrent preeclampsia- may identify a subgroup of women with a higher risk of future morbility and mortality correlated to cardiovascular diseases: myocardial acute heart attack, ictus, thromboembolic events. Unfortunately, the pathogenic mechanisms that undergo to such relationship are still unclear. During pregnancy complicated by hypertension there are metabolic and vascular alterations similar to those present in cardiovascular disease. Therefore we can hypothesize that such conditions subtend shared factor of risk, which lead now to hypertension in pregnancy, now to cardiovascular disease, according to the different ages of women.

**Table 1. Preeclampsia and maternal cardiovascular risk/maternal death.**

| Author, year | Group of Study | sample (n) | Follow-up (years) | Pathology | RR/OR/HR (CI: 95%CI) |
|---|---|---|---|---|---|
| Chesley 1976 | E vs general population | 270 | 22-43 | Death<br>– Primipara<br>– Multipara | <br>3.0<br>5.0 |
| Sibai 1991 | PE vs PP | 125 | 5.4 | Hypertension<br>– PE mild vs PP<br>– PE severe vs PP | <br>34% vs 4%<br>67% vs 4% |
| Jonsdottir 1995 | PE, GH, E vs PP | 7.543 | 50 | Death per AMI<br>– GH<br>– PE<br>– E | <br>1.47 (1.05-2.02)<br>1.90 (1.02-3.52)<br>2.61 (1.11-6.12) |
| Hannaford 1997 | PE vs PP | 23.000 | 33 | – Hypertension<br>– AMI<br>– CH<br>– All isch disease. | 2.35 (2.08-2.65)<br>2.24 (1.42-3.53)<br>1.74 (1.06-2.86)<br>1.65 (1.26-2.16) |
| Irgens 2001 | PE vs general population | 626.272 | 9-35 | Death<br>– PE: 37 week<br>– PE: 16-36week | <br>1.65 (1.01-2.07)<br>8.12 (4.31-15.33) |
| Smith 2001 | PE, IUGR, SGA vs PP | 129.290 | 15-19 | AMI<br>– PE<br>– SGA<br>– PE + IUGR + SGA | <br>2.0 (1.5-2.5)<br>1.9 (1.5-2.4)<br>7.0 (3.3-14.5) |
| Kestenbaum 2003 | GH, PE mild/severe vs PP | 807.010 | 6-15 | Cardiovascular disease<br>– GH<br>– PE mild<br>– PE severe | <br>2.8 (1.6-4.8)<br>2.2 (1.3-3.6)<br>3.3 (1.7-6.5) |
| Wilson 2003 | PE mild/severe vs PP | 3.593 | 33-52 | – Hypertension<br>– Ictus | 2.3 (1.40-3.98)<br>3.59 (1.04-12.04) |
| Funai 2005 | PE vs PP | 37.061 | 24-36 | – death *sine causa*<br>– death per AMI | 2.0 (1.63-2.46)<br>3.07 (2.18-4.34) |
| Ray 2005 | PE + IUGR/fetal death vs PP | 1,03 mln | ≤ 15 | Cardiovascular diseases<br>– PE<br>– PE + IUGR<br>– PE + fetal death | <br>2.0 (1.7-2.2)<br>3.1 (2.2-4.5)<br>4.4 (2.4-7.9) |
| Wikstrom 2005 | GH, PE mild/severe vs PP | 403.550 | 23-32 | AMI<br>– IG<br>– PE mild<br>– PE severe | <br>1.6 (1.3-2.0)<br>1.9 (1.6-2.2)<br>2.8 (2.2-3.7) |
| Brown 2006 | PE vs PP | 682 | 10-14 | Ictus | 1.63 (1.02-2.62) |

RR, relative risk; OR, odds ratio; HR, hazard ratio.

E, eclampsia; PE, preeclampsia; PP, physiological pregnancy; GH, gestation hypertension; AMI acute myocardial infarction; CH chronic hypertension; IUGR, intrauterine growth restriction; SGA, "small for gestational age".

Modifiied by: Harskhamp RE and Zeeman GG. Preeclampsia: at risk for remote cardiovascular disease. Am J Med Sci 2007; 334 (4): 291-295.

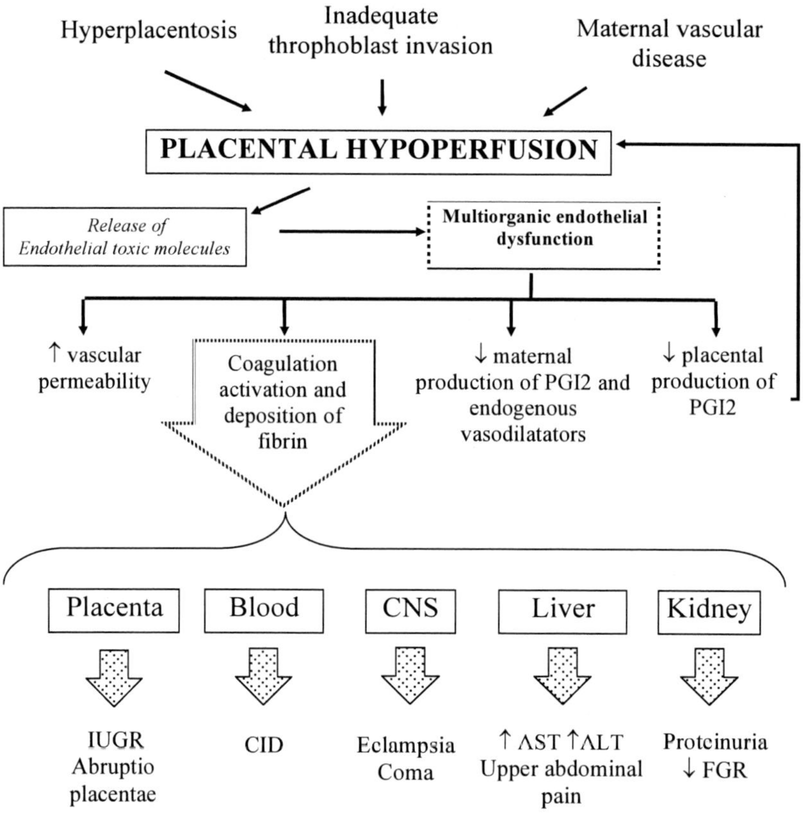


Figure 3. Etiopathogenesis of preeclampsia.

# Hypertensive Disorders in Pregnancy and Cardiovascular Disease: Common Etiopathogenical Mechanisms

## Endothelial Dysfunction

As before underlined, endothelial dysfunction has a crucial role for the pathogenesis of both preeclampsia and cardiovascular disease (Figure 3).

Oxidative stress, release of cytokine from the immune competent cells, a generalized intravascular inflammatory respond (due to the release of fragments of syncytiothrophoblast) determine an increased permeability of the endothelial cells, peroxydation of lipids, blood platelet and coagulation cascade activation and, ultimately, the shift of equilibrium towards vasoconstrictor mediators:

- increase of factor VIII-antigen and of fibronectin;
- increase of the relation between thromboxan (TXA2, vasoconstrictor and proaggregant) and prostacyclin (PGI2, vasodilatator and antiaggregant platelet);
- increase of endothelin (vasoactive mediator);

- reduction of nitric oxide (NO, vasodilatator and antiaggregant platelet).

In pregnancies complicated by preeclampsia, as well in conditions of atherosclerosis, the oxidative stress stimulates the production of free radical which amplifies more the endothelial dysfunction. This mechanism in confirmed by an increased lipoperoxidation associated to a reduced activity of antioxidant enzymes (superoxide-dismutase and glucose-6-fosphate dehydrogenase), by the reduced levels of plasma ascorbic acid and by an increased capacity to generate oxygen free radical from the placental cells of preeclamptic women.

Clinical studies show haw a relative deficit of nitric oxide and an over – expression of several mediator of endothelial cell dysfunction, such as fibronectin factor, von Willebrand factor, the cell adhesion molecule and some cytokine (IL-6 e TNF) could aggravate the state of generalized vasoconstriction characteristic of preeclampsia [33],. It is not well understood whether the endothelial damage is the consequence of the increase of these vasoconstrictor mediators or if their over-expression is a consequence of endothelial dysfunction. Overall all these abnormalities lead to a *condition of systemic vasoconstriction with generalized ischemia and multiorganic dysfunction.*

Recently other new vasoactive mediators have emerged to be associated to preeclampsia [34]:

- vascular endothelial growth factor (VEGF) → pro angiogenic protein produced by glomerular podocyte and of which the most part of the receptors is situated on the endothelial cells,
- soluble fms-like tyrosine kinase-1 (sFlt1) → VEGF membrane receptor which, is a strong antagonist either of the VEGF or of the placenta growth factor (PIGF, pro-angiogenic protein). Since in condition of preeclampsia the placenta produces high concentration of sFlt1, the levels of VEGF and the PIGF would result reduced;
- endoglin (Eng) → co-receptor for the TGF-β1 and TGF-β3, highly expressed from the vascular endothelium and by the syncytiothrophoblast cells. Similarly sFlt1, the soluble endoglin (sEng) is an anti-angiogenic factor which, significantly increases before the clinical manifestation of preeclampsia.

Whatever the cause of endothelial dysfunction, when present, its three main functions are compromised:

- maintenance of the integrity of the vascular system,
- prevention of coagulation,
- modulation of the vascular tone.

## Inflammatory Response

As the atherosclerosis, the adhesion of the leukocyte at the endothelium has a leading role in obtaining an inflammatory response, which may contribute to the development of preeclampsia. Inflammatory response is one of the physiological adaptation which establish in physiological pregnancy and may reflect a maternal immune reaction to the fetal antigens.

Such inflammatory response results abnormal in pregnancy complicated by preeclampsia, that shows high levels of leukocyte activation markers with respect to physiological pregnancy [35]. Among the leukocyte activation molecules elastase (which may compromise the vascular integrity damaging the vascular basal membrane), TNF (mediator of the adherence of the neutrophils to the endothelium), IL-6 (that stimulates the superoxide ion, contributing to the increase of the oxidative stress) and LDL molecules (which are quickly oxidate, promoting the endothelial leukocyte adhesion) are the more investigated. Finally, similarly to the cardiovascular disease, high levels of PCR are associated to a high risk of preeclampsia.

## Prothrombotic State

The physiological prothrombotic state typical of pregnancy is increased in preeclamptic women, as demonstrated by the abnormal reduced ratio between fibrinolysis and coagulation. Different studies have shown in preeclamptic women an increase of the expression of procoagulant proteins, as the tissutal plasminogen activator, PAI1, von Willebrand factor, fibronectin, homocysteine and the thrombomodulin, as well as the contextual reduction of the anticoagulant proteins, as antithrombin III, protein C and protein S. The interaction between prothrombotic state and the endothelial dysfunction is quite complex, given that such mechanisms tend to potentiate each other, leading a generalized vascular damage. Thus endothelial dysfunction and the consequent endothelial cell activation lead to release the procoagulant factors and, consequently, to a hypercoagulability plasmatic state. It is interesting to note that the maternal prothrombotic condition, may be a risk factor for fibrin deposition and placental thrombosis, with subsequent ischemia and, in turn, the release of vasoactive factors. Consistent with these mechanisms, it has been showed that in women with previous preeclampsia there is an increased prevalence of activated protein C resistance, deficit of protein S, anticardiolipin antibody, factor V Leiden and hyperhomocysteinemia compared to women with past physiologic pregnancy [36].

Similarly, high levels of procoagulant factors, specifically homocysteine and PAI1, are associated to a high risk of cardiovascular disease.

## Metabolic Alterations

As previously stated, there are close analogies between metabolic alterations associated to a high cardiovascular risk –among there are obesity, insulin-resistance and dyslipidemia- and those found in patients with hypertension in pregnancy. For this reason the "metabolic syndrome", that is the cluster of the above mentioned metabolic abnormalities, is considered, the real link between preeclampsia and cardiovascular disease. On the other hand the already described alterations – i.e. endothelial dysfunction and inflammatory response – are associated to the metabolic syndrome in the determinism of both preeclampsia and atherosclerosis (Figure 4).

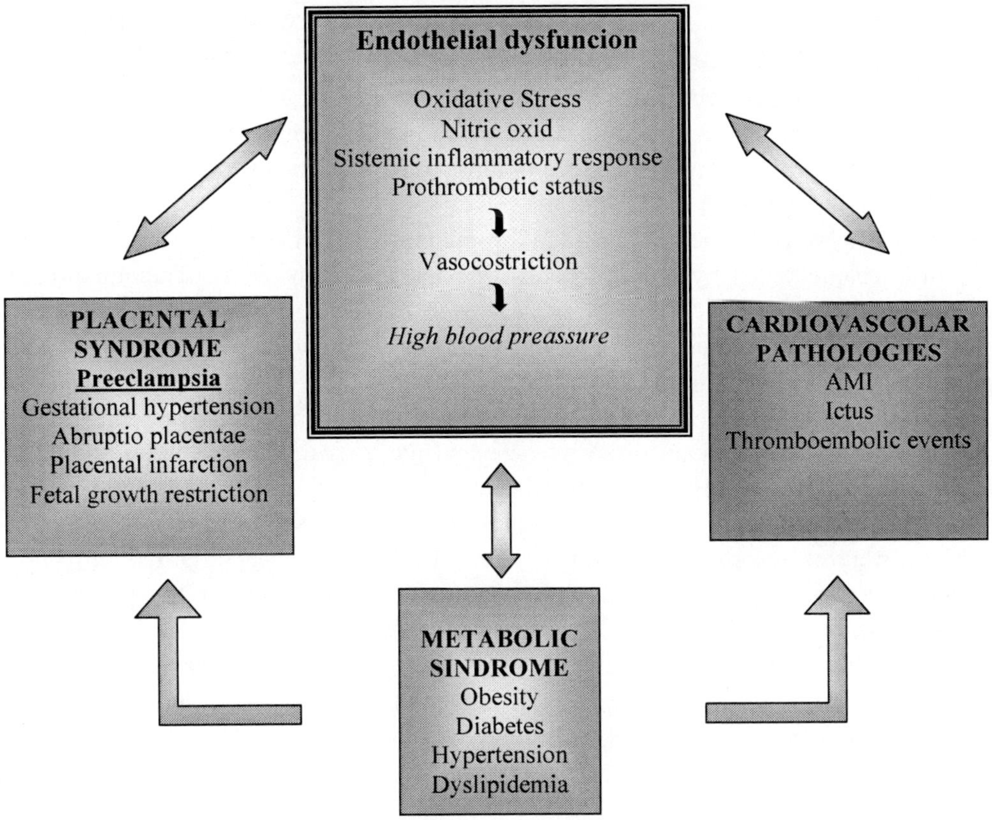


Figure 4. Endothelial dysfunction, preeclampsia, metabolic syndrome, metabolic and cardiovascular diseases.

Different studies sustain this hypothesis. A first remark is the epidemiological data of high risk of hypertension in obese women. Moreover, in pregnancy complicated with diabetes the prevalence of hypertension or preeclampsia is doubled compared to controls [37]. A proatherogenic lipid pattern, characterized by the increasing levels of LDL and triglyceride, has been found either in patients with coronary disease or in women with preeclampsia [38]. In both the pathologies we observe a fast oxidation of LDL and increased levels of lipoperoxide with a subsequent oxidation of the LDL particle by the macrophages. The consequence is an "acute atherosis" at the placental bed level, which is characteristic of preeclampsia and resemble to the typical atherosclerotic plate.

Recent studies have identified leptin, a hormone produced from adopocyte tissue that stimulates surfeit and suppresses appetite, as a marker of increased cardiovascular risk [39]. High levels of leptin are associated to platelet hyperaggregation in obese population. It is interesting to note that an hyperleptinemia is present also in preeclamptic women, thus adding an additional procoagulant risk factor in these women [40].

## Conclusions

It is well known that hypertension-preeclampsia disappear with delivery. Recent studies have shown that despite the normalization of the blood pressure levels, these women apparently in good health continue instead to have some abnormalities that may increase the risk of cardiovascular disease in the later life.

Women with story of preeclampsia tend to maintain, out of pregnancy, an unfavourable lipid profile characterized by reduced levels of HDL and high levels of apolipoprotein B, LDL and cholesterol [41].

On the basis of available data it is not possible to establish whether hypertension in pregnancy is an independent risk factor for cardiovascular disease in the future years. In fact, several confounding factors, such as diabetes, obesity and dyslipidemia can account for the increased cardiovascular risk in these women, and the goal of future studies should be to demonstrated that the association is significant even after the settlement for proved risk factors. The gynaecologist has an important role of counselling for all women with obstetrician story of hypertensive disorders; he must inform about the high risk of recurrence of such diseases in pregnancy as well as of a future development of cardiovascular disease. On this regard, of great importance is primary prevention which is to lead an appropriate lifestyle abolishing smoking, increasing physical exercises, a correct nutrition and to loose weight in the case of obesity or overweigh. Early diagnosis is also crucial for the correct management of these patients, thus reducing morbility and mortality for cardiovascular disease among them [42].

## References


[1] Sibai, BM. Hypertension. In: S. G. Gabbe, J. R. Niebyl, & J. L. Simpson (Eds.), *Obstetrics. Normal and Problem Pregnancies*. Fifth Edition. Churchill Livingstone Elsevier, 2007, 863-912.

[2] *Report of the Working Group on Research on Hypertension During Pregnancy*. Meeting Held April 27, 2001. National Heart, Lung, and Blood Institute

[3] Garovic, VD; Hayman, SR. Hypertension in pregnancy: an emerging risk factor for cardiovascular disease. *Nat Clin Pract Nephrol*, 2007 Nov, 3(11), 613-622.

[4] Paradisi, G; Biaggi, A; Savone, R; Ianniello, F; Tomei, C; Caforio, L; Caruso, A. Cardiovascular risk factors in healthy women with previous gestational hypertension. *J Clin Endocrinol Metab*, 2006 Apr, 91 (4), 1233-1238.

[5] Jonsdottir, LS; Arngrimsson, R; Geirsson, RT; Sigvaldason, H; Sigfusson, N. Death rates from ischemic heart disease in women with a history of hypertension in pregnancy. *Acta Obstet Gynecol Scand*, 1995, 74, 772-776.

[6] Ray, JG; Vermeulen, MJ; Schull, MJ; Redelmeier, DA. Cardiovascular health after maternal syndromes (CHAMPS): population-based retrospective cohort study. *Lancet*, 2005, 366, 1797-1803.

[7] Manten, GTR; Sikkema, MJ; Voorbji, HAM; Visser, GHA; Bruinse, HW; Franx, A. Risk factors for cardiovascular disease in women with a history of pregnancy

complicated by preeclampsia or intrauterine growth restriction. *Hypertension in Pregnancy*, 2007, 26, 39-50.

[8] Berends, AL; de Grot, CJM; Sijbrands, EJ; Sie, MPS; Benneheij, SH; Pal, R; Heydanus, R; Oostra, BA; van Duijn, CM; Steegers, EAP. Shared constitutional risks for maternal vascular-related pregnancy complications and future cardiovascular disease. *Hypertension*, 2008, 51, 1034-1041.

[9] Report of the National High Blood Pressure Education Program. Working group Report on High Blood Pressure in Pregnancy. *Am J Obstet Gynecol*, 2000, 183, S1-S22.

[10] Herrick, WW; Tillman, AJB. The mild toxemias of pregnancy: their relation to cardiovascular and renal disease. *Am J Obstet Gynecol*, 1936, 31, 832-844.

[11] Adams, EM; MacGillivray, I. Long-term effect of preeclampsia on blood pressure. *Lancet*, 1961, 2, 1373-1375.

[12] Singh, MM; MacGillivray, I; Mahaffy, RG. A study of the long-term effects of preeclampsia on blood pressure and renal function. *J Obstet Gynaecol British Commonwealth*, 1974, 81, 903-906.

[13] Lindeberg, S; Axelsson, O; Jorner, U; Malmberg, L; Sandström, B. A prospective controlled five-year follow-up study of primiparas with gestational hypertension. *Acta Obstet Gynecol Scand*, 1988, 67, 605-609.

[14] Kotchen, JM; McKean, HE Blood pressure of young mothers and their children after hypertension in adolescent pregnancy: six- to nine-year follow-up. *Am J Epidemiol*, 1982, 115, 861-867.

[15] Selvaggi, L; Loverro, G; Schena, FP Long-term follow-up of women with hypertension in pregnancy. *Int J Gynaecol Obstet*, 1988, 45-49.

[16] Carleton, H; Forsythe, A; Flores, R. Remote prognosis of preeclampsia in women 25 years hold and younger. *Am J Obstet Gynecol*, 1988, 159, 156-160.

[17] Sibai, MB; et al. Severe preeclampsia-eclampsia in young primigravid women: subsequent pregnancy outcome and remote prognosis. *Am J Obstet Gynecol*, 1986, 155, 1011 1016.

[18] Wilson, BJ; Watson, MS Hypertensive diseases of pregnancy and risk of hypertension and stroke in later life: results from cohort study. *BMJ*, 2003, 326, 845-851.

[19] Stepan, H; Nordmeyer, AK; Faber, R. Proteinuria in hypertensive pregnancy diseases is associated with a longer persistence of hypertension postpartum. *J Human Reproduction*, 2006, 20, 125-128.

[20] Chesley, LC; Annitto, JE; Cosgrove, RA. Long-term follow-up study of eclamptic women. *Am J Obstet Gynecol*, 1976, 124, 446-459.

[21] Smith, GD; Harding, S; Rosato, M. Relation between infants' birth weight and mothers' mortality: prospective observational study. *BMJ*, 2000, 320, 839-840.

[22] Smith, GD; Whitley, E; Gissler, M; Hemminki, E. Birth dimensions of offspring, premature birth and the mortality of mothers. *Lancet*, 2000, 356, 2066-2067.

[23] Smith, GC Pregnancy complications and maternal risk of ischaemic heart disease: a retrospective cohort study of 129.290 births. *Lancet*, 2001, 357, 2002-2006.

[24] Harskhamp, RE; Zeeman, GG. Preeclampsia: at risk for remote cardiovascular disease. *Am J Med Sci*, 2007, 334 (4), 291-295.

[25] Sibai, BM; Mercer, B; Sarinuglu, C. Severe preeclampsia in the second trimester: recurrence risk and long-term prognosis. *Am J Obstet Gynecol*, 1991, 165 (5 Pt 1), 1408-1412.

[26] Irgens, HU; reisaeter, L; Irgens, LM; Lie, RT. Long term mortality of mothers and fathers after pre-eclampsia: population based cohort study. *BMJ*, 2001 Nov 24, 323(7323), 1213-7.

[27] Hannaford, P; Ferry, S; Hirsch, S. Cardiovascular sequelae of toxaemia of pregnancy. *Heart*, 1997, 77, 154-158.

[28] Funai, EF; Friedlander, Y; Paltiel, O; Tiram, E; Xue, X; Deutsch, L; Harlap, S. Long-term mortality after preeclampsia. *Epidemiology.*, 2005 Mar, 16 (2), 206-15.

[29] Kestenbaum, B; Seliger, SL; Easterling, TR; Gillen, DL; Critchlow, CW; Stehman-Breen, CO; Schwartz, SM. Cardiovascular and thromboembolic events following hypertensive pregnancy. *Am J Kidney Dis.*, 2003 Nov, 42 (5), 982-9.

[30] Wikstrom, A; Haglund, B; Olovsson, M; et al. The risk of maternal ischaemic heart disease after gestational hypertensive disease. *Br J Obstet Gynaecol*, 2005, 112, 1486-1491.

[31] Brown, DW; Dueker, N; Jamieson, DJ; et al. Preeclampsia and the risk of ischemia stroke among young women: results from the Stroke Prevention in Young Women Study. *Stroke*, 2006, 37, 1055-1059.

[32] Luoto, R; Kharazmi, E; Whitley, E; Raitanen, J; Gissler, M; Hemminki, E. Systolic hypertension in pregnancy and cardiovascular mortality: a 44-year follow-up study. *Hypertension in Pregnancy*, 2008, 27, 87-94.

[33] Lowe, DT. Nitric oxide dysfunction in the pathophysiology of preeclampsia. *Nitric oxide*, 2000, 4, 441-458.

[34] Baumwell, S; Karumanchi, SA. Pre-eclampsia: Clinical Manifestations and Molecular Mechanisms. *Nephron Clin Pract*, 2007, 106 (2), c72-c81.

[35] Clark, P; Boswell, F; Greer, IA. The neutrophyl and preeclampsia. *Semin Reprod Endocrinol*, 1998, 16, 57-64.

[36] Kupferminc, MJ; Fait, G; Many, A; Gordon, D; Eldor, A; Lessing, JB; et al. Severe preeclampsia and high frequency of genetic thrombophilic mutations. *Obstet Gynecol*, 2000, 96, 45-49.

[37] Dunne, F; Brydon, P; Smith, K; Gee, H. Pregnancy in women with type 2 diabetes: 12 years outcome data 1990-2002. *Diabet Med*, 2003, 20, 734-738.

[38] Sattar, N; Bendomir, A; Berry, C; Shepherd, J; Greer, IA; Packard, CJ. Lipoprotein subfraction concentration in preeclampsia: pathogenic parallels to atherosclerosis. *Obstet Gynecol*, 1997, 89, 403-408.

[39] Wallace, AM; McMahon, AD; Packard, CJ; Kelly, A; Shepherd, J; Gaw, A; Sattar, N. Plasma leptin and the risk of cardiovascular disease in the West of Scotland Coronary Prevention Study (WOSCOPS). *Circulation*, 2001, 104, 3052-3056.

[40] Teppa, RJ; Ness, RB; Crombleholme, WR; Roberts, JM. Free leptin is increased in normal pregnancy and further increased in preeclampsia. *Metabolism*, 2000, 49, 1043-1048.

[41] Hubel, CA; Snaedal, S; Ness, RB Dyslipoproteinaemia in post-menopausal women with a history of eclampsia. *BJOG*, 2000, 107, 776-784.

[42] Mosca, L; Banka, CL Evidence-based guidelines for cardiovascular disease prevention in women: 2007 update. *J Am Coll Cardiol.*, 2007 Mar 20, 49(11), 1230-50. Review.

In: Advances in Cardiovascular Research, Volume 1
Editors: L. Schmitt, T. Konig, pp. 321-341
ISBN: 978-1-60741-720-0


*Chapter XIV*

# Optical Mapping of Intramural Reentry

***Nachaat Mazeh and Bradley J. Roth***
Department of Physics, Oakland University, Rochester, MI, USA

## Abstract

In monitoring complex arrhythmias, optical mapping is used to study the signals obtained from the cardiac tissue surface. Most studies have assumed that the fluorescent signal is emitted from the surface layer of cells. However, recent experiments have proved that the optical signal is the averaged response of the transmembrane potential over depth rather than only the surface. It is important to understand how to interpret the measured transmembrane potential resulting from electric stimulation in terms of the fluorescent signal emitted from the tissue. The objective of this chapter is to compare the results of the optical signal from the surface and averaged over depth.

We use a computer simulation of the bidomain model of the cardiac tissue and the Beeler-Reuter model of the ion channel kinetics to investigate the difference between the surface and the averaged transmembrane potentials. The bidomain model, which consists of intracellular and extracellular domains, approximates the cardiac tissue as a continuum and is a set of two coupled partial differential equations, solved using numerical methods. The Beeler-Reuter model uses Hodgkin-Huxley-like equations to represent four ionic currents in the cardiac membrane.

We use an electrode situated in a bath just above the cardiac tissue to stimulate the tissue, producing an activation wave front and inducing intramural reentry. We analyze potentials at the surface and below, and our results indicate that depth-weighted optical signals may provide important information about cardiac activation dynamics, such as the type of reentry, the direction of the propagation, and the spatial distribution of depolarization or repolarization. Our results show that averaging over depth has a significant impact on the interpretation of optical signals and that many of the poorly-understood features of optical mapping signals--such as double-hump action potentials, slow rates of rise and smaller than predicted polarization during the stimulus--can be explained by merely averaging over depth to obtain the optical signal.

## Introduction

Optical mapping has been used widely for studying and monitoring complex cardiac arrhythmias (Rosenbaum and Jalife, 2001), and it has been a powerful experimental tool for detecting cardiac activation patterns. Used both in isolated single cell (Sharma and Tung, 1999; Knisley et al., 1993) and whole heart (Choi and Salama, 2000; Bray et al., 2000) preparations, the method is based on the cell or tissue being stained with a voltage-sensitive fluorescent dye that emits signals indicative of the membrane potential changes. Electrical activity with temporal resolution on the order of microseconds (Salzberg et al., 1993) and spatial resolution on the scale of 50–100 μm (Grinvald et al., 1986) can be recorded.

The phenomenon of how electric stimulation alters the transmembrane potential is central to electrophysiology (Roth and Krassowska, 1998) and most studies have assumed that the fluorescent signal is emitted from the surface layer of cells. But the effects of signal attenuation with depth on signal interpretation are still unclear (Bray and Wikswo, 2003). It was generally assumed that the epifluorescent signal emanates from the superficial layer of cells in a tissue preparation. For some preparations of single cell layers (Entcheva et al., 2000) this assumption may faithfully reproduce the epicardial distribution of the transmembrane potential. But for more realistic thicknesses of the myocardium, optical mapping does not measure the transmembrane potential distribution at the tissue surface but rather it averages the transmembrane potential over depth (Gray, 1999; Janks and Roth, 2002). Several experiments have provided different results for the depth from which the signals arise, varying from 0.3 mm to 1 mm (Knisley, 1995; Girouard et al., 1996; Al-Khadra et al., 2000; Baxter et al., 2001). Our results suggest that the transmembrane potential weighted average over depth is different from that on the tissue surface.

The electrical stimulation of cardiac tissue in a three-dimensional model simulates an implantable pacemaker (Latimer and Roth, 1998). The typical pacemaker electrode is located on the endocardial surface, near the interface between the cardiac tissue and the blood that fills the atria and the ventricles. Our main goal is to understand how averaging over depth affects optical signals during bipolar electrode stimulation. Although a three-dimensional model is necessary to accurately describe all aspects of the behavior, we will only use a two-dimensional simulation as done previously (Trayanova and Roth, 1993; Trayanova, 1994) to reduce computational time. Our results indicate that depth-weighted optical signals may provide important information about cardiac activation dynamics, such as the type of reentry, the direction of the propagation, and the spatial distribution of depolarization or repolarization.

## Methods

The Beeler-Reuter model with accelerated calcium channel kinetics is used to represent the active membrane, and the bidomain model represents a two-dimensional slab of the cardiac tissue. The equations of the bidomain model (Henriquez, 1993), including the Beeler-Reuter ionic currents (Beeler and Reuter, 1977) are solved using a finite difference method (Langrill Beaudoin and Roth, 2006; Mazeh, 2008; Mazeh and Roth, 2009). The two-dimensional rectangular tissue is adjacent to a conductive bath in which lies a unipolar line electrode (the cathode) at mid horizontal section and 1.1 mm above the tissue (Figure 1). The reference electrode (the anode) is at the upper limit of the bath. The stimulation is induced by the electrode situated in the bath and the reference electrode. This creates an electric field that stimulates the tissue inducing, above some threshold, activation wave fronts and reentry. The tissue and the bath, both uniform, have the same size and dimensions, 40 mm length by 4 mm depth. The coordinate system is chosen so that the principal axes are parallel and perpendicular to the fiber direction. The y direction is perpendicular and downward into the tissue and the x direction is horizontal and parallel to the fiber direction. The origin is just below the electrode at mid-horizontal length of the tissue on the separation line between the tissue and the bath.

The passive bidomain (inactive ion channels) is governed by the following coupled partial differential equations,

$$\nabla \cdot \tilde{g}_i \nabla V_i = \beta\left[G_m(V_i - V_e) + C_m \frac{\partial}{\partial t}(V_i - V_e)\right], \tag{1}$$

$$\nabla \cdot \tilde{g}_e \nabla V_e = -\beta\left[G_m(V_i - V_e) + C_m \frac{\partial}{\partial t}(V_i - V_e)\right], \tag{2}$$

where $V_i$ and $V_e$ are the intracellular and extracellular potentials (V), $\tilde{g}_i$ and $\tilde{g}_e$ are the intracellular and extracellular conductivity tensors (S/m), $\beta$ is the ratio of membrane surface area to tissue volume (the surface-to-volume ratio, 1/m), $C_m$ is the membrane capacitance per unit area (F/m$^2$) and $G_m$ is the membrane conductance per unit area (S/m$^2$).

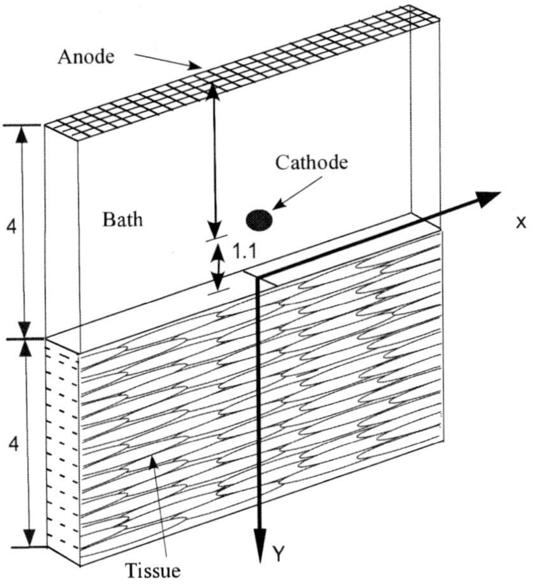


Figure 1. Tissue and bath representation, all units are in mm. When a potential difference is placed between the two electrodes, an electric field extends into the tissue. Only part of the tissue is shown, the tissue actually extends 40 mm the x-direction.

Activation of the ion channels is introduced in the model by replacing the term $G_m$ ($V_i$ – $V_e$) by $J_{ion}$, the active membrane current (A/m$^2$). In the Beeler-Reuter model, $J_{ion}$ consists of four terms: a sodium current, a calcium current, a time-independent potassium current, and a time-dependent potassium current (Beeler and Reuter, 1977). Because of the unequal anisotropy ratios, the bidomain Equations 1 and 2 cannot be decoupled. This is resolved by setting $V_m = V_i - V_e$ and suppressing the time dependence in one of the equations leading to Equations 3 and 4. The equations can be rewritten as an equation for the transmembrane potential and an equation for the extracellular potential (Roth, 1995),

$$C_m \frac{\partial V_m}{\partial t} = -J_{ion} - \frac{1}{\beta} \nabla \cdot \tilde{g}_e \nabla V_e , \qquad (3)$$

$$\nabla \cdot (\tilde{g}_i + \tilde{g}_e) \nabla V_e = -\nabla \cdot \tilde{g}_i \nabla V_m . \qquad (4)$$

The bidomain equations are equivalent to the continuity of current equations,

$$\nabla \cdot J_i = -I_m , \qquad (5)$$

$$\nabla \cdot J_e = I_m , \qquad (6)$$

where $I_m$ is the transmembrane current and is represented by the following:

$$I_m = \beta [C_m \frac{\partial V_m}{\partial t} + G_m V_m] . \qquad (7)$$

For an active membrane such as the Beeler-Reuter model, $G_m$ is replaced by the ionic currents such that

$$I_m = \beta [C_m \frac{\partial V_m}{\partial t} + I_{Jion}(V_m, t)] , \qquad (8)$$

where $I_{Jion}$ is a function of the transmembrane potential and time. The bidomain equations become,

$$\nabla \cdot (\tilde{g}_i + \tilde{g}_e) \nabla V_e = -\nabla \cdot \tilde{g}_i \nabla V_m , \qquad (9)$$

$$\nabla \cdot \tilde{g}_e \nabla V_e = -\beta [C_m \frac{\partial V_m}{\partial t} + I_{Jion}(V_m, t)] . \qquad (10)$$

We apply a stimulus voltage at the electrode placed inside the conductive bath and above the tissue. The electrode is at $(0, y_e)$ and the bath potential is governed by

$$V_b(x, -4) = 0 , \qquad (11)$$

$$V_b(0, y_e) = V_{stim} \quad (12)$$

where $V_{stim}$ is the applied voltage (V) at the electrode with values of $V_1$=-1.0 V for S1-stimulus and $V_2$=-30.0 V for S2-stimulus. $V_b$ is the potential inside the bath (V). The voltage obeys Laplace's equation in the bath, where the conductivity $g_b$ is homogeneous and isotropic. The boundary conditions of the bath-air and tissue-air boundaries are sealed (Latimer and Roth, 1998); no current can flow normal to the boundary planes

$$\frac{\partial V_i(x,y)}{\partial n} = 0, \quad \frac{\partial V_e(x,y)}{\partial n} = 0, \quad (13)$$

where $\partial/\partial n$ is the directional derivative normal to the boundary. At the tissue-bath interface, the boundary conditions are described by Krassowska and Neu (1994) and Roth (1991). The normal component of the current in the bath equals the normal component of current in the interstitial space in the tissue

$$g_b \frac{\partial V_b(x,0)}{\partial y} = g_{eT} \frac{\partial V_e(x,0)}{\partial y}, \quad (14)$$

where $g_{eT}$ is the transverse interstitial conductivity. Also the potential of the bath is equal to the potential of the interstitial space and the intracellular current density normal to the surface is zero

$$V_b(x,0) = V_e(x,0), \quad (15)$$

$$\frac{\partial V_i(x,0)}{\partial y} = 0. \quad (16)$$

The bidomain Equations 9 and 10 are solved numerically (Langrill Beaudoin and Roth, 2006; Mazeh, 2008; Mazeh and Roth, 2009) with successive overrelaxation applied to Equation 9 and Euler's method to solve the time-dependent bidomain equation, Equation 10 (Puwal and Roth, 2007). The bath extends 4 mm above the surface of the tissue and we use the space step $\Delta x = \Delta y = 0.100$ mm both in the tissue and the bath. This yields a discretized grid consisting of 400 x 40 nodes for both the bath and the tissue, measuring 40 mm x 4 mm each. We use a time step of 5 μs leading to a total run time of 500 ms or 100,000 time steps. The computer program, written in FORTRAN (Mazeh, 2008), was executed on a mini-supercomputer Beowulf cluster, containing 100 nodes, at Oakland University leading to a standard computation time of approximately 5 hours. The bidomain parameters are taken from Latimer and Roth (1998) and given in Table 1.

**Table 1. Standard bidomain parameters.**

| Bidomain Parameters | | |
|---|---|---|
| Surface-to volume ratio | $\beta$ | 0.3000 $\mu m^{-1}$ |
| Membrane Capacitance | $C_m$ | 0.0100 $F/m^2$ |
| Bath Conductivity | $g_b$ | 2.0000 S/m |
| Intracellular Longitudinal Conductivity | $g_{ix}$ | 0.1863 S/m |
| Intracellular Transverse Conductivity | $g_{iy}$ | 0.0186 S/m |
| Interstitial Longitudinal Conductivity | $g_{ex}$ | 0.1863 S/m |
| Interstitial Transverse Conductivity | $g_{ey}$ | 0.0745 S/m |

We used the following weighted average function of the transmembrane potential, $\overline{V}_m$, to represent the optical signal,

$$\overline{V}_m(x) = \frac{\int_0^\infty V_m(x,y)w(y)dy}{\int_0^\infty w(y)dy}, \tag{17}$$

where $y$ is the depth inside the tissue below the interface between the bath and the tissue (Janks and Roth, 2002). A simple form of the weight function is an exponential

$$w(y) = e^{-y/\lambda}, \tag{18}$$

where the decay constant $\lambda$ gives the surface $V_m$ for $\lambda = 0$ and equal weighting of all depths for $\lambda = \infty$.

## Results

The threshold curves for both anodal and cathodal stimulation are shown in Figure 2 as a function of tissue length. For anodal stimulation, the tissue exhibits a minimum threshold of about 2 Volts corresponding to a tissue size of 4 mm. For cathodal stimulation, the tissue exhibits a sharp decrease in the magnitude of the threshold stimulus strength as the tissue length increases for a size of up to about 3 mm. For sizes larger than that, the threshold is approximately constant, -0.78 V, as shown in Figure 2. When we vary the position of the electrode inside the bath, the threshold stimulus strength decreases dramatically as the electrode-tissue distance increases, as shown in Figure 3. In both above cases the stimulus was applied for 2 msec.

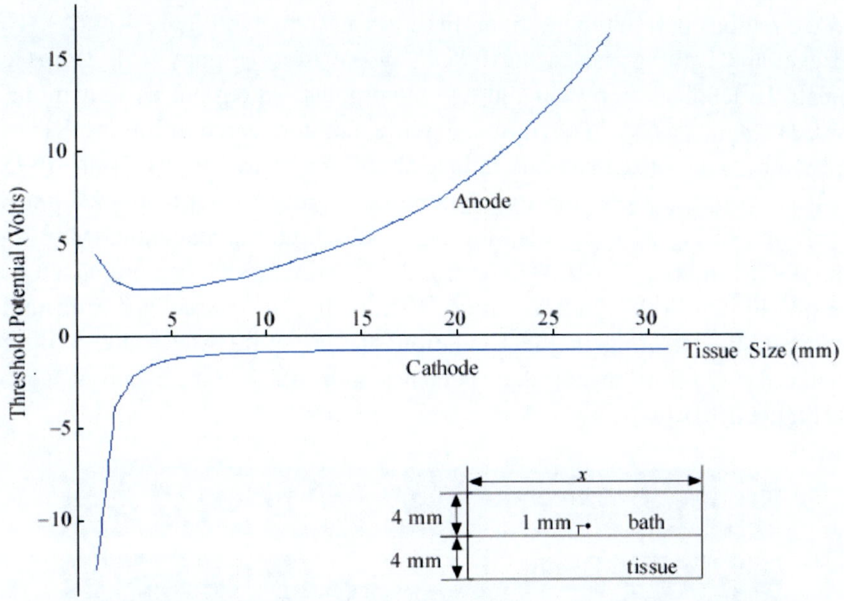


Figure 2. Anodal and cathodal stimulation. Potential threshold values for a tissue and bath depth of 4 mm, the electrode is at 1 mm above the tissue inside the bath. The tissue length is the only variable as shown and the reference electrode is at the top of the bath. The stimulus is applied for 2 msec.

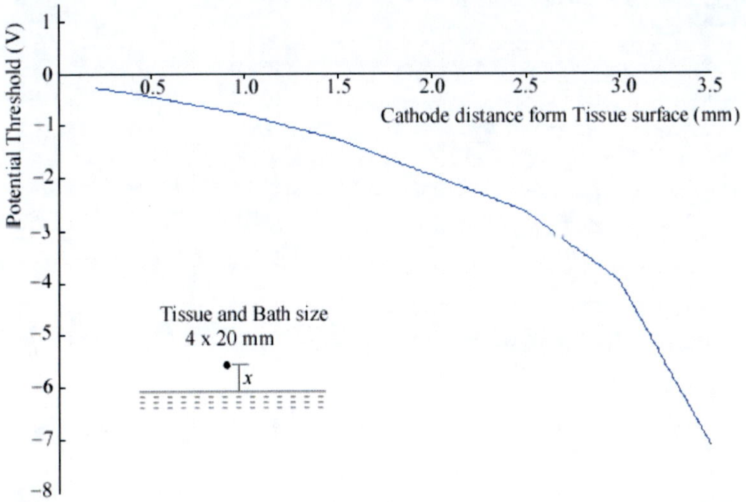


Figure 3. Potential threshold values for a cathode at a distance x from the tissue. The tissue and bath sizes are 4 x 20 mm. The stimulus is applied for 2 msec.

The suprathreshold response of the tissue to S1-S2 stimulation is shown in Figures 4(a) and (b). The first stimulus, S1, of strength -1.0 Volts is applied at 100 μsec for a duration of 2 msec and generates a wave front that propagates downward in the bath as shown in Figure 4(a) from 5 msec to 100 msec. The second stimulus, S2, of strength -30 Volts activated at 105.1 msec and applied for 4 msec, excites the tissue that is still refractory from the S1 wavefront. The S1 stimulus creates a depolarized region under the electrode and two weakly hyperpolarized regions parallel to the fiber direction as shown in Figure 4(c) (A). The tissue is at rest and excitable, giving rise to the first S1 wave front (Figure 4(a), 25 msec). The S2 stimulus creates a depolarized region and two hyperpolarized regions as shown in Figure 4(c) (B) (Sepulveda et al., 1989). The tissue, having not recovered from the S1 wave front, remains refractory. The virtual cathode induces two break wave fronts (Roth, 1995; Wikswo et al., 1995) that propagate into the two symmetric regions of hyperpolarization, the virtual anodes, where the strong hyperpolarization has made the tissue excitable (Saypol and Roth, 1992; Roth, 1997; Lin et al., 1999). Therefore, the S2 wave fronts can propagate outward but not downward (Figure 4(a), 125-150 msec). Eventually (175 msec) the surrounding tissue recovers excitability, resulting in the formation of two spiral waves and a figure-of-eight reentrant pattern (175-200 msec) that persists until 450 msec, when it spontaneously terminates (Figure 4(b)).

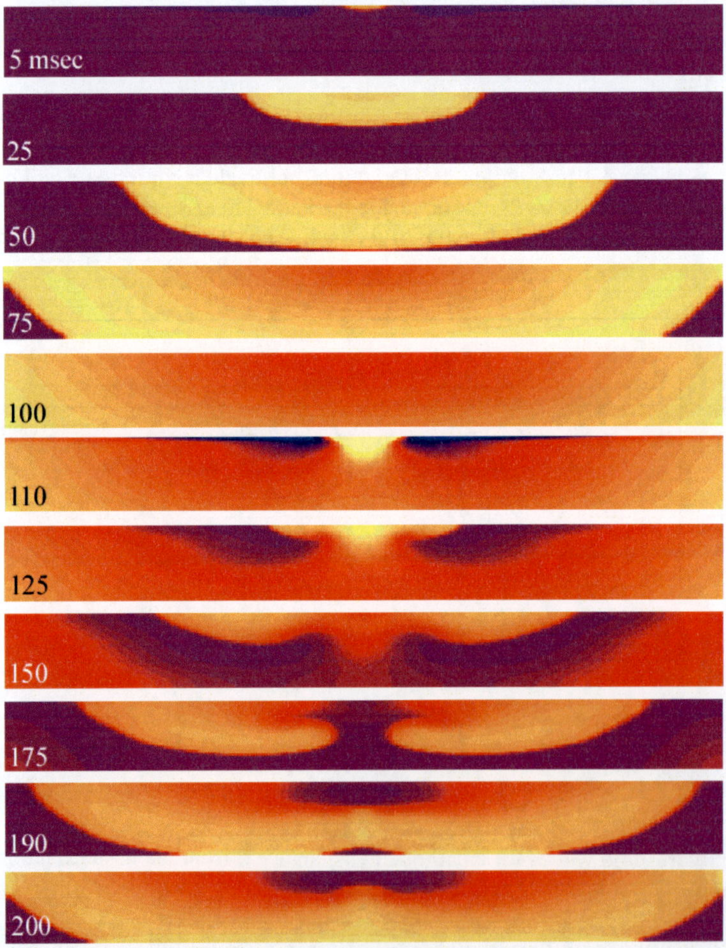


Figure 4(a). Wave front propagation in the tissue (4 x 40 mm) with S1 applied at 0.1 msec and S2 applied at 105.1 msec. The strength and duration of S1 are -1.0 V and 2 msec, for S2 they are -30 V and 4 msec. The numbers shown in the figures are the frame time (msec). The color scale is shown in Figure 4(c).

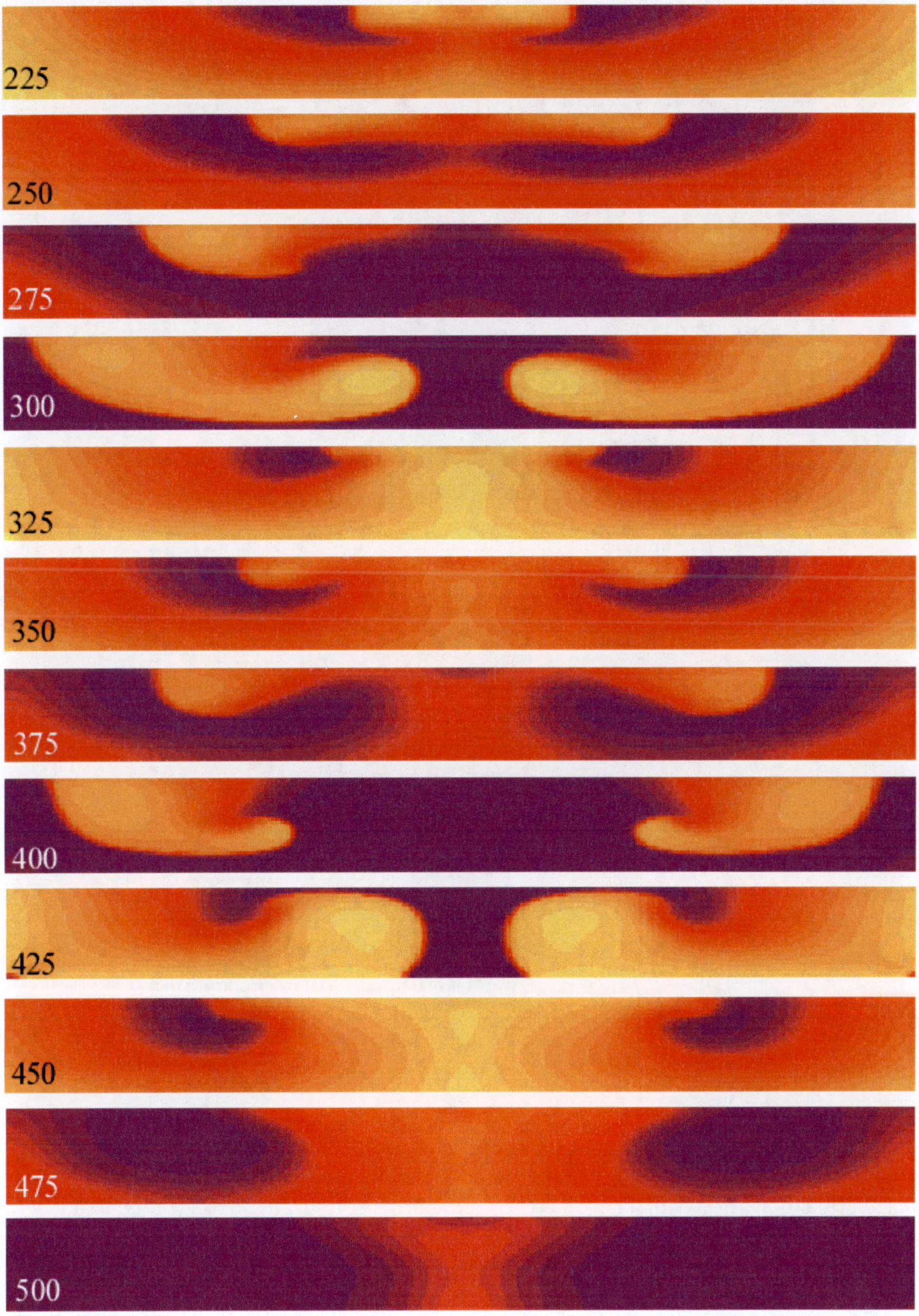


Figure 4(b). Wave front propagation in the tissue (4 x 40 mm). Numbers on frames are time (msec). Three reentries are shown at 225 msec, 325 msec and 450 msec before dying in the tissue between times of 475 to 500 msec.

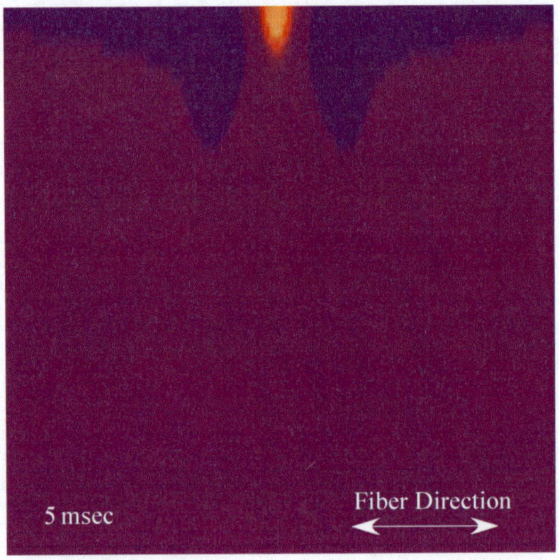


(A) After S1 stimulus

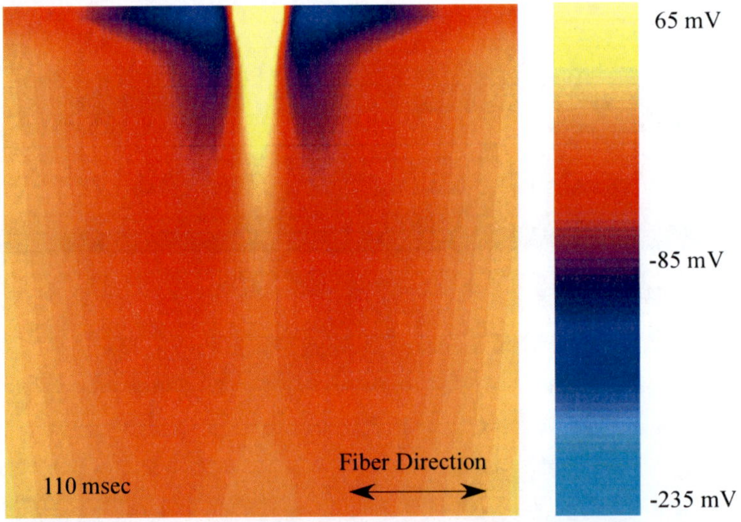


(B) After S2 stimulus

Figure 4(c). Hyperpolarized (blue) and depolarized (yellow) regions in the tissue (4 x 40 $mm^2$). The figure is stretched in the y direction by a factor of 10 to better show the detail. Numbers on frames are time (msec). S1 and S2 are as Figures 4(a) and 4(b). The fiber direction is shown by the arrow.

Figures 5(a) and 5(b) show both the surface recorded and averaged over depth transmembrane potentials for four different locations at the surface and for the decay constant $\lambda = 0.1$ mm. The curves indicate a strong correlation between both measurements. The reentry that was described earlier (Figures 4(a) and 4(b)) is seen in these figures with the multiple action potentials. At the end of the first action potential, the stimulus artifact is clearly seen to be largest closer to the middle of the tissue just underneath the cathode position.

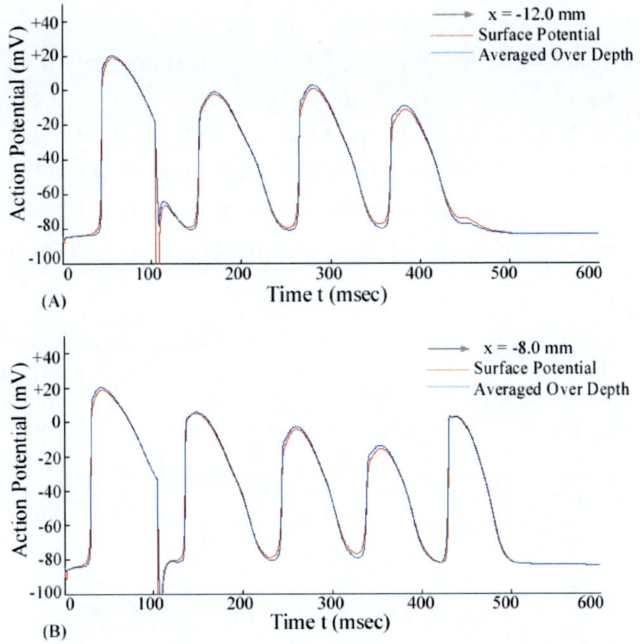


Figure 5(a). Action potentials for both the surface (red curve) and averaged over depth (blue curve). The decay constant is λ=0.1 mm, x is measured from the center at the origin of the x-axis. (A) Measurements at x=-12.0 mm and (B) at x=-8.0 mm from the origin.

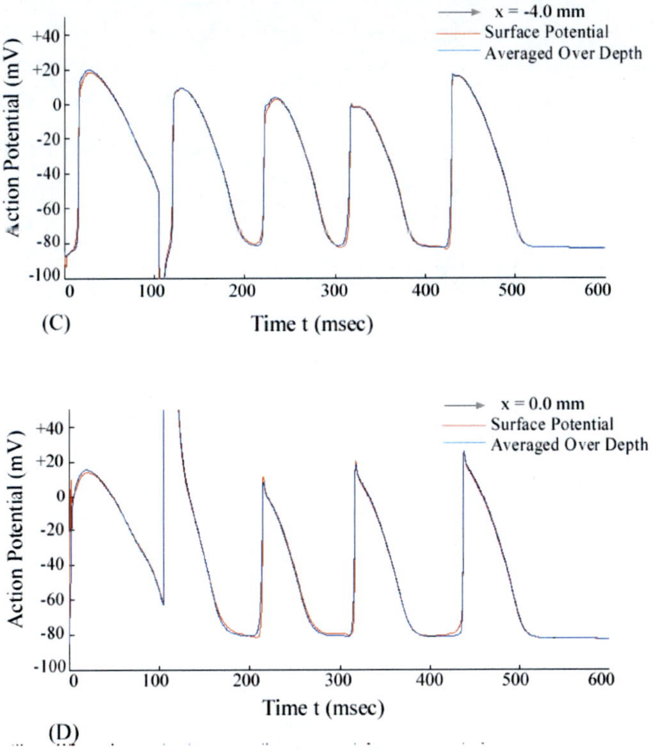


Figure 5(b). Same as 5(a) with λ=0.1 mm for (C) measurements at x=-4.0 mm and (D) at x=0.0 mm at the origin.

Figures 5(a and b) (A), (B) and (C) show the hyperpolarization resulting from the S2 stimulus, just as the tissue recovers from the S1-depolarization, shown at the end of the first AP. The immediate strong depolarization shown in (D) at the end of the first AP appears at x = 0.0 mm just underneath the cathode. Both of these effects during the recovery period of the first AP are the results of the virtual electrodes caused by the S2 stimulus. The strengths of S1 and S2 along with the t1-t2 time, or interval, create the effective protocol parameters for a successful induction of reentry.

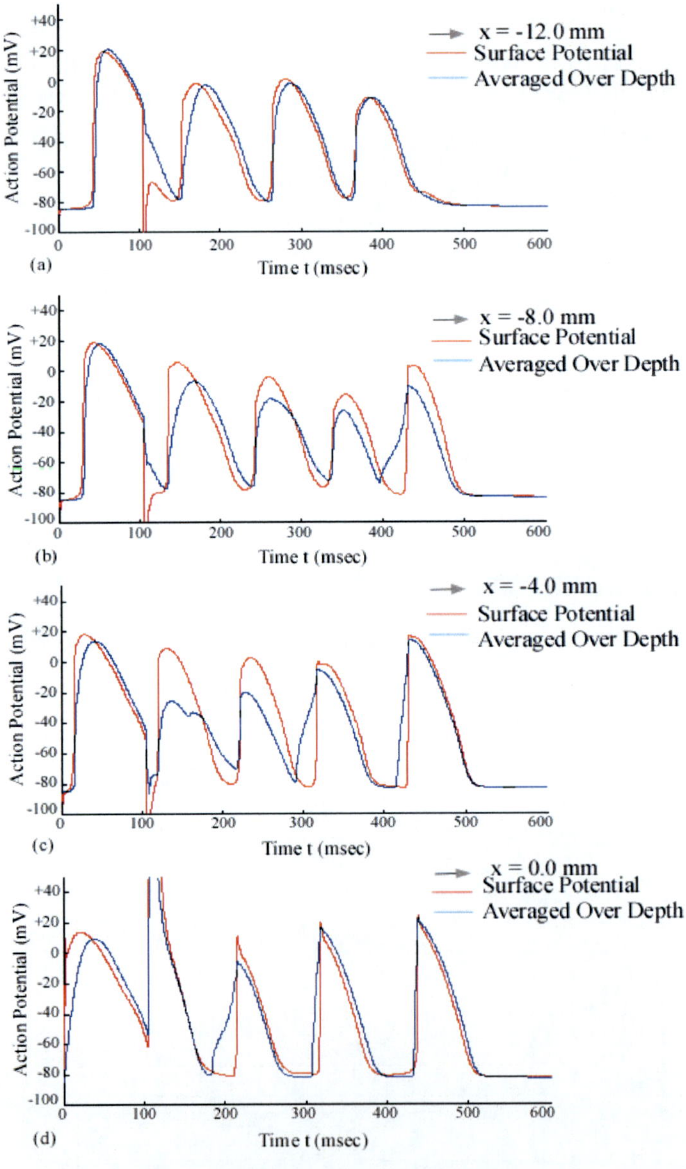


Figure 6. Transmembrane potentials at the surface and averaged over depth for a decay constant λ=1.0 mm, x is measured from the origin at the center of the tissue on the surface.

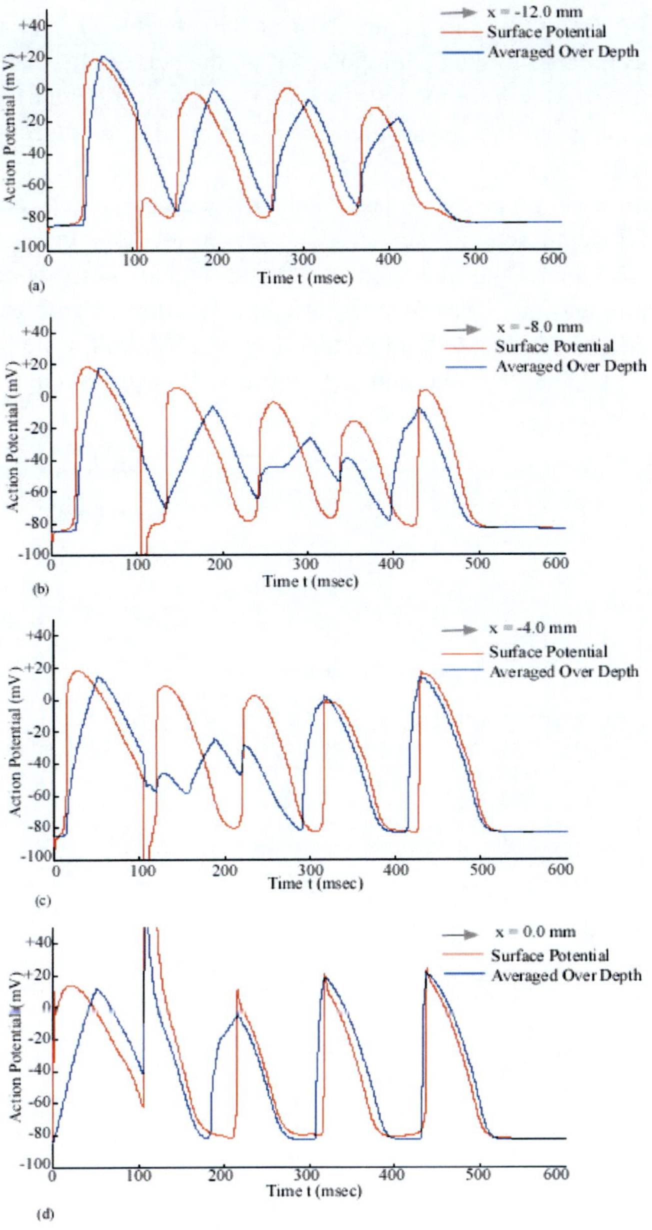


Figure 7. Transmembrane potentials at the surface and averaged over depth for a decay constant $\lambda$=10.0 mm, x is measured from the origin at the center of the tissue on the surface.

Figures 6 and 7, for decay constant values of $\lambda$ = 1.0 mm and $\lambda$ = 10.0 mm, show a poorer correlation between the surface and the averaged over depth action potentials. The surface AP is the same as in Figure 5 and has the same behavior for the same locations (similarity in the AP in red for the same locations). The AP shown in Figure 6(c) at about 150 msec exhibits the double-hump effect as described by Efimov et al. (1999). The reentrant wavefront passes x=-4 mm propagating to the left on the surface (Figure 4A, 125 msec), and then passes the same value of x propagating to the right deeper under the surface (Figure 4A, 175 msec), resulting in two depolarization upstrokes in the averaged signal: a double-hump. Similar double humped APs are evident in Figure 7(b) at 350 msec and 7(c) at 240 msec. The stimulus artifact is compared to the action potential on the surface for decay values of λ=1.0 mm, λ=2.0 mm, and λ=10.0 mm for the location at x = -8.0 mm (Figure 8) and at x = -4.0 mm (Figure 9). The stimulus artifact is smaller or absent in the averaged over depth action potential.

The upstroke of the action potential has a sharper rise on the surface action potential then on the averaged over depth action potential as is seen in all AP's in Figure 10 for lambda λ=1.0 mm at x = -8.0 mm. The averaged over depth signals corresponding to the decay constant of λ=1.0 mm and measured at three different locations, the three figures shown in Figure 11, exhibit clearly the double-hump effect. Figure 11(A) is for the position of x = -6.0 mm, Figure 11(B) for position x = -4.0 mm and Figure 11(C) for position x = -2.0 mm.

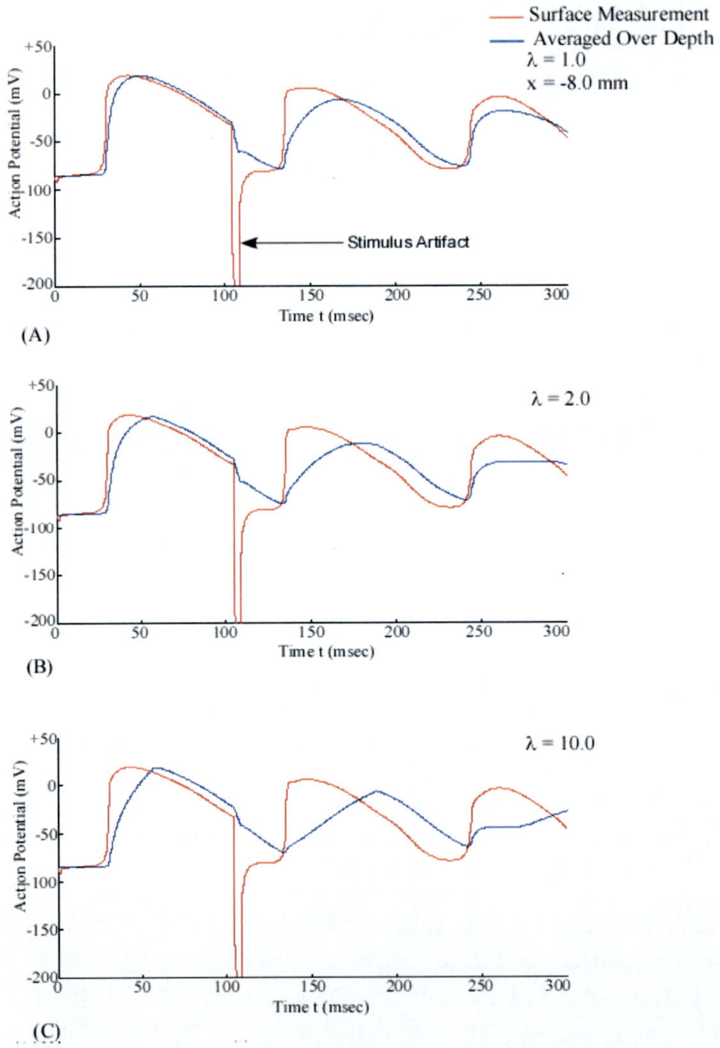


Figure 8. Stimulus artifact compared to the action potential at the location x = -8.0 mm for λ=1.0 mm, 2.0 mm and 10.0 mm.

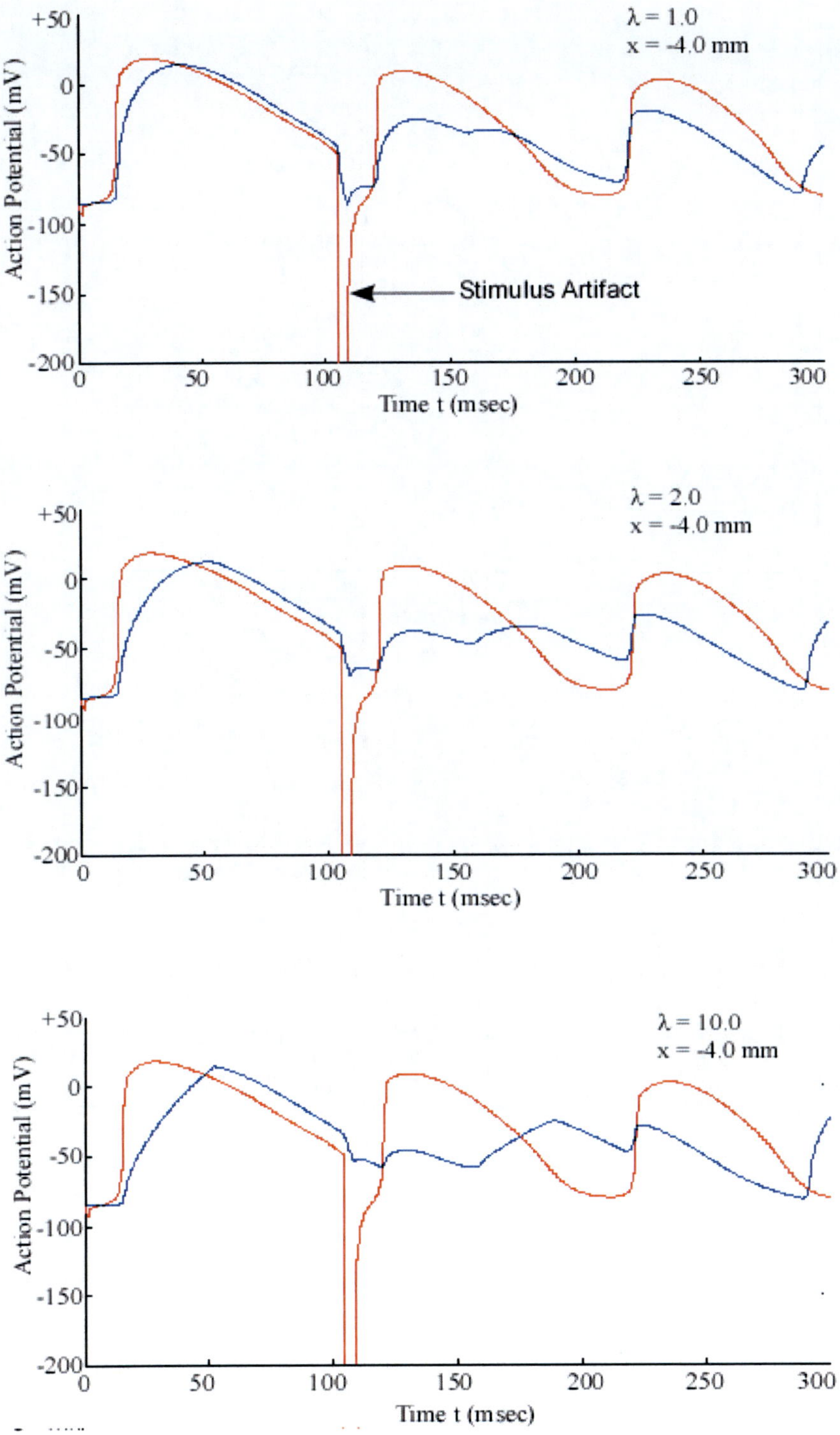


Figure 9. Stimulus artifact compared to the action potential, λ=1.0 mm, 2.0 mm and 10.0 mm with x=-4.0 mm.

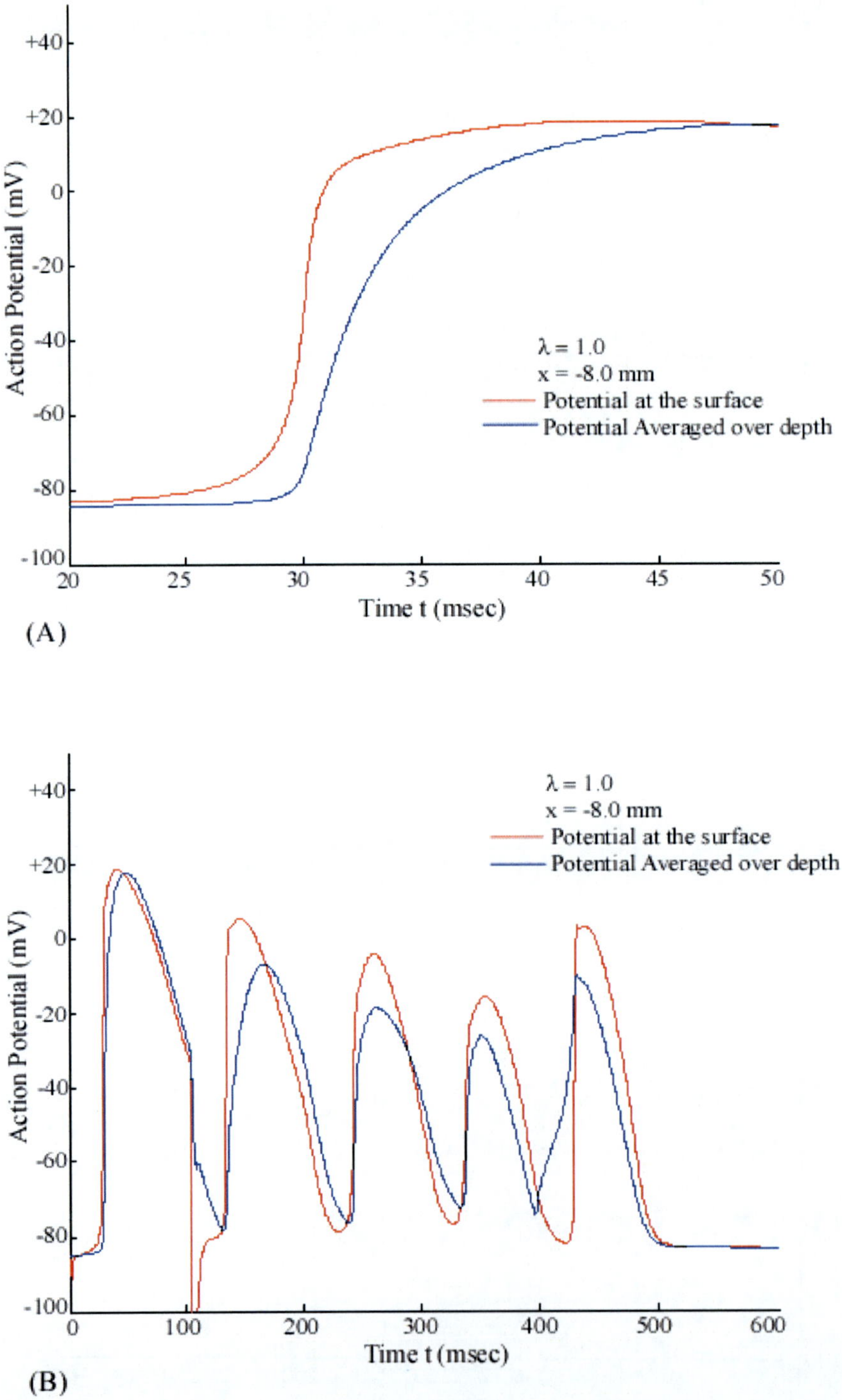


Figure 10. The decay constant is $\lambda$=1.0 mm with x=-8.0 mm. Upstroke of the action potential is shown for (A) 50 msec and (B) in a 600 msec total run time.

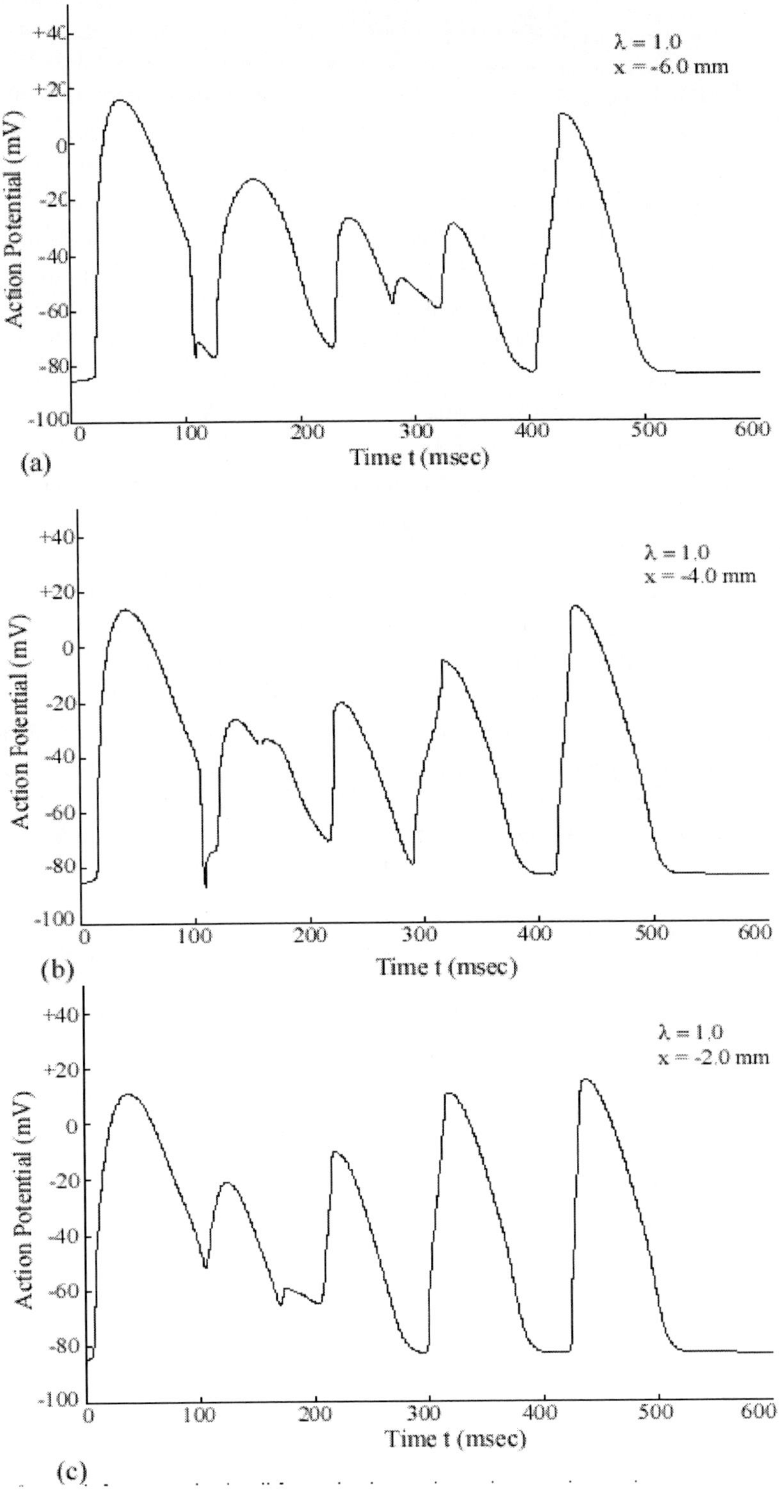


Figure 11. Action potential recorded for a decay constant value of λ=1.0 mm at different positions on the tissue surface, x=-2.0 mm, -4.0 mm and -6.0 mm. The double hump effect is clearly shown.

# Discussion

Our simulations demonstrate that averaging over depth has a significant impact on the interpretation of optical signals during optical mapping experiments of the heart. We were able to induce a reentrant circuit by stimulation through a cathode in the adjacent bath. From the surface, this reentant circuit appeared to be a periodic signal originating from the region below the cathode. However, examination of the transmembrane potential as a function of depth in Figure 4 indicates that the periodic signal arises from an intramural reentrant circuit that exists primarily below the tissue surface. One indication of such an intramural reentrant circuit is double-humped action potentials in the optical signal when averaged over depth.

Our results are consistent with several previous studies. Efimov et al. (1999) observed double-humped action potentials experimentally, and Bray and Wikswo (2003) observed them in their computational simulations. Our results indicated that the tissue polarization during a stimulus is underestimated during optical mapping compared to the surface response, as shown by Janks and Roth (2002). We observed that the upstroke of the averaged action potential is slow, consistent with Hyatt et al. (2003, 2005).

Our simulation has several limitations. We considered only a two-dimensional model, and therefore we do not capture the full three-dimensional behavior of the tissue. The transmembrane potential directly below the stimulus electrode is very large, but our model does not include electroporation (the opening of holes in the cell membrane) known to occur at very strong polarizations. The Beeler-Reuter model (Beeler-Reuter, 1977) is a good approximation to the cardiac membrane behavior, but more detailed models exist. These issues, and others, are discussed in Roth (2002).

Perhaps the most important limitation is that we represented the process of optical mapping as merely averaging over depth (Janks and Roth, 2002; Bray and Wikswo, 2003), but in fact photons in tissue obey a diffusion equation that results in lateral as well as depth averaging. Recently, several authors have analyzed photon diffusion during optical mapping (Hyatt et al., 2003, 2005; Bishop et al., 2006; 2007; Prior and Roth, 2008; Roth, 2008), and use of a more sophisticated model may improve the agreement between our results and experiments. Techniques are being developed that may even allow one to determine the transmembrane as a function of depth from optical measurements (Roth and Pertsov, in press; Prior and Roth, in press).

In conclusion, our results show that many of the poorly-understood features of optical mapping signals--such as double-hump action potentials, slow rates of rise, and smaller than predicted polarization during the stimulus--can be explained by merely averaging over depth to obtain the optical signals. Solving the full optical diffusion equation should provide an even better understanding of these phenomena.

# Acknowledgments

This research was supported by a grant from the National Institutes of Health.

## References


Al-Khadra, A., Nikolski, V. & Efimov, I. R. (2000). The role of electroporation in defibrillation. *Circ Res*, *87*, 797-804.

Baxter, W. T., Mironov, S. F., Zaitsev, A. V., Jalife, J. & Pertsov, A. M. (2001). Visualizing excitation waves inside cardiac muscle using transillumination. *Biophys J*, *80*, 516-530.

Beeler, G. W. & Reuter, H. (1977). Reconstruction of the action potential of ventricular myocardial fibres. *J Physiol*, *268*, 177-210.

Bishop, M. J., Rodriguez, B., Eason, J., Whiteley, J. P., Trayanova, N. & Gavaghan, D. J. (2006). Synthesis of voltage-sensitive optical signals: Application to panoramic optical mapping. *Biophys J*, *90*, 2938-2945.

Bishop, M. J., Rodriguez, B., Qu, F., Efimov, I. R., Gavaghan, D. J. & Trayanova, N. A. (2007). The role of photon scattering in optical signal distortion during arrhythmia and defibrillation. *Biophys J*, *93*, 3714-3726.

Bray, M. A., Lin, S. F. & Wikswo, J. P. Jr. (2000). Three-dimensional surface reconstruction and fluorescent visualization of cardiac activation. *IEEE Trans Biomed Eng*, *47*, 1382-1391

Bray, M. A. & Wikswo, J. P. (2003). Examination of optical depth effects on fluorescence imaging of cardiac propagation. *Biophys J*, *85*, 4134-4145.

Choi, B. R. & Salama, G. (2000). Simultaneous maps of optical action potentials and calcium transients in guinea-pig hearts: mechanisms underlying concordant alternans. *J Physiol*, *529*, 171-188.

Efimov, I. R., Sidorov, V., Cheng, Y. & Wollenzier, B. (1999). Evidence of three-dimensional scroll waves with ribbon-shaped filament as a mechanism of ventricular tachycardia in the isolated rabbit heart. *J Cardiovasc Electrophysiol*, *10*, 1452-1462.

Entcheva, E., Lu, S. N., Troppman, R. H., Sharma, V. & Tung, L. (2000). Contact fluorescent imaging of reentry in monolayers of cultured neonatal rat ventricular myocytes. *J Cardiovasc Electrophysiol*, *11*, 665-676.

Girouard, S. D., Pastore, J. M., Laurita, K. R., Gregory, K. W. & Rosenbaum, D. S. (1996), Optical mapping in a new guinea pig model of ventricular tachycardia reveals mechanisms for multiple wavelengths in a single reentrant circuit. *Circulation*, *93*, 603-613.

Gray, R. A. (1999). What exactly are optically recorded 'action potentials'. *J Cardiovasc Electrophysiol*, *10*, 1463-1466.

Grinvald, A., Lieke, E., Frostig, R. D., Gilbert, C. D. & Wiesel, T. N. (1986). Functional architecture of cortex revealed by optical imaging of intrinsic signals. *Nature*, *324*, 361-364.

Henriquez, C. S. (1993). Simulating the electrical behavior of cardiac tissue using the bidomain model. *Crit Rev Biomed Eng*, *21*, 1-77.

Hyatt, C. J., Mironov, S. F., Wellner, M., Berenfeld, O., Popp, A. K., Weitz, D. A., Jalife, J. & Pertsov, A. M. (2003). Synthesis of voltage-sensitive fluorescence signals from three-dimensional myocardial activation patterns. *Biophys J*, *85*, 2673-2683.

Hyatt, C. J., Mironov, S. F., Vetter, F. J., Zemlin, C. W. & Pertsov A.M. (2005). Optical action potential upstroke morphology reveals near-surface transmural propagation direction. *Circ Res*, *97*, 277-284.

Janks, D. L. & Roth, B. J. (2002). Averaging over depth during optical mapping of unipolar stimulation. *IEEE Trans Biomed Eng*, *49*, 1051-1054.

Knisley, S. B. (1995). Transmembrane voltage changes during unipolar stimulation of rabbit ventricle. *Circ Res*, *77*, 1229-1239.

Knisley, S. B., Blitchington, T. F., Hill, B. C., Grant, A. O., Smith, W. M., Pilkington, T. C. & Ideker, R. E. (1993). Optical measurements of transmembrane potential changes during electric field stimulation of ventricular cells. *Circ Res*, *72*, 255-270.

Krassowska, W. & Neu, J. C. (1994). Effective boundary conditions for syncytial tissues. *IEEE Trans Biomed Eng*, *41*, 143-150.

Langrill Beaudoin, D. & Roth, B. J. (2006). The effect of the fiber. *PACE*, *29*, 496-501.

Latimer, D. C. & Roth, B. J. (1998). Electrical stimulation of cardiac tissue. *IEEE Trans Biomed Eng*, *45*, 1449-1458.

Lin, S. F., Roth, B. J. & Wikswo, J. P. Jr. (1999). Quatrefoil reentry in myocardium: An optical imaging study of the induction mechanism. *J Cardiovasc Electrophysiol*, *10*, 574-586.

Mazeh, N. & Roth, B. J. (2009). A Mechanism for the upper limit of vulnerability. *Heart Rhythm*, *6*, 361-367.

Mazeh, N. (2008). The Upper Limit of Vulnerability of the Heart. *PhD dissertation*. Rochester, MI: Oakland University.

Prior, P. W. & Roth, B. J. (2008). Calculation of optical signal using three dimensional bidomain/diffusion model reveals distortion of the transmembrane potential. *Biophys J*, *95*, 2097-2102.

Prior, P. W. & Roth, B. J. (2009). Development of an imaging modality utilizing 2-D optical signals during an epifluorescent optical mapping experiment. *Phys Med Biol.* 54, 3015-3030.

Puwal, S. & Roth, B. J. (2007). Forward Euler stability of the bidomain model of cardiac tissue. *IEEE Trans Biomed Eng*, *54*, 951-953.

Rosenbaum, D. S. & Jalife, J. (2001). Optical Mapping of Cardiac Excitation and Arrhythmias. (*Futura, New York*).

Roth, B. J. & Krassowska, W. (1998). The induction of reentry in cardiac tissue. The missing link: How electric fields alter transmembrane potential. *Chaos*, *8*, 204-220.

Roth, B. J. & Pertsov, A. M. (2009). Hybrid modeling of electrical and optical behavior in the heart. *Physica D: Nonlinear Phenomena,* 238, 1019-1027.

Roth, B. J. (1991). A comparison of two boundary conditions *Annals Biomed Eng*, *19*, 669-678.

Roth, B. J. (1995). A mathematical model of make and break electrical stimulation of cardiac tissue by a unipolar anode or cathode. *IEEE Trans Biomed Eng*, *42*, 1174-1184.

Roth, B. J. (1997). Nonsustained reentry following successive stimulation of cardiac tissue through a unipolar electrode. *J Cardiovasc Electrophysiol*, *8*, 768-778.

Roth, B. J. (2002). Artifacts, assumptions, and ambiguity: Pitfalls in comparing experimental results to numerical simulations when studying electrical stimulation of the heart. *Chaos*, *12*, 973-981.

Roth, B. J. (2008). Photon density measured over a cut surface: Implications for optical mapping of the heart. *IEEE Trans Biomed Eng*, *55*, 2102-2104.

Salzberg, B. M., Obaid, A.L., & Benzanilla, F. (1993). Microsecond response of a voltage-sensitive merocyanine dye: Fast voltage-clamp measurements of squid giant axon. *Jpn J Physiol,* 43, 37-41.

Saypol, J. M. & Roth, B. J. (1992). A mechanism for anisotropic reentry in electrically active tissue. *J Cardiovasc Electrophysiol*, *3*, 558-566.

Sepulveda, N. G., Roth, B. J. & Wikswo, J. P. Jr. (1989). Current injection into a two-dimensional anisotropic bidomain. *Biophys J*, *55*, 987-999.

Sharma, V. & Tung, L. (1999). Transmembrane responses of single guinea pig Ventricular cell to uniform electric field stimulus. *J CardiovascElectrophysiol*, *10*, 1296.

Trayanova, N. & Roth, B. J. (1993). Mechanisms for cardiac stimulation. *Proc 15th Annual IEEE/EMBS Conf*, 817-818.

Trayanova, N. (1994). Virtual electrode effects in a model of cardiac stimulation. *Proc 16th Annual IEEE/EMBS Conf*, 61-62.

Wikswo, J. P. Jr., Lin, S. F. & Abbas, R. A. (1995). Virtual electrodes incardiac tissue: a common mechanism for anodal and cathodal stimulation. *Biophys J*, *69*, 2195-2210.

In: Advances in Cardiovascular Research, Volume 1
Editors: L. Schmitt, T. Konig, pp. 343-366
ISBN: 978-1-60741-720-0


*Chapter XV*

# Role of Percutaneous Interventions in the Management of Adult Congenital Heart Diseases

***Mukesh Singh*, Sarabjeet Singh, Neyaz Ahmed, Rohit Arora and Sandeep Khosla***

Rosalind Franklin University of Medicine & Science, The Chicago Medical School, North Chicago, and Mount Sinai Hospital, Chicago, Illinois, USA

## Abstract

The advancements of cardiac surgery over the last decades led to larger numbers of patients with operated congenital heart diseases surviving into adulthood. The traditional treatment of congenital heart defects in adults has been surgical correction. Percutaneous interventional treatments for such conditions have rapidly advanced in last two decades. The availability of transcatheter devices has revolutionized the management of patients with congenital heart and vascular disease. The adult congenital heart disease patient, at baseline or in need of intervention, presents unique challenges to caregivers.We discuss the current applications of interventional treatment in adults with congenital heart defects and conclude that it is safe and feasible, that the indications for this approach to treatment are increasing, that it can be undertaken in patients of any age including high-risk patients.

## Background

About 35,000 infants [1 out of every 125] are born with heart defects each year in the United States [1]. In the United States, about 1.4 million children and adults live with congenital heart defects [unrepaired, repaired and palliative] today [2]. Almost all are able to

* Sarabjeet Singh M.D. , Department of Internal Medicine / Division Cardiology, Chicago Medical School, 3333 Green Bay Road, North Chicago, IL 60064, Email: sarabjeetsingh_2000@yahoo.com

lead active, productive lives [1]. Congenital heart defects [CHD] are among the most common birth defects and are the leading cause of birth defect-related deaths [3]. However, advances in diagnosis and surgical treatment have led to dramatic increases in survival for children with serious heart defects. Since the advent of neonatal repair of complex lesions in the 1970s, an estimated 85% of patients survive into adult life. Prior to the advent of surgery, less than 20% of children born with CHD survived to adult life [4]. Now, most deaths from congenital heart disease occur in adults. From 1994 to 2004 death rates for congenital cardiovascular defects declined 31.6 percent, while the actual number of deaths declined 25.4 percent. Given modern surgical mortality rates of less than 5%, one would expect that in the next decade, almost 1 in 150 young adults will have some form of CHD. There is an increase not only in the size of the population but also in the proportion of patients with complex lesions. In particular, there are a substantial number of young adults with single-ventricle physiology, systemic right ventricles [RVs], or complex intracardiac baffles who are now entering adult life and starting families.

**Table 1. Pathophysiological classification of CHD in adults.**

| | | |
|---|---|---|
| A) | left to right shunt lesions. | |
| | a. | Osteum secundum ASD |
| | b. | Patent foramen ovale |
| | c. | Ventricular septal defect. |
| | d. | Patent ductus arteriosus |
| | e. | Coronary arterio-venous fistula |
| B) | Right to left shunt lesions. | |
| | a. | Pulmonary arteriovenous fistula. |
| | b. | Baffle leaks in Mustard / Senning repair. |
| C) | Right heart obstructive lesions. | |
| | a. | Pulmonary stenosis |
| | b. | Tricuspid stenosis |
| D) | Left heart obstructive lesions. | |
| | a. | Aortic stenosis |
| | b. | Mitral stenosis |
| | c. | Coarctation of aorta. |
| E) | Miscellaneous: | |
| | a. | Post- TOF repair. |
| | b. | Post- fontan repair. |
| | c. | Post-mustard / senning operation |
| | d. | Post-arterial switch operation. |

The traditional treatment of congenital heart disease in adults has been surgery. Since the interatrial septostomy described by Rashkind and Miller [5], coronary angioplasty and valvuloplasty by Grüntzig [6], the non-surgical intervention in CHD have developed rapidly. Over the last years, endovascular interventions have become an important part of treatment in adult CHD patients. Currently a large number of catheterization procedures are being performed to treat adult CHD. The objective of this presentation is to analyze the therapeutic possibilities of interventional cardiology in the adult congenital heart disease, previously treated or untreated, and to explore their role in the management of CHD in adult patients. A classification of CHD in adult patients based on pathophysiology is illustrated in table 1.

# Diagnostic Cardiac Catheterization Vs Imaging in Adult Patients with CHD

There has been a shift form cardiac catheterization to non-invasive imaging modalities for adult patients with CHD, which is similar to that which has occurred in pediatric cardiology over the last two decades. The heart, once accessible only by surgeons, angiocardiographers, and pathologists, now can be imaged, sliced safely and accurately, rotated, and examined with minimal discomfort to patients. These tools include echocardiography [transthoracic and transesophageal] and MRI, which are essential in specialist centers. Cardiac catheterization is now reserved for resolution of specific anatomical or physiological questions [coronary arteries, pulmonary vascular resistance] or for intervention.

Echocardiography always will play an important role in the care of patients who have ACHD. Its availability, portability, and familiarity to most recently trained cardiologists is a strength. Echo provides important structural and physiologic information and is the noninvasive reference standard for valvular assessment. Transthoracic echo in adults is less effective than in children at describing complex intracardiac and extracardiac anatomy and physiology. Transesophageal echocardiography often provides definitive information but has the disadvantage of usually requiring sedation or anesthesia. More recently, intracardiac echocardiography has proven to be extremely helpful especially during interventional procedures.

MRI and CT are critical imaging modalities for clinicians. MRI is increasingly becoming the investigation of choice for adult CHD patients providing 3D reconstruction of anatomy, improved temporal and special resolution as well as physiological information. It has proved particularly useful for evaluation of right ventricular volume and mass, right ventricle to pulmonary artery conduit/ valve function as well as for the study of pulmonary arteries, coarctation and systemic and pulmonary venous anomalies [8,9]. Interventional procedures such as balloon dilatation and radio frequency ablation can now be carried out using MRI/catheter fluoroscopy techniques, further extending the role of this imaging modality. Until recently, computed tomography [CT] played only a minor role in the evaluation of congenital heart disease. Newer technologies however, such as ultra fast CT and spiral CT have reduced scanning time and provide excellent imaging which can be seen as complementary to echo-cardiography and MRI [10].

# Interventional Catheterization

There has been a spectacular increase in the number and range of interventional catheter techniques for congenital cardiac malformations. The rapid increase in the type and application of interventional techniques in congenital heart disease of childhood has been mirrored in the adult population. Many of the techniques developed in children were subsequently adapted to the treatment of grown-ups with congenital heart disease. However, the decision to perform an intervention should undergo a similar process of peer-review, and multidisciplinary discussion as with surgery.

Most adult congenital catheterization practices consist of approximately 70% intracardiac device implantation and approximately 30% other interventions [11]. Percutaneous interventions in patients with CHD may be categorized as: percutaneous balloon angioplasty; percutaneous balloon angioplasty and stenting; percutaneous occlusion of shunt lesions; and percutaneous balloon valvotomy or valvuloplasty. Various interventional techniques and their indications have been listed in table 2.

**Table 2. Catheter Interventions in Adult Congenital Heart Defects**

| Catheter Intervention | Adult CHD |
|---|---|
| Balloon Dilatation | Congenital Aortic Stenosis;<br>Congenital Pulmonary Stenosis. |
| Balloon Dilatation with Stent Implantation | Branch and distal pulmonary arterial stenosis (129).<br>Resistant stenoses in surgical venous pathways (130) (Mustard/Senning/Fontan). |
| Occlusion & Embolization Techniques | Secundum ASD<br>PFO<br>VSD<br>PDA<br>Others: Baffle leaks; systemic arterial; coronary; and venous fistulas communications |
| Percutaneous Valve Insertion | Pulmonary Regurgitation in Adults following TOF repair in childhood. |

# Percutaneous Occlusion of Shunt Lesions

## Atrial Septal Defects

Atrial septal defect [ASD] is the most common CHD encountered in adults [excluding mitral valve prolapse and bicuspid aortic valve], accounting for up to 15% of all adults with CHD. ASDs are present in approximately 0.317 of every 1000 live births [12]. Most patients with hemodynamically significant ASD are asymptomatic during first decade of life. It is estimated that most patients with an ASD with significant shunt flow [i.e., pulmonary to systemic flow more than 2:1] will be symptomatic and require surgical correction by the age of 40 [13]. However, some patients have been reported not becoming symptomatic until 60 years of age or older [14,15].

Small ASDs with a diameter of less than 5 mm and no evidence of RV volume overload do not impact the natural history of the individual and thus may not require closure unless associated with paradoxical embolism. Larger defects with evidence of RV volume overload on echocardiography usually only cause symptoms in the third decade of life, and closure is usually indicated to prevent long-term complications such as atrial arrhythmias, reduced exercise tolerance, hemodynamically significant TR, right to-left shunting and embolism during pregnancy, overt congestive cardiac failure, or pulmonary vascular disease that may develop in up to 5% to 10% of affected [mainly female] individuals [16].

Percutaneous closure of an atrial septal defect was first described in 1976 by King et al [17]. Since then, it is estimated that more than 30,000 percutaneous closure procedures have been performed in patients with patent foramen ovale [PFO] and atrial septal defects [ASD]. Continued evolution of device design and operator experience have resulted in remarkably low complication rates for these procedures. The development of percutaneous transcatheter closure techniques has provided an alternative method of closure for uncomplicated secundum ASDs with appropriate morphology [18-20]. The surgery has been the traditional treatment of ASDs in past, and although they have a mortality rate near zero, but carry overall 70% of minor complications, 5-10% of serious complications and a 8-17% of arrhythmia [21-23]. For these reasons percutaneous device closure of the defect has been developed as a safer, quicker option [24-32]. Currently, the majority of secundum ASDs can be closed with a percutaneous catheter technique. The emergence of Amplatzer device has revolutionized the treatment since it allows the closure of communications of up to 40 mm in diameter with minimal complications [19, 33-36]. Also more than one device can be inserted to close multiple ASDs [37,38]. The United States Food and Drug Administration's Center for Devices and Radiological Health has approved two devices for percutaneous ASD closure [39,40]. These are the Amplatzer Septal Occluder and the CardioSEAL Septal Occlusion System.

Latest ACC/AHA guidelines recommend surgical closure when percutaneous closure is not feasible or is not appropriate [16]. Sinus venosus, coronary sinus, and primum defects are not amenable to device closure. The ideal lesion for percutaneous closure is considered to be a defect less than 30 mm in diameter with a rim of tissue around the defect of at least 5 mm to prevent obstruction of the coronary sinus, right pulmonary veins, vena cavae, or atrioventricular valves. Approximately half to two-thirds of ASDs in adults meet these criteria [41,42]. An ASD with a large septal aneurysm or a multifenestrated atrial septum requires careful evaluation by and consultation with interventional cardiologists before device closure is selected as the method of repair. Similarly European society of cardiology task force on management of grown up CHD recommends closure of large ASD [>10 mm] unless pulmonary vascular disease [PVR>8 $Um^2$, L-R shunt <1.5, no response to pulmonary vasodilators] and paradoxical embolism are present when smaller ASD may be considered for closure [11].

Favorable outcomes have been described by various clinical studies, in the great majority of patients treated with percutaneous closure, most of whom have been children [35-37,43-47]. Defect closure has been shown to cause a reduction in left atrial volume and improvements in right and left ventricular function [45]. Giardini et al demonstrated that percutaneous ASD closure improves functional capacity, even in asymptomatic patients as illustrated in their study of 32 adults who underwent ASD closure at a mean age of 43 years [47]. The limited data comparing surgical and percutaneous closure of a secundum ASD suggest that the rate of procedural success is comparable or possibly better than with surgery, but that the rate of complications and length of hospital stay may be reduced with the percutaneous approach. It is likely that percutaneous closure will replace surgical closure in many patients, especially those with significant operative risks. The complications of device closure of osteum secundum ASDs are described in table 3.

**Table 3. Complications of ASD percutaneous device closure**

| | | |
|---|---|---|
| **A.** | **Early:** | |
| | a. | Device embolisation. |
| | b. | Device malposition. |
| | c. | Arrhythmias (usually atrial). |
| | d. | Cardiac perforation (leading to hemopericardium; pericardial effusion; cardiovascular collapse; or sudden death). |
| **B.** | **Late:** | |
| | a. | Device erosion. |
| | b. | Thrombus formation. |
| | c. | Sudden death. |

Follow-up with echocardiography at 24 hours, 1 month, 6 months, and 1 year and at regular intervals thereafter is recommended for patients after device closure along with clinical assessment of symptoms of arrhythmia, chest pain, or embolic events and echocardiographic surveillance for device position, residual shunting, and complications such as thrombus formation or pericardial effusion [16].

## Patent Foramen Ovale

The patent foramen ovale [PFO] is a congenital cardiac lesion that can persist into adulthood [48-50]. Embryologically, PFO is a flap like communication in which the septum primum covering the fossa ovalis overlaps the superior limbic band of the septum secundum. The prevalence of PFO in different studies has been estimated in the range of 25 to 30 percent [48,51-53].

Although most patients with a PFO are asymptomatic, a variety of clinical manifestations may be seen, including cryptogenic stroke. The association between PFO and cryptogenic stroke has been described in observational clinical trials [54,55]. Patients with documented PFO and previous embolic events are at increased risk for recurrent stroke of up to 4.2% per year, even in the context of therapeutic anticoagulation [56-59]. However, appropriate therapy for these patients is still undetermined.

Migraine and vascular headache may be associated with PFO and right-to-left cardiac shunting. As a result, PFO closure has been evaluated as a treatment for migraine headache. Decompression sickness in scuba divers can result in air embolism through a PFO. The risk is increased with larger PFOs and in patients who travel by air within 12 to 48 hours after diving.

Some data also suggest that specific PFO parameters, such as the degree of right-to-left shunting, the presence of atrial septal aneurysm, and PFO tunnel length, may increase the risk for thromboembolic events and may represent the cohort of patients who will receive the greatest benefit from device closure [60,61]. Percutaneous transcatheter closure is a potential option for such patients with PFO and thromboembolic phenomena that avoids the morbidity associated with surgical closure or lifelong anticoagulation [56]. However, the optimal therapy of patients with a patent foramen ovale [PFO] or secundum atrial septal defect [ASD] who have had a cerebrovascular event is not well defined because definitive controlled trials specifically addressing this issue have not been completed. Although it seems intuitive that closure of the defect would provide optimal protection, at present there is no clear evidence that closure is better than medical therapy, at least in part because not all recurrent cerebral events are due to paradoxical embolization [62]. Consensus guidelines from American Academy of Neurology [AAN], the American Heart Association/American Stroke Association [AHA/ASA], and the American College of Chest Physicians [ACCP] have concluded that there is insufficient evidence to evaluate the efficacy of surgical or percutaneous closure compared with medical therapy [63-65].

The platypnea-orthodeoxia syndrome is a rare disorder characterized by both dyspnea [platypnea] and arterial desaturation in the upright position with improvement in the supine position [orthodeoxia] [40,66]. An elevation in right atrial pressure causing right-to-left shunting is usually required, although blood may flow from right to left even with normal right atrial pressure, as is typically seen with persistence of eustachian valves [40,67-68]. The definitive treatment for these patients is closure of the atrial shunt [69,70].

## Ventricular Septal Defect

VSD is the most common congenital heart defect at birth [71] and presents in approximately 3.0 to 3.5 infants per 1000 live births. Because there is a high incidence of spontaneous closure of small VSDs, the incidence is much less in older infants and particularly in adults [72,73]. Although VSD is most often an isolated lesion, it is a common component of complex abnormalities such as conotruncal defects [eg, tetralogy of Fallot, transposition of great arteries]. VSD can also be associated with left-sided obstructive lesions such as subvalvular aortic stenosis and coarctation of the aorta. A subpulmonary [supracristal] VSD is often associated with progressive aortic valve regurgitation caused by prolapse of the aortic cusp [usually right] through the defect. VSDs are classified as inflow, muscular, or perimembranous depending on location in the septum. A classification scheme suggested by the Society for Thoracic Surgery's Congenital Heart Surgery Database Committee and representatives from the European Association for Cardiothoracic Surgery [74] is shown in table 4. Patients with sizable VSD can develop cardiac left-sided volume overload, subsequent ventricular failure, and pulmonary hypertension, typically at younger ages than patients with atrial-level defects.

**Table 4. Classification of Ventricular Septal Defects***

| | |
|---|---|
| **Type 1:** | Lies beneath semilunar valves in conal or outlet septum. |
| **Type 2:** | Peri- or paramembranous; may extent into inlet or outlet area. |
| **Type 3:** | Involves the inlet of ventricular septum immediately inferior to AV valve apparatus. |
| **Type 4:** | Muscular |

* Modified from Jacobs et al (74).

Percutaneous closure of VSD offers an attractive alternative to surgical management in patients with increased surgical risk factors, multiple previous cardiac surgical interventions, poorly accessible muscular VSDs, or "Swiss cheese"–type VSDs. At present, US Food and Drug Administration approval for device closure of VSDs in the United States is limited to closure of muscular VSDs. Experience with percutaneous closure of other types of VSDs has been obtained at centers outside the United States or in centers with investigational protocols.

Devices used for VSD closure have included the Rashkind double umbrella device, the Sideris button device, and more recently the CardioSEAL/STARFlex system and the Amplatzer muscular VSD occluder device. The most commonly used devices are of Amplatzer family. They involve the presence of two self expanding discs developed from a network of nitinol filaments united by a cylindrical segment of variable thickness, whose diameter corresponds to the VSD diameter. The two lateral discs have a diameter larger than the central cylinder in order to avoid the displacement of device. The type of occluding disc varies depending on the type of VSD [75,76].

It is important to carefully select patients for transcatheter closure. Patients selected for transcatheter closure should also meet the criteria for surgical correction. Thus, patients with small defects who have normal left heart volumes and right ventricular pressures are not candidates for surgical or interventional therapy. Patient selection is based upon the size of the patient, location and size of defect, and surrounding anatomical considerations. Transcatheter closure of VSDs is difficult and should be performed only in centers with considerable experience and expertise in interventional catheterization techniques and specialized surgical backup [77,78]. Indications for catheter device closure of VSD include residual defects after prior attempts at surgical closure, restrictive VSDs with a significant left-to-right shunt, trauma, or iatrogenic artifacts after surgical replacement of the aortic valve. Indications for closure of restrictive VSDs in the adult population include a history of bacterial endocarditis or a hemodynamically significant left-to-right shunt [Qp/Qs greater than 1.5:1]. ACC/AHA guidelines [16] recommend device closure of a muscular VSD may be considered, especially if the VSD is remote from the tricuspid valve and the aorta, if the VSD is associated with severe left-sided heart chamber enlargement, or if there is PAH [Class IIb]. [*Level of Evidence: C*]

Success rates of the procedure are high, with closure rates with the membranous device of up to 92% at 15 minutes after device implantation and a 92% rate of complete closure at the 12-month follow-up for device closure of muscular VSD. These results, unfortunately, are not matched in patients undergoing closure of a postinfarct VSD because of the often moribund status of these patients and the tendency of the VSD to enlarge over time owing to ongoing necrosis [16]. Ventricular arrhythmia, heart block, considerable blood loss, and valvular damage are all potential complications of transcatheter closure [77]. Complications have been reported in as many as 10.7% of patients and most frequently include rhythm and conduction abnormalities, as well as hypotensive episodes or blood loss [79]; however, complications are significantly associated with a lower patient weight [below 10 kg], and therefore the adult population is likely to represent a lower-risk group for percutaneous closure of muscular VSDs. Complications after closure of perimembranous VSDs predominantly include rhythm and conduction abnormalities, as well as the potential for new or increased AR or TR, which is usually of a trivial or mild degree.

Adults with no residual VSD, no associated lesions, and normal pulmonary artery pressure do not require continued follow-up at a regional ACHD center except on referral from their cardiologist or physician. Patients who develop bifascicular block or transient trifascicular block after VSD closure are at risk in later years for the development of complete heart block and should be followed up yearly by history and ECG and have periodic ambulatory monitoring and/or exercise testing [16]. Closure of perimembranous defects is particularly associated with complete heart block [80], which is thought to be due to overlapping of the ventricular conduction system by the right ventricular retention disk as it passes above or anterosuperiorly to the defect. Affected patients require a permanent pacemaker post-procedure [81].

## Patent Ductus Arteriosus

The ductus arteriosus [DA], which is present in all mammalian species, is a vascular connection between the main pulmonary artery and the aorta. PDA is the persistence of this communication between the aorta and the pulmonary artery. It can be isolated or may be present in association with all forms of CHD. The most common associated lesions are VSDs or ASDs. The incidence of PDA has increased dramatically over the last two decades due to the improved survival rate of premature infants. The incidence is approximately 0.02 to 0.04 percent among term infants born at sea level, with a slight female predominance, but is higher in children born at high altitude [82] and in premature infants. The estimated incidence is as high as 60 percent in infants born before 28 weeks gestation [83] due to immature development of the DA, which fails to constrict normally [84].

If the PDA is large and nonrestrictive, the patient may present with Eisenmenger physiology, including differential cyanosis and clubbing. Patients are at an increased risk of developing endarteritis, heart failure, and pulmonary vascular disease. It is important to note that individuals with PDA have increased morbidity and mortality, primarily due to HF and infective endocarditis [IE] [85].

In adults, the ductus is frequently calcified, is friable and can have aneurysmal dilation. For all these reasons, surgical ligation is a procedure of risk. Percutaneous closure of patent ductus is a quick, simple, involving less than 24 hours of hospitalization, and that leaves no scar. The most frequent complication is the device embolization that usually can be resolved in the same procedure [86]. Also the mortality and morbidity is very low in comparison to surgical closure [86-92]. The procedure can be performed without anesthesia and often as an outpatient.

A variety of devices have been used for percutaneous closure of a PDA. Percutaneous coil occlusion has achieved widespread acceptance for the treatment of small to medium sized PDAs and is rapidly becoming the treatment of choice for most children and adults [93,94]. A variety of different coil deployment methods have been described; all are designed to position embolization coils across the PDA and achieve complete permanent occlusion [95]. The efficacy of coil occlusion was demonstrated in a series of 1258 patients from the European Registry [96]. The immediate occlusion rate following coil insertion was 59 percent and was 95 percent at one year.

The Amplatzer duct occluder is an effective therapy for a PDA [92,97]. Occlusion can also be successfully achieved with this device in patients with large PDAs and systemic or near-systemic pulmonary artery pressures [98]. However, there is a potentially increased risk of device embolism into the aorta in such patients. The Rashkind umbrella occlusion device has also been successfully used for percutaneous closure of a PDA, although the outcome appears to be better with coil occlusion or surgery [94,99,100].

Thus, adults with PDA are better suited for percutaneous closure with either the occlusion device or coils because of its high success and few complications [101]. If the PDA is associated with other conditions that require surgical correction, the ductus may be closed during the same operation, although percutaneous closure of the PDA before other cardiac surgery may decrease the risk of cardiopulmonary bypass. Follow-up approximately every 5 years for patients who received a device is recommended because of the lack of long-term data on device closure with the occlusion device.

# Percutaneous Angioplasty and Stenting

## Coarctation of Aorta

Coarctation of the aorta is a common malformation, accounting for 6 to 8 percent of all congenital heart defects, occurring two to five times more frequently in males than females. Discrete coarctation of the aorta consists of short-segment narrowing in the region of the ligamentum arteriosum adjacent to the origin of the left subclavian artery. In some cases, there is also narrowing of the aortic arch or isthmus. Extensive collateral vessels may arise proximal to the obstruction. The presence of abundant collaterals may reduce the gradient across the coarctation and mask the severity of the obstruction. An associated intrinsic abnormality in the aortic wall predisposes to dissection or rupture in the ascending aorta or the area of the coarctation.

The adult who had surgical repair of coarctation of the aorta as an infant is more likely to have associated cardiac lesions with bicuspid aortic valve, subvalvular aortic stenosis, VSD, and varying degrees of arch hypoplasia. Residual hemodynamic problems from any of these defects may complicate the clinical course and may require more detailed evaluation and follow-up. Coarctation of the aorta in the adult patient has an increased risk of left ventricular dysfunction, persistent hypertension, coronary atherosclerosis and cerebral premature chance of breakage or aortic dissection or vessel cerebrales [102].

Surgery carries the risk of paraplegia, and in adults, a major bleeding due to the very presence of increased collateral circulation. On the other hand, percutaneous angioplasty has a significant rate of restenosis and aneurysms [103]. McCrindle et al reported the recurrence rate after balloon angioplasty of primary coarctation in adults at approximately 7%, with a further 7% of patients having a suboptimal primary outcome [104]. However, with stenting these risks have been minimized. Implantation of a stent after balloon angioplasty limits the risks associated with angioplasty, results in a minimal residual gradient, improves luminal diameter, and sustains hemodynamic benefit. The coated stent has helped reduce the risk when the coarctation is very severe or treat associated pathology such as patent ductus arteriosus or aneurysms. Angioplasty with stent implantation is now the preferred technique for the treatment of native coarctation of the aorta as well as post-surgery adult [105-109].

For recurrent aortic coarctation [coarctation after surgical repair], the prevailing opinion now is that catheter-based intervention [balloon or stent] is generally safe and the preferred alternative to surgery in the absence of confounding features [e.g., aneurysm or pseudo aneurysm formation, or significant coarctation that affects the adjoining arch arterial branches] [109-112]. The initial success rate, defined as a gradient ≤20 mmHg across the coarctation, is approximately 80 to 90 percent in the largest studies [108,109,113,114].

In many ACHD centers, surgery is reserved for patients who are unsuitable for percutaneous treatment or who have undergone unsuccessful percutaneous treatment. The role of balloon dilatation of native or postoperative aortic coarctation remains controversial [115]. Dilatation of previous patch aortoplasty carries the highest risk of aortic rupture and should be performed with surgical standby. Balloon dilatation of native aortic disease can often be achieved with excellent results, although failure to relieve stenosis [10–20%] aneurysm formation [5–10%] and restenosis [5–10%] have all been reported [116]. For this reason, there has been an increase in vogue towards balloon dilatation with simultaneous stent implantation.

Major long-term complications of repair include recoarctation, aortic aneurysm, and systemic hypertension with or without exercise [117]. Patients should be monitored with periodic clinical examinations and an imaging procedure. MRI may be most cost-effective for detecting both recoarctation and aneurysm formation [118]. All patients with either interventional catheterization or surgical repair of coarctation of the aorta should have close follow-up and aggressive management of blood pressure and other risk factors for cardiovascular disease. This should include at least yearly cardiology evaluations. Consultation with a cardiologist with special expertise in ACHD should be obtained on initial contact to determine risk factors specific for the patient's anatomy and the presence of associated lesions. Evaluation of the repair site by MRI/CT should be repeated at intervals of 5 years or less, depending on the specific anatomic findings before and after repair. Consideration should be given to cumulative lifetime radiation exposure with multiple CT examinations.

## Percutaneous Valvuloplasty and Valve Insertion

Percutaneous valve replacement is a potentially extremely beneficial procedure for ACHD patients who have been subjected to multiple operations and may have premature aging of multiple organ systems, raising the risk of recurrent surgeries. The largest group to potentially benefit from such advances, at present, includes patients with tetralogy of Fallot with postoperative residual pulmonary insufficiency [40].

## Post TOF Repair

TOF consists of subpulmonary infundibular stenosis, a VSD, an aorta that overrides the VSD, and right ventricular hypertrophy. It accounts for approximately 10 percent of all cases of congenital heart disease and is one of the most common cyanotic congenital heart defects [119]. It is also the most common cyanotic malformation to reach adulthood without surgical repair. Reparative surgery, which is usually performed electively in the first year of life [120], permits over 85 percent of children with TOF to survive to adulthood [121]. With improving surgical techniques and improved survival more and more post-TOF repair patients are likely to be encountered in clinical practice. Although long-term outcomes are generally good in patients with TOF but there is a risk of complications such as sudden cardiac death [SCD] and heart failure [122-124]. SCD is an important cause of mortality after intracardiac repair of TOF. In three large series of patients followed for 21 to 36 years, SCD occurred in 2.0, 2.7, and 9 percent of patients [123,125,126].

After repair of tetralogy, echocardiography is usually very helpful in assessing for the presence and severity of residual RVOT obstruction and pulmonary regurgitation along with the presence or absence of TR. Recent data suggests MRI as the reference standard [127,128] for assessment of RV volume and systolic function. It can also help in assessing the severity of pulmonary regurgitation and associated pathology, especially involving the pulmonary arteries and the ascending aorta.

Recently published latest ACC / AHA guidelines [16] recommend catheterization to assess the potential for repair for the unusual case of a patient with tetralogy of Fallot who has undergone palliation with a surgical shunt. The presence or absence of additional muscular VSDs may be determined, as well as the course and anatomy of the epicardial coronary arteries. The pulmonary architecture and vascular pressure and resistance should be delineated, because pulmonary artery distortion and PAH are frequent sequelae of palliative surgical shunts. Potential catheter interventions include elimination of collateral vessels or systemic–pulmonary artery shunts, dilation/stent implantation of obstructed pulmonary arteries, and, more recently, the possibility of percutaneous pulmonary valve implantation.

Cardiac catheterization is not used routinely in the assessment of patients who have undergone repair, except when surgery or other therapy is being considered or for the evaluation of the pulmonary and coronary arteries. As per latest ACC / AHA guidelines [16], in adults with repaired tetralogy of Fallot, catheterization may be considered to better define potentially treatable causes of otherwise unexplained LV or RV dysfunction, fluid retention, chest pain, or cyanosis [Class IIb indication]. In these circumstances, transcatheter interventions may include: a. Elimination of residual shunts or aortopulmonary collateral vessels. [*Level of Evidence: C*] b. Dilation [with or without stent implantation] of RVOT obstruction. [*Level of Evidence: B*] c. Elimination of additional muscular or patch margin VSD. [*Level of Evidence: C*] d. Elimination of residual ASD. [*Level of Evidence: B*] [16].

Percutaneous valve implantation offers the exciting prospect of non-surgical management of pulmonary regurgitation after repair of Tetralogy of Fallot and related conditions. It is now possible to insert into the right ventricular outflow, a stent mounted bovine jugular venous valve, via a cardiac catheter [129]. Further work is required to develop a valve, which is suitable for the dilated outflow tract found in many adult patients. An implantable valve that can be used in the systemic circulation also appears possible.

## Pulmonary Valve Stenosis

Pulmonary valve stenosis in adults is usually of congenital origin and rarely acquired. Valvular PS is usually an isolated lesion, occurs in approximately 7% to 12% of all CHD, and accounts for 80% to 90% of all lesions that cause RVOT obstruction [130]. Its inheritance rate is low, ranging from 1.7% to 3.6% [131,132]. Approximately 20% of patients with valvular PS have a dysplastic valve [133,134], and if part of Noonan syndrome, these patients have an autosomal dominant trait with variable penetrance that has been mapped to chromosome 12 [135,136]. Most patients with PS who reach adulthood are asymptomatic and require no specific therapy.

Balloon valvotomy is recommended for asymptomatic patients with a domed pulmonary valve and a peak instantaneous Doppler gradient greater than 60 mm Hg or a mean Doppler gradient greater than 40 mm Hg [in association with less than moderate pulmonic valve regurgitation]. [*Level of Evidence: B*] Since the initial successful report of percutaneous balloon valvotomy for pulmonary valve stenosis in 1982 [137], the procedure has evolved to become the treatment of choice for patients with classic domed valvular PS. Balloon valvotomy produces relief of the gradient by commissural splitting. As might be expected from the morphology, results in patients with a dysplastic pulmonary valve are less impressive. In the Valvuloplasty and Angioplasty of Congenital Anomalies [VACA] registry, in 784 cases, the mean transvalvular gradient declined from 71 to 28 mm Hg in patients with typical PS and from 79 to 49 mm Hg in patients with a dysplastic valve [138].

PPV is highly technically successful and safe in the adult population with results comparable to those of surgical valvotomy. A significant reduction in gradient is obtained in up to 80% of procedures [influenced by annulus size, valve morphology, or operator technique], and most patients are free of events in the long term after a single procedure. Further reduction in residual gradients may be seen over time because of resolution of residual hypertrophic subvalvular stenosis. Long-term follow-up of adults who underwent PPV in their youth suggests that, similar to results with surgical valvotomy, late moderate or greater pulmonary regurgitation is increasingly recognized,7 and preprocedural counseling and surveillance for such are recommended.

In general, acute complications from the procedure have been minimal. During the acute performance of the valvotomy, vagal symptoms predominate, along with catheter-induced ventricular ectopy and occasionally right bundle-branch block. Other complications include pulmonary valve regurgitation, pulmonary edema [presumably from increasing pulmonary blood flow to previously underperfused lungs], cardiac perforation and tamponade, high-grade AV nodal block, and transient RVOT obstruction. The latter is sometimes referred to as a "suicidal right ventricle" and is due to abrupt infundibular obstruction once the pulmonary valve obstruction has been relieved [139]. This may be alleviated by volume expansion and beta blockade. This postprocedural infundibular obstruction tends to regress over time.

## Peripheral Pulmonary Artery Stenosis

Abnormal narrowing of the main pulmonary artery, the major pulmonary arterial branches, and the peripheral pulmonary arteries can all lead to obstruction of RV outflow. Pulmonary artery stenosis [PAS] in patients with congenital heart disease may occur anywhere in the pulmonary vascular tree from the main pulmonary artery to the distal-most branches. Peripheral pulmonary artery stenoses tend to occur in multiple tertiary branches of the pulmonary tree and are progressive; by the time patients are seen as adults, there may be considerable loss of lung parenchyma due to totally occluded segmental pulmonary arteries. With PAH, pulmonary valve regurgitation may be expected.

Percutaneous treatment of branch pulmonary artery stenosis remains a challenge for the interventional cardiologist. In general, indications for percutaneous intervention for branch pulmonary artery stenosis include a marked asymmetry of the pulmonary blood flow or a significant increase in right ventricular pressure. According to the latest ACC/AHA guidelines [16], percutaneous interventional therapy is recommended as the treatment of choice in the management of appropriate focal branch and/or peripheral pulmonary artery stenosis with greater than 50% diameter narrowing, an elevated RV systolic pressure greater than 50 mm Hg, and/or symptoms. [*Level of Evidence: B*]. The use of high pressure balloon has significantly improved the outcome of pulmonary angioplasty. The success rate of primary pulmonary angioplasty has been reported to be approximately 60%, with up to 10% of patients developing a recurrent branch pulmonary artery stenosis [140]. Stent implantation is indicated for any stenosis unresponsive to conventional management or tortuous / long segment stenosis / pulmonary artery stenosis secondary to extrinsic compression. Palmer-Genesis stent has superior flexibility which is of benefit in advancing stents around very tight angles into stenotic segments of branch pulmonary arteries. Data on long term results after stenting branch pulmonary arteries in adults is virtually non-existent [141]. Redilatation of stent has been reported to be required in up to 11 out of 29 pediatric patients, but is likely to be significantly less in the adult population, where outgrowing the stent is not an issue [142].

## Aortic Stenosis

Congenital aortic stenosis is most frequently secondary to congenital fusion of one or more comissures, typically resulting in a bicuspid or even unicuspid aortic valve. BAV is one of the most common congenital cardiovascular malformations, with an estimated incidence of 1% to 2% of the population. The prevalence of AS is harder to calculate because, unlike many other congenital heart lesions, a BAV may develop significant obstruction or regurgitation after midlife, with a peak age range for surgical intervention between 60 and 80 years [143,144]. There is male preponderance for AS. A BAV may be inherited, and family clusters have been studied [144,145].

A BAV can be predominately obstructive or regurgitant, depending on the degree of commissural fusion. According to most recent ACC/AHA guidelines [16], aortic balloon valvotomy is indicated in young adults and others without significantly calcified aortic valves and no AR who fulfil following criteria: a. Those with symptoms of angina, syncope, dyspnea on exertion, and peak-to-peak gradients at catheterization greater than 50 mm Hg. [*Level of Evidence: C*] b. Asymptomatic adolescents or young adults who demonstrate ST or T-wave abnormalities in the left precordial leads on ECG at rest or with exercise and a peak-to-peak catheter gradient greater than 60 mm Hg. [*Level of Evidence: C*]

## Miscalleneous Conditions

Several other miscalleneous congenital conditions offer new avenues for transcatheter interventions like occlusion of coronary artery fistulae, and occlusion of major aortopulmonary collaterals along with some post-operative conditions. Transcatheter balloon dilatation with or without stent implantation is used for post-Mustard or post-Senning operative patients with stenosis of surgical conduits and baffles which is seen in about 5-10%

cases, most commonly involving the superior vena caval baffles [146]. Dilatation of Fontan circuit stenoses due either to anastomotic narrowing or kinking of a conduit has also been performed by transcatheter route [147].

## Conclusion

The number of adult patients with congenital heart disease, surviving from interventions in infancy, is rising. Longevity increases also the number of patients with mild disease [small ASD, bicuspid valves and mild coarctation], who reach adulthood untreated. Currently there are more adults than children in the US living with CHD. Intervention can be carried out for various conditions and carry low risk and very high success rate. With ongoing advances in the technology, the future is very promising with increasing prospects for successful percutaneous interventions in the management of adult patients with CHD.

## References


[1] National Heart, Lung and Blood Institute. Congenital Heart Defects. December 2007.

[2] Pierpont, ME; et al. Genetic Basis for Congenital Heart Defects: Current Knowledge: A Scientific Statement From the American Heart Association Congenital Cardiac Defects Committee, Council on Cardiovascular Disease in the Young. *Circulation,* volume 115, June 12, 2007, pages 3015-3038.

[3] Congenital Cardiovascular Defects: Current Knowledge: A Scientific Statement From the American Heart Association Council on Cardiovascular Disease in the Young. *Circulation*, volume 115, June 12, 2007, pages 2995-3014.

[4] MacMahon, B; McKeown, T; Record, RG. The incidence and life expectation of children with heart disease. *Br Heart J* 1953; 15:121.

[5] Rashkind, WJ; Miller WW. Creation of an atrial septal defect without thoracotomy. *JAMA* 1966;196:991-2.

[6] Grüntzig A. Die perkutane Rekanalisation chronischer arterieller Verschisse (Dotter-Prinzip) mit einem doppellumigen Dilatations-Katheter. *Forstchr Rontgenstr* 1976;124:80-6.

[7] Kan, JS; White, RI Jr; Mitchell, SE; Gardner, TJ. Percutaneous balloon valvuloplasty: A new method for treating congenital pulmonary valve stenosis. *N Engl J Med* 1982;307:540-2.

[8] Carr-White, GS; Kilner, PJ; Hon, JK; et al. Incidence, location, pathology and significance of pulmonary homograft stenosis after the Ross operation. *Circulation* 2001;104(12 Suppl (1);I16–120.

[9] Wood, NB; Weston, SJ; Kilner, PJ; et al. Combined MR imaging and CFD simulation of flow in the human descending aorta. *J Magn Reson Imaging* 2001;13(5):699–713.

[10] Kaemmerer, H; Stern, H; Fratz, S; et al. Imaging in adults with congenital cardiac disease (ACCD). *Thoracic Cardiovasc Surg* 2000;48(6):328–35.

[11] Management of Grown Up Congenital Heart Disease: The Task Force on the Management of Grown Up Congenital Heart Disease of the European Society of Cardiology. *European Heart Journal* (2003) 24, 1035–1084.

[12] Ferencz, C; Rubin, JD; McCarter, RJ; et al. Congenital heart disease: prevalence at livebirth. The Baltimore- Washington Infant Study. *Am J Epidemiol* 1985;121:31–6.

[13] Rostad, H; Sorland, S. Atrial septal defect of secundum type in patients under 40 years of age. A review of 481 operated cases. Symptoms, signs, treatment and early results. *Scand J Thorac Cardiovasc Surg* 1979; 13: 123-127.

[14] John Sutton, MG; Tajik, AJ; McGoon, DC. Atrial septal defect in patients aged 60 years or older: operative results and long term postoperative follow up. *Circulation* 1981;64:402-409.

[15] Konstantinides, S; Geibel, A; Olschewski, M; et al. A comparison of surgical and medical therapy for atrial septal defect in adults. *N Eng J Med* 1995; 333:469-473.

[16] ACC/AHA 2008 Guidelines for the Management of Adults With Congenital Heart Disease: A Report of the American College of Cardiology/American Heart Association Task Force on Practice Guidelines (Writing Committee to Develop Guidelines on the Management of Adults With Congenital Heart Disease). *J. Am. Coll. Cardiol.* 2008;52;e1-e121.

[17] King, TD; Thompson, SL; Steiner, C; Mills, NL. Secundum atrial septal defect. Nonoperative closure during cardiac catheterization. *JAMA* 1976;235:2506–9.

[18] Fischer, G; Stieh, J; Uebing, A; Hoffmann, U; Morf, G; Kramer, HH. Experience with transcatheter closure of secundum atrial septal defects using the Amplatzer septal occluder: a single centre study in 236 consecutive patients. *Heart* 2003;89:199 –204.

[19] Du, ZD; Hijazi, ZM; Kleinman, CS; Silverman, NH; Larntz, K. Comparison between transcatheter and surgical closure of secundum atrial septal defect in children and adults: results of a multicenter nonrandomized trial. *J Am Coll Cardiol* 2002;39:1836–44.

[20] Dhillon, R; Thanopoulos, B; Tsaousis, G; Triposkiadis, F; Kyriakidis Redington, A. Transcatheter closure of atrial septal defects in adults with the Amplatzer septal occluder. *Heart* 1999;82:559–62.

[21] Murphy, JG; Gersho, BJ; McGoon, MD; Mair, DD; Porter, CJ; Ilstrup, DM; et al. Long term outcome after surgical repair of isolated atrial septal defect: follow-up at 27 to 32 years. *N Engl J Med* 1990; 323:1645-50.

[22] Attie, F; Rosas, F; Granados, NC; Zabal Buendia, AJ. Calderon. Surgical treatment for secundum atrial septal defect in patients> 40 years old. A randomized clinical trial. *J Am Coll Cardiol* 2001; 38:2035-42.

[23] Pastorek, JS; Allen, HD; Davis, JT. Current outcomes of surgical closure of secundum atrial septal defect. *Am J Cardiol* 1994; 74: 75-7.

[24] Rao, PS; Sideris, EB; Hausdorf, G; King, C; Lloyd, TR; Beekman, RH; et al. International experience with secundum atrial septal defect occlusion by the Botton device. *Am Heart J* 1994; 128: 1022-35.

[25] Hausdorf, G; Schneider, M; Franzbach, B; Kampmann, C; Kargus, KB. Goeldner. Transcatheter closure of secundum atrial septal defects with the atrial septal defect occlusion system (ASDOS): initial experience in children. *Heart* 1996; 75:83-8.

[26] Kaulitz, R; Paul, T; Hausdorf, G. Extending the limits of transcatheter closure of atrial septal defects with the double umbrella device (CardioSEAL). *Heart* 1998; 80:54-9.

[27] Justo, RN; Nykanen, DG; McCrindle, BW; Boutin, C; Benson, LN. The clinical impact of catheter closure of secundum atrial septal defects with the double umbrella device: up to 56 months follow-up. *Circulation* 1995; 92 (Suppl): 308.

[28] Zahn, EM; Benson, LN; Hellenbrand, WE; Latson, THE; Lock, JE; Moore, P; et al. Transcatheter closure of secundum ASDs with the CardioSEAL septal occlusion system: early results of the North American trial [abstract]. *Circulation* 1997; 96 (Suppl):1-568.

[29] Das, GS; Shrivastava, S; O'Laughlin, MP; Salmon, AP; Mendelsohn, AM; Hijazi, ZM; et al. Intermediate-term follow up of patients after percutaneous closure of atrial septal defects with the DAS Angel Wings device [abstract]. *Circulation* 1996; 95:1-56.

[30] Latson, LA; Benson, LN; Hellenbrand, WF; Mullins, CE; Lock, JF. Transcatheter closure of ASD early results of Multicenter trial of the Bard Clamshell septal occluder [abstract]. *Circulation* 1991; 84 (Suppl 11): 544.

[31] Babic, UU; Grujicic, S; Popovic, Z. Double umbrella device for transvenous closure of patient ductus arteriosus and atrial septal defect. First experience. *Intervention J Cardiol* 1991; 4:283-94.

[32] Rickers, C; Hamm, C; Stern, M; Hofmann, T; Franzen, O; Schrader, R; et al. Percutaneous closure of secundum atrial septal defect with a new self-Centering device ("angel wings"). *Heart* 1998; 80: 517-21.

[33] Masur, J; Gavora, P; Formanek, A; Hijazi, ZM. Transcatheter closure of secundum atrial septal defects using the new self-Centering Amplatzer septal occluder: initial human experience. *Catheter Cardiavasc Diagn* 1997; 42:388-93.

[34] Thanopoulos, BD; Laskari, CV; Tsaousis, GS; Zarayelyan, A; Vekiou, A; Papadopoulos, GS. Closure of atrial septal defects with the Amplatzer occlusion device: preliminary results. *J Am Coll Cardiol* 1998; 31:1110-6.

[35] Chan, KC; Godman, MJ; Walsh, K; Wilson N; Redington A; Gibbs JL. Transcatheter closure of atrial septal defect and interatrial communications with a new self-expanding nitinol double disc device (Amplatzer septal occluder): Multicenter UK experience. *Heart* 1999; 82:300-6.

[36] Fischer, G; Kramer, M; Stieh, J; P Harding, O. Jung. Transcatheter closure of secundum atrial septal defects with the new self-Centering Amplatzer septal occluder. *Eur Heart J* 1999; 20:541-9.

[37] Carminati, M; Chessa, M; Butera, G et al. Transcatheter closure of atrial septal defects with the STARFlex device: early results and follow-up. *J Interv Cardiol* 2001;14:319-324.

[38] Cao, Q; Radtke, W; Berger, F et al. Transcatheter closure of multiple atrial septal defects. Initial results and value of two- and three-dimensional transoesophageal echocardiography. *Eur Heart J* 2000;21:941-947.

[39] Schwetz, BA. Congenital heart defect devices. From the Food and Drug Administration. *JAMA* 2002; 287:578.

[40] Inglessis, I; Landzberg, MJ. Interventional catheterization in adult congenital heart disease. *Circulation* 2007; 12: 1622-1633.

[41] Ferreira, SM; Ho, SY; Anderson, RH. Morphological srudy of defects of the atrial septum within the oval fossa: Implications for transcatheter closure of the left-to-right shunt. *Br Heart J* 1992;67:316-320.

[42] Prokselj, K; Kozeli, M; Zadnik, V; Podnar, T. Echocardiographic characteristics of secundum-type atrial septal defects in adult patients: Implications for percutaneous closure using amplatzer septal occluders. *J Am Soc Echocardiogr* 2004;17:1167-1172.
[43] Chessa, M; Carminati, M; Butera, G et al. Early and late complications associated with transcatheter occlusion of secundum atrial septal defect. *J Am Coll Cardiol* 2002;39:1061-1065.
[44] Masura, J; Gavora, P; Podnar, T. Long-term outcome of transcatheter secundum-type atrial septal defects closure using Amplatzer septal occluders. *J Am Coll Cardiol* 2005;45:505-507.
[45] Salehian, O; Horlick, E; Schwerzmann, M et al. Improvements in cardiac form and function after transcatheter closure of secundum atrial septal defects. *J Am Coll Cardiol* 2005;45:499-504.
[46] Pedra, CA; Pihkala, J; Lee KJ et al. Transcatheter closure of atrial septal defects using the Cardio-Seal implant. *Heart* 2000;84:320-326.
[47] Giardini, A; Donti, A; Formigari, R et al. Determinants of cardiopulmonary functional improvement after transcatheter atrial septal defects closure in asymptomatic adults. *J Am Coll Cardiol* 2004;43:1886-1891.
[48] Hara, H; Virmani, R; Ladich, E et al. Patent foramen ovale: current pathology, pathophysiology; and clinical status. *J Am Coll Cardiol* 2005;46:1768-1776.
[49] Wu, LA; Malouf, JF; Dearani, JA et al. Patent foramen ovale in cryptogenic stroke: current understanding and management options. *Arch Intern Med* 2004;164:950-956.
[50] Kerut, EK; Norfleet, WT; Plotnick, GD; Giles, TD. Patent foramen ovale: a review of associatedconditions and the impact of physiological size. *J Am Coll Cardiol* 2001;38:613-623.
[51] Hagen, PT; Scholz, DG; Edwards, WD. Incidence and size of patent foramen ovale during the first 10 decades of life: an autopsy study of 965 normal hearts. *Mayo Clin Proc* 1984;59:17-20.
[52] Meissner, I; Whisnant, JP; Khandheria, BK et al. prevalence of potential risk factors for stroke assessed by transesophageal echocardiography and carotid ultrasonography: the SPARC study. Stroke Prevention: Assessment of risk in a community. *Mayo Clin Proc* 1999;74:862-869.
[53] Pinto, FJ. When and how to diagnose patent foramen ovale. *Heart* 2005;91:438-440.
[54] Overell, JR; Bone, I; Lees, KR. Interatrial septal abnormalities and stroke: a meta-analysis of case-control studies. *Neurology* 2000;55: 1172–1179.
[55] Di Tullio, M; Sacco, RL; Gopal, A; Mohr, JP; Homma, S. Patent foramen ovale as a risk factor for cryptogenic stroke. *Ann Intern Med* 1992; 117:461– 465.
[56] Chatterjee, T; Petzsch, M; Ince, H; Rehders, TC; Korber, T; Weber, F; Schneider, H; Auf der Maur, C; Nienaber, CA. Interventional closure with Amplatzer PFO occluder of patent foramen ovale in patients with paradoxical cerebral embolism. *J Interv Cardiol* 2005;18:173–179.
[57] Hanna, JP; Sun, JP; Furlan, AJ; Stewart, WJ; Sila, CA; Tan, M. Patent foramen ovale and brain infarct. Echocardiographic predictors, recurrence and prevention. *Stroke* 1994;25:782–786.
[58] Mas, JL; Zuber, M. Recurrent cerebrovascular events in patients with patent foramen ovale, atrial septal aneurysm, or both and cryptogenic stroke or transient ischemic

attack. French Study Group on Patent Foramen Ovale and Atrial Septal Aneurysm. *Am Heart J* 1995;130: 1083–1088.

[59] De Castro, S; Cartoni, D; Fiorelli, M; Rasura, M; Anzini, A; Zanette, EM; Beccia, M; Colonnese, C; Fedele, F; Fieschi, C; Pandian, NG. Morphological and functional characteristics of patent foramen ovale and their embolic implications. *Stroke* 2000;31:2407–2413.

[60] Agmon, Y; Khandheria, BK; Meissner, I; Gentile, F; Whisnant, JP; Sicks, JD; O'Fallon, WM; Covalt, JL; Wiebers, DO; Seward, JB. Frequency of atrial septal aneurysms in patients with cerebral ischemic events. *Circulation* 1999;99:1942–1944.

[61] Windecker, S; Wahl, A; Nedeltchev, K; Arnold, M; Schwerzmann, M; Seiler, C; Mattle, HP; Meier, B. Comparison of medical treatment with percutaneous closure of patent foramen ovale in patients with cryptogenic stroke. *J Am Coll Cardiol* 2004;44:750 –758.

[62] Holmes, DR Jr; Cabalka, A. Was your mother right--do we always need to close the door?. *Circulation* 2002; 106:1034.

[63] Messe, SR; Silverman, IE; Kizer, JR et al. Practice parameter: recurrent stroke with patent foramen ovale and atrial septal aneurysm: report of the Quality Standards Subcommittee of the American Academy of Neurology. *Neurology* 2004;62:1042-1050.

[64] Sacco, RL; Adams, R; Albers, G et al. Guidelines for prevention of stroke in patientswith ischemic stroke or transient ischemic attack: a statement for healthcare professionals from the American Heart Association / American Stroke Association Council on Stroke: co-sponsored by the Council on Cardiovascular Radiology and Intervention. *Stroke* 2006;37:577-617.

[65] Albers, GW; Amarenco, P; Easton, JD et al. Antithrombotic and thrombolytic therapy for ischemic stroke: American College of Chest Physicians Evidence Bases Clinical Practice Guidelines (Eighth Edition). *Chest* 2008;133:630S-669S.

[66] Bruch, L; Parsi, A; Grad, MO et al. transcatheter closure of interatrial communicatios for secondary prevention of paradoxical embolism: single center experience. *Circulation* 2002;105:2845-2848.

[67] Information for physicians and patients on the withdrawal of two humanitarian device exemptions (HDEs) for patent foramen ovale (PFO) occluders. U.S. Food and Drug Administration Center for Devices and Radiological health. www.fda.gov/cdrh/ode/h000007-h990011withdraw.html (Accessed on September 25; 2008).

[68] Windecker, S; Wahl, A; Nedeltchev, K et al. Comparison of medical treatment with percutaneous closure of patent foramen ovale in patients with cryptogenic stroke. *J AM Coll Cardiol* 2004;44:750-758.

[69] Spies, C; Strasheim, R; Timmermanns, I; Schraeder, R. Patent foramen ovale closure in patients with cryptogenic thrombo-embolic events using the Cardia PFO occluder. *Eur heart J* 2006;27:365-371.

[70] Thomson, JD. Percutaneous PFO closure, further data but many unanswered questions. *Eur Heart J* 2006; 27:258.

[71] Hoffman, JI; Kaplan, S. The incidence of congenital heart disease. *J Am Coll Cardiol* 2002;39:1890 –900.

[72] Du, ZD; Roguin, N; Wu, XJ. Spontaneous closure of muscular ventricular septal defect identified by echocardiography in neonates. *Cardiol Young* 1998;8:500 –5.

[73] Kidd, L; Driscoll, DJ; Gersony, WM; et al. Second natural history study of congenital heart defects. Results of treatment of patients with ventricular septal defects. *Circulation* 1993;87:I38-I51.

[74] Jacobs, JP; Burke, RP; Quintessenza, JA; Mavroudis, C. Congenital heart surgery nomenclature and database project: ventricular septal defect. *Ann Thorac Surg* 2000;69:S25–S35.

[75] Amin, Z; Gu, X; Berry, JM; Bass, JL; Titus, JL; Urness, M et al. New device for closure of muscular ventricular septal defect in a canine model. *Circulation* 1999; 100: 320-328.

[76] Bass, JL; Kalra, GS; Arora, R; Masura, J; Gavora, P; Thanapolous, BD et al. Initial human experience with the Amplatzer perimembranous ventricular septal occluder septal device. *Catheter Cardiovasc Interv* 2003; 58: 238-245.

[77] Rudolph, AM. Ventricular Septal Defect. In: Congenital Diseases of the Heart: Clinical-Physiological Considerations, Rudolph, AM (Ed), Futura Publishing Company, New York 2001. p.197.

[78] Gumbiner, CH; Takao, A. Ventricular septal defect. In: The Science and Practice of Pediatric Cardiology, 2nd ed, Garson, A, Bricker, JT, Fisher, DJ, Neish, SR (Eds), Williams & Wilkins, Baltimore, 1998. p. 1119.

[79] Holzer, R; Balzer, D; Cao, QL; Lock, K; Hijazi, ZM. Device closure of muscular ventricular septal defects using the Amplatzer muscular ventricular septal defect occluder: immediate and mid-term results of a US registry. *J Am Coll Cardiol* 2004;43:1257– 63.

[80] Thanopoulos, BD; Rigby, ML. Outcome of transcatheter closure of muscular ventricular septal defects with the Amplatzer ventricular septal defect occluder. *Heart* 2005;91:513-516.

[81] Butera, G; Carminati, M; Chessa, M et al. Transcatheter closure of perimembranous ventricular septal defects: early and long-term results. *J Am Coll Cardiol* 2007;50:1189-1195.

[82] Mullins, CE. Patent ductus arteriosus. In: The Science and Practice of Pediatric Cardiology Garson, A, Bricker, JT, McNamara, DG (Eds), Lea & Febiger, Philadelphia 1990. p.1055.

[83] Freedom, RM; Benson, LN; Smallhorn, JF. Neonatal Heart Disease. Springer-Verlag, New York 1992. p.593.

[84] Gittenberger-de Groot, AC; van Ertbruggen, I; Moulaert, A; Harinck, E. The ductus arteriosus in the preterm infant: Histologic and clinical observations. *J Pediatr* 1980;96:88-93.

[85] Campbell, M. Natural history of persistent ductus arteriosus. *Br Heart J* 1968; 30:4.

[86] Faella, HJ; Hijazi, ZM. Closure of the patent ductus arteriosus with the Amplatzer PDA device: immediate results of the international clinical trial. Catheter Cardiovasc Interv 2000;51:50-4. Cerrar [Medline] [Descargar cita] 57. Faella HJ; Hijazi ZM.. Closure of the patent ductus arteriosus with the Amplatzer PDA device: immediate results of the international clinical trial. *Catheter Cardiovasc Interv* 2000;51:50-4.

[87] Chessa, M; Mohamed, B; Giusti, S; Butera, G; Bini, RM; Carano, M; et al. Transcatheter treatment of patent ductus arteriosus. *Ital Heart J* 2002;3(II Suppl):1092-7.

[88] Hong, TE; Hellenbrand, WE; Hijazi, ZM. Amplatzer investigators. Transcatheter closure of patent ductus arteriosus in adults using the Amplatzer duct occluder: initial results and follow-up. *Indian Heart J* 2002;54:384-9.

[89] Thanopoulos, BD; Hakim, FA; Hiari, A; Tsaouris, GS; Paphitis, C; Hijazi, ZM. Patent ductus arteriosus equipment and technique. Amplatzer duct occluder: intermediate-term follow-up and technical considerations. *J Interv Cardiol* 2001;14:247-54.

[90] Wang, JK; Lian, CS; Huang, JJ; Hsu, KL; Lo, PH; Hung, JS; et al. Transcatheter closure of patent ductus arteriosus using Gianturco coils in adolescents and adults. *Catheter Cardiovasc Interv* 2002; 55:513-8.

[91] Lee, CH; Leung, YL; Chow, WH. Transcatheter closure of the patent ductus arteriosus using an Amplatzer duct occluder in adults. *Jpn Heart J* 2001;42:533-7.

[92] Bilkis, AA; Alwi, M; Hasri, S; Haifa, AL; Geetha, K; Rehman, MA; et al. The Amplatzer duct occluder experience in 209 patients. *J Am Coll Cardiol* 2001;37:258-61.

[93] Shim, D; Fedderly, RT; Beekman, RH 3rd et al. Follow-up of coil occlusion of patent ductus arteriosus. *J Am Coll Cardiol* 1996;28:207-211.

[94] Janorkar, S; Goh, T; Wilkinson, J. Transcatheter closure of patent ductus arteriosus with the use of rashkind occluders and / or gianturco coils: long-term follow-up in 123 patients and special reference to comparison, residual shunts, complications, and technique. *Am Heart J* 1999;138:1176-1183.

[95] Ebeid, MR; Gaymes, CH; Smith, JC; Braden, DS. Gianturco-Grifka vascular occlusion device for closure of patent ductus arteriosus. *Am J Cardiol* 2001;87:657-660.

[96] Mage, AG; Huggon, IC; Seed, PT; Qureshi, SA. Transcatheter coil occlusion of the arterial duct. Results of the European Registry. *Eur Heart J* 2001;22:1817-1821.

[97] Thanopoulos, BD; Hakim, FA; Hiari, A; Goussous, Y. Further experience with transcatheter closure of the patent ductus arteriosus using the Amplatzer duct occluder. *J Am Coll Cardiol* 2000;35:1016-1021.

[98] Pass, RH; Hijazi, Z; Hsu, DT et al. Multicenter USA Amplatzer patent ductus arteriosus occlusion device trial: initial and one year results. *J Am Coll Cardiol* 2004;44:4513-519.

[99] Jaeggi, ET; Fasnacht, M; Arbenz, U; Beghetti, M. Transcatheter occlusion of the patent ductus arteriosus with a single device technique: comparison between the Cook detachable coil and the Rashkind umbrella device. *Int Cardiol* 2001;79:71-76.

[100] Gray, DT; Fyler, DC; Walker, AM; Weinstein, MC. Clinical outcomes and cost of transcatheter as compared with surgical closure of patent ductus arteriosus. The Patent Ductus Arteriosus Closure Comparative Study Group. *N Eng J Med* 1993;329:1517-1523.

[101] Celermajer, DS; Sholler, GF; Hughes, CF; Baird, DK. Persistent ductus arteriosus in adults. A review of surgical experience with 25 patients. *Med J Aust* 1991;155:233–6.

[102] Zabal C. Cerdeira. The therapeutic catheterization. In: Faus Attie; editor. Congenital heart disease in adults. Madrid: Elsevier Science; 2003; p. 281-3.

[103] Tyagui, S; Arora, R; Kane, UA; Sethi, KK; Gambhir, DS; Khalilullah, M. Balloon Angioplasty of native coarctation of the aorta in adolescents and young adults. *Am Heart J* 1992; 123:674-80.

[104] McCrindle, BW; Jones, TK; Morrow, WR; et al. Acute results of balloon angioplasty of native coarctation versus recurrent aortic obstruction are equivalent. Valvuloplasty and Angioplasty of Congenital Anomalies (VACA) Registry Investigators. *J Am Coll Cardiol* 1996;28:1810 –7.

[105] Bulbul, ZR; Bruckheimer, E; Love, JC; Fahey JT; Hellenbrand WE. Implantation of balloon-expandable stent for coarctation of the aorta: attainment data and short term results. *Catheter Cardiovasc Diagn* 1996; 39:36-42.

[106] Rosenthal, E; Qureshi, SA; Tynan, M. Aortic Stent attainment for recoarctation. *Am Heart J* 1995; 129:1220-1.

[107] Harrison, DA; McLaughlin, PR; Lazzam, C; Connelly, M; Beson, LN. Endovascular stents in the management of coarctation of the aorta in the adolescent and adult: one year follow-up. *Heart* 2001; 85:561-6.

[108] Fawzy, ME; Awad, M; Hassan, W et al. Long-term outcome (up to 15 years) of balloon angioplasty of discrete native coarctation of aorta in adolescents and adults. *J Am Coll Cardiol* 2004;43:1062-1067.

[109] Hellenbrand, WE; Allen, HD; Golinko, RJ et al. Balloon angioplasty for aortic recoarctation: results of Valvuloplasty and Angioplasty of Congenital Anomalies Registry. *Am J Cardiol* 1990;65:793-797.

[110] Cooper, SG; Sullivan, ID; Wren, C. Treatment of recoarctation: balloon dilatation angioplasty. *J Am Coll Cardiol* 1989;14:413-419.

[111] Hijazi, ZM; Fahey, JT; Kleinman, CS; Hellenbrand, WE. Balloon angioplasty for recurrent coarctation of aorta. Immediate and long-term results. *Circulation* 1991;84:1150-1156.

[112] Anjos, R; Qureshi, SA; Rosenthal, E et al. Deteminants of hemodynamic results of balloon dilatation of aortic recoarctation. *Am J Cardiol* 1992;69:665-671.

[113] Yetman, AT; Nykanen, D; McCrindle, BW et al. Balloon angioplasty of recurrent coarctation: a 12 year review. *J Am Coll Cardiol* 1997;30:811-816.

[114] Fletcher, SE; Nihill, MR; Grifka, RG et al. Balloon angioplasty of native coarctation of aorta: midterm follow-up and prognostic factors. *J Am Coll Cardiol* 1995; 25:730-734.

[115] Rosenthal, E. Stent implantation for aortic coarctation: The treatment of choice in adults? *J Am Coll Card* 2001;138(5):1524–7.

[116] Patel, HT; Madani, A; Paris, YM et al. Balloon angioplasty of native coarctation of the aorta in infants and neonates: Is it worth the hassle? *Paed Cardiology* 2001;22(1):53–7.

[117] Stewart, AB; Ahmed, R; Travill, CM; Newman, CG. Coarctation of the aorta life and health 20-44 years after surgical repair. *Br Heart J* 1993;69:65-70.

[118] Therrien, J; Thorne, SA; Wright, A et al. Repaired coarctation: a "cost-effective" approach to identify complications in adults. *J Am Coll Cardiol* 2000;35:997-1002.

[119] Hoffman, JI. Incidence of congenital heart disease: I. Postnatal incidence. *Pediatric Cardiol* 1995;16:103-113.

[120] Report of the New England Regional Infant Cardiac Program. *Pediatrics* 1980; 65:375.

[121] Murphy, JG; Gersh, BJ; Mair, DD. Long-term outcome in patients undergoing surgical repair of tetrology of Fallot. *N Eng J Med* 1993;329:593-599.

[122] Hokanson, JS; Moller, JH. Significance of early transient complete heart block as a predictor of sudden death late after operative correction of tetrology of Fallot. *Am J Cardiol* 2001;87:1271-1277.

[123] Nollert, G; Fischlein, T; Bouterwek, S et. Long-term survival in patients with repair of tetrology of Fallot: 36-year follow up of 490 survivors of the first year after surgical repair [see comments]. *J Am Coll Cardiol* 1997;30:1374-1383.

[124] Engelfriet, P; Boersma, E; Oechslin, E et al. The spectrum of adult congenital heart disease in Europe: morbidity and mortality in a 5 year follow-up period. The Euro Heart Survey on adult congenital heart disease. *Eur Heart J* 2005;26:2325-2333.

[125] Gatzoulis, MA; Balaji, S; Webber, SA et al. Risk factors for arrhythmia and sudden cardiac death late after repair of tetrology of Fallot: a multicentre study. *Lancet* 2000;356:975-981.

[126] Garson, A Jr; McNamara, DG. Sudden death in a pediatric cardiology population; 1958-1983: relation to prior arrhythmias. *J Am Coll Cardiol* 1985;5:134B-137B.

[127] Davlouros, PA; Kilner, PJ; Hornung, TS; et al. Right ventricular function in adults with repaired tetralogy of Fallot assessed with cardiovascular magnetic resonance imaging: detrimental role of right ventricular outflow aneurysms or akinesia and adverse right-to-left ventricular interaction. *J Am Coll Cardiol* 2002;40:2044 –52.

[128] van Straten, A; Vliegen, HW; Hazekamp, MG; de Roos, A. Right ventricular function late after total repair of tetralogy of Fallot. *Eur Radiol* 2005;15:702–7.

[129] Bonhoeffer, P; Boudjemline, Y; Saliba, Z et al. Percutaneous replacement of pulmonary valve in a right-ventricle to pulmonary-artery prosthetic conduit with valve dysfunction. *Lancet* 2000;356:1403–5.

[130] Cheatham, JP; Coe, JY; Kugler, JD; Fletcher, SE; Tower AJ. Successful transcatheter perforation of the atretic pulmonary valve membrane in a newborn using the new Coe radiofrequency end hole catheter. *Cathet Cardiovasc Diagn* 1998;45:162– 6.

[131] Driscoll, DJ; Michels, VV; Gersony, WM; et al. Occurrence risk for congenital heart defects in relatives of patients with aortic stenosis; pulmonary stenosis; or ventricular septal defect. *Circulation* 1993; 87(suppl II):I114 –20.

[132] Nora, JJ; Nora, AH. Recurrence risks in children having one parent with a congenital heart disease. *Circulation* 1976;53:701–2.

[133] Mendez, HM; Opitz, JM. Noonan syndrome: a review. *Am J Med Genet* 1985;21:493–506.

[134] Noonan, J. Noonan syndrome—then and now. *Cardiol Young* 1999;9: 545–6.

[135] Tramboo NA; Iqbal K; Dar, MA; Malik, RA; Naikoo, BA; Andrabi, MA. Unusual dysmorphic features in five patients with Noonan's syndrome: a brief review. *J Paediatr Child Health* 2002;38:521–5.

[136] Fryns, JP. The cardio-facio-cutaneous (CFC) syndrome and Robertsonian 15/22 translocation. *Ann Genet* 1992;35:186–8.

[137] Kan, JS; White, RI Jr; Mitchell, SE; Gardner, TJ. Percutaneous balloon valvuloplasty: a new method for treating congenital pulmonary-valve stenosis. *N Engl J Med* 1982;307:540 –2.

[138] Stanger, P; Cassidy, SC; Girod, DA; Kan, JS; Lababidi, Z; Shapiro, SR. Balloon pulmonary valvuloplasty: results of the Valvuloplasty and Angioplasty of Congenital Anomalies Registry. *Am J Cardiol* 1990;65: 775–83.

[139] Ben-Shachar, G; Cohen, MH; Sivakoff, MC; Portman, MA; Riemenschneider, TA; Van Heeckeren, DW. Development of infundibular obstruction after percutaneous pulmonary balloon valvuloplasty. *J Am Coll Cardiol* 1985;5:754–6.

[140] Boudjemline, Y; Agnoletti, G; Bonnet, D; Sidi, D; Bonhoeffer, P. Percutaneous pulmonary valve replacement in a large right ventricular outflow tract: an experimental study. *J Am Coll Cardiol* 2004; 43: 1082-1087.

[141] Gentles, TL; Lock, JE; Perry, SB. High pressure balloon angioplasty for branch pulmonary artery stenosis: early experience. *J Am Coll Cardiol* 1993; 22: 867-872.

[142] Holzer, R; Cao, Qi-Ling; Hijazi, ZM. State of the art catheter interventions in adults with congenital heart disease. *Expert Rev Cardiovasc Ther* 2004; 2(5):699-711.

[143] Fogelman, R; Nykanen, D; Smallhorn, JF; McCrindle, BW; Freedom, RM; Benson, LN. Endovascular stents in pulmonary circulation. Clinical impact on management and medium term follow up. *Circulation* 1995; 92: 881-885.

[144] Hoffman, JI; Kaplan, S. The incidence of congenital heart disease. *J Am Coll Cardiol* 2002;39:1890 –900.

[145] Basso, C; Maron, BJ; Corrado, D; Thiene, G. Clinical profile of congenital coronary artery anomalies with origin from the wrong aortic sinus leading to sudden death in young competitive athletes. *J Am Coll Cardiol* 2000;35:1493–501.

[146] Fedak, PW; Verma, S; David, TE; Leask, RL; Weisel, RD; Butany, J. Clinical and pathophysiological implications of a bicuspid aortic valve. *Circulation* 2002;106:900–4.

[147] Bu'Lock, FA; Tometzki, AJ; Kitchiner, DJ et al. Balloon expandable stents for systemic venous pathway stenosis late after Mustard's operation. *Heart* 1998; 79:225-229.

[148] Hornung, TS; Benson, LN; McLaughlin, PR. Catheter interventions in adult patients with congenital heart disease. *Current Cardiol Reports* 2002; 4: 54-62.

In: Advances in Cardiovascular Research, Volume 1
Editors: L. Schmitt, T. Konig, pp. 367-379
ISBN: 978-1-60741-720-0


*Chapter XVI*

# Aortic Stenosis and Systemic Arterial Hypertension: See beyond the Valve

***L. Kadem****

Laboratory for Cardiovascular Fluid Dynamics, Department of Mechanical and Industrial Engineering, Concordia University; Montreal; Quebec; Canada.

## Abstract

Aortic stenosis is the most frequently occurring valvular heart disease and cardiovascular disease after systemic arterial hypertension and coronary artery disease. Contrary to old assumptions, the coexistence of aortic stenosis and systemic arterial hypertension is highly significant (32 to 50%). In this case, the overloaded left ventricle has to support, at the same time, the increase in pressure due to systemic arterial hypertension as well as the increase in transvalvular pressure gradient due to the aortic stenosis. Knowing which overload is the most significant, valvular or arterial, is a difficult problem. However, this information is essential to determine which medical treatment is more beneficial to the patient: valve replacement or reduction of arterial pressure. Indeed, replacing the native valve while the most significant load supported by the left ventricle is systemic arterial hypertension will not necessarily improve patient's condition. In the same way, reducing arterial pressure in severe aortic stenosis can compromise coronary circulation (mainly if the hypertension results from a significant decrease in arterial compliance). This chapter deals with the interaction between aortic stenosis and systemic arterial hypertension and their combined effect on the left ventricle. More specifically, the impact of systemic arterial hypertension on the assessment of aortic stenosis severity, in terms of transvalvular pressure gradients and effective orifice areas, will be addressed. Then, new parameters such as "valvulo-arterial impedance" and "hypertensive equivalent effective orifice area", introduced to determine the overall load supported by the left ventricle, will be explained and discussed. Furthermore, recommendations on how markers of aortic stenosis severity in hypertensive patients should be interpreted will be issued.

* Corresponding author: Laboratory for Cardiovascular Fluid Dynamics; Department of Mechanical and Industrial Engineering; Concordia University; 1455 de Maisonneuve Blvd W; Montreal QC Canada H3G 1M8, Email: kadem@encs.concordia.ca, Telephone number: 514-848-2424 (ext. 3143), Fax number: 514-848-3175.

Aortic stenosis (AS) is considered the most common cardiac disease in developed countries after coronary artery disease and systemic arterial hypertension (Braunwald et al. (2001)). It is usually a degenerative disease that produces an obstruction to flow passing from the left ventricle (LV) to the ascending aorta. Its prevalence in industrialized countries ranges between 2 to 7% (Stewart et al. (1997); Lindroos et al. (1993)) and it is responsible for around 100,000 valve replacements and 20,000 deaths per year in North America (Pibarot et al. (2007)). However, only few patients develop an isolated AS. This shows that AS is a component of a more global group of pathologies affecting not only the valve itself but also the proximal arteries. Among all of the pathologies associated with AS, systemic arterial hypertension has a very high prevalence. Systemic arterial hypertension is defined as an abnormal increase in blood pressure (systolic pressure > 140 mmHg and/or diastolic pressure > 90 mmHg). It may result from an increase in systemic arterial resistance (systolo-diastolic hypertension), a decrease in systemic arterial compliance (systolic hypertension), or both.

Table 1 shows the classification of aortic stenosis and hypertension severities as evaluated using systolic pressure, diastolic pressures and effective orifice area, respectively.

## Coexistence of Aortic Stenosis and Systemic Arterial Hypertension

One of the first large studies dealing with the coexistence of AS and systemic arterial hypertension was published in 1934 by McGinn and White. They reported a prevalence of 27% of systemic arterial hypertension (systolic pressure higher than 150 mmHg) in a cohort of 236 patients with AS. Ikram et al. (1979) showed that systemic arterial hypertension was present in 14% of the 50 patients with concomitant systemic arterial hypertension and AS. Some more recent studies have reported an even higher prevalence; indeed, Antonini-Canterin et al. (2003) reported a prevalence of 32% of systolic hypertension in a series of 193 patients with severe symptomatic AS, and Briand et al. (2005) showed that this prevalence can reach up to 50%. Table 2 summarizes different studies related to the coexistence of systemic arterial hypertension and AS.

**Table 1. Classification of systemic arterial hypertension and aortic stenosis severities. Adapted from (Garcia et al. 2007).**

| | Systemic Arterial Hypertension | | Aortic Stenosis |
|---|---|---|---|
| | Systolic Pressure (mmHg) | Diastolic Pressure (mmHg) | Effective Orifice Area ($cm^2$) |
| NORMAL | 120-129 | 80-84 | ≥ 3 |
| HIGH NORMAL | 130-139 | 85-89 | - |
| MILD | 140-159 | 90-99 | > 1.5 |
| MODERATE | 160-179 | 100-109 | 1.0-1.5 |
| SEVERE | ≥ 170 | ≥ 110 | ≤ 1.0 |

**Table 2. Prevalence of concomitant systemic arterial hypertension in patients in aortic stenosis.**

| Authors | Year | Number of patients with aortic stenosis | % of patients with aortic stenosis AND systemic arterial hypertension |
|---|---|---|---|
| Christian | 1931 | 57 | 1% |
| McGinn and White | 1934 | 236 | 27% |
| Contralto and Levine | 1937 | 180 | 9% |
| Ikram et al. | 1979 | 50 | 14% |
| Antonini-Canterin | 2003 | 193 | 32% |
| Briand et al. | 2005 | 208 | 50% |

The presence of systemic arterial hypertension affects clinical decision in two ways (Otto 2006):

(1) systemic arterial hypertension may mask the severity of aortic stenosis.
(2) the presence of aortic stenosis may affect the optimal treatment of hypertension.

## Impact of Systemic Arterial Hypertension on the Evaluation of Aortic Stenosis Severity

The apparition of symptoms in patients with AS having a larger effective orifice area when concomitant systemic arterial hypertension was present (Antonini-Cantarin et al. 2003), raises a question on the validity of current diagnosis parameters to evaluate AS severity. Indeed, the clinical decision regarding valve replacement in patients with AS is mainly based on two criteria: 1) an effective orifice area (EOA) lower than 1.0 $cm^2$ and 2) the apparition of symptoms. It is not necessarily true that patients with severe AS (1.0 $cm^2$) will develop symptoms. Predicting the presence or the absence of symptoms in patients with AS is still a challenging issue. However, it is quite unexpected for a patient to develop symptoms with a moderate AS. Then, under such conditions the following question raises: Does systemic arterial hypertension lead to an underestimation of the severity of AS? In other words, how sensitive are AS evaluation parameters (transvalvular pressure gradient, effective orifice area and energy loss coefficient) to a variation in blood pressure?

Laskey et al. (1995) tried to address the above interrogation using a mathematical model applied to in vivo data. They found that transvalvular pressure gradient (TPG) may decrease irrespective of flow as a direct consequence of an increase in blood pressure, resulting from an increase in systemic arterial resistance. Contrastingly, Razzolini et al. (1999) showed, using an experimental model, that TPG increases linearly with systemic arterial resistance.

To resolve these discrepancies, Kadem et al. (2005) performed an animal study in which they created supravalvular stenoses of varying severities and simulated systemic arterial hypertension by a distal constriction of the aorta or phenylephrine perfusion. They showed, using this model, that systemic arterial hypertension induces significant decreases in TPG and an increase in EOA. Figure 1 shows a sample of left ventricle (LV) and aortic waveforms obtained from their animal model for a severe supravalvular AS and different stages of systemic arterial hypertension induced by banding of the aorta and then after severe systemic arterial hypertension induction using administration of phenylephrine. They showed that the observed reduction in TPG can be attributed to: 1) a decrease in cardiac output resulting from systemic arterial hypertension; 2) an increase in blood pressure, which can lead to an increase in EOA due to an expansion of the aortic root; 3) a decrease in systemic arterial compliance, which has an independent effect on peak-to-peak TPG but not on mean and maximal TPGs.

Some of these findings have been confirmed in in vivo study on the impact of blood pressure on Doppler echocardiographic assessment of AS severity (Little et al. 2007). In this study, the authors were able to increase blood pressure using a handgrip exercise or phenylephrine infusion in 22 patients with AS. They confirmed that systemic arterial hypertension may interfere with the assessment of AS, which is not directly related to the increase in systemic arterial resistance and the decrease in systemic arterial compliance induced by systemic arterial hypertension, but rather to the change in mean transvalvular flow rate. This variation in mean transvalvular flow rate induces a variation in EOA and TPGs, which lead to an overestimation or an underestimation of the severity of AS dependent on the direction of the variation in mean transvalvular flow rate. They also explained that the calcification of the aortic annulus in patients with AS may limit its expansion as a result of an increase in blood pressure, leaving, in these patients, the variation in mean flow rate as the only independent contributor to the variation in TPGs. This was further confirmed by Mascherbauer et al. (2008) using in vitro and computational fluid dynamics studies.

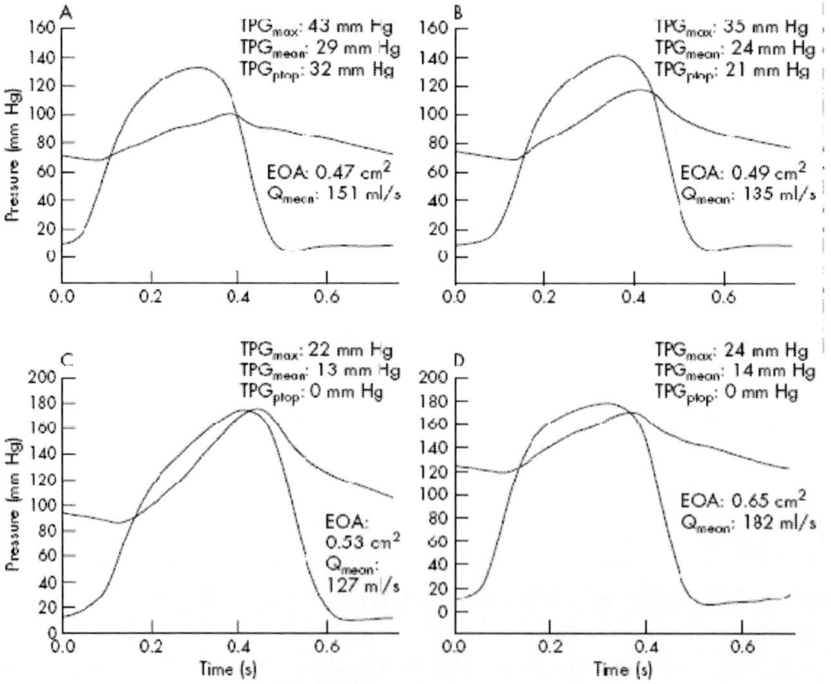


Figure 1. Effect of concomitant systemic arterial hypertension on the evaluation of the severity of aortic stenosis (from Kadem et al. (2005) with permission).

**Table 3. Recommendations for optimal treatment of patients with aortic stenosis and concomitant systemic arterial hypertension.**

| | |
|---|---|
| 1) | Blood pressure should be recorded systematically during echocardiography in patients evaluated for aortic stenosis. |
| 2) | Serial evaluations should take into account whether the patient's blood pressure level is within the same range as in the previous evaluation. |
| 3) | Doppler echocardiographic evaluation should be performed when blood pressure control is optimal. If the blood pressure is elevated at the time of examination, it would be preferable to repeat the measurements after optimization of blood pressure treatment. |
| 4) | Peak to peak transvalular pressure gradient should not be used in patients with AS and concomitant systemic hypertension because it is highly dependent on systemic arterial compliance independently of AS severity. |

Finally, it should be noted that even though AS is underestimated due to a reduction in TPGs resulting from a decrease in mean transvalvular flow rate, ventricular systolic wall stress increases significantly with induced systemic arterial hypertension, showing that this apparent reduction in TPGs should not be interpreted as reflecting a reduction in ventricular afterload. Furthermore, this demonstrates that the investigation of the severity of AS and its impact on LV load should not be limited to the stenotic valve but rather be more global and thus include the arteries. This will allow a larger view of all loads that have to be supported by the LV, which may provide a better understanding of the complex relation between the severity of AS and the apparition of symptoms.

Table 3 summarizes some recommendations for optimal treatment of patients with aortic stenosis and concomitant systemic arterial hypertension.

## Impact of Aortic Stenosis and Systemic Arterial Hypertension: Double Loaded Ventricle

When systemic arterial hypertension coexists with AS, it imposes an additional afterload that should be supported the left ventricle. This results in a double loaded ventricle: aortic stenosis load + systemic arterial hypertension load. The adaptive response of the left ventricle to both loads is a myocardial concentric hypertrophy (Jolobe (2008)) and a reduction in exercise capacity (Cremariuc et al. (2006)). Furthermore, Antonini-Canterin et al. (2003) showed that a concomitant systemic arterial hypertension can lead to the apparition of symptoms with a larger effective orifice area and lower stroke work loss as a response to the additional overload resulting from systemic arterial hypertension.

These loads on the left ventricle can be reduced by a valve replacement (reduction of the valvular load) and restoration of normal blood pressure (reduction of arterial load). However, in clinical practice, hypertension usually remains untreated (Jolobe (2008)). As a consequence, patients with AS and concomitant systemic arterial hypertension have reduced LV hypertrophy reduction and exercise capacity improvement even after a valve replacement.

Garcia et al. (2007) investigated, using a theoretical model, the impact of AS load and systemic arterial hypertension load on LV hypertrophy. The use of theoretical models allowed the simulation of several pathological conditions which are difficult to investigated clinically and to decouple the loads due to hypertension and to AS. They used their clinically validated mathematical ventricular-valvular-vascular ($V^3$) model (Garcia et al. 2005) to determine AS and systemic arterial hypertension loads, and then upgraded it using Art's model of myofiber stress (Arts et al. 1991) to determine LV wall volume. They showed that for a fixed AS severity, LV wall volume increases linearly with systemic arterial hypertension severity. The increase becomes "exponential" for fixed systemic arterial hypertension severity and various AS severities. By fitting their results, they were able to express the variation in LV wall volume as a function of AS load and systemic arterial hypertension load using the following formulation:

$$V_w = \underbrace{0.781\left(\frac{A}{EOA}-1\right)^{2.35}}_{AS\ component} + \underbrace{214\left(\frac{SAP}{P_{ref}}-1\right)}_{Hypertension\ component} + \underbrace{120}_{\substack{LV\ wall\ volume \\ under\ normal\ conditions}}$$

where, A is the aortic cross-sectional area measured at the sinutubular junction, EOA is the effective orifice area, SAP is the systolic arterial pressure (peak aortic pressure) and $P_{ref}$ is the systolic pressure in normotensive condition (120 mmHg). The main conclusions from their work were that the effect of a mild to moderate systemic arterial hypertension on the LV wall volume is more important than the impact of a mild to moderate AS, but when AS becomes severe, its impact is the most preponderant.

Finally, it should be noted that although systemic arterial hypertension represents an additional load on the LV, it usually remains untreated in such patients because it is commonly believed that lowering arterial pressure may increase transvalvular pressure gradient, putting the patient at higher risks of heart failure or syncopal attacks (Beevers et al. (1983)). However, recent studies showed that systemic arterial hypertension can be treated in patients with moderate to severe AS using a rennin-angiotensin blockade and an aldosterone blockade using eplerenone (Jimenez-Candil et al. (2005), Krum et al. (2002)).

## Characterization of the Double Loaded Ventricle

Initial studies on the coexistence of AS and systemic arterial hypertension focused mainly on their impact on the evaluation of AS severity and on ventricular afterload. However, these studies were not designed to determine, for a specific patient, which load: AS or systemic arterial hypertension, is the most preponderant for the LV. This issue is extremely important since it determines which load should be targeted with higher priority: AS (valve replacement) or systemic arterial hypertension (medication).

The first attempt was proposed by Briand et al. (2005). Through an in vivo study on 208 patients with AS and systemic arterial hypertension, the authors proposed a new non-invasive parameter: valvulo-arterial impedance ($Z_{va}$) to determine the total afterload supported by the LV. This new parameter includes both AS and systemic arterial hypertension loads and is calculated as:

$$Z_{va} = \frac{SAP + TPG_{net}}{SV_i}$$

where, SAP is the systolic arterial pressure, $SV_i$ is the indexed stroke volume and $TPG_{net}$ is net mean transvalvular pressure gradient:

$$TPG_{net} = TPG_{mean\ Doppler} - 4V^2\left(2\frac{EOA}{A}\right)\left(1-\frac{EOA}{A}\right)$$

where, A is the aortic cross sectional area at the sinotubular junction, V is the maximal continuous-wave Doppler velocity across the stenotic valve. $TPG_{net}$ takes into account pressure recovery downstream of the AS.

In addition, the authors showed that a valvulo-arterial impedance ≥ 5 mmHg/ml/$m^2$ is a strong predictor of risk of LV systolic dysfunction. It should be noted, however, that valvulo-arterial impedance indicates the importance of the total afterload (AS + systemic arterial hypertension) but does not allow the determination of the independent load produced by each disease. A first attempt to resolve this complex problem is done through the introduction of the notion of equivalent hypertension – effective orifice area.

## Equivalent Hypertension – Effective Orifice Area

To introduce this new concept, the ventricular-valvular-vascular coupling model ($V^3$ model) recently developed by Garcia et al. (2005) was used. This model allows the computation of the instantaneous left ventricular pressure and volume, the aortic pressure and the transvalvular flow rate using data, non-invasively, measured in patients.

Briefly below are the $V^3$ model results from the combination of the following three models:

### Ventricular Model

The pressure ($P_v$)-volume (V) relationship in the left ventricle is defined using the LV time-varying elastance E(t):

$$E(t) = \frac{P_V(t)}{V(t) - V_0} \tag{1}$$

where, $V_0$ is the unloaded ventricular volume.

## Aortic Valve Model

Recently, Garcia et al. (2005) developed a semi-analytical model of the instantaneous transvalvular net pressure gradient across the aortic valve ($TPG_{net}$). This explicit model expresses $TPG_{net}$ as a function of flow rate and its first derivative, and the energy loss coefficient $E_LCo$:

$$TPG_{net}(t) = \frac{2\pi\rho}{\sqrt{E_LCo}} \frac{\partial Q}{\partial t} + \frac{\rho}{2} \frac{Q(t)}{E_LCo^2} \tag{2}$$

$$E_LCo = \frac{A \times EOA}{A + EOA}$$

where ρ is the fluid density, Q is the transvalvular flow rate, A is the aortic cross-sectional area at the level of the sinotubular junction, and EOA is the effective orifice area.

## Vascular Model

The flow (Q)-pressure ($P_A$) relationship in the arterial tree was modeled using the well-known three-element windkessel model (Westerhof et al. (1971)):

$$\frac{\partial P_A}{\partial t} + \frac{P_A(t)}{R \times C} = \frac{Z_0 + R}{R \times C} Q(t) + Z_0 \frac{\partial Q}{\partial t} + \frac{P_{VE}}{R \times C} \tag{3}$$

where, R is the systemic arterial resistance, C is the systemic arterial compliance, $Z_0$ is the characteristic impedance (R/15) and $P_{VE}$ is the central venous pressure (=5 mmHg).

## Hypertensive Equivalent Effective Orifice Area

To compare the load induced by the AS to the one induced by systemic arterial hypertension in patients with AS and concomitant systemic arterial hypertension, the concept of "hypertensive equivalent effective orifice area" (EEOA) was introduced. This parameter considers the load induced by systemic arterial hypertension as equivalent to an additional AS and, therefore, can be represented by its "effective orifice area". As defined, the EEOA is a very interesting parameter since it allows the comparison of the load induced by the two pathologies (AS and systemic arterial hypertension) using the same terminology (effective orifice area). It is indeed, more convenient to state for example that a patient has an AS with an EOA of 1.00 $cm^2$ and must support an additional load due to systemic arterial hypertension equivalent to a more severe AS of 0.75 $cm^2$, than to compare an AS effective orifice area with an increase in systemic arterial pressure.

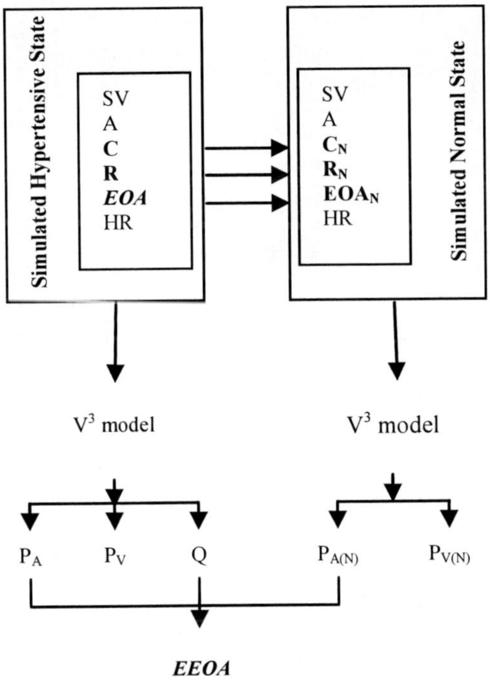


Figure 2. Schematic representation of the calculation of the hypertensive equivalent effective orifice area (EEOA) using the $V^3$ model.

Figure (2) shows how the EEOA is computed using the $V^3$ model. To summarize, data are recorded non-invasively in a patient with AS and concomitant systemic arterial hypertension (stroke volume (SV); aortic cross-sectional area (A); systemic arterial compliance (C); systemic arterial resistance (R); effective orifice area (EOA); heart rate (HR)). Then, using these data, the instantaneous flow rate, and ventricular and aortic pressures ($P_A$; $P_V$; Q) are computed using the $V^3$ model. Now if the same patient with the same (SV; A and HR) is considered under normal conditions, with a normal EOA ($EOA_N$) (no AS) and a normal systemic arterial resistance ($R_N$) and systemic arterial compliance ($C_N$) (no systemic arterial hypertension), it is then possible to compute using the $V^3$ model its hypothetical normal state: normal ventricular pressure ($P_{V(N)}$) and normal aortic pressure ($P_{A(N)}$). Finally, using hypertensive aortic pressure ($P_A$) and the normal aortic pressure ($P_{A(N)}$), a mean equivalent transvalvular pressure gradient (ETPG) is computed and the equivalent effective orifice area is therefore obtained using:

$$EEOA = \left( \frac{1}{A} + \sqrt{\frac{2}{\rho} \frac{ETPG}{\overline{Q}^2}} \right)^{-1}$$

where A is the aortic cross-sectional area; ETPG is the hypertensive equivalent transvalvular pressure gradient and $\overline{Q}^2$ is the mean squared transvalvualr flow.

Figure (3) shows typical ventricular ($P_V$) and aortic ($P_A$) pressure curves obtained using the $V^3$ model. It also shows the simulated normal aortic pressure ($P_{A(N)}$). These curves were obtained for an EOA of 1.00 $cm^2$, a stroke volume of 70 ml, a systemic arterial compliance of 0.98 ml/mmHg, a systemic arterial resistance of 1.53 mmHg s/$cm^2$, an aortic cross sectional area of 7 $cm^2$, and a heart rate of 70 bpm.

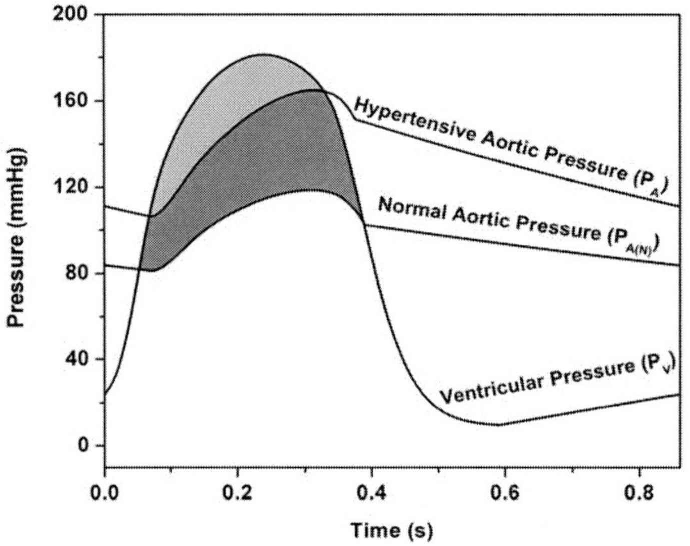


Figure 3. Hypertensive aortic pressure ($P_A$), ventricular pressure ($P_V$) and normal aortic pressure ($P_{A(N)}$) computed using the $V^3$model. The light grey area represents the transvalvular pressure gradient due to a stenosis and the dark grey area represents the hypertensive equivalent pressure gradient. Simulation parameters (EOA: 1.00 $cm^2$; SV: 70 mL; C: 0.98 mL/mmHg; R: 1.53 mmHg s/$cm^5$; A: 7 $cm^2$)

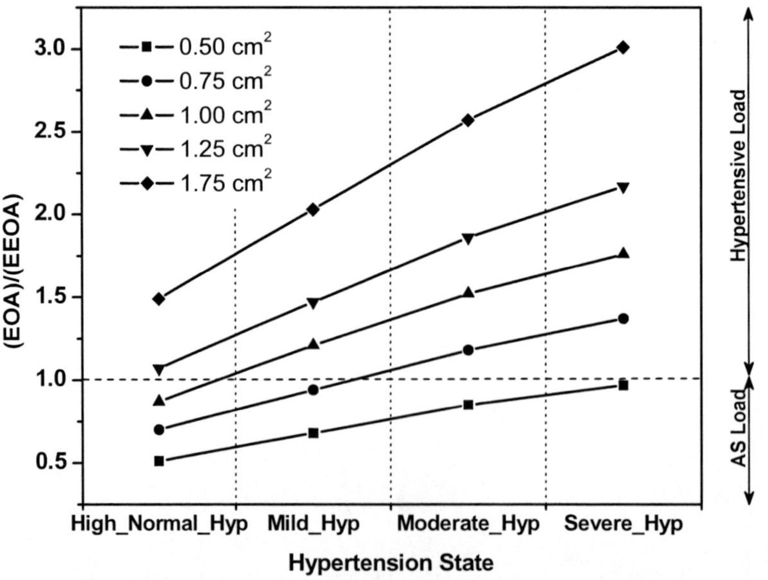


Figure 4. Variation in the ratio of effective orifice area (EOA) to equivalent effective orifice area (EEOA) with systemic hypertension, for AS severity from 0.5 $cm^2$ to 1.75 $cm^2$.

Figure (4) shows the variation in the ratio of effective orifice area (EOA) to equivalent effective orifice area (EEOA) with different states of hypertension (from high normal hypertension: SBP [130 139] mmHg; DBP [85 89] mmHg to severe hypertension: systolic blood pressure (SBP) > 180 mmHg; diastolic blood pressure (DBP) > 110 mmHg). These simulations were performed for different levels of aortic stenosis severity from 0.5 to 1.75 $cm^2$. It appears that for an EOA=0.5 $cm^2$, AS is the predominant load on the left ventricle, no matter how severe the systemic arterial hypertension. For an AS severity of 0.5 $cm^2$ to 1.0 $cm^2$, the stenosis load will still be the predominant load for high normal hypertension and mild hypertension, however, when hypertension severity increases (moderate to severe) it becomes the most important load that the LV must face compared to stenosis load. For stenosis with EOA higher than 1.0 $cm^2$, systemic arterial hypertension is always the predominant load, even if only high normal.

Then, by using the ratio of EOA to EEOA (valvular load/ vascular load), we once again showed that hypertension is always the most significant load supported by the left ventricle if the AS severity is > 1.0 $cm^2$. This result is in a good agreement with the study of Garcia et al. (2005), in which they showed that systemic arterial hypertension is the most important determinant of the left ventricular stroke work for AS with effective orifice areas > 1.0 $cm^2$.

It should be noted, however, that some limitations are associated with the ratio of EOA to EEOA. Indeed, the major limitation is that the ratio between effective orifice area (EOA) and hypertensive equivalent orifice area (EEOA) is flow dependent. In fact, even if the EOA is flow dependent only for moderate stenosis at low flow rate (Kadem et al. (2006)), the EEOA is flow dependent for all flow rates. However, the usefulness of the ratio (EOA/EEOA) is not to compare different patient populations, but rather it must be considered a patient specific parameter to compare a patient's actual valvular load to actual vascular load.

Another limitation is this ratio (EOA/EEOA) must be measured before and after a valve replacement in patients with AS and concomitant hypertension to determine if it is correlated with a reduction in heart stroke work: patients with a low (EOA/EEOA) ratio, should have more benefit from valve replacement than patients with a high (EOA/EEOA) ratio.

## Conclusion

Aortic stenosis is often associated with systemic arterial hypertension. Systemic arterial hypertension can interfere with AS leading to an underestimation or an overestimation of AS severity through variations in flow rate. Furthermore, when AS coexists with systemic arterial hypertension, the left ventricle has to face two loads: valvular load (aortic stenosis) and vascular load (systemic arterial hypertension). It is very important to determine which of these two loads is the most significant to help the clinician target proper treatment. This can be achieved using valvulo-arterial impedance, allowing the determination of the total load supported by the left ventricle and/or by using an equivalent hypertensive effective orifice area allowing the determination of which load (AS or systemic arterial hypertension) is the more significant for the LV.

# References


Antonini-Canterin, F; Huang, G; Cervesato, E; et al. Symptomatic aortic stenosis: does systemic hypertension play an additional role? *Hypertension.*, 2003, 41, 1268-72.

Arts, T; Bovendeerd, PH; Prinzen, FW; et al. Relation between left ventricular cavity pressure and volume and systolic fiber stress and strain in the wall. *Biophy J.*, 1991, 59, 93-102.

Beevers, DG; Sloan, PJM; Mackinnon, J. Aortic stenosis and systemic hypertension. *Br Med J.*, 1983, 286, 1960-1961.

Braunwald, E. *Valvular heart disease*; W.B. Saunders Company: London, 2001, 1643-1713.

Briand, M; Dumesnil, JG; Kadem, L; et al. Reduced systemic arterial compliance impacts significantly LV afterload and functions in aortic stenosis: Implications for diagnosis and treatment. *J Am Coll Cardiol.*, 2005, 46, 291-8.

Christian, HA. Aortic stenosis with calcification of the cusps. *JAMA.*, 1931, 97, 158-61.

Contralto, AW; Levine, SA. Aortic stenosis with special reference to angina pectoris and syncope. *Ann Intern Med.*, 1937, 10, 1636-53.

Cramariuc, D; Gerdts, E; Segadal, L; et al. Impact of hypertension on left ventricular hypertrophy regression and exercise capacity in patients operated for aortic valve stenosis. *Scand Cardiovasc J.*, 2006, 40, 167-174.

Garcia, D; Barenbrug, PJ; Pibarot, P; et al. A ventricular-vascular coupling model in presence of aortic stenosis. *Am J Physiol Heart Circ Physiol.*, 2005, 288(4), 1874-1884.

Garcia, D; Pibarot, P; Durand, LG. Analytical modeling of the instantaneous pressure gradient across the aortic valve. *J Biomech.*, 2005, 38(6), 1303-1311.

Garcia, D; Pibarot, P; Kadem, L; et al. Respective impacts of aortic stenosis and systemic hypertension on the left ventricular hypertrophy. *J Biomech.*, 2007, 40 (5), 972-980.

Ikram, H; Marshall, DE; Moore, SM; et al. Hypertension in valvular aortic stenosis. *NZ Med J.*, 1979, 89, 204-207.

Jimenez-Candil, J; Bermejo, J; Yotti, R; et al. Effects of angiotensina converting enzyme inhibitors in hyopertensive patients with aortic valve stenosis: a drug withdrawal study. *Heart.*, 2005, 91, 1311-1318.

Jolobe, OM. Systolic hypertension is also the neglected stepsister of aortic stenosis. *Am J Med.*, DOI: 10.1016/j.amjmed.2008.03.047.

Kadem, L; Dumesnil, JG; Rieu, R; et al. Impact of systemic hypertension on the assessment of aortic stenosis. *Heart.*, 2005, 91, 354-61.

Kadem, L; Rieu, R; Dumesnil, JG; et al. Flow dependent changes in Doppler derived aortic valve effective orifice area are real and not due to artifact. *J Am Coll Cardiol.*, 2006, 47(1), 131-137.

Krum, H; Nolly, H; Workman, D; et al. Efficacity of eplerenone added to rennin-angiotensin blockade in hypertensive patients. *Hypertension.*, 2002, 40, 117-123.

Laskey, WK; Kussmaul, WG; Noordergraaf, A. Valvular and systemic arterial hemodynamics in aortic valve stenosis. *Circulation.*, 1995, 92, 1473-8.

Lindroos, M; Kupari, M; Heikkila, J; et al. Prevalence of aortic valve abnormalities in the elderly: an echocardiographic study of random population sample. *J Am Coll Cardiol.*, 1993, 21, 1220-1225.

Little, SH; Chan, KL; Burwash, IG. Impact of blood pressure on the Doppler echocardiographic assessment of severity of aortic stenosis. *Heart.*, 2007, 93, 848-55.

Mascherbauer, J; Fuchs, C; Stoiber, M; et al. Systemic pressure does not directly affect pressure gradient and valve area estimates in aortic stenosis in vitro. *Eur Heat J.*, 2008, DOI: 10.1093/eurheartj/ehn209.

McGinn, S; White, PD. Clinical observations on aortic stenosis. *Am J Med Sci.*, 1934, 188, 1-15.

Otto, CM. Valvular aortic stenosis: Disease severity and timing of intervention. *J Am Coll Cardiol.*, 2006, 47, 2141-2151.

Pibarot, P; Dumesnil, JG; Mathieu, P. Nouveautés sur le rétrécissement valvulaire aortique. *Medecine/Sciences.*, 2007, 23, 81-87.

Razzolini, R; Gerosa, G; Leoni, L; et al. Transaortic gradient is pressure-dependent in a pulsatile model of the circulation. *J Heart Valve Dis.*, 1999, 8, 279-83.

Stewart, BF; Siscovick, D; Lind, BK; et al. Clinical factors associated with calcific aortic stenosis. *J Am Coll Cardiol.*, 1997, 29, 630-634.

Westerhof, N; Elzinga, G; Sipkema, P. An artificial arterial system for pumping hearts. *J Appl Physiol.*, 1971, 31, 776-781.

In: Advances in Cardiovascular Research, Volume 1
Editors: L. Schmitt, T. Konig, pp. 381-390
ISBN: 978-1-60741-720-0


*Chapter XVII*

# Minimally Invasive Aortic Valve Surgery: Port Access or Catheter-Based?

***Edgar G. Chedrawy**, Sunil M. Prasad, Ahmed Tarakji and Malek G. Massad***

Divisions of Cardiothoracic Surgery; Departments of Surgery;
L. Weiss Memorial Hospital, Mt. Sinai Hospital and the University of Illinois Medical Center and College of Medicine, Chicago, Illinois 60612, USA

## Abstract

Median sternotomy with central cannulation is the standard approach to the aortic valve for repair or replacement. Over the last decade, surgical exposure options other than a full sternotomy such as a "J" or "T" partial-sternotomy, or a right "mini" anterior thoracotomy and peripheral cannulation methods have captured the interest of cardiac surgeons in search of a "less invasive, minimal access" approach. Less invasive surgical approaches have reduced peri-operative mortality, ventilatory support time, intensive care unit and hospital stays and total hospital costs. Over the last five years, catheter-based technologies have emerged as viable options for aortic valve replacement in patients previously considered to be too high risk for conventional or minimally invasive aortic valve (MIAV) surgery. Implantation of catheter-mounted prostheses may be performed via the antegrade (femoral vein), retrograde (femoral artery) or transapical (left ventricular apex) route. Each delivery route has potential advantages and disadvantages as well as technical, vascular and mechanical limitations. As technology improves, current and future devices and delivery systems being evaluated should overcome these limitations and provide catheter-based prostheses as a viable therapeutic option for aortic valve replacement.

**Keywords:** Aortic valve; Replacement; Port Access; Catheter based.

* Corresponding author: Division of Cardiothoracic Surgery, University of Illinois at Chicago College of Medicine, 840 S. Wood Street, CSB Suite 417 (MC 958), Chicago, Illinois 60612, E-mail: echedrawy@hotmail.com, Phone 312-996-4942; Fax 312-996-2013.

# Introduction

Surgery of the aortic valve dates back to 1913 when Tuffier dilated a stenotic aortic valve by invaginating the aorta[1]. Numerous experimental studies, over the following 40 years, led to the development of the heart-lung machine by Gibbon ushering in the "modern era" of open heart surgery and allowing Harken to implant the first successful mechanical aortic valve in a patient with severe aortic insufficiency, in 1960[1]. The following decades focused more on the development of a variety of types and shapes of valvular prostheses (including mechanical vs. biologic, stented vs. stentless, autograft vs. xenograft) and less on modifications of the implantation technique. The standard implantation technique consisted of full median sternotomy, cardiopulmonary bypass and cardioplegic arrest. The sternotomy incision allows access to the heart and great vessels for central cannulation and excellent valve exposure. Cardiopulmonary bypass is usually instituted with aortic and right atrial cannulation. Cardioplegia is delivered antegrade through the aortic root or retrograde through a cannula inserted through the right atrial wall and advanced into the coronary sinus, or through both the antegrade and retrograde routes. The left ventricle is decompressed through the aortic root or through a vent advanced through the right superior pulmonary vein across the mitral valve into the left ventricle. After institution of cardiopulmonary bypass and cardioplegic arrest, the aorta is opened through a standard "lazy s" or "Hockey stick" shaped aortotomy about an inch superior to the aortic valve annulus to allow full visualization of the aortic valve and root. The standard approach is safe, efficient and applicable in almost all cases.

In the early 1990s, the success of laparoscopy and thoracoscopy-based techniques demonstrated clear benefits, compared with traditional open surgery, and captured the interest of surgeons and patients alike. These minimally invasive approaches led to a surge in the development of less invasive techniques for open heart surgery. The development of peripheral-vessel based cannulation techniques and of peripherally inserted catheters for venting and delivering cardioplegia stimulated the interest in searching for smaller, more focused, incisions specifically targeting the region of the heart or valve of interest. Many "minimal-access" or "port-access" incisions were explored as an alternative route to the aortic valve[2,3]. Also, peripheral cannulation methods were needed for these "direct-access" incisions to provide cardiopulmonary bypass support during the valve repair or replacement. The ultimate goal of minimally invasive aortic valve (MIAV) surgery is to minimize surgical trauma and thereby reduce operative morbidity and mortality, increase patient satisfaction and lower costs while still providing safe, durable and efficient valve repair or replacements. In the last five years, some patients deemed too high risk for valve repair or replacement under cardiopulmonary bypass (by any approach) might have benefited from catheter-based valve replacement[4]. Implantation of catheter-mounted prostheses has emerged as a viable option for patients that were previously considered inoperable. The limitations of catheter-based techniques relate to the delivery system and vascular anatomy of the individual patients. The results, so far, are very encouraging.

## Operative Approaches and Techniques

The "minimally invasive" revolution has stressed the importance of a multidisciplinary approach to heart valve surgery[5,6]. Unlike the standard approach, some essential components of the operative strategy are completely under the control of the anesthesiologist and perfusionist. Specialized techniques and training are required for minimal access incisions, peripheral-vessel based cannulation and peripherally inserted cannulae for venting of the right and left ventricle and for cardioplegia delivery. Also, catheter-based strategies require proficiency in endovascular techniques and some interventional cardiology maneuvers such as aortic valvuloplasty and imaging.

## Intraoperative Anesthetic Management

The conventional approach to aortic valve replacement requires general anesthesia, single-lumen endotracheal intubation, systemic arterial and pulmonary artery Swan-Ganz pressure monitoring. MIAV surgery requires additional preparation on behalf of the anesthesiologist. Transcutaneous defibrillator pads are placed before skin preparation and draping. While internal pediatric defibrillator pads will generally fit through a small incision and can be carefully guided around the ventricles to defibrillate the heart, this may prove to be difficult around a distended heart and external pads greatly facilitate defibrillation in this scenario. Depending on the incision, the anesthesiologist may have to position a double-lumen endotracheal tube for (right) lung isolation. The anesthesiologist, depending on the cannulation strategy, may be responsible for positioning the retrograde coronary sinus cardioplegia delivery catheter under transesophageal and /or fluoroscopic guidance. Also, via the internal jugular vein catheter, the anesthesiologist may insert the pulmonary artery venting cannula to decompress the left heart from systemic venous return[6].

## Perfusion Techniques

Various cannulation methods are available ranging from central to peripheral with various permutations in between. Minimally invasive incisions have forced surgeons to abandon central cannulation where the various cannulae and perfusion adjuncts are in the operative field and adapt peripheral cannulation methods leaving the main incision as a portal to the operative site only. A pure peripheral approach would entail femoral arterial and femoral venous cannulation for cardiopulmonary bypass. The left ventricle will be decompressed through a peripheral pulmonary arterial vent. Cardioplegia will be delivered through a peripheral retrograde coronary sinus cardioplegia catheter placed by the anesthesiologist. This approach minimizes the amount of perfusion adjuncts needed to be placed through the incision albeit at the expense of time, effort and cost[5,6].

## Surgical Approaches

The ideal incision for aortic valve surgery is one that is versatile, simple to perform, has low morbidity and mortality and allows adequate exposure of the valve and root. Since the first report of minimally invasive aortic valve replacement by Cosgrove[2] in 1996 many techniques of minimally invasive approaches and peripheral cannulation have been described. These techniques include right anterior thoracotomy, right parasternal incision and "J" or "T" partial sternotomy.

Benetti[7] first reported the right anterior thoractomy through the third intercostal space for exposure of the aortic valve. Benetti reported adequate exposure of the aortic valve and root and claimed that this procedure caused less post operative pain because no cartilage was resected and no rib was fractured as he used an adaptive wound spreader in a 6 to 7 cm incision. Cardiopulmonary bypass was established through femoral arterial and right atrial cannulation with venting through the right superior pulmonary vein. Cardioplegia was administered antegrade down the aortic root.

The parasternal incision was first described by Cosgrove and Sabik[2]. A 10 cm incision is made from the lower edge of the second costal cartilage to the superior edge of the fifth costal cartilage. This incision provides exposure of the second through fifth intercostal spaces after resection of the third and fourth costal cartilages and at the expense of ligating the right internal mammary artery. The femoral artery and vein were cannulated. This incision resulted in significant post operative pain as two cartilages were resected and the internal mammary artery was ligated resulting in poor wound healing. This technique for the most part has been abandoned.

The first report of a partial sternotomy was described by Konertz[8] and eventually popularized by Gundry[9]. The "T" mini sternotomy consists of a 6 to 10 cm midline incision with partial upper sternotomy for the upper half with "teeing" off of the sternum to either the third or fourth intercostal space. This divides the sternum without disturbing the surrounding soft tissues and, in most instances, preserves the internal mammary arteries. The ascending aorta and right atrium are used for cannulation. Cardioplegia is delivered retrograde and the heart is vented through the right superior pulmonary vein. The surgeon stands over the patient's right shoulder to perform aortic valve surgery.

Svensson[10] in 1997 described the "J" incision as a 7 to 8 cm skin incision with vertical split of the manubrium down the midline from the sternal notch to end as a horizontal cut in the fourth intercostal space. The aorta and right atrium are used for cannulation with the venous drainage brought out through a subxyphoid wound that becomes an exit site for the mediastinal drainage tube before sternotomy closure. Cardioplegia is delivered retrograde and the heart is vented through the right superior pulmonary vein.

## Aortotomy Exposure

Regardless of the skin incision or type of sternotomy or thoracotomy, optimal aortotomy exposure of the aortic valve and root is best achieved through a curvilinear incision across the aortic root and partly into the noncoronary sinus of valsalva. Partial thickness aortic traction silk sutures are then placed through the top of each commissure and secured firmly to the drape with a clamp. At this point aortic valve repair or replacement can proceed as per the standard operative approach[1-3].

## Deairing and Closure

Deairing of the heart is undoubtedly more difficult without manual access to the left ventricle[6]. Deairing is facilitated by carbon dioxide insuflalation into the field. Transesophageal echocardiography is essential to guide deairing and should be used as deairing maneuvers such as volume loading of the heart, ventilating the lungs, and weaning from gradual weaning from cardiopulmonary bypass are performed. Epicardial pacing wires and thoracostomy tubes should be placed while the heart is decompressed on cardiopulmonary bypass. Occasionally, when weaning from bypass, transesophageal echocardiography may detect what appears to be an under filled right ventricle. This is caused by compression of the anterior wall of the right ventricle by the undivided lower sternum. The compression is relieved by releasing the pericardial traction sutures[6].

## The Catheter-Based Approach

As the population ages, the burden of aortic valve disease (mostly aortic stenosis) seems to be on the rise[11]. Already the United States has more than 50,000 open surgical aortic valve replacements performed every year. The associated in-hospital death rate is 8.8% in patients over the age of 65 and as high as 13% in low volume centers[12]. The steady increase in the number of patients, the high surgical risk in some patients, the reluctance of some patients to undergo the trauma and pain associated with open heart surgery via sternotomy and cardio pulmonary bypass has driven the development of catheter-based techniques forward. Lung[12] recently showed that 33% of patients over the age of 75 were deemed too high risk for open heart surgery and the aortic valve pathology was left untreated. The idea of percutaneous treatment was first brought into clinical practice in 1985 when Cribier[13] performed an aortic balloon valvuloplasty. Percutaneous aortic valve replacement was first reported in 1992, using a closed chest pig model[14]. In 2002, the first successful percutaneous aortic valve replacement in a human was reported[15,16].

Three prosthetic valves have been used in clinical trials: The Cribier-Edwards[17,18] valve, the CoreValve[19-21] and the Edwards SAPIEN[22,23] valve. The Cribier-Edwards[17,18] valve (Edwards Lifesciences) is an equine, pericardial, stainless steel mounted, balloon-expandable tissue valve used in the antegrade, retrograde and transapical routes and has reached Phase III trials in the USA. The Corevalve Revalving System[19-21] (CoreValve) is a bovine, pericardial, nitinol stent mounted, self-expanding tissue valve used exclusively in the retrograde route and is approved for use in Europe (Phase III in USA). The Edwards SAPIEN[22,23] valve (Edwards Lifesciences) is a bovine, pericardial, stainless steel mounted, balloon expandable tissue valve used in the retrograde and transapical routes and is approved for use in Europe (Phase III in the USA).

The three techniques to implant the catheter-based valves include the antegrade, the retrograde and the transapical approaches. In the antegrade[17,18] approach, access to the femoral vein is obtained and the prosthetic valve is advanced traversing the interatrial septum and the mitral valve, and is positioned within the diseased aortic valve. The main advantage of this technique is that the femoral vein accommodates a large catheter sheath and it is relatively easy to manage this peripheral access site. The disadvantage of this technique includes possible injury to the interatrial septum and the mitral valve and the challenge of positioning the mounted valve in the correct anatomic site. This technique has been abandoned.

In the retrograde[19-21] transfemoral technique, access to the femoral artery is gained and the prosthetic valve is advanced up the aortoiliac tree to the diseased aortic valve. This approach is faster, technically easier than the antegrade approach, but has the disadvantage of being potentially damaging to the aortoiliac vessels and crossing the diseased aortic valve may be challenging.

In the transapical technique[22,23] a small left anterior thoracotomy incision is made and carried down between the ribs. The apex of the left ventricle is punctured with a needle and the prosthetic valve is positioned within the diseased aortic valve. The main advantage of this technique is that access to the valve is more direct and eliminates the need for large peripheral access in patients with peripheral vascular disease, small tortuous vessels or a history of major vascular problems. One potential disadvantage is the fact that this technique requires general anesthesia, chest tube placement, apical puncture of the left ventricle and its complications including possible development of left ventricular aneurysm or pseudoaneurysm.

The position of final deployment of the catheter based valve is defined by the patient's native valvular structure and anatomy and is optimized by using fluoroscopic imaging of the native aortic valve calcification, as an anatomical marker, along with guidance from angiography and transesophageal echocardiography[17-23]. The prosthesis is placed in the same plain as the patient's aortic valve taking care not to impinge on the coronary ostia or to impede the motion of the anterior mitral valve leaflet. In all three techniques, the prosthesis is deployed by maximally inflating, rapidly deflating and immediately withdrawing the delivery system. This step is carried out using temporary, high-rate, rapid right ventricular apical pacing which produces heart rates of 180 to 220 beats per minute for up to 10 seconds. This leads to an immediate decrease in stroke volume resulting in minimal forward flow through the aortic valve to facilitate precise positioning of the prosthetic valve[17-23].

## Clinical Outcomes of MIAVS

A recent meta-analysis by Murtuza[24] *et al* questioned the clinical outcomes in patients undergoing conventional versus minimal access aortic valve replacement. The meta analysis identified 89 published reports between 1998 and 2006. Of these, 26 comparative studies were included in the meta-analysis: 4 were randomized controlled trials and 22 were retrospective or prospective comparative studies. The total number of patients in these 26 studies was 4891 with 2249 in the minimally invasive group and 2642 in the conventional group. The meta-analysis did not show any significant quantitive difference between conventional and minimal approaches for perioperative mortality or other primary outcome event such as stroke, renal failure, or respiratory failure. Sensitivity analysis suggested that there was a small but statistically significant benefit for surrogate outcomes of ventilation times, ICU stay and total length of stay in the minimally invasive group; however, cardiopulmonary bypass time and total operating times were longer in this group. Meta-analysis of all other secondary outcome events did not demonstrate any significant difference between the minimally invasive and conventional techniques.

Detter[25] and Mihaljevic[26] separately reported mid-term and long-term results in MIAVS compared to conventional aortic valve surgery. Detter reported freedom from re-operation of 98% versus 100% (for MIAVS versus conventional surgery group) and freedom from endocarditis of 100% versus 97%. Mihaljevic reported, in one thousand patients, an actuarial survival of 98%, 94% and 82% at 1, 3 and 5 years respectively for MIAVS versus 94%, 90% and 86% for conventional surgery. These results, although not randomized, suggest that MIAVS may be performed with comparable mid-term and long-term results when compared to conventional aortic valve surgery.

## Results of Catheter-Based Approaches

As the standard aortic valve surgery carries a death rate of 15% in patients age 80 to 84 and 18% for patients over 85 years old[12], catheter-based techniques have focused on the elderly population or the high-risk surgical population. In the RECAST trial[17] (Registry of Endovascular Critical Aortic Stenosis Treatment) all patients were formally evaluated by two surgeons and deemed inappropriate candidates for surgical aortic valve replacement. The Cribier-Edwards valve was implanted successfully in 85% of the patients using the antegrade approach and in 57% of the patients using the retrograde approach. The main complications included prosthesis migration or embolisation, failure to cross the stenotic aortic valve and paravalvular aortic regurgitation[17]. At 24 months, there was a significant improvement in aortic valve area, left ventricular ejection fraction and New York Heart Association (NYHA) functional class. Lichtenstein[27] implanted the Cribier-Edwards valve through a transapical approach in a high-risk elderly population with poor functional status and peripheral vascular disease, deemed ineligible for a transfemoral approach due to severe aortoiliac disease. The mid and long-term results were favorable. To date, more than 500 Cribier-Edwards valves have been implanted worldwide with greater than 95% technical success rate. As the experience grows, the previously reported complications (prosthesis migration, embolization, and paravalvular aortic regurgitation) have been reduced with the use of larger prostheses (> 26 mm).

The CoreValve[19-21] is implanted exclusively in the retrograde route and may be used in aortic insufficiency and other non-calcified valvular conditions due to its self-expanding nature which allows it to conform to different aortic sizes and anchor well in the annulus[19-21]. Grube[21] and colleagues reported a short term (30 day) success rate of 88% in 86 elderly patients with poor functional class and severe aortic stenosis. Post-procedure the mean aortic valve gradient decreased significantly, the functional class improved significantly and no patient had more than moderate aortic insufficiency[19-21]. TheCoreValve[19-21] was approved for clinical use in Europe in May 2007.

The Edwards SAPIEN[22,23] valve is a modification of the initial Cribier-Edwards valve and is available in 23 mm and 26 mm sizes. The multicenter Placement of Aortic

Transcatheter Valves (PARTNER) trial in North America is continuing to enroll patients. The surgical arm of this randomized prospective trial compares the Edwards SAPIEN valve to standard surgical therapy and the medical arm compares the Edwards SAPIEN valve against medical therapy or balloon valvuloplasty in high-risk patients. The first 100 patients[22] (74 transfemoral, 26 transapical route) who underwent Edwards SAPIEN valve implantation, for compassionate use, were reported by Pasupati[22] et al in 2007. Of those, 74 were performed through a transfemoral route and 26 through a transapical route. Survival rates were reported as 85%, 78% and 60% at 30 days, 6 months and 2 years, respectively. Aortic valve size, left ventricular hemodynamics, mitral regurgitation and functional class were all significantly improved at 6 months. In early 2008, Walther[23] reported outcomes on their first 50 patients whose devices were all delivered through the transapical route. The overall survival rate was 92% at 30 days and 80% at 1 year. The prosthesis was implanted in all 50 patients but three patients required conversion to open sternotomy. In September 2007, the Edwards SAPIEN[22,23] valve was approved for clinical use in Europe with the Retroflex transfemoral delivery system and the Ascendra transapical delivery system. Approval is still pending for clinical use in North America.

## Conclusion

The conventional, open, approach to the aortic valve remains the gold standard for aortic valve surgery. The search for minimally invasive alternatives has led to many combinations of surgical exposure and peripheral cannulation methods that have reduced peri-operative mortality, ventilatory support time, intensive care unit and hospital stays and total hospital costs. Over the last five years, catheter-based technologies have emerged as a viable option for aortic valve replacement in patients previously considered to be too high risk for conventional or minimally invasive aortic valve replacement. The results, to date, have been encouraging. Catheter-based prostheses have been limited by technical, vascular and mechanical limitations. As technology improves, future devices and delivery systems should overcome the current limitations and provide catheter-based prostheses as a viable therapeutic option for aortic valve replacement not only in the high risk and elderly patient population but in the lower risk and younger patients as well.

## References

[1] Soltesz, EG; Cohn, LH. Minimally invasive valve surgery. *Cardiology in review.*, 2007, 15, 109-115.

[2] Cosgrove, DM; Sabik, JF. Minimally invasive approach for aortic valve operations. *Ann Thorac Surg.*, 1996, 62, 596-597.

[3] Cohn, LH; Adams, DH; Couper, GS; *et al.* Minimally invasive aortic valve replacement. *Semin Thorac Cardiovasc Surg.*, 1997, 9, 331-336.

[4] Singh, IM; Shishehbor, MH; Christofferson, Rd; *et al.* Percutaneous treatment of aortic valve stenosis. *Cleveland Clinic Journal of Medicine.*, 2008, 75, 805-812.

[5] Estrera, AL; Reardon, MJ. Current approaches to minimally invasive aortic valve surgery. *Current opinion in cardiology.*, 2000, 15, 91-96.

[6] Woo, YJ; Seeburger, J; Mohr, FW. Minimally invasive valve surgery. *Semin Thorac Cardiovasc Surg.*, 2007, 19, 289-298.

[7] Benetti, FJ; Mariani, MA; Rizzardi, JL; *et al.* Minimally invasive aortic valve replacement. *J Thorac Cardiovasc Surg.*, 1997, 113, 806-807.

[8] Konertz, W; Waldenberger, F; Schmutzler, M; *et al.* Minimal access valve surgery through superior partial sternotomy: a preliminary study. *J Heart Valve Dis.*, 1996, 5, 638-640.

[9] Gundry, SR; Shattuck, OH; Razzouk, AJ; et al. Facile minimally invasive cardiac surgery via ministernotomy. *Ann Thorac Surg.*, 1996, 65, 1100-1104.

[10] Svensson, LG; D'Agostino, RS. "J" incision minimal access valve operations. *Ann Thorac Surg.*, 1998, 66, 1110-1112.

[11] Bonow, RO; Carabello, BA; Kanu, C; *et al.* ACC/AHA 2006 guidelines for the management of patients with valvular heart disease. *Circulation*, 2006, 114, e84-231.

[12] Lung, B; Cachier, A; Baron, G; *et al.* Decision making in elderly patients with severe aortic stenosis: why are so many denied surgery? *Eur Heart J.*, 2005, 26, 2714-2720.

[13] Cribier, A; Savin, T; Saoudi, N; Rocha, P; Berland, J; Letac, B. Percutaneous transluminal valvuloplasty of acquired aortic stenosis in elderly patients: an alternative to valve replacement? *Lancet*, 1986, 1, 63-67.

[14] Bonhoeffer, P; Boudjemline, Y; Saliba, Z; *et al.* Percutaneous replacement of pulmonary valve in a right ventricle to pulmonary artery prosthetic conduit with valve dysfunction. *Lancet*, 2000, 356, 1403-1405.

[15] Anderson, HR; Knudsen, LL; Hasenkam, JM. Transluminal implantation of artificial heart valves. Description of a new expandable aortic valve and initial results with implantation by catheter technique in closed chest pigs. *Eur Heart J.*, 1992, 13, 704-708.

[16] Cribier, A; Eltchaninoff, H; Bash, A; *et al.* Percutaneous transcatheter implantation of an aortic valve prosthesis for calcific aortic stenosis: first human case description. *Circulation*, 2002, 106, 3006-3008.

[17] Cribier, A; Eltchaninoff, H; Tron, C; et al. Treatment of calcific aortic stenosis with the percutaneous heart valve: mid-term followup from the intial feasibility studies: The French experience. *J Am Coll Cardiol*, 2006, 47, 1214-1223.

[18] Ye, J; Cheung, A; Lichtenstein, SV; *et al.* Six month outcome of transapical transcatheter aortic valve implantation in the initial seven patients. *Eur J Cardiothorac Surg.*, 2007, 31, 16-21.

[19] Grube, E; Laborde, JC; Gerckens, U; *et al.* Percutaneous implantation of the CoreValve self-expanding valve prosthesis in high-risk patients with aortic valve disease: the Siegburg first-in-man study. *Circulation*, 2006, 114, 1616-1624.

[20] Grube, E; Laborde, JC; Zickmann, B; *et al.* First report on a human percutaneous transluminal implantation of a self-expanding valve prosthesis for interventional treatment of aortic valve stenosis. *Catheter Cardiovasc Interv*, 2005, 66, 465-469.

[21] Grube, E; Schuler, G; Buellesfeld, L; et al. Percutaneous aortic valve replacement for severe aortic stenosis in high risk patients using the second and current third generation self-expanding CoreValve prosthesis: device success and 30-day clinical outcome. *J Am Coll Cardiol*, 2007, 50, 69-76.

[22] Pasupati, S; Humphries, K; AlAli, A; *et al.* Balloon expandable aortic valve (BEAV) implantation. The first 100 Canadian patients. *Circulation*, 2007, 116 (suppl), 357.

[23] Walther, T; Falk, V; Kempfert, J; *et al.* Transapical minimally invasive aortic valve implantation; the initial 50 patients. *Eur J Cardioth Surg*, 2008, 33, 983-988.

[24] Murtuza, B; Pepper, JR; Stanbridge, RD; et al. Minimal access aortic valve replacement: Is it worth it? *Ann Thorac Surg*, 2008, 85, 1121-1131.

[25] Detter, C; Deuse, T; Boehm, DH; Reichenspurner, H; Reichart, B. Midterm results and quality of life after minimally invasive vs. conventional aortic valve replacement. *Thorac Cardiovasc Surg.*, 2002, 50, 337-341.

[26] Mihaljevic, T; Cohn, LH; Unioc, D; Aranki, SF; Couper, GS; Byrne, JG. One thousand minimally invasive valve operations: early and late results. *Ann Surg*, 2004, 240, 529-534.

[27] Lichtenstein, SV; Cheung, A; Ye, J; *et al.* Transapical transcatheter aortic valve implantation in humans: initial clinical experience. *Circulation*, 2006, 114, 591.

In: Advances in Cardiovascular Research, Volume 1
Editors: L. Schmitt, T. Konig, pp. 391-398 ISBN: 978-1-60741-720-0


*Chapter XVIII*

# Aorto-Enteric Fistulas: Our Choices

***F. Chierichetti*[*]*, B. Campanati, E. Costantini, L. Miglierina, U. Rosanna, L. Rosati, S. Belletti and A. Tori***
O.U. of Vascular Surgery, H. Busto Arsizio., Via A.da Brescia, 1, 21052 Busto Arsizio (VA), Italy.

## Summary

In this case report authors analyse their own experience in the treatment of aortoenteric fistulas (AEF), consequently to the last technical improvements. They have favoured amongst others, arterial allografts, axillo-femoral bypasses and endografts. For the purpose of this report, their surgical activities between January 1994 and December 2008 have been analysed and obtained datas have proved that allografts are an efficacious technical option for the treatment of AEFs. Extra-anatomical bypasses are an alternative whether a lack of prosthetic material is encountered; endografts, in spite of their wide diffusion in literature, remain a limited and definite indication in few cases or one way to solve a severe haemorrhage, carrying the patients to better conditions to be operated on consequentially.

It is also underlined how the complexity of clinical manifestations of AEFs needs a wide selection of treatments and technical choices available to operators.

## Introduction

AEF is a rare event following the evolution of non-operated abdominal aortic aneurysms (AAA) or heterologous grafts used in aortic procedures.

AEFs are classified as primary, due to the erosion of an AAA into a segment of intestine (usually the duodenum) or secondary, when they develop between a synthetic vascular graft

[*] Corresponding author: O.U. Vascular Surgery Hospital Busto Arsizio, via varzi 3, 21052 Busto Arsizio Varese, Italy, E-mail: fabiochierichetti@libero.it

or a suture line into a loop of bowel. Sir Astley Cooper firstly described the primitive ones in 1927 [1,2] as a natural complication of AAA.

Broke in 1953 described the second ones, as a complication of an allograft happened one year after its implantation [2]; three years after, Clayton outlined the first case due to a synthetic graft [2].

Recently some events of secondary AEFs after an implantation of endografts have been described in literature; this kind of grafts have been used to solve a massive haemorrhage but not the enteric lesion nor the infection of the contiguous tissues [3,4].

In spite of different surgical techniques have been described to solve AEFs, these fistulas represent a catastrophic complication with high mortality and morbidity rates. AEFs' rates vary from 0,5-2,5% of all abdominal aorta graft-replacement operations. The time from the operation and the development of an AEF differs from 2 weeks to more than 10 years [5].

# Secondary Aorto-Enteric Fistula

## Clinical Manifestation

Although it is an infrequent event, it is pivotal to take into count a secondary AEF possible onset, because it needs a quick diagnosis and an early therapy.

At the O.U. of Vascular Surgery in the Hospital of Busto Arsizio, Italy, 39 patients with an abdominal graft infection have been hospitalized between January 1994 to December 2008; 27 out of 39 were affected from AEFs. The mean time for a clinical manifestation of AEF was 1- 132 months. The symptomatology was very different: high or low acute lumbar pain and abdominalgia, fever or slight fever, gastro-enteric bleeding (GEB) as well as occult blood or melena or haematemesis and sometimes sepsis. Septic embolization is a very rare event while 36% of the patients refers general discomfort [2].

Seriousness of symptoms depends on the erosion of the enteric wall until the development of a link from the aortic graft and the enteric lumen where a valve mechanism often causes an intermittent haemorrhage in the intestine.

As a consequence, blood test results appear unbalanced: leukocytosis, increase of RCP, platelets and fibrinogen. Hypotension is frequently due to haemorrhage rather than sepsis.

Our 27 patients with AEFs were carriers of 22 aorto-bifemoral grafts, 2 aorto-biliac grafts and 3 aorto-aortic grafts, all Dacron knitted.

In 15 patients an AEF developed itself on the aortic suture line and in 2 cases over a pseudoaneurysm which lately eroded the third portion of the duodenum. In 10 cases there was only a perigraft erosion with a beginning of ischemic lesion of the enteric wall.

Gastro-enteric segments involved were studied to be 22 out of 27 affecting the duodenum and only 5 concerning the ileum.

Whenever a patient holds an aortic graft, it is therefore recommended to suspect of an AEF, especially if the patient himself suffers from occult blood, general indisposition, increased levels of RCP and severe to mild leukocytosis. Some patients have indeed referred mild discomfort and a stable haemodynamic frame.

The primary cause of AEFs is an infection of the graft which can take place after direct contamination whilst being implanted or after a fortuitous contact of the surgical line, a difficult wound healing (due to dehiscences or infections) or through direct aerial contact during operations that last over 4 hours. Later on in time, infections through haematogenous or lymphatic lines can take place.

Bacterial flora which has been isolated during surgical procedures was 45% polymicrobical with nearly 13% of funguses; 39% developed only one etiologic agent and in 16% of the cases no agents have been found.

In more than 50% of the patients, Gram+ Cocci, S. Aurei, S. Epidermidis and S. Haemolyticus have been isolated, most of which were resistant to more drugs. Only two cases were affected by Salmonella and Proteus Mirabilis; infections developed through those agents or Klebsiella, Pseudomonas or Enterobacter seem to be more frequent in early infections associated with massive intestinal haemorrhages resulting from a wider contact with the intestine itself.

Late infections are to be related mostly to coagulase negative Gram+ bacteria as S. Epidermidis which might delay the immune response of the host.

## Screenings

Screenings are basically related to the symptoms the patients show during recovery.

During an emergency where a GEB is suspected, an angio Computed Tomography (TC) is highly recommended, as well as a duodenogastroscopy which inspects the 3rd and 4th segments of the duodenum. If the above-mentioned exams are impossible to be performed, a simple explorative laparoscopy is to be executed.

Whether an AEF is identified, the first step is to remove the graft; if the conditions of the patients are stable, an extra-anatomical axillo-femoral bypass will then be performed. Otherwise it will be necessary to suspend temporarily the operation and observe the severeness of the ischaemia developing afterwards [6].

In the last few years, a new endovascular technique has been developed giving the possibility to stop aorto-enteric bleeding and to avoid lower limbs' ischaemia, stabilizing the haemodynamic condition of the patient even though it does not vary the seriousness of infections and the intestinal perforation is not solved. This technique has been chosen by our team to assist aged patients with occult haemorrhage and hazardous conditions or in those cases there was the intent of preparing the patient himself to a conventional surgical procedure in better conditions.

In those events where a haemodynamic situation is stable, more screenings are encouraged: angio CT or a MRI, marked leukocytes scintigraphy, PET and also FluoroDesossiGlucose (FDG) which can be detected through PET or CT techniques in the related infections sites [7].

AEFs do not require an arteriography, even though it can be helpful to evaluate the anastomosis margins of the graft that has to be removed.

The EsophagoGastroDuodenoscopy (EGD) is a very important screening method which has not to be interrupted in case of gastric bleeding because the duodenum needs to be investigated closely; however through this exam it is unusual to display directly the graft through the fistula and only 50% or slightly more of the EGD will result positive [8].

CT is another useful method 2-3 months after the procedure where a perigraft air mass can easily be associated with a developing infectious phlogistic process [9]. The CT itself does not represent the first choice amongst screening methods, even though it can underline abnormality datas diagnosis-related (perigraft fluids, an increase of the perigraft soft tissue, the presence of a pseudoaneurysm, a lack of continuity on the aortal internal tissue and a thinness of the intestine wall adjacent to the graft [8,9,10].

A marked leukocytes scintigraphy, as well as other exams revealing leukocytes masses and therefore potentially infectious sites, does not represent a diagnostic procedure in AEF, but it is highly recommended in clinical stable situations whether an infection is to be investigated.

In all patients with important bleeding and unstable vital signs, it is necessary to perform an EGD and, if possible, an angio CT as well as actuating all resuscitating techniques to reach the surgery room on time.

## Operative Menagement

We have treated 28 patients, 4 women and 24 men, 54 to 78 years of age; 22 of the abovementioned patients were in stable haemodynamic conditions and therefore have been operated 6 hours after the first observation.

### *The Stable Patient*

Stable patients have been operated on as follows: 16 patients with direct revascularization with homograft and 6 with endografts. The average age was 61,75 years, the patients were all ASA II and ASA III where a homograft has been privileged for the possibility to remove the infected graft, to perform a surrounding tissues debridement and to get direct vascularization with a low amputation risk. Whenever a donator graft is not promptly available and therefore once implanted, reactions such as dilatations, thrombosis, rips, calcifications, fistulas and secondary atheromasia may develop [11]. For these reasons, allografts have been figured out to be a temporary solution and to be later on replaced when the patients clinical status would have improved.

Through a constant observation of the operated patients, it has been estimated that complications related to a homograft wall degeneration were primarily precocious and might have been due to technical reasons or a persistent local infection consequent to a high virulence of germs themselves and/or a poor debridement. Another cause could have been the donors arteries preservation technique, in which those cryopreserved seem to be the most resistant and the only ones used since 1998 [11, 12, 13, 14, 15, 16].

We have prepared 13 aorto-femoral, 2 aorto-aortic and 1 aorto-biliac grafts. A mortality of 27% within 30 days after the operation has been registered with 2 cases of homograft-intestine fistulization, 2 myocardial infarctions and 1 intestinal infarction. After 12 months, the mortality rates increased to 38,8% (16,6% of which homograft-related) and after 24 months, it was registered to be 50% homograft non-related. Homograft-related causes of death were: 2 homograft-enteric fistulas, 1 septic shock and 1 graft occlusion.

Those 6 endograft-treated patients were the most recent out of all cases; studies of other case reports and a chance to highly critical conditions have brought our team to choose for an endograft solution. The average age was 70,66 years and all 6 patients referred severe melena. All of them were classified as ASA III or IV and a quick response to haemorrage was primarily important.

We've been using 1 arto-rectal, 4 aorto-uniliac with a simultaneous femoro-femoral bypass and 2 aorto-biliac grafts (66% Talent, 27% Zenith, 14% Vanguard). The mortality rate during surgery procedures was 12,5%, due to persistent intestinal bleedings; 37,5% referred worsening of both vital and infection signs, while we have not encountered technical complications endografts-related. One year mortality rate has been registered to be 25% (Figure 1).

Three endografts have been replaced with homografts after 15 to 180 days.

### *The Unstable Patient*

Unstable patients are those with poor haemodynamic conditions, referring hypovolaemic and/or haemodynamic shock and that includes 4 elderly patients for whom an axillo-bifemoral graft has been chosen to be implanted being a homograft unavailable promptly.

As a whole, 4 patients out of 6 were treated with an axillo-bifemoral bypass and AEF treatment, while 2 with an aorto-uniliac endograft and suprapubic bypasses.

In the first group 67 to 70 years-old subjects (68,25 avarage) were included, with the following clinical signs: abdominal pain, persistent feverish state, severe melena several times per day and needs of reanimation therapies. An axillo-bifemoral bypass implant has promptly been chosen after removal of the infected graft, periaortic tissues debridement and AEF treatment. All interventions have been executed at once according to the sufficient clinical stability of all patients while several-step operations would have stressed even more patients conditions.

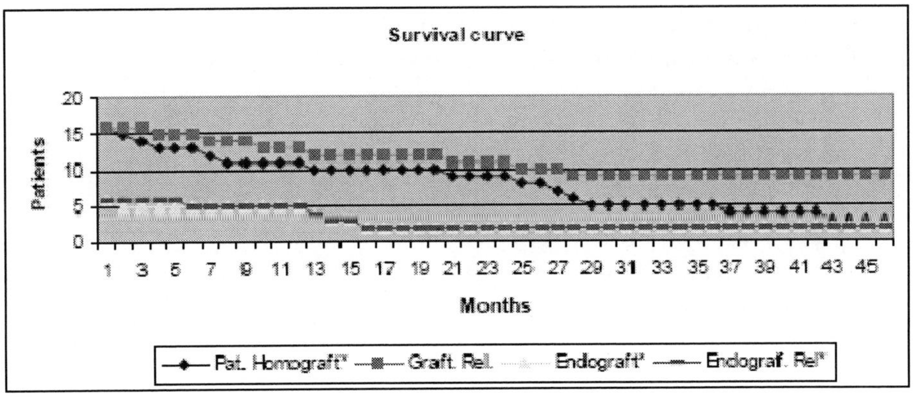


Figure 1.

Two direct duodenum suture interventions and 2 ileum resections have been performed. One patient had undergone a thigh amputation because of a bypass branch thrombosis. Within 40 days after interventions, 2 people have deceased further to cardiologic and nephrologic complications.

In the second group 2 recently operated patients were involved, 63 and 68 years of age. Symptoms shown were abdominal pain, haematemesis, melena, hypotension, luekocytosis and CRP high score. Two aorto-uniliac endograft with suprapubic bypasses have been implanted.

One patient is at present alive and in good health, while the other deceased 24 hours after the operation following a haemorragic shock.

Amongst all patients, both clinically stable or unstable, the amputation rate was 19%.

## Results

Above all we have privileged homografts, even though we have considered other recently introduced techniques; this has helped us to acquaint a larger range of options which could be useful when facing AEFs treatments.

According to our results, the elective solution comprises a first surgical treatment to remove the infected graft, a periaortic tissues debridement and then the AEF treatment itself. Homografts respond perfectly to our necessities, adding the possibility to revasculate directly through a biologic graft.

Evaluating the efficacy of homograft, some authors have initially compared those cryopreserved and the fresh ones finding no relevant differences [15]; other authors referred a highly resistance to infections of cryopreserved grafts [13, 16], due to a higher physicalchemical stability, an immune reactions resistance as well as an infection resistance consequent to an antibiotic charge [16, 17].

According to our survey, graft-related morbidity and mortality rates, vary constantly in the first 30 days to 2 years after surgery (30 days: 27%; 12 months: 38,8%; 24 months: 50%, graftrelated: 16,6%); after 24 months, primary causes are to be ascribed to a normal atherosclerosis course and its complications, depending on the arterial segment origins and an initial atheromasic involvement. All this has brought us to evaluate that grafts-related causes are precocious and then general conditions of each patient will settle the survival issue.

Aortic endografts are simple and rapid to implant, even though underneath there might be doubts about their AEFs treatment efficacy. According to our experience, 30 days mortality rate was significantly lower compared to those patients treated with conventional surgery procedures; after 12 months, though, death causes were similarly comparable, registering a higher incidence of those grafts-type related (total grafts mortality rate: 37,5%, 25% of which graft-related); reinfections rate was 37,5 % despite a prolonged and intense antibiotic therapy.

This technique is better suitable for elderly patients who suffer from a massive bleeding which needs to be plugged in order to rebalance the haemodynamic asset. Being this procedure less invasive, it helps surgeons to overcome a critical event and investigate further options.

A graft implant is not technically demanding, since a previous graft generally supplies an adequate implant site. In spite of this, it was our preference to use endografts suprarenal connected in order not to stress the anastomosis involved in the infective diastase or where a pseudoaneurysm may have developed.

If on one side endografts lead to immediate mortality and morbidity lower rates, on the other do not solve problems related to infections or to enteric fistulas; an antibiotic therapy might halt modestly aggressive bacteria and only an incomplete fistulization gives healing guarantees. Graft substitution problems, enteric wound treatment and infective tissues debridement are therefore generally postponed.

In any case, bleedings have seem to stop and patients general conditions have been optimized to better deal with the operation.

We do have also evaluated that 12 months mortality rates are frequently related to highly infective grafts. This would then qualify endografts for emergencies, in order to settle conditions for an optimal conventional operation.

Grafts removal and axillo-bifemoral bypasses were not frequently chosen in our experience; this intervention requires a strong vascular situation in order to avoid a precocious failure. Furthermore inguinal regions are not always infections-free and some risks related to the aortic stump tightness need to be considered.

We believe anyway that this is an historically consolidated technique which appears to be very useful in those situations whcrc unstableness of patients and a lack of other alternatives, require its use.

## Conclusions

Our experience brought us to privilege allografts according to Kieffer's experience since 1991. This choice has been determined following a good resistance to infections, a valid immune stability and the possibility to get an anatomical revascularization. On the other side, it has been evaluated that immune problems may arise, due to a particularly aggressive infection and to the allograft type involved; as other authors have shown, segments of descendent thoracic aorta are not utilized anymore [16].

Endografts are therefore a good alternative since they may promptly resolve bleeding problems in elderly patients with other severe illnesses. In certain conditions of a low infective charge, endografts might also be resolving.

Extra-anatomical bypasses, which limits have been widely studied, are historically proved options where no others are available.

We have not used Dacron-medicated grafts because we do not believe there are scientific evidences about their resistance to infections. We also consider venous allografts to be hazardous for our patients, because of vascular consequences after femoral veins removal; being this kind of operations effortful and enduring, we have privilieged other options.

At last, since AEFs may display multiple clinical manifestations, it is pivotal to take into count their possible onset in order to arrange a wide selection of treatments suitable for each single patient.

## References

[1] Cooper, A. The Lectures of Sir Astley Cooper on the Priciples and Practice of Surgery with Additional Notes and cases by Tyrell F. 5fth. Ed. Philadelphia: Haswell, Barrington and Haswell,1939.

[2] Santilli, S; Goldstone, J. Aortoenteric fistula. In Arterial Surgery:management of challenging problems, In: J. S. T. Jao, & W. H. Pearce (Eds.), Appleton e Lange, Stanford, 1996, 209-21.

[3] Burks, JA; Faries, PL; Gravereaux, EC; Hollier, LH; Marin, ML. Endovascular repair of bleeding aortoenteric fistulas: a 5-year experience. J Vasc Surg, 2001, 34, 1055-1059

[4] Eskandari, MK ; Makaroun, MS ; Abu-Elmagd, KM ; Billiar, TR. Endovascular repair of aortoduodenal fistula. J. Endovasc. Ther.2000, 7, 328-332.
[5] Busuttil, SJ; Goldstone, J. Diagnosis and management of aortoenteric fistulas. Semin. Vasc. Surg. 2001, 14, 302-311.
[6] O'Brian, SP; Ernst, CB. Aortoenteric fistula. In "Decision making in vasular surgery" Cronenwett Rutherforded WB SaundersPhyladelphia, 2001, 112-117.
[7] Keidar, Z; Nitecki, S. FDG-PET for the detection of infected vascular grafts. 2009 Mar, 53(1), 35-40.
[8] Reilly, LM. Aortic graft-enteric fistola. In Current Therapy in vascular surgery. 4th Ed. Ernst-Stanley, ed. Mosby St.Luois, 2001, 428-31.
[9] Kuestner, LM; Reilly, LM; Jicha, DJ; et al. secondary aoertoenteric fistula: contemporary outcome using extra-anatomic bypass and infected graft excision. J. Vasc. Surg., 21, 1995, 184-196.
[10] Low, RN; Wall, SD; Jeffrey, RB; et al. Durability of cross-femoral grafts following aortic graft infection:evaluated with CT, Radiology. 175, 1990, 157-162.
[11] Kieffer, E; Gomes, D; Plissonnier, D; Koskas, F; Bahnini, A. "Current use of allografts for infrarenal sortic graft infection" In Modern vascular surgery Yao JST & Pearce WH, edMcGrowHill 2000, 27, 297-308.
[12] Nevelsteen, A. Feryn TlacroixH et al. Experience with cryopreserved arterial allografts in the treatment of prosthetic graft infections. Cardiovasc. Surg., 1998, 6, 178-383.
[13] Voght, PR; Brunner-LaRocca, HP; Carrel, T; et al. Cryopreserved arterial allografts in the treatment of majorvascular infection:a comparison with conventional surgical techniques. J. Thorac. Cardiovasc. Surg., 1998, 116, 965-972.
[14] Lehalle, B; Geschier, C; Fieve, G; Stoltz, JF. Early rupture and degeneration of cryopreserved arterial allografts. J. Vasc. Surg. 1997, 25, 751-752.
[15] Chiesa, R; Astore, D; Piccolo, G; et al. Fresh and cryopreserved arterial homografts in the treatment of prosthetic graft infections:experience of the Italian Collaborative vascular Homograft Group. Ann. Vasc. Surg., 1998, 12, 583-588.
[16] Kieffer, E; Gomes, D; Chiche, L; et al. Allograft replacement for infrarenal aortic graft infection: Early and late results in 179 patients. JVS. 2004, 39(5), 1009-17.
[17] Chiesa, R; Astore, D; Frigerio, S; et al. Vascular prosthetic graft infection: epidemiology, bacteriology, pathogenesis and treatment. Acta Chir. Belg., 2002 Aug., 102(4), 238-47.
[18] Allaire, E ; Allaire, E ; Guettier, C ; Bruneval, P ; Plissonnier, D ; Michel, JB. Cell free arterial grafts: morphologic characteristics of aortic isografts, allografts and xenografts in rats. J. *Vasc. Surg.* 1994, 19, 446-56.

In: Advances in Cardiovascular Research, Volume 1
Editors: L. Schmitt, T. Konig, pp. 399-405
ISBN: 978-1-60741-720-0


*Chapter XIX*

# Cardiac Sympathetic Nervous System Denervation and Sudden Cardiac Death: Studies with Iodine-123 Metaiodobenzylguanidine Scintigrphy

***Yasushi Akutsu** * and Youichi Kobayashi***
Division of Cardiology, Department of Medicine, Showa University School of Medicine. Japan

## Abstract

It is well known that sympathetic nervous system innervation is important in the genesis of ventricular fibrillation. Loss of protective vagal reflex measured using heart rate variability or baroreflex sensitivity is also associated with sudden cardiac death because of reflecting sympathetic hyperinnervation. However, recent studies propose the close relationship between cardiac sympathetic denervation and occurrence of ventricular tachyarrhythmias. Sympathetic hyperinnervation caused by heart diseases or arrhythmogenesis itself results in cardiac sympathetic rejuvenation (hyperplasia, reduced norepinephrine uptake, reduced norepinephrine synthesis, and fetal gene expression) into the heart. Thus, rejuvenated and hyperinnervated neurons progress to cardiac sympathetic nervous system denervation. Recently, these co-existences have been suggested to be a trigger of ventricular tachyarrhythmia. Beta-adrenergic blockade has been shown not only to decrease sudden cardiac death but also to improve cardiac sympathetic nervous system denervation in patients with myocardial ischemia or heart failure. Iodine-123 metaiodobenzylguanidine ($^{123}$I-MIBG) represents an analog of norepinephrine, and $^{123}$I-MIBG scintigraphy can assess the magnitude of catecholamine re-uptake into heart, and impairment of cardiac sympathetic nervous system. Recent investigators and we have evaluated using cardiac uptakes of $^{123}$I-MIBG whether cardiac sympathetic nervous

* Corresponding author: Yasushi Akutsu, MD, PhD. Division of Cardiology, Department of Medicine, Showa University School of Medicine, 1-5-8 Hatanodai, Shinagawaku, Tokyo 142-8666, Japan, E-mail: hzn01233@s02.itscom.net.

system denervation is associated with the occurrence of ventricular tachyarrhythmia and sudden cardiac death. $^{123}$I-MIBG scintigraphy was performed in patients with ventricular tachyarrhythmias, and these patients were followed up. These studies found that the cardiac sympathetic nervous system denervation is predictive of sudden cardiac death in both patients with structural heart disease and idiopathic ventricular tachyarrhythmia. These results may explain that cardiac sympathetic nervous system denervation is one of the triggers of life-threatening ventricular tachyarrhythmias.

## Introduction

The sympathetic nervous system can play an important pathogenic role as a trigger of ventricular tachyarrhythmias and sudden cardiac death. Hyperinnervation of sympathetic nervous system has been focused as a cause of fatal arrhythmia[1], and the inhibition or blunting of sympathetic neural activity has been found to be associated with reduced mortality or arrhythmogenesis[2]. Heart rate profile that is represented as the value of sympathetic nervous system activity predicts mortality[3,4] and sudden cardiac death[5]. Instead of sympathetic nervous system activity, loss of protective vagal reflex measured using heart rate variability or baroreflex sensitivity has also reported to be associated with a greater susceptibility to ventricular fibrillation in human and animal models of myocardial infarction during and after ischemic episode[6-8]. However, recent studies propose that cardiac sympathetic nervous system denervation is associated with the occurrence of life threatening ventricular tachyarrhythmias.

## Structural Heart Disease and Sudden Cardiac Death

More than 90% of sudden cardiac death occurs in patients with coronary artery disease or cardiomyopathy, and severe left ventricular dysfunction or history of cardiac arrest also increases a risk of sudden cardiac death or sustained ventricular tachyarrhythmic event[9]. When the compensatory support is needed to meet the demands of organ perfusion due to reduced myocardial contractility or hemodynamic overload by structural heart diseases, the cardiac adrenergic system becomes maladaptive and can cause change that increase occurrences of ventricular tachyarrhythmias[10]. Kimura et al.[11] demonstrated that mechanical stretch or pressure overload into heart caused by structural heart disease with left ventricular dysfunction not only caused sympathetic hyperinnervation but also result in rejuvenation (hyperplasia, reduced norepinephrine uptake, reduced norepinephrine synthesis, and fetal gene expression) of cardiac sympathetic nerve system, which leads to cardiac denervation. Recently, these co-existences have been suggested to be a trigger of ventricular tachyarrhythmias[12]. Iodine-123 metaiodobenzylguanidine ($^{123}$I-MIBG) represents an analog of norepinephrine, and $^{123}$I-MIBG scintigraphy can assess the magnitude of catecholamine re-uptakes on the whole of left ventricle, and impairment of cardiac sympathetic nervous system[13,14]. Recently, cardiac sympathetic nervous system denervation measured by $^{123}$I-MIBG scintigraphy has been described for the occurrences of ventricular tachyarrhythmias associated with myocardial ischemia, infarction[15], dilated and hypertrophic cardiomyopathies[16], or heart failure[13]. Beta-adrenergic blockade has been shown not only to decrease sudden cardiac death but also to improve cardiac sympathetic nervous system denervation in patients with myocardial ischemia or heart failure[17]. These results indicate the significance of cardiac sympathetic nervous system denervation for the occurrence of fatal arrhythmia. Nagahara et al.[18] showed the close relationship between recurrent ventricular tachycardia or fibrillation and cardiac sympathetic denervation for 15 months follow-up in 54 patients who were diagnosed as high-risk group and were implanted Cardioverter Defibrillator. Seventeen of 21 patients with recurrent ventricular tachycardia or fibrillation, or sudden death (81%) had cardiac sympathetic denervation whereas 18 of 33 patients without the events (54.5%) did not have cardiac denervation. Tamaki et al.[19] also reported that cardiac sympathetic denervation was associated with sudden cardiac death in 106 patients with a history of heart failure who had left ventricular ejection fraction less than 40%. The prediction of sudden cardiac death was 78% in sensitivity and 56% in specificity using cardiac sympathetic denervation. The value of cardiac sympathetic denervation was powerful predictive of sudden cardiac death with adjusted hazard ratio of 4.8 [95% Confidence Interval 1.6-14.8, $p<0.01$]. Those results support that cardiac sympathetic denervation is associated with occurrence of ventricular tachyarrhythmias in high-risk group with left ventricular dysfunction.

## Idiopathic Ventricular Tachyarrhythmias and Sudden Cardiac Death

Preliminary data suggest that ventricular tachyarrhythmia without proven structural heart disease is associated with 25%-30% risk of recurrence of cardiac arrest[20]. Further, patients who underwent heart transplantation and had denervated hearts did not show left ventricular dysfunction, but about 10 % of the patients developed sudden cardiac death, presumably due to ventricular tachyarrhythmias[21]. Those results support that primary involvement of cardiac sympathetic denervation is considered to be directly associated with arrhythmogenesis in patients without left ventricular dysfunction[22-24]. Further, the patients with ventricular tachyarrhythmias in apparently normal heart or slight left ventricular dysfunction who were not found structural heart disease go from bad to worse of cardiac function by masked or pre-heart disease, and may have a high risk of sudden cardiac death finally[25]. Recent studies demonstrated that the patients without left ventricular dysfunction who were diagnosed as arrhythmogenic right ventricular cardiomyopathy[26], long-QT syndrome[27], or Brugada syndrome showed cardiac sympathetic denervation[28]. Schafers et al. reported in 1999 that $^{123}$I-MIBG uptake into left ventricle reduced significantly in 45 patients with a history of cardiac arrest caused by idiopathic ventricular fibrillation[29]. Their group demonstrated in 2006 that reduced $^{123}$I-MIBG uptakes into left ventricle were associated with ventricular tachyarrhythmic events during a follow-up of 7 years in 20 patients with idiopathic ventricular fibrillation[30]. Of those, reduced MIBG uptakes were observed in 13 patients, and 18 episodes of ventricular fibrillation or fast polymorphic ventricular tachycardia occurred in 4 idiopathic ventricular fibrillation patients with cardiac sympathetic denervation whereas only 2 episodes of monomorphic ventricular tachycardia (and no ventricular fibrillation) occurred in a single idiopathic ventricular fibrillation patient with normal cardiac sympathetic nervous system activity. We also reported that cardiac sympathetic denervation is a readily available and powerful predictor of recurrent ventricular tachyarrhythmic events for 11 years follow-up in 50 patients with ventricular tachycardia who did not have conventional risk of sudden cardiac death[31]. The prediction of recurrent ventricular arrhythmic events or sudden cardiac death was 75% of sensitivity and 71% of specificity in patients with idiopathic ventricular tachycardia (adjusted hazard ratio of 5.3 [95% Confidence Interval 1.4-20.8, p<0.05]). These results suggest that cardiac sympathetic denervation play an important role for evaluating long-term prognosis of patients with ventricular tachyarrhythmia who seem to be low risk of sudden cardiac death.

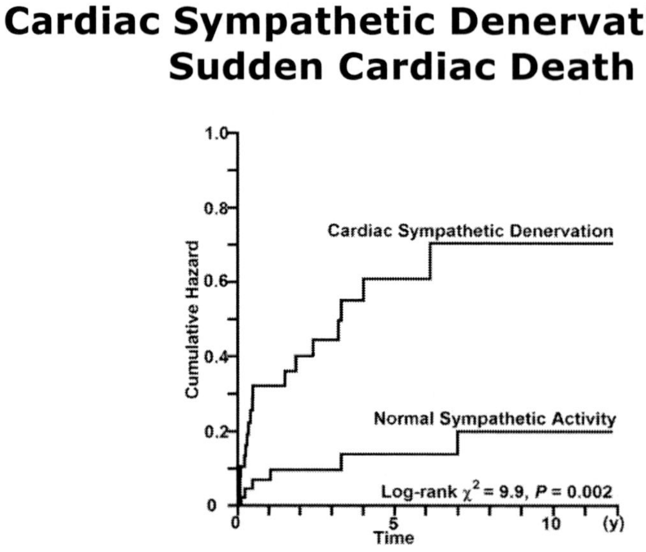


Figure 1. Kaplan-Meier cumulative hazard of sudden cardiac death or occurrence of recurrent ventricular tachyarrhythmic events according to cardiac sympathetic nervous system denervation in 86 patients with a history of ventricular tachyarrhythmias. Over 11 years follow up, cardiac sympathetic denervation was predictive of sudden cardiac death or occurrence of ventricular arrhythmic events with hazard ratio of 4 times compared to normal cardiac sympathetic activity (4 [95% Confidence Interval 1.6 to 10, p<0.005]) in no relation to whether these patients had a history of structural heart disease (Cardiac sympathetic denervation was associated with follow-up events with hazard ratio of 9.4 [95% Confidence Interval 1.1 to 74, p=0.033] when only patients with structural heart disease were considered).

We recently reported that cardiac sympathetic denervation had a powerful prognostic power of sudden cardiac death despite of the random cardiac population with arrhythmic disorder[32] (Figure 1). These study patients included 44 patients with cardiovascular process and 42 patients with idiopathic ventricular tachycardia or fibrillation. Eighteen of 24 patients with recurrent ventricular tachyarrhythmias or sudden death (75%) had cardiac sympathetic denervation whereas 40 of 62 patients without the events (64.5%) did not have cardiac denervation. The value of cardiac denervation was powerful predictive of recurrent ventricular tachyarrhythmic events or sudden cardiac death with adjusted hazard ratio of 3.6 [95% Confidence Interval 1.4-9.2, p<0.01] although cardiac sympathetic denervation was more associated with follow-up events with hazard ratio of 9.4 in only patients with structural heart disease compared to random cardiac population including idiopathic arrhythmic disorder.

The results of these studies which were obtained using $^{123}$I-MIBG scintigraphy indicate strongly that cardiac denervation of sympathetic nervous system is associated with sudden cardiac death in no relation to whether cardiac denervation was caused directly or secondary.

# References


[1] Cao, JM; Fishbein, MC; Han, JB; et al. Relationship between regional cardiac hyperinnervation and ventricular arrhythmia. *Circulation.*, 2000, 101, 1960-69.

[2] The Norwegian Multicenter Study Group. Timolol-induced reduction in mortality and reinfarction in patients surviving acute myocardial infarction. *N Engl J Med.*, 1981, 304, 801-7.

[3] Cole, CR; Blackstone, EH; Pashkow, FJ; Snader, CE; Lauer, MS. Heart-rate recovery immediately after exercise as a predictor of mortality. *N Engl J Med.*, 1999, 341, 1351-7.

[4] Akutsu, Y; Gregory, SA; Kardan, A, et al. Delayed heart rate recovery after adenosine stress testing with supplemental arm; exercise predicts mortality. *J Nucl Cardiol.*, 2009, 16, 54-62.

[5] Jouven, X; Empana, JP; Schwartz, PJ; Desnos, M; Courbon, D; Ducimettiere, P. Heart-rate profile during exercise as a predictor of sudden death. *N Engl J Med.*, 2005, 352, 1951-8.

[6] Schwarts, PJ; Vanoli, E; Stramba-Badiale, M; et al. Autonomic mechanisms and sudden death new insights from analysis of baroreceptor reflexes in conscious dogs with and without a myocardial infarction. *Circulation.*, 1988, 78, 969-79.

[7] Adamson, PB; Huang, MH; Vanoli, E; et al Unexpected interaction between beta-adrenergic blockade and heart rate variability before and after myocardial infarction. A longitudinal study in dogs at high and low risk for sudden death. *Circulation.*, 1994, 90, 976-82.

[8] La Rovere, MT; Bigger, JT Jr.; Marcus, FL; et al. Baoreflex sensitivity and heart-rate variability in prediction of total cardiac mortality after myocardial infarction ATRAMI (Autonomic Tone and Reflexes After Myocardial Infarction) investigators. *Lancet.*, 1998, 351, 478-84.

[9] Bloomfield, DM; Steinman, RC; Namerow, PB; et al. Microvolt T-Wave Alternans distinguishes between patients likely and patients not likely to benefit from implanted cardiac defibrillator therapy. A solution to the multicenter automatic defibrillator implantation trial (MADIT) II conundrum. *Circulation.*, 2004, 110, 1885-9.

[10] Anderson, KP. Sympathetic nervous system activity and ventricular tachyarrhythmias: recent advances. *Ann Noninvasive Electrocardiol.*, 2003, 8, 75-89.

[11] Kimura, K; Ieda, M; Kanazawa, H; et al. Cardiac sympathetic rejuvenation. A link between nerve function and cardiac hypertrophy. *Circ Res.*, 2007, 100, 1755-64.

[12] Chen, PS; Chen, LS; Cao, JM; et al. Sympathetic nerve sprouting, electrical remodeling and the mechanism of sudden cardiac death. *Cardiovasc Res.*, 2001, 50, 409-16.

[13] Merlet, P; Valette, H; Dubois-Rande, JL; et al. Prognostic Value of Cardiac Metaiodobenzylguanidine Imaging in Patients with Heart Failure. *J Nucl Med.*, 1992, 33, 471-7.
[14] Yamashina, S; Yamazaki, J. Neuronal imaging using SPECT. *Eur J Nucl Med Mol Imaging.*, 2007, 34, 939-50.
[15] Wakabayashi, T; Nakata, T; Hashimoto, A; et al. Assessment of underlying etiology and cardiac sympathetic innervation to identify patients at high risk of cardiac death. *J Nucl Med.*, 2001, 42, 1757-67.
[16] Terai, H; Shimizu, M; Ino, H; et al. Cardiac sympathetic nerve activity in patients with hypertrophic cardiomyopathy with malignant ventricular tachyarrhythmias. *J Nucl Cardiol.*, 2003, 10, 304-10.
[17] Toyama, T; Hoshizaki, H; Seki, R; et al. Efficacy of carvedilol treatment on cardiac function and cardiac sympathetic nerve activity in patients with dilated cardiomyopathy: comparison with metoprolol therapy. *J Nucl Med.*, 2003, 44, 1604-11.
[18] Nagahara, D; Nakata, T; Hashimoto, A; et al. Predicting the need for an implantable cardioverter defibrillator using cardiac metaiodobenzylguanidine activity together with plasma natriuretic peptide concentration or left ventricular function. *J Nucl Med.*, 2008, 49, 225-33.
[19] Tamaki, S; Yamada, T; Okuyama, Y; et al. Cardiac iodine-123 metaiodobenzylguanidine imaging predicts sudden cardiac death independently of left ventricular ejection fraction in patients with chronic heart failure and left ventricular systolic dysfunction. *J Am Coll Cardiol.*, 2009, 53, 426-35.
[20] No authors listed. Survivors of out-of-hospital cardiac arrest with apparently normal heart. Need for definition and standardized clinical evaluation. Consensus statement of the joint steering committees of the unexplained cardiac arrest registry of Europe and of the idiopathic ventricular fibrillation registry of the United States. *Circulation.*, 1997, 95, 265-72.
[21] Chantranuwat, C; Blakey, JD; Kobashigawa, JA; et al. Sudden, unexpected death in cardiac transplant recipients: an autopsy study. *J Heart Lung Transplant.*, 2004, 23, 683-9.
[22] Ieda, M; Kanazawa, H; Kimura, K; et al. Sema3a maintains normal heart rhythm through sympathetic innervation patterning. *Nat Med.*, 2007, 13, 604-12.
[23] Kienzle, MG; Martins, JB; Constantin, L; Aschoff, A. Effect of direct, reflex and exercise-provoked increases in sympathetic tone on idiopathic ventricular tachycardia. *Am J Cardiol.*, 1992, 69, 1433-38.
[24] Zipes, DP. Sympathetic stimulation and arrhythmias. *N Engl J Med.*, 1991, 325, 656-7.
[25] Wichter, T; Breithardt, G; Borggrefe, M. Ventricular tachycardia in the normal heart. In: Pordrin PJ, Kowery PR, eds. Cardiac arrhythmia: mechanism, diagnosis and management. Baltimore, MD: *Williams & Wilkins.*, 1995, 1219-38.
[26] Wichter, T; Schafer, M; Rhodes, CG; et al. Abnormalities of cardiac sympathetic innervation in arrhythmogenic right ventricular cardiomyopathy : quantitative assessment of presynaptic norepinephrine reuptake and postsynaptic beta-adrenergic receptor density with positron emission tomography. *Circulation.*, 2000, 101, 1552-8.
[27] Chevalier, P; Rodriquez, C; Bontemps, L; et al. Non-invasive testing of acquired long QT syndrome: evidence for multiple arrhythmogenic substrates. *Cardiovasc Res.*, 2001, 50, 386-98.

[28] Wichter, T; Matheja, P; Eckardt, L; et al. Cardiac autonomic dysfunction in Brugada syndrome. *Circulation.*, 2002, 105, 702-6.

[29] Schafers, M; Wichter, T; Lerch, H; et al. Cardiac $^{123}$I-MIBG uptake in idiopathic ventricular tachycardia and fibrillation. *J Nucl Med.*, 1999, 40, 1-5.

[30] Paul, M; Schafers, M; Kies, P; et al. Impact of sympathetic innervation on recurrent life-threatening arrhythmias in the follow-up of patients with idiopathic ventricular fibrillation. *Eur J Nucl Med Mol Imaging.*, 2006, 33, 866-70.

[31] Akutsu, Y; kaneko, K; Kodama, Y; et al. Cardiac sympathetic nerve abnormality predicts ventricular tachyarrhythmic events in patients without conventional risk of sudden death. *Eur J Nucl Med Mol Imaging.*, 2008, 35, 2066-73.

[32] Akutsu, Y; Kaneko, K; Kodama, Y; et al. The significance of cardiac sympathetic nervous system abnormality in the long-term prognosis of patients with a history of ventricular tachyarrhythmia. *J Nucl Med.*, 2009, 50, 61-7.

In: Advances in Cardiovascular Research, Volume 1
Editors: L. Schmitt, T. Konig, pp. 407-412
ISBN: 978-1-60741-720-0


*Chapter XX*

# Low Birth Weight Is a Risk Factor for Cardiovascular Disease

***Peter J. Giannone, Juli M. Richter and John A. Bauer***
Nationwide Children's Hospital, Columbus, OH, USA

The impact of the fetal environment on the frequency of cardiovascular disorders in adults was first noted in a report by Dr. David Barker.[1] In this seminal report, it was shown that individuals, who were small at birth, had substantially increased risk of death from cardiovascular disease and stroke. This concept has since been coined the 'Barker Hypothesis' and numerous studies and texts have described the phenomenon of fetal imprinting of adult cardiovascular disease.[2] Similar findings have been published by many other investigators, and the main focus of this field of research to date has been on the impact of poor fetal nutrition leading to long term impact on cardiovascular system structure and/or function[3]. Low birth weight has been associated with increased rates of coronary heart disease and the related disorders of stroke, hypertension and type 2 diabetes.[4] Although caloric (and especially protein) restriction leads to reduced fetal growth and development, an additional major cause for delivery of low birth weight infants, particularly preterm infants, is maternal infection and inflammation.[5, 6] Although the mechanisms involved are not well defined, the significance of this problem will expand, as the incidence of preterm birth and the survival of low birth weight babies continues to increase throughout the world.

Infants born at low birth weights have nearly an equivalent risk of developing later onset cardiovascular disease as adults who smoke tobacco. If you are born weighing less than 2.5 kilograms, your risk of dying from heart disease is more than 1.5 times the risk as compared to an appropriately weighing term infant. In addition, the risk of developing cardiovascular disease appears to be inversely proportional to birth weight.[1] It is now not uncommon for infants with birth weights as low as 0.5 kilograms to survive.[7] Smoking is considered a major risk factor for developing cardiovascular disease.[8] It is our opinion that the American Heart Association should also consider being born low birth weight a major risk factor for developing cardiovascular disease.

Although improvements in clinical care have greatly increased the survival of infants born prematurely, preterm birth remains a major cause of infant mortality and morbidity.[14] The mechanisms responsible for preterm birth have not been clearly defined but an association with maternal inflammation has been recently proposed as an important contributor. For example, infections, including chorioamnionitis, gingivitis, and systemic inflammation, have been shown to be strongly associated with increased risk of preterm labor.[9, 10] Many of these infants who are born prematurely may have been exposed to low-grade inflammation for prolonged periods. These exposures may not only be infectious in nature, but may include environmental toxins as well. For reasons that are presently unknown, these pregnancies usually do not present with preterm labor before 20 weeks gestation, even if the amniotic fluid was positive for pro-inflammatory cytokines or organisms prior to the preterm labor.[11] These exposures to intrauterine infections/inflammation may result in more serious injury than just preterm delivery alone, including brain and lung injuries that manifest during infancy.[12, 15] Also, antenatal insults, such as infections and inflammation, have been implicated in alterations of development leading to increased incidences and/or severities of diseases of later onset, but these mechanisms remain poorly understood.[1, 13, 16]

The associations between preterm births and developmental defects may arise from common variables. The relationship between maternal infection and preterm labor is well recognized.[9, 17] Animal models of maternal inflammation have been used to induce preterm labor.[18-20] The use of established models has allowed us to evaluate the effect of prenatal inflammation on the development and function of specific organ systems. The association between chorioamnionitis and infant morbidities, such as lung and brain injury, is well documented.[11, 21] However, subclinical infections are believed to play a role in preterm delivery and neonatal outcome as well.[22] Buhimschi et al. reported that administration of lipopolysaccharide (LPS) to pregnant C57BL/6 mice caused fetal demise and premature delivery without signs of sepsis in the dams.[18] Hepatic reduced glutathione (GSH) levels in the dams and in the pups were decreased 16 h post LPS administration, and administration of N-Acetyl Cysteine (NAC) 30 min before and 2 h after LPS prevented the LPS-induced decline in GSH levels, prolonged latency to delivery, and improved fetal survival. The authors concluded that the effects of LPS were mediated by oxidative stress mechanisms. Fetal death represents an obvious and extreme form of toxicity arising from an intrauterine exposure, but less severe treatments, as with lower doses and less sensitive subjects, can result in premature delivery and/or altered fetal and postnatal development. It is conceivable that prenatal exposure to infection and/or inflammation, which may lead to premature delivery and low birth weight infants, may alter the programming of the immune response to subsequent antigens. This enhanced immune response may contribute to the development of disease states later in life.

Inflammation has also been shown to be a contributing factor in many settings of adult cardiovascular disease.[24, 25] For example, acute myocardial infarction, coronary artery disease, arrhythmias, and acute heart failure are all associated with increases in inflammatory cytokines, elevated C-reactive protein and other acute phase response proteins, and evidence of reactive oxygen or nitrogen species.[26] In addition to acute settings of ischemia, other more protracted forms of heart disease (non-ischemic cardiomyopathy, viral myocarditis, diabetic cardiomyopathy) have also often been shown to each have an inflammatory component in adult disease.[27-32] Some studies have also shown similar phenomena in pediatric settings of heart failure and cardiomyopathy.

Innate immunity driven inflammatory responses may have beneficial influences that preserve myocardial function in the short term but may be maladaptive in chronic states. Given the narrow margin for benefit of cardiac inflammation, special regulatory mechanisms likely raise the threshold, compared to other tissues, for the induction and persistence of adaptive immune responses.[33] These mechanisms include strong central and peripheral T cell tolerance to heart antigens and induction of anti-inflammatory feedback mechanisms.[34] However, it is possible that early fetal imprinting alters these regulatory pathways disabling the myocardium's ability to attenuate inflammation either under conditions of acute stress or chronically. At this crucial time of cardiac development, not only could analtered inflammatory response damage the heart, it could alter the myocardium's ability to repair and/or regenerate itself leading to cardiovascular dysfunction. It is likely this imprinting would not become evident until adulthood since this may be the first time the individual may be presented with a severe cardiac stress.

Humans and other animals are sensitive to environmental conditions that modulate ontogenic pathways thus, exerting persistent influences on diverse functional outcomes.[35, 36] This concept of imprinting discrete biological responses has been well studied in regards to adult immune system performance. For example, presenting the immature immune system with antigen in prenatal or early postnatal life can permanently alter the long-term performance of the immune system[37, 38] and permanently enhance the immune response to a systemic challenge[39]. While this more vigorous response to a secondary antigen presentation may be an advantage to immunity, there is potential that related inflammatory activation could cause a greater degree of parenchymal organ damage and dysfunction. This concept has not been addressed in previous investigations, perhaps since much of the literature has focused on immune competence rather than immune system mediated toxicities and pathogenesis. We postulate that a prenatal imprinting of cardiac myocyte responses to inflammatory stimuli contribute to later cardiac abnormalities in adulthood. These abnormalities may not be readily apparent under 'basal' conditions, but may require additional stressors or secondary challenges to manifest evidence of disease or dysfunction. These concepts are strongly supported by various observations, especially those with specific focus on immunity mechanisms.

There is now enough evidence to warrant naming low birth weight as a major risk factor for developing cardiovascular disease as defined by the American Heart Association. However, although the 'Barker Hypothesis' (also known as the Fetal Origins of Disease Hypothesis) has been substantiated by numerous epidemiological studies, the mechanisms involved remain poorly defined. Since preterm birth and low birth weight have been linked to perinatal infection, inflammation and innate immune pathways, and now also environmental toxic exposures, it is plausible that these contribute to, or are responsible for, cardiovascular disease in adulthood. Further mechanistic studies, leading to the rational development of potential therapeutic or preventive strategies would be beneficial to this vulnerable population.

# References

[1] Barker, DJ. The fetal and infant origins of adult disease. *Bmj*, 1990, 301(6761), 1111.

[2] Barker, DJ; Osmond, C; Law, CM. The intrauterine and early postnatal origins of cardiovascular disease and chronic bronchitis. *J Epidemiol Community Health*, 1989, 43(3), 237-40.

[3] McMillen, IC; Robinson, JS. Developmental origins of the metabolic syndrome: prediction, plasticity, and programming. *Physiol Rev*, 2005, 85(2), 571-633.

[4] Barker, DJ. The developmental origins of adult disease. *J Am Coll Nutr*, 2004, 23(6 Suppl), 588S-95S.

[5] Goldenberg, RL; Andrews, WW; Faye-Petersen, O; Cliver, S; Goepfert, AR; Hauth, JC. The Alabama Preterm Birth Project: placental histology in recurrent spontaneous and indicated preterm birth. *Am J Obstet Gynecol*, 2006, 195(3), 792-6.

[6] Hagberg, H; Mallard, C; Jacobsson, B. Role of cytokines in preterm labour and brain injury. *Bjog*, 2005, 112 Suppl 1, 16-8.

[7] Fanaroff, AA; Stoll, BJ; Wright, LL; Carlo, WA; Ehrenkranz, RA; Stark, AR; et al. Trends in neonatal morbidity and mortality for very low birthweight infants. *Am J Obstet Gynecol*, 2007, 196(2), 147 e1-8.

[8] Prugger, C; Wellmann, J; Heidrich, J; Brand-Herrmann, SM; Keil, U. Cardiovascular risk factors and mortality in patients with coronary heart disease. *Eur J Epidemiol*, 2008.

[9] Goldenberg, RL; Hauth, JC; Andrews, WW. Intrauterine infection and preterm delivery. *N Engl J Med*, 2000, 342(20), 1500-7.

[10] Han, YW; Redline, RW; Li, M; Yin, L; Hill, GB; McCormick, TS. Fusobacterium nucleatum induces premature and term stillbirths in pregnant mice: implication of oral bacteria in preterm birth. *Infect Immun*, 2004, 72(4), 2272-9.

[11] Jobe, AH; Ikegami, M. Antenatal infection/inflammation and postnatal lung maturation and injury. *Respir Res*, 2001, 2(1), 27-32.

[12] Alexander, JM; Gilstrap, LC; Cox, SM; McIntire, DM; Leveno, KJ. Clinical chorioamnionitis and the prognosis for very low birth weight infants. *Obstet Gynecol*, 1998, 91(5 Pt 1), 725-9.

[13] Barker, DJ. In utero programming of chronic disease. *Clin Sci (Lond)*, 1998, 95(2), 115-28.

[14] Parker, RA; Lindstrom, DP; Cotton, RB. Improved survival accounts for most, but not all, of the increase in bronchopulmonary dysplasia. *Pediatrics*, 1992, 90(5), 663-8.

[15] Alexander, JM; McIntire, DM; Leveno, KJ. Chorioamnionitis and the prognosis for term infants. *Obstet Gynecol*, 1999, 94(2), 274-8.

[16] Gillman, MW. Developmental origins of health and disease. *N Engl J Med*, 2005, 353(17), 1848-50.

[17] Goldenberg, RL; Culhane, JF. Infection as a cause of preterm birth. *Clin Perinatol*, 2003, 30(4), 677-700.

[18] Buhimschi, IA; Buhimschi, CS; Weiner, CP. Protective effect of N-acetylcysteine against fetal death and preterm labor induced by maternal inflammation. *Am J Obstet Gynecol*, 2003, 188(1), 203-8.

[19] Kajikawa, S; Kaga, N; Futamura, Y; Kakinuma, C; Shibutani, Y. Lipoteichoic acid induces preterm delivery in mice. *J Pharmacol Toxicol Methods*, 1998, 39(3), 147-54.

[20] Mitsuhashi, Y; Otsuki, K; Yoda, A; Shimizu, Y; Saito, H; Yanaihara, T. Effect of lactoferrin on lipopolysaccharide (LPS) induced preterm delivery in mice. *Acta Obstet Gynecol Scand*, 2000, 79(5), 355-8.

[21] Goldenberg, RL; Culhane, JF; Johnson, DC. Maternal infection and adverse fetal and neonatal outcomes. *Clin Perinatol*, 2005, 32(3), 523-59.

[22] Goldenberg, RL; Culhane, JF. Preterm birth and periodontal disease. *N Engl J Med*, 2006, 355(18), 1925-7.

[23] Giannone, PJ; Schanbacher, BL; Bauer, JA; Reber, KM. Effects of prenatal lipopolysaccharide exposure on epithelial development and function in newborn rat intestine. *J Pediatr Gastroenterol Nutr*, 2006, 43(3), 284-90.

[24] Chaves, AA; Baliga, RS; Mihm, MJ; Schanbacher, BL; Basuray, A; Liu, C; et al. Bacterial lipopolysaccharide enhances cardiac dysfunction but not retroviral replication in murine AIDS: roles of macrophage infiltration and toll-like receptor 4 expression. *Am J Pathol*, 2006, 168(3), 727-35.

[25] Zhang, J; Liu, Y; Shi, J; Larson, DF; Watson, RR. Side-stream cigarette smoke induces dose-response in systemic inflammatory cytokine production and oxidative stress. *Exp Biol Med (Maywood)*, 2002, 227(9), 823-9.

[26] Suleiman, M; Khatib, R; Agmon, Y; Mahamid, R; Boulos, M; Kapeliovich, M; et al. Early inflammation and risk of long-term development of heart failure and mortality in survivors of acute myocardial infarction predictive role of C-reactive protein. *J Am Coll Cardiol*, 2006, 47(5), 962-8.

[27] Westermann, D; Rutschow, S; Van Linthout, S; Linderer, A; Bucker-Gartner, C; Sobirey, M; et al. Inhibition of p38 mitogen-activated protein kinase attenuates left ventricular dysfunction by mediating pro-inflammatory cardiac cytokine levels in a mouse model of diabetes mellitus. *Diabetologia*, 2006, 49(10), 2507-13.

[28] Haidara, MA; Yassin, HZ; Rateb, M; Ammar, H; Zorkani, MA. Role of oxidative stress in development of cardiovascular complications in diabetes mellitus. *Curr Vasc Pharmacol*, 2006, 4(3), 215-27.

[29] Diamant, M; Lamb, HJ; Smit, JW; de Roos, A; Heine, RJ. Diabetic cardiomyopathy in uncomplicated type 2 diabetes is associated with the metabolic syndrome and systemic inflammation. *Diabetologia*, 2005, 48(8), 1669-70.

[30] Calabrese, F; Angelini, A; Carturan, E; Thiene, G. Myocarditis and inflammatory cardiomyopathy: histomorphological diagnosis. *Ernst Schering Res Found Workshop*, 2006(55), 305-21.

[31] Kan, H; Finkel, MS. Inflammatory mediators and reversible myocardial dysfunction. *J Cell Physiol*, 2003, 195(1), 1-11.

[32] Szalay, G; Sauter, M; Hald, J; Weinzierl, A; Kandolf, R; Klingel, K. Sustained nitric oxide synthesis contributes to immunopathology in ongoing myocarditis attributable to interleukin-10 disorders. *Am J Pathol*, 2006, 169(6), 2085-93.

[33] Taqueti, VR; Mitchell, RN; Lichtman, AH. Protecting the pump: controlling myocardial inflammatory responses. *Annu Rev Physiol*, 2006, 68, 67-95.

[34] He, H; Stone, JR; Perkins, DL. Analysis of differential immune responses induced by innate and adaptive immunity following transplantation. *Immunology*, 2003, 109(2), 185-96.

[35] Waterland, RA; Garza, C. Potential mechanisms of metabolic imprinting that lead to chronic disease. *Am J Clin Nutr*, 1999, 69(2), 179-97.

[36] Klein, SL; Rager, DR. Prenatal stress alters immune function in the offspring of rats. *Dev Psychobiol*, 1995, 28(6), 321-36.

[37] Fagoaga, OR; Nehlsen-Cannarella, SL. Maternal modulation of neonatal immune system development. *Dev Immunol*, 2002, 9(1), 9-17.

[38] Bilbo, SD; Levkoff, LH; Mahoney, JH; Watkins, LR; Rudy, JW; Maier, SF. Neonatal infection induces memory impairments following an immune challenge in adulthood. *Behav Neurosci*, 2005, 119(1), 293-301.

[39] Williams, AE; Edwards, L; Humphreys, IR; Snelgrove, R; Rae, A; Rappuoli, R; et al. Innate imprinting by the modified heat-labile toxin of Escherichia coli (LTK63) provides generic protection against lung infectious disease. *J Immunol*, 2004, 173(12), 7435-43.

In: Advances in Cardiovascular Research, Volume 1
Editors: L. Schmitt, T. Konig, pp. 413-417
ISBN: 978-1-60741-720-0


*Chapter XXI*

# Disorders of the Haemostatic System in Patients with Solid Malignancies

***Géza Bozóky and Éva Ruby***
Department of Pulmonology, Municipal Hospital of Bács-Kiskun County, Kecskemét, Hungary.

We performed a retrospective study on the occurrence of haemostatic disorders in 1381 patients with various malignant tumours between 1996 and 2004 (Table 1). The mean age of the 872 male and 509 female patients was 57.8 (37 to 79) years. In the majority or our patients we diagnosed a malignancy of primary pulmonary localisation (1140 patients) including 790 patients with non-small cell lung cancer (NSCLC), mostly adenocarcinoma and squamous cell carcinoma (70 %). In the other cases large cell carcinoma, bronchioloalveolar or mixed type malignant tumour was diagnosed (Table 1). 68 of the 790 patients with NSCLC were in an operable stage, 346 patients belonged to Stages IIIA and IIIB, while 274 have proven to be of clinical Stage IV.

Of the 350 patients with SCLC, 185 and 165 were of extended or limited clinical stage, respectively. The other patients with tumours of non-bronchopulmonary localisation (n = 241) had advanced, metastasising mammary, colorectal, renal or vesical carcinoma (Table 1).

*Of the 1381 patients, we found haemostatic disorders with abnormal clinical manifestations in a total of 397 patients (28.7 %) (Table 1)*. DVT and APE have proven to be the most frequent ones (n = 305; 22 %). Other types of haemostatic disorders (migrating superficial thrombophlebitis, aDIC, septic thrombosis, microangiopathic haemolytic anaemia) occurred in 71 patients with neoplastic diseases (6.7 %). More than 90 % of all haemostatic disorders have proven to be VTE. In nearly 30 % of our patients (400/1381) we found various not neoplastic co-morbidities. A non-malignant co-morbidity occurred in 40 % of patients with malignancies and associated VTE. In the majority of our patients various diseases of cardiac origin (congestive cardiac failure, history of an acute coronary syndrome, cardiomyopathy, valvular heart defects) were found; chronic obstructive pulmonary disease occurred in a somewhat smaller proportion. In nearly 10 % of the 397 patients with haemostatic disorder, the significant tumour mass (mediastinal 'bulky' metastatic lymph node conglomerate located in the superficial regions) also contributed to the development of venous circulation disorder.

In cases of *clinically suspected DVT*, in addition to the laboratory D-dimer examination, we also performed compression Doppler sonography which confirmed the thrombosis that developed in the venous system with great accuracy (D-dimer determination happened to be negative in 24 of 305 cases): the venous thrombosis was of femoropopliteal localisation in nearly 80 % of cases, and ileofemoral in the remaining ones. When the clinical signs raised the *suspicion of APE with high probability*, we performed ventilation-perfusion lung scintigraphy after the D-dimer examination. If this result was not of diagnostic value, or when the patient had severe COPD, HR-CT and echocardiography were performed. Of the 58 patients with APE, the D-dimer examination was negative in 6 cases. Ventilation-perfusion lung scintigraphy gave unequivocally positive diagnoses in 24 patients, and HR-CT examination provided the diagnosis in the remaining cases. *Acute massive pulmonary embolism* occurred in 5 of the 58 patients with APE; the underlying malignancy was in a very advanced stage in these patients, and severe co-morbidity and pulmonary infection was also found in all cases. A *migrating thrombophlebitis* was diagnosed in 56 patients. We performed compression Doppler sonography in all patients in order to exclude DVT.

*Acute diffuse (disseminated) intravascular coagulation (aDIC)* was diagnosed in 11 patients on the basis of the co-existing thrombotic and haemorrhagic symptoms. The clinical suspicion was raised by an increased haemorrhage from the injection site in all cases. In addition to the cutaneous haemorrhages, diffuse bleeding of mucous membranes, as well as multi-organ (pulmonary, hepatic, renal, CNS) function disorder due to thrombotic disturbances of microcirculation could be observed. We found very low platelet count, delayed prothrombin and thrombin times in our patients, without any exception. Fragmentocytes could be seen in the peripheral blood smear, D-dimer values were elevated, and fibrinogen levels were significantly decreased. Clinically the severe coagulation disorder had an acute, fulminant course in all cases. In all of these patients the malignant disease was in a very advanced stage, and the clinical picture was deteriorated also by severe non-malignant co-morbidity. *Septic thrombosis* was diagnosed in four patients. Septic course of fever, leucocytosis, shift to the left in the peripheral differential leucocyte count, and increased erythrocyte sedimentation rate (ESR) could be observed in these cases. Bacteraemia caused by Pseudomonas aeruginosa and by Klebsiella pneumoniae has been demonstrated in two cases each. Infected thrombus could be detected in the brachiocephalic veins by colour Doppler sonography in all four patients. The underlying malignancy was SCLC of advanced stage in all cases, and no other source of sepsis was found except the infected thrombosis. *Thrombotic thrombocytopenic purpura (thrombotic microangiopathy)*, observed in three patients, manifested itself in an acute form associated with fever, thrombocytopenia, fluctuating central neurological symptoms, non-immune haemolytic anaemia and renal function disorder. Fragmentocytes could be seen in the peripheral blood smear, severe thrombocytopenia, very high serum lactate dehydrogenase (LDH) levels and impaired renal function could be observed, and the clinical course was fulminant in all patients. The clinical diagnosis of *superficial thrombophlebitis* causes no difficulties in the everyday practice. Having observed the characteristic clinical symptoms of recurrent or migrating thrombophlebitis, the possibility of malignancy emerges, and detailed extensive research is required /1/. In our series, migrating thrombophlebitis occurred in 4 % (56 patients). The primary role of compression Doppler sonography is exclusion of deep vein thrombosis in these patients.

In cases of clinical *suspicion for VTE*, in addition to the determination of D-dimer, compression Doppler sonography gives a result of verifying or excluding force; in the small number of uncertain cases performance of lower limb phlebography is justified. In cases with marked clinical signs of *suspicion for APE* (acute, otherwise unexplained dyspnoea, chest pain, cough, and haemoptysis) clinical information raising suspicion can be obtained from the possible changes of ECG (sinus tachycardia, suddenly occurring atrial fibrillation, and signs of a load on the right half of the heart), the alterations seen on thoracic x-ray picture (higher positioned diaphragm, presence of pleural fluid, development of inhomogeneous or homogeneous infiltrative elements within 24 or 48 hours following the appearance of APE), as well as the determination of D-dimer /2, 26, 32/. Ventilation-perfusion lung scintigraphy and compression Doppler sonography of the lower limb is of diagnostic value in the majority of cases; in uncertain cases or in severe COPD the spiral CT angiography provides an exact diagnosis (specificity = 100 %, sensitivity = 63 to 100 %). Pulmonary angiography that provides specificity and sensitivity of nearly 100 % (the 'gold standard') has to be performed rarely; in case of an acute massive PE transthoracic or transoesophageal echocardiography assures an exact diagnosis /2, 34/.

*Septic thrombosis, thrombophlebitis* of the deep venous system is almost always associated with an underlying malignancy. The diagnosis of septic thrombosis can be based on the presence of septic clinical symptoms, the exclusion of other infectious origin and on the result of the compression Doppler sonography /33/. HR-CT and – according to the most recent data of the literature – positron emission tomography may help in differentiating from a non-infected deep vein thrombosis /5/.

*Thrombotic thrombocytopenic purpura (TTP)* is a severe coagulation disorder associated with fever, undulating CNS symptoms, renal function impairment, microangiopathic haemolytic anaemia and thrombocytopenia. In the background of the clinical syndrome there lies the development of systemic microvascular thromboses (CNS, lung, myocardium, kidneys). The suspicion of TTP is raised by the severe non-immune microangiopathic anaemia and thrombocytopenia (without leucopenia). Fragmented RBCs (schizocytes) can be seen in the peripheral blood smear, elevated serum LDH and unconjugated bilirubin levels, as well as impaired renal function can be observed. In the development of TTP a central role is played by the depletion or inhibition of ADAMTS-13 (A Disintegrin-like And Metalloprotease with ThromboSpondin type 1 repeats). ADAMTS-13 is a von Willebrand factorcleaving protease with adhesive properties secreted by the endothelial cells; and in a part of the cases severe deficiency develops due to autoantibody production and reaction. In lack of ADAMTS-13, ultra-large multimers of von Willebrand factor are present in the patient's plasma, and their increased reacting capacity with platelets leads to the formation of thrombi /6/.

**Table 1. Clinical characteristics of our patients with malignant tumours and occurrence of the associated haemostatic disorders.**

| Primary type of tumour | Number of cases | Migrating thrombo-phlebitis | Deep vein thrombosis; acute pulm. embolism | Acute DIC | Septic thrombo-phlebitis | TTP |
|---|---|---|---|---|---|---|
| NSCLC | n = 790 | 9 | 138/34 | 1 | 1 | 2 |
| SCLC | n = 350 | 16 | 68/13 | 4 | 3 | 1 |
| Breast | n = 128 | 5 | 19/7 | 3 | | |
| Colorectal | n = 64 | 8 | 7/3 | 2 | | |
| Kidney | n = 13 | 7 | 6/1 | | | |
| Bladder | n = 18 | 6 | 4 | 1 | | |
| Thyroid | n = 6 | - | 1 | | | |
| Panceras | n = 6 | 5 | 3 | | | |
| Mesothelioma | n = 6 | 1 | | | | |
| n = 1381 | n = 56 (4 %) | n = 305 (22 %) | n = 11 | n = 4 | n = 3 | |

NSCLC = Non-Small Cell Lung Cancer; SCLC = Small Cell Lung Cancer; DIC = Diffuse Intravascular Coagulation; TTP = Thrombotic Thrombocytopenic Purpura.

*Clinical recognition of aDIC* is possible based on the severe diffuse haemorrhagic diathesis (bleeding from the injection sites, haemorrhages of the mucous membranes, haematuria, haematochezia, haemoptysis) and the concurrently occurring multi-organ (renal, hepatic, pulmonary, CNS) function disorder. The multi-organ function disorder is the consequence of the diffuse intravascular thrombosis. In cases of aDIC fragmentocytes can be seen in the peripheral blood smear, there is very low platelet number, elevated D-dimer level, delayed thrombin and prothrombin time, elevated LDH, and decreased fibrinogen level /7/.

Based on our experiences, observations as well as on the data of the literature, the development of VTE is certainly to be expected more frequently in patients with solid malignancies, primarily in those in an advanced clinical stage. In cases of idiopathic VTE detailed examinations are required in order to prove or preclude an asymptomatic (occult) malignancy, and 1- to 3-year-long follow-up is necessary after a negative result of these examinations. Non-neoplastic comorbidity represents a further risk factor for the development of VTE. In patients with malignancies of advanced clinical stage, in addition on the most frequently occurring DVT, acute massive pulmonary embolism should also be kept in mind. The most recent clinical data and research indicate that the activation of coagulation system also promotes the local invasiveness of tumour cells and the development of metastases /8,9, 10/.

## Abbreviations

aDIC = acute diffuse intravascular coagulation
APE = acute pulmonary embolism
DVT = deep vein thrombosis
VTE = venous thromboembolism
TTP = thrombotic thrombocytopenic purpura
CNS = central nervous systeme
SCLC = small-cell lung cancer

NSCLC = non-small-cell lung cancer
COPD = chronic obstructive pulmonary disease

## References

[1] Varki, A. Trousseau syndrome: multiple definition and multiple mechanism. *Blood*, 2007, 110, 1723-1729.

[2] Sorensen, HT; Mellemkjaer, L; Steffensen, FH; et al. The risk of a diagnosis of cancer after primary deep venous thrombosis or pulmonary embolism. *N Eng I*, 1998, 338, 1169-1173.

[3] Hirsch, J; Lee, AY. How we diagnose and treat deep vein thrombosis. *Blood*, 2002, 99, 3102-3110.

[4] Baron, IA; Gridley, G; Weiderpass, M; et al. Venous thromboembolism and cancer. *Lancet*, 1998, 351, 1077-1080.

[5] Miceli, M; Atoni, R; Walker, R; et al. Diagnosis of deep septic thrombophlebitis in cancer patients by fluorine-18 fluordeoxyglucose positron emission tomography scanning: a preliminary report. *J Clin Oncol*, 2004, 22, 1949-1956.

[6] George, IN. Thrombotic thrombocytopenic purpura. *N Eng J Med*, 2006, 354, 1927-1935.

[7] Colman, R; Rubin, RN. Disseminated intravascular coagulation due to malignancy. *Semin Oncol*, 1990, 17, 172-186.

[8] Francis, IL; Biggerstaff, J; Amirkhosravi, A. Haemostasis and malignancy. *Semin Thromb Hemost*, 1998, 24, 93-108.

[9] Sallah, S; Wan, IY; Nguyen, NP. Venous thrombosis in patients with solid tumors: determination of frequency and characteristic. *Thromb Hemost*, 2002, 87, 575-579.

[10] Lugassy, G; Yoffe, B. Thrombotic complications of overt cancer. In G. Lugassy, A. Falanga, A. K. Kakkar, & F. Rickles (Eds.), *Thrombosis and Cancer*. Taylor R and Francis Group, London, 2004, 109-115.

In: Advances in Cardiovascular Research, Volume 1
Editors: L. Schmitt, T. Konig, pp. 419-430
ISBN: 978-1-60741-720-0


*Chapter XXII*

# Vascular Associations of Pseudoexfoliation Syndrome

***Sergio Pinar Sueiro*[*1], *Nerea Martínez-Alday*[2]**
***Lorea Martínez Indart*[2], *Nora Muruzabal Zaldíbar*[2]**
***Maialen López Aritza*[2] *and Miguel Rueda Gutiérrez*[2]**
[1]University of the Basque Country
[2]Hospital de Cruces, Barakaldo Spain

## Abstract

### Purpose

To determine if there is an association between the presence of abdominal aortic aneurysm and the prevalence of ocular pseudoexfoliation syndrome (PEX).

### Methods

We studied 120 eyes of 60 patients, distributed into two groups according to whether they had been diagnosed with abdominal aortic aneurysm in the past 5 years (n=30) or not (n=30). A complete ophthalmologic examination was performed, classifying patients in whom pseudoexfoliation was found into 3 levels according to its severity, and serum concentrations of folic acid, vitamin B12 and homocysteine were determined.

### Results

* Correspondence: Dr. Sergio Pinar Sueiro, Departamento de Oftalmología, Hospital de Cruces, Plaza de Cruces s/n, C.P. 48903, Baracaldo, Vizcaya, Spain., E- mail: luengonosvemos@yahoo.es, Tel: +34-615-005-389

The prevalence of pseudoexfoliation syndrome in patients with abdominal aortic aneurysm was 3.3% versus 13.3% in the control group. A higher prevalence of ischemic heart disease (50%) was found in the group of patients with pseudoexfoliation than in the rest of the study subjects (7.5%) (p=0.09). Mean homocysteine levels in patients without pseudoexfoliation were lower (13.3 μmol/l) than in the group of patients with pseudoexfoliation (31.98 μmol/l) (p=0.001).

### Conclusions

This study raises the need to screen for hyperhomocysteinemia in patients in whom pseudoexfoliation is detected, because high homocysteine levels could be related to the higher incidence of ischemic heart disease in this patient group. In these cases, treatment with vitamin B group supplements could prevent the development of cardiovascular disease.

**Key Words:** Abdominal aortic aneurysm, folic acid, homocysteine, pseudoexfoliation syndrome, vitamin B12.

## Introduction

Pseudoexfoliation syndrome (PEX) is a systemic disorder of unknown cause characterized by the accumulation of specific fibrillar substance that affects the eye and other tissues, which is clinically significant because it is associated with the development of senile cataract and is the primary cause of chronic secondary open-angle glaucoma. Its prevalence varies widely depending on the geographical area and is related to age, occurring in 0.6% of patients aged 52-64 years, 2.6% of patients aged 65-74 years and 5.0% of patients aged 75-85 years.(1)

The spectrum of vascular disease associated with pseudoexfoliation syndrome is increasingly wide,(2) and pseudoexfoliation syndrome has also been associated with signs of ocular ischemia such as iris neovessels,(3) altered blood flow and central retinal vein occlusion,(4,5) cardiovascular and cerebrovascular disorders(2,6-8) and asymptomatic myocardial dysfunction.(9) There is also a suggested association between pseudoexfoliation syndrome and abdominal aortic aneurysms, (10) as well as with large vessel dysfunction.(11)

A possible association has also been reported with other cardiovascular risk factors, such as higher levels of homocysteine(12) and lower levels of vitamin B6, B12 and folates,(13) but these results could not be reproduced in other studies.(14)

The primary aim of this study was to analyze the association between the presence of abdominal aortic aneurysms and the prevalence of pseudoexfoliation syndrome. We also analyzed the differences in the levels of other factors associated with vascular risk (homocysteine, vitamin B12 and folate) between patients with abdominal aneurysms and the control group, as well as between patients with pseudoexfoliation syndrome and the rest of the study subjects.

# Materials and Methods

A cross-sectional observational design was used in this study, which was conducted under the supervision and with the prior approval of the clinical research ethics committee (CREC) of Hospital de Cruces. All study subjects were informed and gave their written consent.

## Patient Selection

Patients were selected who had a confirmed diagnosis of abdominal aorta aneurysm after imaging tests (CT, angiography) and who had been registered in the database of the Vascular Surgery Department for the last four years. The control group included patients from the General Surgery Department (outpatient clinic) who had undergone an abdominal CT scan as part of their routine clinical care and in whom the presence of abdominal aortic aneurysm had been excluded.

Patients over 40 years of age from the two groups described above who had been appropriately informed and had voluntarily given their consent to participate were included in the study.

The exclusion criteria considered were Marfan syndrome and other connective tissue disorders predisposing to the development of an aneurysm, aneurysms of traumatic origin and arteritis.

We studied 120 eyes of 60 patients included in the abdominal aortic aneurysm group (n=30) or in the control group (n=30).

## Ophthalmologic Study

After collecting epidemiological data from their medical records, a systematic ophthalmologic examination of the patients was made.

Best-corrected far visual acuity was measured in all patients. A biomicroscopic study of the anterior segment was also performed in all cases, describing the main features associated with the pseudoexfoliation syndrome, which was classified into three severity levels [*mild, 1*: unilateral with a single pseudoexfoliation rim, not associated with iris abnormalities; *moderate, 2*: unilateral with $\geq 1$ pseudoexfoliation rims, and iris abnormalities (peripupillary atrophy/pupil diameter <5 mm after three instillations of tropicamide + phenylephrine); *severe, 3*: bilateral pseudoexfoliation associated with the previously mentioned pupillary abnormalities].

Intraocular pressure was recorded and a fundus examination was performed.

Endothelial cell count was also done using a noncontact specular microscope (Konan SP-6000).

### Biochemical Study

A blood chemistry test was performed in all subjects to assess vitamin B12, folic acid and homocysteine levels.

Quantitative determination of homocysteine levels was performed by fluorescence polarization immunoassay (FPIA) using the IMx analyzer (Abbott). Samples were drawn into chilled EDTA tubes, centrifuging and separating the plasma before 30 minutes. These samples were then frozen to -20°C until their processing.

Vitamin B12 and folic acid levels were measuring in serum samples by direct competitive chemiluminescent assay using the ADVIA Centaur XP system (Siemens).

### Statistical Analysis

Each variable was described using frequency distributions and percentages for qualitative (categorical) variables and measures of central tendency and dispersion (mean, median, standard deviation (SD), minimum and maximum values) for quantitative variables, depending on their distribution characteristics. In other words, the mean and standard deviation were used if the data did not have a very skewed distribution, or otherwise the median and minimum and maximum values.

Comparison of proportions between qualitative (categorical) variables was done using the chi-square test or its corresponding corrections, such as Fisher's correction when the expected frequencies were <5.

Comparison between two groups with a continuous variable was done using the nonparametric Mann-Whitney U test because the number of cases was small.

These analyses were performed using the SPSS version 16.0 software.

## Results

### General Descriptive Statistics

In the study sample, 23.3% were women and 76.7% were men. Mean age was 71.67 ± 9.18 years, mean visual acuity of the sample in the decimal system was 0.71 ± 0.23, mean intraocular pressure was 15.14 ± 3.03 mm Hg, and mean epithelial cell density was 2017.84 ± 507.14 cels/mm$^2$ (Table 1). The incidence of glaucoma was 5% (n=3), and 71.7% of the sample had some type of associated vascular disease (Table 2).

Mean vitamin B12 levels for the study sample were 449.07 ± 160.75 pg/ml, with normal vitamin B12 levels (220-980 pg/ml) in 92.9% (n=42) of subjects and diminished levels in 7.1%.

**Table 1. Description of main quantitative variables in the study sample.**

| | N | MINIMUM | MAXIMUM | MEAN | STANDARD DEVIATION |
|---|---|---|---|---|---|
| AGE | 57 | 54 | 93 | 71,67 | 9,18 |
| ANEURYSM SIZE | 22 | 2,5 | 8,7 | 5,61 | 1,38 |
| MEAN FVA | 59 | 0,12 | 1,12 | 0,71 | 0,23 |
| MEAN IOP | 58 | 9 | 23 | 15,14 | 3,03 |
| MEAN ENDOTHELIAL COUNT | 53 | 1015,50 | 3115 | 2017,85 | 507,15 |
| VITAMIN B12 | 42 | 172 | 930 | 449,07 | 160,75 |
| FOLIC ACID | 46 | 2,9 | 25 | 9,73 | 5,14 |
| HOMOCYSTEINE | 40 | 6,3 | 49,7 | 14,77 | 7,17 |

**Table 2. Frequency distribution of cardiovascular disease in abdominal aortic aneurysm groups versus the control group. (HT: Arterial hypertension; DM: Diabetes Mellitus; DLP: Dyslipidemia; PVD: Peripheral vascular disease; IHD: Ischemic heart disease).**

| ABDOMINAL AORTIC ANEURYSM | VASCULAR DISEASE | FREQUENCY | PERCENTAGE (%) |
|---|---|---|---|
| NO | None | 8 | 26,7 |
| | HT | 7 | 23,3 |
| | DM | 3 | 10 |
| | DLP | 2 | 6,7 |
| | PVD | 2 | 6,7 |
| | IHD | 2 | 6,7 |
| | Cardiac arrhythmia | 2 | 6,7 |
| | HT+DM | 2 | 6,7 |
| | HT+IHD | 2 | 6,7 |
| | ***TOTAL*** | ***30*** | ***100*** |
| YES | None | 9 | 30 |
| | HT | 5 | 16,7 |
| | DM | 3 | 10 |
| | DLP | 3 | 10 |
| | PVD | 6 | 20 |
| | IHD | 1 | 3,3 |
| | HT+DM | 1 | 3,3 |
| | HT+IHD | 2 | 6,7 |
| | ***TOTAL*** | ***30*** | ***100*** |

Mean folic acid levels of the sample (n=46) were 9.73 ± 5.14 ng/ml, with normal folic acid levels (3.4-20 ng/ml) in 91.3% of subjects and raised levels in 8.7%.

Mean homocysteine levels of the sample (n=40) were 14.76 ± 7.16 μmol/l. Of note was the presence of raised homocysteine levels (5-15 μmol/ml) in 39.5% of subjects and normal levels in 60.5%.

## Abdominal Aortic Aneurysm Group Versus Control Group

Nearly all patients (96.7%) with abdominal aortic aneurysms were male. The mean aneurysm size at diagnosis was 5.61 ± 1.38 cm. The prevalence of systemic vascular disease was similar in the abdominal aortic aneurysm group (30%) and in the control group (26.7%).

The best-corrected far visual acuity (FVA) was greater in patients diagnosed with abdominal aortic aneurysm than in the control group (p=0.012). The prevalence of glaucoma in the control group was 3.3% versus 6.7% in those with a history of abdominal aortic aneurysm.

The prevalence of pseudoexfoliation syndrome in patients with abdominal aortic aneurysm was 3.3% versus 13.3% in the control group (Figure 1).

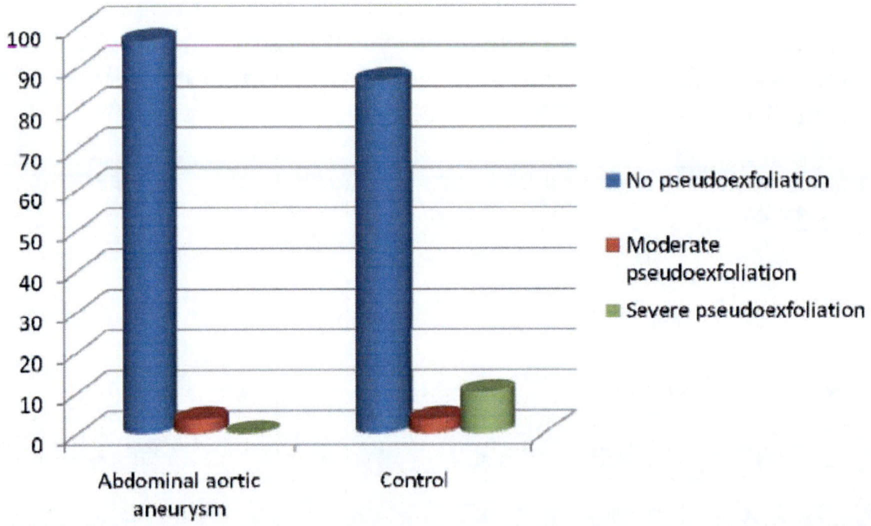


Figure 1. Prevalence of pseudoexfoliation syndrome classified by severity in the abdominal aortic aneurysm groups and the control group.

Although folic acid levels were raised in 15% of control subjects versus 3.8% of patients with abdominal aortic aneurysm, the latter had higher mean folic acid levels than the control group, and these differences were statistically significant (p=0.022).

Vitamin B12 levels were normal in 93.8% of controls without abdominal aortic aneurysms and diminished in 6.2%. This percentage of patients with diminished vitamin B12 levels was 7.7% in the group of patients with abdominal aortic aneurysm.

Considering the normal range for homocysteine levels, 37.5% of patients in the aneurysm group had raised levels versus 42.9% in the control group.

## Pseudoexfoliation Group versus Control Group

Pseudoexfoliation syndrome (PEX) was diagnosed in 8.3% of the study subjects. According to our classification of pseudoexfoliation, 91.7% of subjetc did not have PEX, 3.3% had moderate PEX and 5% had severe PEX in both eyes. Sixty percent of subjects with PEX were female.

The higher frequency of ischemic heart disease among patients with pseudoexfoliation (50%) and severe pseudoexfoliation (65.5%) compared to the rest of the study subjects (7.5%) was notable, and these differences were statistically significant between the group of patients with pseudoexfoliation and the group of subjects without pseudoexfoliation (p=0.09) (Figure 2).

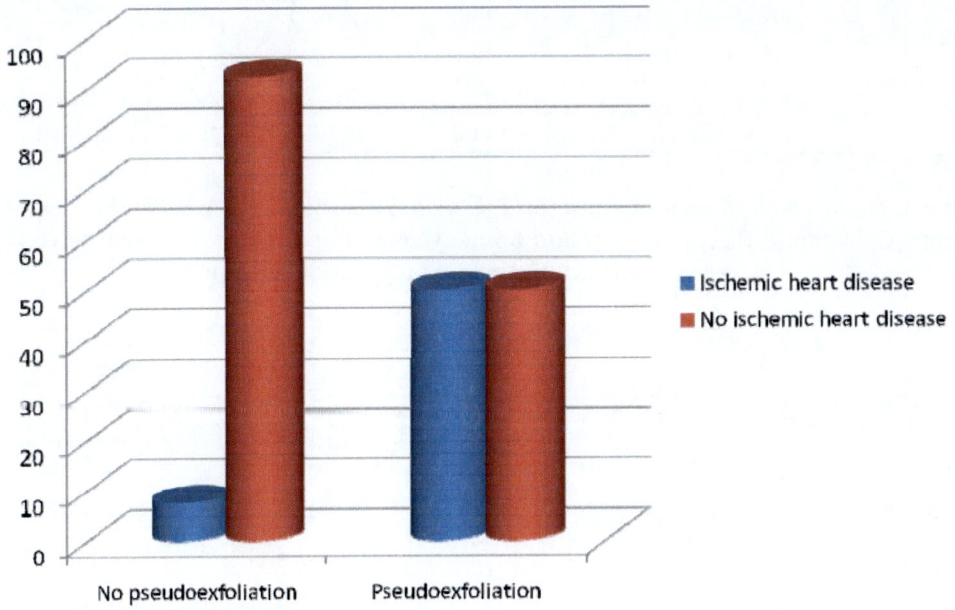


Figure 2. Prevalence of ischemic heart disease in the group of patients with pseudoexfoliation versus the rest of subjects in the study sample. A higher prevalence of ischemic heart disease was shown in patients with pseudoexfoliation, and these differences were statistically significant (p=0.09) by Fisher's exact test.

The group of subjects without PEX had a higher mean FVA (0.73 ± 0.21) than patients with PEX (0.4062 ± 0.2) and patients with severe PEX (0.25 ± 0.17) (p=0.01) (Table 3).

**Table 3. Description of main quantitative variables studied in the sample in the group of patients with pseudoexfoliation versus the rest of study subjects. (FVA: Far visual acuity; IOP: Intraocular pressure, Mean EC: Mean endothelial count).**

| PSEUDOEXF. | VARIABLE | N | MINIMUM | MAXIMUM | MEAN | STANDARD DEVIATION |
|---|---|---|---|---|---|---|
| NO | AGE | 52 | 54 | 93 | 70,90 | 9,03 |
| | MEAN FVA | 55 | 0,32 | 1,12 | 0,73 | 0,21 |
| | MEAN IOP | 55 | 9 | 23 | 15,05 | 3,08 |
| | MEAN EC | 49 | 1015,50 | 3115 | 2022,49 | 520,02 |
| | VIT. B12 | 38 | 177 | 930 | 455,05 | 156,43 |
| | FOLIC ACID | 42 | 2,9 | 25 | 9,43 | 5,05 |
| | HOMOCYSTEINE | 37 | 6,3 | 25 | 13,371 | 3,95 |
| YES | AGE | 5 | 71 | 89 | 79,6 | 7,47 |
| | MEAN FVA | 4 | 0,12 | 0,6 | 0,41 | 0,21 |
| | MEAN IOP | 3 | 16 | 18 | 16,67 | 1,15 |
| | MEAN EC | 4 | 1432 | 2196 | 1961 | 355,89 |
| | VIT. B12 | 4 | 172 | 580 | 392,25 | 215,82 |
| | FOLIC ACID | 4 | 7,5 | 20,3 | 12,80 | 5,82 |
| | HOMOCYSTEINE | 3 | 21,8 | 49,7 | 31,98 | 15,43 |

**Table 4. Description of mean values for age, visual acuity (mean VA), endothelial count (mean EC), vitamin B12, folic acid and homocysteine in patients with pseudoexfoliation, severe pseudoexfoliation or no pseudoexfoliation.**

| | NO PEX | | | PEX | | | Severe PEX | | |
|---|---|---|---|---|---|---|---|---|---|
| | N | Mean | S.D. | N | Mean | S.D. | N | Mean | S.D. |
| **Age** | 52 | 70,90 | 9,03 | 5 | 79,60 | 7,47 | 3 | 82,67 | 7,71 |
| **Mean VA** | 55 | 0,73 | 0,21 | 4 | 0,41 | 0,21 | 2 | 0,25 | 0,18 |
| **Mean EC** | 49 | 2022,49 | 520,02 | 4 | 1961 | 355,89 | 2 | 1784,50 | 498,51 |
| **Vit. B12** | 38 | 455,05 | 156,43 | 4 | 392,25 | 215,82 | 3 | 329,67 | 215,33 |
| **Folic acid** | 42 | 9,43 | 5,04 | 4 | 12,80 | 5,82 | 3 | 14,09 | 6,39 |
| **Homocysteine** | 37 | 13,37 | 3,96 | 3 | 31,98 | 15,44 | 3 | 31,98 | 15,44 |

We did not find statistically significant differences in endothelial cell density between the control group (2022.48 ± 520.02 cells/mm$^2$) and the group of patients with PEX (1961 ± 355.88 cells/mm$^2$) ($p=0.808$) or severe PEX (1432.3 ± 498.51 cells/mm$^2$) ($p=0.444$).

Folic acid levels were increased in 7.1% of subjects without PEX and in 25% of patients with PEX.

Vitamin B12 was decreased in 5.3% of control subjects without PEX versus 25% of patients with PEX and 33.3% with severe PEX.

Homocysteine was altered in 34.3% of patients without PEX and in 100% of patients with PEX. Mean homocysteine levels were lower in patients without PEX (13.3 μmol/l) than in patients with PEX (31.98 μmol/l) (p=0.001) (Tables 3 and 4).

## Discussion

Pseudoexfoliation syndrome is characterized by deposits of a specific fibrillar material with a complex composition of glycoproteins/proteoglycans, as well as a high content in elastic microfibrillar components. In extraocular locations, pseudoexfoliation material is primarily found in the connective tissue of organs, often in the periphery of blood vessels, derived from connective tissue fibroblasts, smooth and striated muscle, and cardiac muscle cells, which has led to this syndrome being considered as an elastosis, which would explain a possible association of this syndrome with abdominal aortic aneurysms.(15) However, and despite previous studies in which pseudoexfoliation syndrome came to be considered as the etiologic agent of systemic vascular disease.(2-7;10,11) this study does not allow some of these results to be reproduced as a higher prevalence of pseudoexfoliation syndrome was not found among patients with abdominal aortic aneurysms.

However, we did find interesting clinical differences between the group of patients diagnosed with pseudoexfoliation and the rest of the study subjects. Mean age was lower in this latter group, while it was found to increase according to the severity of pseudoexfoliation. Endothelial cell density also decreased in the group of patients with pseudoexfoliation, and this decrease was more marked as the severity of pseudoexfoliation increased. The same phenomenon was observed to occur with visual acuity. In this regard, the association of older age with the severity of pseudoexfoliation syndrome could be considered a confounding factor when analyzing the other two variables, because this older age of the patients could be associated with a higher prevalence of ophthalmologic comorbidities (AMD, cataracts, etc.) and the natural progressive reduction in endothelial cell density.

Perhaps the most interesting finding is the higher prevalence of ischemic heart disease in patients with pseudoexfoliation, which increased according to the severity of pseudoexfoliation. We should also consider that these patients had decreased folic acid and vitamin B12 levels and increased homocysteine levels, the latter being an independent cardiovascular risk factor.(16)

The origin of this increased risk of ischemic heart disease in patients with pseudoexfoliation syndrome is due to the endothelial dysfunction caused by the accumulation of pseudoexfoliation material in the adventitial and subendothelial connective tissue of the vessel walls. The pathophysiological mechanism of this endothelial dysfunction could be related to the increase in fibrosis and elastosis of the tunica media, as well as an alteration in the self-regulatory mechanisms mediated by nitric oxide (NO), increasing oxidative stress.(15,17) This increase in oxidative stress seems to be related to a decrease in lipid-soluble B type vitamins (folic acid, vitamin B6, B12), which are essential in mediation of vasodilatory factors such as nitric oxide synthase, maintenance of homocysteine levels, and have clear antithrombotic and antioxidant effects. As a result of this alteration in correct endothelial metabolism and function, homocysteine levels are increased, resulting in an increase in oxidative stress and platelet aggregation.

As a conclusion, we think that screening for hyperhomocysteinemia should be considered in patients with pseudoexfoliation, and especially in those with grade 3 severity according to our classification. We found that high levels of homocysteine were a risk factor for the development of ischemic heart disease in this patient group. Treatment with vitamin B group supplements can be considered if altered homocysteine levels are detected in this risk group.

## Acknowledgments

Jesús Gangoiti Barrera Foundation, Dr. Elena Vecino Cordero (Head of Department of Cell Biology, University of the Basque Country), Dr. José Ignacio Pijoan (Section Head of Research Unit, Hospital de Cruces), Amaia Martínez Galarza (Department of Epidemiology, Hospital de Cruces), Dr. Juan Antonio García Alonso (Head of Department of Vascular Surgery, Hospital de Cruces), Dr. Andoni Junquera Landeta (Ophthalmology Resident, Hospital de Cruces), Dr. Iñaki Aldasoro Cáceres (Ophthalmology Resident, Hospital de Cruces), Dr. Cristina Prieto Valtuille (Pharmacist Resident, Hospital de Cruces), Idoia Beramendi Eraso (Graduate Nurse, Hospital de Cruces), Milagros Bahillo Franco (Graduate Nurse, Hospital de Cruces), Mª Teresa Prieto Luis (Graduate Nurse, Hospital de Cruces).

## Responsible Institution

Department of Ophthalmology, Hospital de Cruces, Barakaldo, Spain.

*"Patients were informed by the research team both orally and in writing about the nature of the study and were able to ask as many questions and clarify any doubts they considered appropriate. They also had as much time as they considered necessary to think about their decision before giving their informed consent to participate in the study.*

*All patients gave their informed consent in writing prior to the start of the study.*

*The protocol, information sheet and informed consent and all other study documents were previously submitted to the clinical research ethics committee (CREC) of Hospital de Cruces for their approval."*

## Conflicts of Interest

This study was funded by the Jesús de Gangoiti Barrera Foundation.

# References


[1] Hiller R, Sperduto RD, Krueger DE. Pseudoexfoliation, intraocular pressure and senile lens changes in a population-based survey. *Arch Ophthalmol* 1982; 100: 1080-1082.

[2] Tarkkanen A. Is exfoliation syndrome a sign of systemic vascular disease? *Acta Ophthalmol* 2008; 86: 832-836.

[3] Ringvold A, Davanger M. Iris neovascularisation in eyes with pseudoexfoliation syndrome. *British Journal of Ophthalmology* 1981; 65, 138-141.

[4] Yüksel N, Karabaş VL, Demirci A, Arslan A, Altintaş Ö, Çağlar Y. Comparison of blood flow velocities of the extraocular vessels in patients with pseudoexfolitaion or primary open-angle glaucoma. *Ophthalmologica* 2001; 215: 424-429.

[5] Cursiefen C, Hammer T, Küchle M, Naumann GOH, Schlötzer-Schrehardt U. Pseudoexfoliation syndrome in eyes with ischemic central retinal vein occlusion. *Acta Ophthalmol Scand* 2001; 79: 476-478.

[6] Shrum KR, Hattenhauer MG, Hodge D. Cardiovascular and cerebrovascular mortality associated with ocular pseudoexfoliation. *Am J Ophthalmol* 2000; 129: 83-86.

[7] Yüksel N, Anik Y, Kiliç A, Karabaş V, Demirci A, Çağlar Y. Cerebrovascular blood flow velocities in pseudoexfoliation. *Graefe's Arch Clin Exp Ophthalmol* 2006; 244: 316-321.

[8] Yüksel N, Anik Y, Altintaş O, Onur I, Cağlar Y, Demirci A Magnetic resonance imaging of the brain in patients with pseudoexfoliation syndrome and glaucoma. *Ophthalmologica* 2006; 220(2):125-30.

[9] Bojić L, Ermacora R, Polić S, et al. Pseudoexfoliation syndrome and asymptomatic myocardial dysfunction. *Graefe's Arch Clin Exp Ophthalmol* 2005; 243: 446–449.

[10] Schumacher S, Schlötzer-Schrehardt U, Martus P, Lang W, Naumann GOH. Pseudoexfoliation syndrome and aneurysms of the abdominal aorta. *Lancet* 2001; 357: 359 –360.

[11] Visontai Z, Merisch B, Kollai M, Holló G. Increase of carotid artery stiffness and decrease of baroreflex sensitivity in exfoliation syndrome and glaucoma. *Br J Ophthalmol* 2006; 90: 563-567.

[12] Altintaş O, Maral H, Yüksel N, Karabaş VL, Dillioğlugil MO, Cağlar Y. Homocysteine and nitric oxide levels in plasma of patients with pseudoexfoliation syndrome, pseudoexfoliation glaucoma, and primary open-angle glaucoma. *Graefes Arch Clin Exp Ophthalmol 2005;* 243(7): 677-83.

[13] Roedl JB, Bleich S, Reulbach U, et al. Vitamin deficiency *J Neural Transm* 2007; 114(5):571-5.

[14] Puustjärvi T, Blomster H, Kontkanen M, Punnonen K, Teräsvirta M. Plasma and aqueous humour levels of homocysteine in exfoliation syndrome. *Graefe's Arch Clin Exp Ophthalmol* 2004; 242: 749-754.

[15] Atalar PT, Atalar E, Kilic H, et al. Impaired systemic endothelial function in patients with pseudoexfoliation syndrome. *Int Heart J* 2006; 47: 77-84.

[16] Moens AL, Christiaan J, Vrints CJ, et al. Mechanisms and potential therapeutic targets for folic acid in cardiovascular disease. *Am J Physiol Heart Circ Physiol* 294: 1971–1977, 2008.

[17] Kobayashi N, DeLano FA, Geert W. Schmid-Schönbein, GW. Oxidative stress promotes endothelial cell apoptosis and loss of microvessels in the spontaneously hypertensive rats. *Arterioscler Thromb Vasc Biol* 2005; 25:2114-2121.

# Index

## A

## B

## C

## D

## E

## F

## G

## H

## J



## K



## L

## M

## N

## O



## P

## Q



## R

## S

## T

## U



## V

## W



## X



## Y